Bioengineering Innovations for Surgery

Bioengineering Innovations for Surgery

Editor: Amina Fowler

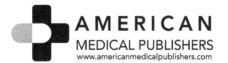

AMERICAN
MEDICAL PUBLISHERS
www.americanmedicalpublishers.com

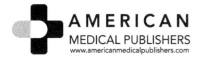

Cataloging-in-Publication Data

Bioengineering innovations for surgery / edited by Amina Fowler.
   p. cm.
Includes bibliographical references and index.
ISBN 978-1-63927-918-0
1. Surgical technology. 2. Bioengineering. 3. Surgery--Technological innovations.
4. Biomedical engineering. 5. Surgical instruments and apparatus. I. Fowler, Amina.
RD32.3 .B56 2023
610.736 77--dc23

American Medical Publishers,
41 Flatbush Avenue,
1st Floor, New York,
NY 11217, USA

ISBN 978-1-63927-918-0 (Hardback)

Contents

Preface

It is often said that books are a boon to mankind. They document every progress and pass on the knowledge from one generation to the other. They play a crucial role in our lives. Thus I was both excited and nervous while editing this book. I was pleased by the thought of being able to make a mark but I was also nervous to do it right because the future of students depends upon it. Hence, I took a few months to research further into the discipline, revise my knowledge and also explore some more aspects. Post this process, I begun with the editing of this book.

Surgery is a branch of medicine that uses operative manual and instrumental techniques to investigate or treat a pathological condition such as a disease or injury. There are several surgical procedures commonly categorized by urgency, type of procedure, body system involved, the degree of invasiveness and special instrumentation. Some of the most important advances in surgery include minimally invasive surgeries and robotics, which have been possible due to contributions of both engineers and surgeons. Minimally invasive surgery is a surgical technique characterized by small incisions, quicker healing, lower pain and reduced risk of infection. These surgeries are guided by laparoscopic or arthroscopic devices, large scale display panel, and remote-control manipulation of instruments. Refractive eye surgery, cryosurgery, keyhole surgery and stereotactic surgery are some examples of minimally invasive surgical procedures. This book is compiled in such a manner, that it will provide in-depth knowledge about bioengineering innovations for surgery. It aims to present researches that have transformed this area of medicine and aided in its advancement. This book is a resource guide for experts as well as students.

I thank my publisher with all my heart for considering me worthy of this unparalleled opportunity and for showing unwavering faith in my skills. I would also like to thank the editorial team who worked closely with me at every step and contributed immensely towards the successful completion of this book. Last but not the least, I wish to thank my friends and colleagues for their support.

Editor

How 3D Printing is Reshaping Translational Research

Elizabeth A. W. Sigston [1,2,3]*

[1]Monash Institute of Medical Engineering, Monash University, Melbourne, VIC, Australia, [2]Department of Surgery, School of Clinical Sciences at Monash Health, Monash University Melbourne, Melbourne, VIC, Australia, [3]Department of Otolaryngology, Head and Neck Surgery, Monash Health, Melbourne, VIC, Australia

*Correspondence:
Elizabeth A. W. Sigston
elizabeth.sigston@
monashhealth.org

"Translational Research" has traditionally been defined as taking basic scientific findings and developing new diagnostic tools, drugs, devices and treatment options for patients, that are translated into practice, reach the people and populations for whom they are intended and are implemented correctly. The implication is of a unidirectional flow from "the bench to bedside". The rapidly emergent field of additive manufacturing (3D printing) is contributing to a major shift in translational medical research. This includes the concept of bidirectional or reverse translation, early collaboration between clinicians, bio-engineers and basic scientists, and an increasingly entrepreneurial mindset. This coincides with, and is strongly complemented by, the rise of systems biology. The rapid pace at which this type of translational research can occur brings a variety of potential pitfalls and ethical concerns. Regulation surrounding implantable medical devices is struggling to keep up. 3D printing has opened the way for personalization which can make clinical outcomes hard to assess and risks putting the individual before the community. In some instances, novelty and hype has led to loss of transparency of outcomes with dire consequence. Collaboration with commercial partners has potential for conflict of interest. Nevertheless, 3D printing has dramatically changed the landscape of translational research. With early recognition and management of the potential risks, the benefits of reshaping the approach to translational research are enormous. This impact will extend into many other areas of biomedical research, re-establishing that science is more than a body of research. It is a way of thinking.

Keywords: additive manufacturing, 3D printing, translational research, bioengineering, systems biology, biomedical, design methodology, entrepreneurship

INTRODUCTION

"Translational Research" has been defined as taking basic scientific findings and developing new diagnostic tools, drugs, devices and treatment options for patients, "the bench to bedside" goal of biomedical research. (Woolf 2008; van der Laan and Boenink 2015; Sanders 2020). The implication is of unidirectional flow with the aim of seeking how scientific knowledge can be applied in a clinical setting. (Rubio et al., 2010). This century has seen translational research dramatically rise in prominence, largely driven by the recognition that statistically few discoveries in "bench" science have had any material impact on human health or clinical practice with a considerable lag time for those that do. (Balas and Boren 2000; Contopoulos-Ioannidis et al., 2008; Trochim et al., 2011).

Modern healthcare demands for innovative, faster and more personalized solutions have seen the convergence of engineering and biomedical research, leading to emergence of the rapidly growing field of bioengineering, driven to a large extent through the application of additive manufacturing. (Homes 2018). Additive manufacturing, otherwise known as 3D printing was first created in the 1980s. It refers to creating a three-dimensional object from a digital model or blueprint through the printing of materials in successive layers. (Ventola 2014; Fan et al., 2020). This technique enables a focus on functional design, rapid prototype production and individual customization. (Parthasarathy 2014; Ventola 2014; Paul et al., 2018; Fan et al., 2020).

3D printing has not only been instrumental to the development of new fields of study, it has brought together multidisciplinary teams from across the spectrum of engineering, medicine, biomedical research, information technology with other stakeholders, including consumers and commercial funders. The result is reframing of multiple aspects of translational research, ranging from how translational research is defined, to the role of multidisciplinary teams, to tools that better replicate human biology, to the fundamental philosophies that drive it and, ultimately, to the pace at which it occurs.

EVOLVING DEFINITION OF TRANSLATION RESEARCH

Appreciating the impact of 3D printing on translational research starts with defining what "translational research" means. The term was originally used sporadically during the 1990s in cancer research to describe research that spanned different types or different disciplines of research, such as basic and clinical research, or immunology and molecular genetics. (Rubio et al., 2010). The turn of the century saw increasing concern from medical scientists and public health policy makers that scientific discoveries were failing to generate any tangible human benefit. (Sung et al., 2003) Even though more scientific discoveries were being achieved and at a faster rate, translation into clinical practice was little better than it was 100 years prior. (Balas and Boren 2000). Studies estimated it took 17–24 years for 14% of new scientific discoveries to enter day-to day clinical practice. (Westfall et al., 2007; Contopoulos-Ioannidis et al., 2008). Lag time and lack of practical impact has ramifications not only for biomedical research, patients and the public but also for governments and funding bodies who are accountable for ensuring resources invested into biomedical research will amount to some measurable improvement in health outcomes. (Woolf 2008; Trochim et al., 2011; Schwartz and Macomber 2017; Sanders 2020).

In June 2000 the initial meeting of the Clinical Research Roundtable of the Institute of Medicine (Sung et al., 2003), a body founded under the charter of the National Academy of Sciences in the United States, was convened to address these concerns. (Fallon 2002). From this arose the concept of 'translational research' as the taking of basic scientific findings and developing new diagnostic tools, drugs, devices and

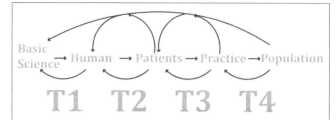

FIGURE 1 | Traditionally translational research was described as the process of taking a basic scientific discovery and working out how that knowledge may be applied at the bedside. The limited progress from discovery to creating an impact on clinical practice and the slow pace at which this occurs has seen an evolution in the way translational research is both defined and approached. Translational research is now considered as a multidirection, cyclic process with starting point being any of the translational phases T1 to T4. Phase T1 represents translation of basic science to application in humans, T2 from human application to patients, T3 from patients into accepted clinical practice and T4 from clinical practice to the population. Each phase can move in either direction and can feedback or feed forward to influence or direct the other phases.

treatment options for patients. (Woolf 2008). Obstacles to this progression were defined as "translational blocks" described as T1, the translation of basic science to human studies, and T2, the translation of new knowledge into clinical practice and healthcare decision making. (Sung et al., 2003).

Over time the "T" has changed from representing a translational block to representing a translational phase. Currently there is general consensus on the definitions of T1 through to T4 (**Figure 1**). (Fort et al., 2017) Additionally, T0 has been proposed to represent genomic-wide association studies and basic science discovery. (Gannon 2014; Fort et al., 2017). T5 is used in some forums to represent international adoption of a clinical practice. (Fort et al., 2017).

The other major shift has been acceptance that translational research needs to be multidirectional, recognizing that data and observations from clinical practice, individual and collective behaviours are critical in creating real world impacts. (Woolf 2008; Cohrs et al., 2015; van der Laan and Boenink 2015; Jia 2016; Smith et al., 2017). The European Society for Translational Medicine (EUSTM) defines translational research as *an interdisciplinary branch of the biomedical field supported by three main pillars: benchside, bedside and community.* (Cohrs et al., 2015). Merging this concept with the translational phases, modern translational biomedical research can be viewed as a multidirectional integrated process (**Figure 1**).

FROM PONDERING TO PROBLEM SOLVING

Biomedical research has been dominated by basic research (Sung et al., 2003; Woolf 2008), that is, research that results in adding to general knowledge and understanding of nature and its laws, but without the practical ends in mind. (Rubio et al., 2010; Patel and Mehta 2016). It follows the fundamental steps of scientific method: observation, hypothesis, experimentation and generalization, favouring a quantitative and analytical

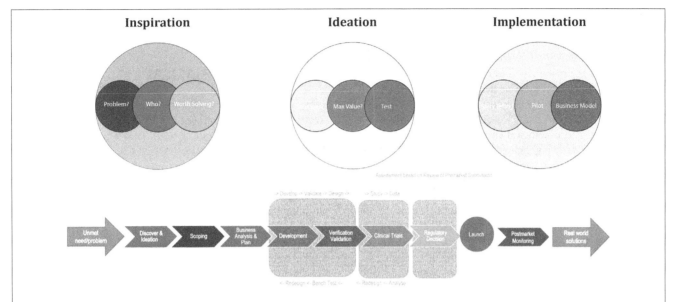

FIGURE 2 | Applying engineering design thinking and entrepreneurial thinking in the translational research process creates a systematic approach to finding a solution to a problem that is worth solving. In biomedical research this starts with identifying an unmet healthcare need or clinical problem. Scoping of the problem and undertaking a business analysis occurs at the beginning, ideas of how the problem may be solved are explored, re-iterated and then progress to implementation and a real world solution. (Flow chart component developed by Monash Institute of Medical Engineering, Monash University.)

approach. (Greenman et al., 2007). Translational research in this methodology, the "bench to bedside" approach, requires working out how that knowledge is then applicable to clinical health scenarios. The implication is of unidirectional flow underpinned by the reductionist philosophy that biology can be explained by breaking it down to chemical or molecular reactions. By simply tying this knowledge together, answers to all clinical questions can be found. As discussed above, translation of biomedical research into clinical practice using this approach has been slow and largely ineffective. (Balas and Boren 2000; Balas and Boren 2000; Westfall et al., 2007; Contopoulos-Ioannidis et al., 2008; Trochim et al., 2011).

In contrast, the engineering method (engineering design) is a systematic approach to finding a solution to a problem. The starting point is identifying and researching the problem, followed by ideation of a solution, planning, development of proof of concept and/or prototyping, testing and re-iterations, then implementation. (Lasser 2013; Greene et al., 2017). The engineering design method compared to traditional biomedical research, deals primarily with something that doesn't yet exist. (Patel and Mehta 2016).

The application of 3D technologies to human biology and medicine in order to improve healthcare and healthcare outcomes has contributed to the rise of the new field of biomedical engineering. (Moffat 2017). Use of problem solving engineering design methodology in biomedical research places an unmet clinical or healthcare need as the problem to be solved, driving translational research in a targeted direction. (**Figure 2**). For example, assessing the clinical problem of high rates of plate extrusion, screw loosening and/or poor osseointegration in mandibular reconstructions in head and neck cancer patients (Shaw et al., 2004; Goh et al., 2008) and finding poor match in

elastic properties of titanium plates to native bone produces stress shielding (Gutwald et al., 2017; Soro et al., 2019), enabled development of an alternative alloy produced through 3D printing with better mechanical properties and improved osteogenic potential. (Soro et al., 2019; Brodie et al., 2021).

A SYSTEMS APPROACH

Complex systems exist everywhere in nature, including the human body. (Van Regenmortel 2004; Mazzocchi 2008; Mesarovic, 2017). They are dynamic and have the ability to self-correct through cyclic feedback loops. A systems approach considers a complex system as a whole and involves understanding interactions and influences between various components in a system to solve complex problems. (Patel and Mehta 2016). At the core are the concepts of emergence and interrelatedness, that a system is more than the sum of its parts. (Patel and Mehta 2016; Greene et al., 2017; Kolodkin, 2017).

Ironically, whilst the engineering field adopted systems thinking generating the fields of cybernetics and system dynamics (Greene et al., 2017), biomedical research followed the reductionist path of molecular biology, identifying the gene as the fundamental unit of biological information and chemistry the effective mechanistic explanation of biological processes. (Nurse 2008; Green 2017). Though this approach has led to significant improvement in understanding of human disease, translation to clinical impact has not been fast or frequent. Increasingly gaps and paradoxes arising from this assumption (Sonnenschein and Soto 2008; Bertolaso et al., 2011; Baker 2012; Bizzarri and Cucina 2014; Bertolaso, 2017) has led to acknowledgement that biological complexity has been overlooked (Nurse 2008) resulting in the rise of "systems biology", a term that describes the quantitative analysis of the dynamic interactions among several components of a biological system with the aim to understand the behavior of the system as a whole.

Systems thinking allows biomedical research and engineering to dovetail into translatable solutions (Chien et al., 2015) and 3D printing is at the heart of it. Two-dimensional monolayer cells cultures do not reflect biological complexity. The importance of 3D culture was initially highlighted by Mina Bissell and her team, demonstrating that both structural and biochemical cues are required for mammary acinar development. (Schmeichel et al., 1998). This led to development of "organoids", miniature organs derived from tissue-resident stem/progenitor cells or embryonic stem cells in the presence of organ-specific cues and matrices in culture dishes. Organoids resemble an organ in both structure and function. (Rawal et al., 2021). 3D printing is now being used to reliability reproduce organoids, tumoroids, and even whole organs that better represent human systems for use in disease and regenerative research with ultimate potential to produce transplantable tissues. (Reid et al., 2018; Mansilla et al., 2021; Rawal et al., 2021).

RISE OF THE PROSUMER

Availability of 3D printers to the wider public has seen the rise of the "prosumer", a person who is involved in the co-creation and innovation of the product they use. (Rayna et al., 2015). In healthcare, prothesis have been the target of prosumers. e-NABLE, an online global community of volunteers is an example of prosumers not waiting for companies or governments to find solutions. The open-source designs created by e-NABLE volunteers allow their community to use personal 3D printers to help those born with missing fingers and hands or who have lost them due to war, natural disaster, illness or accidents. Over 8,000 recipients have been helped. (eNABLE).

The Covid-19 pandemic has also driven prosumers to the fore with 3D printing used widely to fill the need for low-cost, rapid fabrication of medical devices and personal protective equipment as the world faced a short fall from more established production lines. Frontline healthcare workers became actively involved in designing items for personal and peer use. Not only was 3D printing used to crucially help with this shortfall, it demonstrated, in real time, how fast translation can be when problem and outcome focused. (Radfar et al., 2021).

Public awareness of the ability to use 3D printing to customize prothesis, implants and other devices is increasing demand for such products. In turn, this drives innovation and translation. There has been an explosion in prosumer driven custom-made prosthetics, such as Free 3D Hands and Art4Leg, allowing patients to be involved in designing their own limb or casts with an increasing focus on developing better functionality at lower cost. (Ventola 2014; Nawrat 2018; Paul et al., 2018; Aimar et al., 2019). Surgeons commonly use 3D models and templates to plan and improve surgery, resulting in shorter operating times and

better functional outcomes. (Shinomiya et al., 2018; Witjes et al., 2018; Aimar et al., 2019; Fan et al., 2020).

ENTREPRENEURIALISM

Entrepreneurialism seeks creation or extraction of value through creativity and innovation. (Patel and Mehta 2016). The historic lack of return on biomedical research is a prime driving force behind the increased need for entrepreneurial thinking in translational research to continue to attract funding and investment. (Woolf 2008; Molas-Gallart et al., 2016). 3D printing has done that partly because the products are physically tangible and immediate. The healthcare impacts and hence return on investment is visible. A burgeoning industry based on 3D printing has evolved. Established medical device companies, such as Stryker and Medtronic, are investing heavily in 3D printing, for customized implants, training and simulation, and to reduce development time via the use of rapid prototyping. (Medtronic 2017; Sher 2020). Multiple new companies have arisen producing 3D printers, 3D printing material and digital files, creating such products as "organs-on-a-chip". (Jiang et al., 2017; Paul et al., 2018; Aimar et al., 2019; Fan et al., 2020; Wu et al., 2020).

The impact is that the foundations of good business (creating or delivering something of value that people want or need, at a price they are willing to pay, in a way that meets their needs and expectations and that will generate enough profit to make it worthwhile for the owners to continue operations) (Kaufman 2013), need to be worked into the translational research design. Increasingly business management strategies are being employed in translational research to improve efficiency and cost-effectiveness. (Schweikhart and Dembe 2009).

OBSTACLES AND PITFALLS

3D printing is an exciting technology. It fires the imagination, bringing with it the biggest risk: exposing scientific research to public hype. The Gartner Hype Cycle is a graphic representation of the maturity and adoption of technologies and applications, and how they are potentially relevant to solving real world problems. (Gartner 2020). Whilst publicity can be good, hype can inflate public expectations and erode trust, undermining the scientific process and profession. (Rinaldi 2012). In healthcare, public trust is paramount for uptake of new ideas and technologies. They need to be seen to deliver on their promise.

Complex regulatory requirements are seen as a major barrier. (Fudge et al., 2016). New requirements for medical devices introduced in Europe in 2017 and subsequently by other jurisdictions to improve the safety of medically implanted devices (European Parliament and Council on medical devices 2017) followed a significant breast implant issue. (Russell 2017). Whilst appropriate for mass production implants they lack the nuance required for more customized 3D printed products. Legislation for 3D printing of devices in many jurisdictions doesn't distinguish between difference purposes. A 3D model for surgical planning or educating patients can fall into the same regulation as devices for implant. Use of 3D printing across many facets of translational research makes it difficult to produce cohesive regulation. (Christensen and Rybicki 2017). Achieving balance of safety and social responsibility without generating too much stifling red tape is challenging. (Christensen and Rybicki 2017; Adamo et al., 2018; Aimar et al., 2019).

3D printing highlights the need for increased and early multidisciplinary collaboration in translational research. (Fudge et al., 2016; Homes 2018). Whilst a major benefit in ensuring research is directed to a real world need, lack of clear definition of concepts and different language between engineers, clinicians and other stakeholders can create confusion, lack of clarity and direction that can hamper progress. (Woolf 2008; LeClair et al., 2020). Competing demands on clinicians time with lack of protected and funded time for research impedes stakeholder engagement. (LeClair et al., 2020). The application of engineering principles to human biology and medicine in order to improve healthcare and healthcare outcomes brings with it the burden of ethical responsibilities to bioengineers to anticipate the consequences of their technological designs for medical practice in a manner similar to a medical practitioner. These include do no harm, informed consent, confidentiality and dignity. Tissue engineering, use of biomaterials and implants, and neural engineering each generate specific numerous ethical concerns that will need to be addressed. (Moffat 2017).

Commercial partnerships and funding arrangements can generate conflict of interest and pitfalls, through looking for faster, more expedient ways to bring devices or technologies to market, or creating prestige to advance further funding opportunities without paying attention to the way this is achieved. (Molas-Gallart et al., 2016). The disastrous artificial tracheal implant saga highlights this can occur at even the most respected institutes. (Schneider 2016). Repercussions impact not only the individuals and institute involved but undermine public confidence across the medical implant device industry and potentially the view taken by regulators.

Finally, measuring and evaluating progress is unstandardized. Personalization makes outcome measures harder to determine and standardize and risks putting the need of the individual before the community. Many academic organizations reward work based on individual output primarily through publications and grants, rather than team outputs, patents, trade secrets, and impact on health outcomes. This can dissuade collaboration and translation.(Fudge et al., 2016; Smith et al., 2017; Clay et al., 2019).

FUTURE

3D printing has demonstrated that when healthcare needs, such as prosthetic limbs, are the driver, real world outcomes can be achieved at a faster pace with less waste and lower costs. As the cost of 3D printers and materials reduce, these technologies will become more widely available. Use of 3D printed organoids is already seeing the cost of pharmaceutical development being reduced and has potential to reduce, if not eliminate, use of animal experimentation. (Fan et al., 2020; Rawal et al., 2021). Prosumer groups, such as e-NABLE, have demonstrated that it will not necessarily be the wealthiest countries to benefit.

The temptation may be to either overregulate or forgo proper safety assessment. Jurisdictions that are agile in adapting their regulations to ensure a balance of safety whilst not stifling progress will be the big winners.

Those countries or groups who can connect and engage with the end-users, build functioning multi-disciplinary teams across a myriad of disciplines, and maintain focus on meeting the desired healthcare outcomes will achieve faster translation and better return on research, government and commercial funding. Finally, those who are able to grasp how 3D printing technologies can be used in understanding complex systems will be the ones to tap into the wealth of knowledge that has yet to produce healthcare impact.

SUMMARY

In this century, 3D printing has moved from the realm of fiction to generating impact on health outcomes and healthcare across the spectrum. 3D printing has been pivotal in the merging of engineering and biomedical fields. In this way, it has helped shape how translational research is defined, understood and pursued.

AUTHOR CONTRIBUTIONS

ES researched, developed, drafted and wrote the article.

ACKNOWLEDGMENTS

Thank you to both Funding Groups that have enabled the Author to develop expertise in translational research in the bioengineering field.

REFERENCES

1. Adamo, J. E., Grayson, W. L., Hatcher, H., Brown, J. S., Thomas, A., Hollister, S., et al. (2018). Regulatory Interfaces Surrounding the Growing Field of Additive Manufacturing of Medical Devices and Biologic Products. J. Clin. Trans. Sci. 2 (5), 301–304. doi:10.1017/cts.2018.331
2. Aimar, A., Palermo, A., and Innocenti, B. (20192019). The Role of 3D Printing in Medical Applications: A State of the Art. J. Healthc. Eng. 2019, 5340616. doi:10.1155/2019/5340616
3. Baker, S. G. (2012). Paradoxes in Carcinogenesis Should Spur New Avenues of Research: An Historical Perspective. Disruptive Sci. Technol. 1 (2), 100–107. doi:10.1089/dst.2012.0011
4. Balas, E. A., and Boren, S. A. (2000). Managing Clinical Knowledge for Health Care Improvement. Yearb. Med. Inform. 09, 65–70. doi:10.1055/s-0038-1637943
5. Bertolaso, M. (2017). "A System Approach to Cancer. From Things to Relations," in Philosophy of Systems Biology : Perspectives from Scientists and Philosophers. Editor S. Green (Heidelberg, Germany: Springer International Publishing), 37–47. doi:10.1007/978-3-319-47000-9_3
6. Bertolaso, M., Giuliani, A., and De Gara, L. (2011). Systems Biology Reveals Biology of Systems. Complexity 16 (6), 10–16. doi:10.1002/cplx.20353
7. Bizzarri, M., and Cucina, A. (2014). Tumor and the Microenvironment: a Chance to Reframe the Paradigm of Carcinogenesis? Biomed. Res. Int. 2014 (934038), 934038. doi:10.1155/2014/934038

8. Brodie, E. G., Robinson, K. J., Sigston, E., Molotnikov, A., and Frith, J. E. (2021). Osteogenic Potential of Additively Manufactured TiTa Alloys. ACS Appl. Bio Mater. 4 (1), 1003–1014. doi:10.1021/acsabm.0c01450

9. Chien, S., Bashir, R., Nerem, R. M., and Pettigrew, R. (2015). Engineering as a New Frontier for Translational Medicine. Sci. Transl Med. 7 (281), 281fs13. doi:10.1126/scitranslmed.aaa4325

10. Christensen, A., and Rybicki, F. J. (2017). Maintaining Safety and Efficacy for 3D Printing in Medicine. 3d Print Med. 3 (1), 1. doi:10.1186/s41205-016-0009-5

11. Clay, M., Hiraki, L. T., Lamot, L., Medhat, B. M., Sana, S., and Small, A. R. (2019). Developing Reflection and Collaboration in Translational Medicine toward Patients and Unmet Medical Needs. Front. Med. 6, 94. doi:10.3389/fmed.2019.00094

12. Cohrs, R. J., Martin, T., Ghahramani, P., Bidaut, L., Higgins, P. J., and Shahzad, A. (2015). Translational Medicine Definition by the European Society for Translational Medicine. New Horizons Translational Med. 2 (3), 86–88. doi:10.1016/j.nhtm.2014.12.002

13. Contopoulos-Ioannidis, D. G., Alexiou, G. A., Gouvias, T. C., and Ioannidis, J. P. A. (2008). Life Cycle of Translational Research for Medical Interventions. Science 321 (5894), 1298–1299. doi:10.1126/science.1160622

14. eNABLE (). Enabling the Future. Available at: https://enablingthefuture.org/.

15. European Parliament and Council on medical devices (2017). Regulation (EU) 2017/745 of the European Parliament and of the Council of 5 April 2017 on Medical Devices, Amending Directive 2001/83/EC, Regulation (EC) No 178/2002 and Regulation (EC) No 1223/2009 and Repealing Council Directives 90/385/ EEC and 93/42/EEC (Text with EEA relevance)Text with EEA Relevance. (EU) 2017/745. Available at: https://eur-lex.europa.eu/legal-content/EN/TXT/? uri=CELEX%3A32017R0745.

16. Fallon, H. J. (2002). The Institute of Medicine and its Quality of Healthcare in America Reports. Trans. Am. Clin. Climatol Assoc. 113, 119–125. discussion 125.

17. Fan, D., Li, Y., Wang, X., Zhu, T., Wang, Q., Cai, H., et al. (2020). Progressive 3D Printing Technology and its Application in Medical Materials. Front. Pharmacol. 11, 122. doi:10.3389/fphar.2020.00122

18. Fort, D. G., Herr, T. M., Shaw, P. L., Gutzman, K. E., and Starren, J. B. (2017). Mapping the Evolving Definitions of Translational Research. J. Clin. Trans. Sci. 1 (1), 60–66. doi:10.1017/cts.2016.10

19. Fudge, N., Sadler, E., Fisher, H. R., Maher, J., Wolfe, C. D. A., and McKevitt, C. (2016). Optimising Translational Research Opportunities: A Systematic Review and Narrative Synthesis of Basic and Clinician Scientists' Perspectives of Factors Which Enable or Hinder Translational Research. PLoS One 11 (8), e0160475. doi:10.1371/journal.pone.0160475

20. Gannon, F. (2014). The Steps from Translatable to Translational Research. EMBO Rep. 15 (11), 1107–1108. doi:10.15252/embr.201439587

21. Gartner (2020). Gartner Hype Cycle. Available at: https://www.gartner.com/en/ research/methodologies/gartner-hype-cycle.

22. Goh, B. T., Lee, S., Tideman, H., and Stoelinga, P. J. W. (2008). Mandibular Reconstruction in Adults: a Review. Int. J. Oral Maxillofac. Surg. 37 (7), 597–605. doi:10.1016/j.ijom.2008.03.002

23. Green, S. (2017). "Introduction to Philosophy of Systems Biology," in Introduction to Philosophy of Systems Biology. Philosophy of Systems Biology : Perspectives from Scientists and Philosophers. Editor S. Green (Heidelberg, Germany: Springer International Publishing), 1–23. doi:10.1007/978-3-319-47000-9_1

24. Greene, M. T., Gonzalez, R., Papalambros, P. Y., and McGowan, A.-M. (2017). Design Thinking vs. Systems Thinking for Engineering Design: What's the Difference? 21st International Conference on Engineering Design. Vancouver, Canada: University of British Columbia.

25. Greenman, C., Stephens, P., Smith, R., Dalgliesh, G. L., Hunter, C., Bignell, G., et al. (2007). Patterns of Somatic Mutation in Human Cancer Genomes. Nature 446 (7132), 153–158. doi:10.1038/nature05610

26. Gutwald, R., Jaeger, R., and Lambers, F. M. (2017). Customized Mandibular Reconstruction Plates Improve Mechanical Performance in a Mandibular Reconstruction Model. Comp. Methods Biomech. Biomed. Eng. 20 (4), 426–435. doi:10.1080/10255842.2016.1240788

27. Homes, J. W. (2018). Accelerating Health Care Innovation by Connecting Engineering and medicine." the Conversation. Available at: https://theconversation.com/accelerating-health-careinnovation-by-connecting-engineering-and-medicine-107125.

28. Jia, X. (2016). Translational Medicine: Creating the Crucial Bidirectional Bridge between Bench and Bedside. Int. J. Mol. Sci. 17 (11), 1918. doi:10.3390/ijms17111918

29. Jiang, R., Kleer, R., and Piller, F. T. (2017). Predicting the Future of Additive Manufacturing: A Delphi Study on Economic and Societal Implications of 3D Printing for 2030. Technol. Forecast. Soc. Change 117, 84–97. doi:10.1016/j.techfore.2017.01.006

30. Kaufman, J. (2013). The Personal MBA: A World-Class Business Education in a Single Volume GB. London, United Kingdom: Penguin UK.

31. Kolodkin, A. (2017). "Systems Biology through the Concept of Emergence," in Systems Biology through the Concept of Emergence. Philosophy of Systems Biology : Perspectives from Scientists and Philosophers. Editor S. Green (Heidelberg, Germany: Springer International Publishing), 181–191. doi:10.1007/978-3-319-47000-9_17

32. Lasser, R. (2013). Engineering Method. Electrical and Computer Engineering Design Handbook. Massachusetts: Department of Electrical and Computer Engineering, Tufts University.

33. LeClair, A. M., Kotzias, V., Garlick, J., Cole, A. M., Kwon, S. C., Lightfoot, A., et al. (2020). Facilitating Stakeholder Engagement in Early Stage Translational Research. PLoS One 15 (7), e0235400. doi:10.1371/ journal.pone.0235400

34. Mansilla, M. O., Salazar-Hernandez, C., Perrin, S. L., Scheer, K. G., Cildir, G., Toubia, J., et al. (2021). 3D-printed Microplate Inserts for Long Term High-Resolution Imaging of Live Brain Organoids. BMC Biomed. Eng. 3 (1), 6. doi:10.1186/s42490-021-00049-5

35. Mazzocchi, F. (2008). Complexity in Biology. EMBO Rep. 9 (1), 10–14. doi:10.1038/ sj.embor.7401147

36. Medtronic (2017). 3D Printing: A New Frontier. Medtronic News Available at: https://www.medtronic.com/ca-en/about/news/3D-printing-at-Medtronic. html 2020.

37. Mesarovic, M. (2017). "Complexity Organizing Principles: Prerequisites for Life," in Philosophy of Systems Biology : Perspectives from Scientists and Philosophers. Editor S. Green (Heidelberg, Germany: Springer International Publishing), 205–213.

38. Moffat, S. (2017). Ethics of Biomedical Engineering: The Unanswered Questions. Significances Bioeng. Biosci. 1 (1). doi:10.31031/sbb.2017.01.000505

39. Molas-Gallart, J., D'Este, P., Llopis, O., and Rafols, I. (2016). Towards an Alternative Framework for the Evaluation of Translational Research Initiatives. Res. Eval. 25 (3), 235–243. doi:10.1093/reseval/rvv027

40. Nawrat, A. (2018). 3D Printing in the Medical Field: Four Major Applications Revolutionising the Industry. Medical Device Network. Available at: https://www.medicaldevice-network.com/features/3d-printing-in-the-medical-field-applications/.

41. Nurse, P. (2008). Life, Logic and Information. Nature 454 (24), 424–426. doi:10.1038/454424a

42. Parthasarathy, J. (2014). 3D Modeling, Custom Implants and its Future Perspectives in Craniofacial Surgery. Ann. Maxillofac. Surg. 4 (1), 9–18. doi:10.4103/2231-0746.133065

43. Patel, S., and Mehta, K. (2016). Systems, Design, and Entrepreneurial Thinking: Comparative Frameworks. Syst. Pract. Action. Res 30 (5), 515–533. doi:10.1007/ s11213-016-9404-5

44. Paul, G. M., Rezaienia, A., Wen, P., Condoor, S., Parkar, N., King, W., et al. (2018). Medical Applications for 3D Printing: Recent Developments. Mo. Med. 115 (1), 75–81.

45. Radfar, P., Bazaz, S. R., Mirakhorli, F., and Warkiani, M. E. (2021). The Role of 3D Printing in the Fight against COVID-19 Outbreak. J. 3D printing Med. 5 (1), 51–60. doi:10.2217/3dp-2020-0028

46. Rawal, P., Tripathi, D. M., Ramakrishna, S., and Kaur, S. (2021). Prospects for 3D Bioprinting of Organoids. Bio-des. Manuf. 4 (3), 627–640. doi:10.1007/ s42242-020-00124-1

47. Rayna, T., Striukova, L., and Darlington, J. (2015). Co-creation and User Innovation: The Role of Online 3D Printing Platforms. J. Eng. Technol. Manage. 37, 90–102. doi:10.1016/j.jengtecman.2015.07.002

48. Reid, J. A., Mollica, P. A., Bruno, R. D., and Sachs, P. C. (2018). Consistent and Reproducible Cultures of Large-Scale 3D Mammary Epithelial Structures Using an Accessible Bioprinting Platform. Breast Cancer Res. 20 (1), 122. doi:10.1186/ s13058-018-1045-4

49. Rinaldi, A. (2012). To Hype, or Not To(o) Hype. EMBO Rep. 13 (4), 303–307. doi:10.1038/embor.2012.39

50. Rubio, D. M., Schoenbaum, E. E., Lee, L. S., Schteingart, D. E., Marantz, P. R., Anderson, K. E., et al. (2010). Defining Translational Research: Implications for Training. Acad. Med. 85 (3), 470–475. doi:10.1097/acm.0b013e3181ccd618

51. Russell, B. (2017). PIP Breast Implants: French Court Tells TUV to Pay Damages. London, United Kingdom: BBC News Online, BBC News.

52. Sanders, S. (2020). What's in a Name: Innovation Partnerships for 21st century Health Care: The Australian challenge. Science 370 (6514), 2.

53. Schmeichel, K. L., Weaver, V. M., and Bissell, M. J. (1998). Structural Cues from the Tissue Microenvironment Are Essential Determinants of the Human Mammary Epithelial Cell Phenotype. J. Mammary Gland Biol. Neoplasia 3 (2), 201–213. doi:10.1023/a:1018751124382

54. Schneider, L. (2016). Macchiarini and Karolinska: the Biomedical Ethics Meltdown. For Better Science Available at: https://forbetterscience.com/2016/02/21/macchiarini-and-karolinska-the-biomedical-ethics-meltdown/.

55. Schwartz, J., and Macomber, C. (2017). So, You Think You Have an Idea: A Practical Risk Reduction-Conceptual Model for Academic Translational Research. Bioengineering (Basel) 4 (2). doi:10.3390/bioengineering4020029

56. Schweikhart, S. A., and Dembe, A. E. (2009). The Applicability of Lean and Six Sigma Techniques to Clinical and Translational Research. J. Investig. Med. 57 (7), 748–755. doi:10.2310/jim.0b013e3181b91b3a

57. Shaw, R. J., Kanatas, A. N., Lowe, D., Brown, J. S., Rogers, S. N., and Vaughan, E. D. (2004). Comparison of Miniplates and Reconstruction Plates in Mandibular Reconstruction. Head Neck 26 (5), 456–463. doi:10.1002/hed.10343

58. Sher, D. (2020). How Medical Device Companies Use AM Today Part 1: Stryker Additive Manufacturing. 3D Printing Media network Available at: https://www.3dprintingmedia.network/stryker-additive-manufacturing/.

59. Shinomiya, A., Shindo, A., Kawanishi, M., Miyake, K., Nakamura, T., Matsubara, S., et al. (2018). Usefulness of the 3D Virtual Visualization Surgical Planning Simulation and 3D Model for Endoscopic Endonasal Transsphenoidal Surgery of Pituitary Adenoma: Technical Report and Review of Literature. Interdiscip. Neurosurg. 13, 13–19. doi:10.1016/j.inat.2018.02.002

60. Smith, C., Baveja, R., Grieb, T., and Mashour, G. A. (2017). Toward a Science of Translational Science. J. Clin. Trans. Sci. 1 (4), 253–255. doi:10.1017/cts.2017.14

61. Sonnenschein, C., and Soto, A. M. (2008). Theories of Carcinogenesis: an Emerging Perspective. Semin. Cancer Biol. 18 (5), 372–377. doi:10.1016/j.semcancer.2008.03.012

62. Soro, N., Attar, H., Brodie, E., Veidt, M., Molotnikov, A., and Dargusch, M. S. (2019). Evaluation of the Mechanical Compatibility of Additively Manufactured Porous Ti-25Ta alloy for Load-Bearing Implant Applications. J. Mech. Behav. Biomed. Mater. 97, 149–158. doi:10.1016/j.jmbbm.2019.05.019

63. Sung, N. S., Crowley, W. F., Jr., Genel, M., Salber, P., Sandy, L., Sherwood, L. M., et al. (2003). Central Challenges Facing the National Clinical Research enterprise. JAMA 289 (10), 1278–1287. doi:10.1001/jama.289.10.1278

64. Trochim, W., Kane, C., Graham, M. J., and Pincus, H. A. (2011). Evaluating Translational Research: a Process Marker Model. Clin. Transl Sci. 4 (3), 153–162. doi:10.1111/j.1752-8062.2011.00291.x

65. van der Laan, A. L., and Boenink, M. (2015). Beyond Bench and Bedside: Disentangling the Concept of Translational Research. Health Care Anal. 23 (1), 32–49. doi:10.1007/s10728-012-0236-x

66. Van Regenmortel, M. H. V. (2004). Biological Complexity Emerges from the Ashes of Genetic Reductionism. J. Mol. Recognit. 17 (3), 145–148. doi:10.1002/jmr.674 Ventola, C. L. (2014). Medical Applications for 3D Printing: Current and Projected Uses. P T 39 (10), 704–711.

67. Westfall, J. M., Mold, J., and Fagnan, L. (2007). Practice-Based Research-"Blue Highways" on the NIH Roadmap. JAMA 297 (4), 403–406. doi:10.1001/jama.297.4.403

68. Witjes, M. J. H., Schepers, R. H., and Kraeima, J. (2018). Impact of 3D Virtual Planning on Reconstruction of Mandibular and Maxillary Surgical Defects in Head and Neck Oncology. Curr. Opin. Otolaryngol. Head Neck Surg. 26 (2), 108–114. doi:10.1097/moo.0000000000000437

69. Woolf, S. H. (2008). The Meaning of Translational Research and Why it Matters. JAMA 299 (2), 211–213. doi:10.1001/jama.2007.26

70. Wu, Q., Liu, J., Wang, X., Feng, L., Wu, J., Zhu, X., et al. (2020). Organ-on-a-chip: Recent Breakthroughs and Future Prospects. Biomed. Eng. Online 19 (1), 9. doi:10.1186/s12938-020-0752-0

2

Development and Characterization of a Biomimetic Totally Implantable Artificial Basilar Membrane System

Juyong Chung[1], Youngdo Jung[2], Shin Hur[2], Jin Ho Kim[3], Sung June Kim[3], Wan Doo Kim[2], Yun-Hoon Choung[4]* and Seung-Ha Oh[5]*

[1] Department of Otolaryngology, Wonkwang University School of Medicine, Iksan, South Korea, [2] Department of Nature-Inspired System and Application, Korea Institute of Machinery and Materials, Daejeon, South Korea, [3] Nano-Bioelectronics & Systems Laboratory, Department of Electrical and Computer Engineering, Seoul National University, Seoul, South Korea, [4] Department of Otolaryngology, Ajou University School of Medicine, Suwon, South Korea, [5] Department of Otorhinolaryngology, Sensory Organ Research Institute, Seoul National University Medical Research Center, Seoul National University College of Medicine, Seoul, South Korea

*Correspondence:
Yun-Hoon Choung
yhc@ajou.ac.kr
Seung-Ha Oh
shaoh@snu.ac.kr

Cochlear implants (CIs) have become the standard treatment for severe-to-profound sensorineural hearing loss. Conventional CIs have some challenges, such as the use of extracorporeal devices, and high power consumption for frequency analysis. To overcome these, artificial basilar membranes (ABMs) made of piezoelectric materials have been studied. This study aimed to verify the conceptual idea of a totally implantable ABM system. A prototype of the totally implantable system composed of the ABM developed in previous research, an electronic module (EM) for the amplification of electrical output from the ABM, and electrode was developed. We investigated the feasibility of the ABM system and obtained meaningful auditory brainstem responses of deafened guinea pigs by implanting the electrode of the ABM system. Also, an optimal method of coupling the ABM system to the human ossicle for transducing sound waves into electrical signals using the middle ear vibration was studied and the electrical signal output according to the sound stimuli was measured successfully. Although the overall power output from the ABM system is still less than the conventional CIs and further improvements to the ABM system are needed, we found a possibility of the developed ABM system as a totally implantable CIs in the future.

Keywords: hearing loss, sensorineural, biomimetics, basilar membrane, cochlear implant

INTRODUCTION

The human ear consists of the external ear, middle ear, and inner ear. Sound waves enter the external ear and pass through the external ear canal, which reach the ear drum. Eardrum vibrates in response to the sound signal. These vibrations are amplified in the middle ear through the ossicular transmission and sent to the cochlea. The cochlea acts as a transducer that converts mechanical vibration into electrical signals (Kang et al., 2015). The basal membrane in the cochlear has a trapezoid structure, which is narrow and thick in the base, and wide and thin in the apex. Due to its physical and structural features, the basal membrane acts as a frequency analyzer that shows frequency selectivity (Saadatzi et al., 2020). On the base, the maximal displacement of BM is shown for the high frequency sound, and the maximal displacement at the apex is shown for the low frequency sound. The BM separate the vibration according to the frequency. And then, the hair cell react to its movement generating electrical signal. The electrical signal stimulates the auditory nerve and is transmitted to the auditory cortex. Problems in any part of the process of sound transmission from the external ear to the brain can lead to hearing loss, and most of the hearing loss is caused by cochlear impairment.

Cochlear implants (CIs) are universally considered to be the standard of care for the medical treatment of severe-to-profound sensorineural hearing loss. Nevertheless, conventional CIs have some challenges such as problems caused by the use of extracorporeal devices and a very high power consumption of the wireless power transmission, implanted stimulating circuit, and digital signal processor (DSP) (Wang et al., 2008). To overcome these problems, many researchers have focused on developing fully implantable CIs (FICIs). However, even the newly developed FICI had some limitations in its practical application. It has a subcutaneous microphone that produces too much ambient noise, and a battery that requires frequent recharging (Briggs et al., 2008). As a result, an FICI requires ultra-low-power sound processing and energy-efficient neural stimulation (Yip et al., 2014). To solve these two problems, several researchers developed a bioelectronic middle ear microphone to eliminate the need for a subcutaneous microphone and a self-powered piezoelectric device to reduce power consumption.

To eliminate the microphone, some researchers have used the acoustic energy directly from the ossicles. In 1999, Maniglia et al. (1999) developed a bioelectronic middle ear microphone of this kind. More recently, the Envoy Esteem implant uses a "sensor" that is placed on the body of the incus where it can detect tympanic membrane vibration. The sensor converts the vibration to an electrical signal and sends it to the sound processor. Subsequently, the sound processor amplifies, filters, and sends the stimulus to the piezoelectric transducers (the "driver") that converts the electrical signal back to mechanical energy and vibrates the stapes (Pulcherio et al., 2014). Thus, fully implantable middle ear implants typically use an implantable sensor to detect the mechanical motion of the ossicles, using the ear as a natural microphone (Yip et al., 2014).

Besides, to solve the problem of conventional CIs requiring frequent recharging, many studies have tried to reproduce the function of a basilar membrane in the human cochlea and to develop an artificial cochlea. At present, several research groups have been focusing on the development of an artificial basilar membrane (ABM), which is a piezoelectric acoustic nanosensor that mimics the function of human hair cells. In a healthy inner ear, sound waves move hair cells by converting vibrations to electrical signals; likewise, sound waves deform the piezoelectric membrane, generating electrical signals that propagate through the auditory nerve. Frequency selectivity in the ABM is determined by the trapezoidal geometry as it is in a natural basilar membrane. Piezoelectric membranes can self-generate electricity, thereby reducing the need for frequent battery recharging.

There are two types of ABM; the cantilever type and membrane-type ABM. Tanaka et al. (1998) and Xu et al. (2004) proposed a microcantilever array that mimics the mechanical

performance of the BM. Recently, Jang et al. (2015) reported an ABM that was fabricated using a micro-electromechanical system (MEMS)-based piezoelectric cantilever array. However, the cantilever-type ABM has a higher resonant frequency (> 3 kHz) than the human voice band (0.3–3.5 kHz). Our research team has developed a membrane type ABM with resonant frequencies within the human hearing sound range (Jung et al., 2015). In our previous paper (Jung et al., 2015), our teams reported the development of an ABM with frequency separation behaviors within an audible frequency range (450–5,000 Hz), which covers most of the voice band. This ABM can analyze vibratory signal inputs and convert them into electrical signal outputs without an external power source by mimicking the function of the human cochlea. The ABM is composed of a piezoelectric film (polyvinylidene difluoride, PVDF) with 13 electrodes on top. The piezoelectric artificial membrane was assembled with a liquid chamber, which was fixed onto the experimental platform. This membrane structure was adjacent to the liquid chamber, and if the micro-accelerator pushed the base port equivalent to the oval window of the cochlea, membrane displacement occurred, resulting in the generation of an electronic signal from the ABM. We measured the vibration response and voltage production of the ABM throughout the frequency range to analyze the function of the ABM as a sound frequency analyzer (Jung et al., 2015).

However, preexisting ABMs have some limitations for clinical application. First, the electrical output from ABMs is not sufficient to stimulate auditory neurons. To acquire sufficient and effective stimulation of auditory neurons, the electrical output should be amplified throughout the EM. Second, we need to use the acoustic energy directly from the ossicles to eliminate the microphone for totally implantable cochlear implants. An optimal method of connection for transmitting the vibration energy to the coupled piezoelectric ABM is needed.

This study aimed to devise and evaluate the feasibility of a new concept of a totally implantable ABM system using an ABM.

1. To develop an EM for the amplification of electrical output from ABMs and investigate the auditory brainstem responses of deafened guinea pigs, which are stimulated by the amplified output of electricity generated by the combination of the ABM and EM in response to vibration input from the micro-actuator.
2. To study the most suitable connection method for coupling ABMs to the middle ear ossicle and check the possibility of a bioelectronic middle ear microphone.

MATERIALS AND METHODS

Conceptual Design of a Totally Implantable ABM System

The term totally implantable ABM system implies a complete connection system, as shown in **Figure 1**. The system works as thus: the sound vibrates the ossicle, which activates the connected ABM. From there, the ABM converts the sound into electrical output. The output from the ABM is amplified and converted into a biphasic current signal by the EM, which transmits the electrical output to the electrode inserted into the cochlea. This electrode, in turn, stimulates the auditory nerve. This is a schematic of the entire system, implanted in the mastoid cavity. Unlike conventional CIs, there was no external microphone because we used ossicular vibrations. The ABM converts ossicular vibrations into electrical signals, which are transmitted to the inserted electrode array, stimulating the auditory nerve. The EM is located in the temporal area (**Figure 1**). Thus, the ABM is an acoustic sensor that senses the sound stimuli and converts it to an electrical signal and acts as a frequency analyzer.

ABM Packaging and Functional Evaluation of ABM

A detailed description of ABM is provided in a previous paper (Jung et al., 2015). The fabrication process included a microfabrication process that formed patterned line electrodes and electrical pads, a corona polling process to increase piezoelectricity of piezoelectric polymer film, and assembly process of a membrane part and packaging part. In brief, the ABM is composed of a piezoelectric film (PVDF) with 13 electrodes on top (**Figure 2A**). The membrane was designed to have a logarithmic width varying from 0.97 to 8.0 mm along the 28-mm length. The piezoelectric polymer film was made of a 25.4-μm thick PVDF film (Kynar® Film, Professional Plastics, Singapore). The fabricated ABM was assembled with the newly developed package as shown in **Figure 2A**. The package includes a main liquid chamber on which ABM is assembled firmly with liquid sealing layer and ABM fixture. External vibrational stimuli are applied through a base port and the output signals from the ABM are transmitted through a slit on the apex side. All the package was made with biocompatible titanium. The size of ABM packaging was minimized for implantation in the mastoid cavity. The ABM successfully separated low frequency at the apex (distal end) and high frequency at the base (proximal end) from incoming sound stimuli. In a previous paper, we analyzed the voltage production of the ABM throughout the frequency range, and our ABM showed six channels of frequency separation characteristics. The base port of the ABM is the movable area where the vibration input by the piezoactuator (P-883.11, PI Ceramic, Lederhose, Germany) is applied. This area is equivalent to an oval window in the human ear. The piezoactuator generates a displacement of the base port up to 6.5 μm according to the amplified voltage applied to the piezoactuator by the amplifier. Since the blocking force of the piezo actuator is very high (190 N) compared to the force required to move the base port, the displacement of the base port is the same as that of the piezoactuator. The displacement of the piezoactuator (from 0 to 5 μm) showed a linear relationship with the applied voltage input to the piezoactuator amplifier (from 0 to 10 V) (**Figure 2B**). We measured the electrical output from the ABM according to the input voltage of the piezoactuator (**Figure 2C**). We acquired the relationship between the displacement of the base port and the electrical output from ABM using the measured values (**Figure 2D**). The ratio of the electrical output and the displacement of the base port represents the sensitivity (mV/μ M) of the ABM.

Development of the EM and Functional Analysis

The EM is composed of an amplifier module, signal controller, current stimulator, and Bluetooth module to enable recharging (**Figure 3A**).

This module obtains electrical signals from the ABM, amplifies the electrical output from the ABM, and transfers controlled biphasic signals to the electrode inserted into the cochlea. This EM has 16 channels and an amplification ratio of 40.22 to 57.13 db. The stimulation strategy of the current stimulator is the continuous interleaved sampling (CIS) strategy. The conversion ratio (mA/mV) for EM was from 0.05 to 0.53. Thus, an electrical output of 1 mV generated by the ABM was amplified and converted to biphasic signals of at least 0.05 to 0.53 mA.

In the *in vivo* experiment, we used two guinea pigs (Hartley, males, 8 weeks old, 300–350 g in weight). Anesthesia was induced using ketamine (40 mg/kg, intramuscularly) and xylazine (10 mg/kg, intramuscularly). And then, under aseptic conditions, a retroauricular incision was made. And the overlying muscle was dissected to expose the bulla. Bullotomy was performed by drilling a hole through the bulla to expose the round window niche and the basal turn of the cochlea. And cochleostomy was performed on the basal turn of cochlea and saline was irrigated through the cochleostomy site to introduce deafening in both ears (Lee et al., 2017). In order to confirm deafness, we assessed the hearing status of guinea pigs after deafening by measuring ABRs. Then, the subjects were implanted with intracochlear stimulating electrodes into the cochlea. The intracochlear electrode was inserted into scala tympani through the cochleostomy site and then placed about 2 mm deep from the cochleostomy site (**Supplementary Figure 1**). All animal and experimental protocols were approved by the Seoul National University Hospital Institutional Animal Care and Use Committee (SNUH-IACUC, No. 12-0144). All animals were treated in accordance with the Guide for the Care and Use of Laboratory Animals (8th ed., 2010). And electrical auditory brainstem response (eABR) measurements were performed in a sound-attenuated and electrically shielded room. eABRs were recorded in a similar manner to ABR measurements. The stimulus presentations, ABR acquisitions, equipment control and data management were coordinated using the computerized Intelligent Hearing Systems (IHS, Miami, FL, United States) with the Smart EP software. The biphasic current signal from a combination of the microphone and EM were applied. The electrical stimuli stimulated the subjects' auditory nerves and we measured it with an eABR. The data acquisition digitization parameters were identical to the ABR recording parameters (100–1,500-Hz filter, 512 repetitions). When sound stimuli (from 77 to 85 dB SPL) was applied, a conventional microphone to transmit the electrical signal to the EM. The electrical output amplified and modulated by the EM was transmitted to the electrode inserted into the guinea pig's cochlea (**Figure 3B**). The spiral

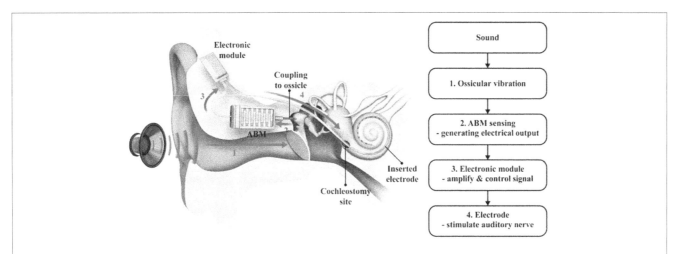

FIGURE 1 | A schematic drawing of the entire ABM system. (1) The sound vibrates the ossicle which activates the connected ABM, (2) The ABM converts the ossicular vibration into electrical output, (3) The output from ABM is amplified and modified by the electronic module, (4) The signal transmitted to the electrode stimulates the auditory nerve. A red arrow indicates the direction in which the signal goes.

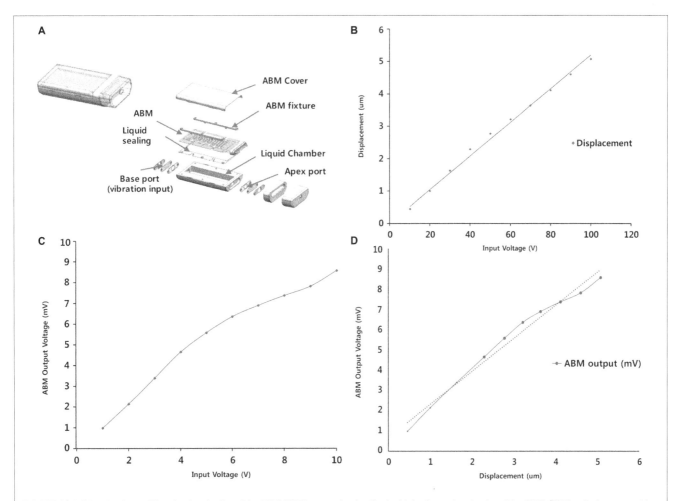

FIGURE 2 | ABM Packaging and functional evaluation of the ABM. (A) The steps involved in the fabrication and packaging of the ABM. (B) The displacement of the base port according to input voltage of piezoactuator. (C) The electrical output from ABM according to the input voltage of the piezoactuator. (D) The relationship between the displacement of the base port and the electrical output from ABM.

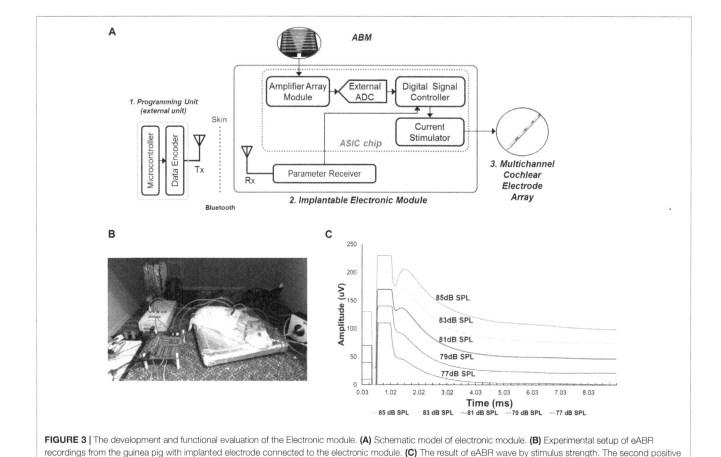

FIGURE 3 | The development and functional evaluation of the Electronic module. **(A)** Schematic model of electronic module. **(B)** Experimental setup of eABR recordings from the guinea pig with implanted electrode connected to the electronic module. **(C)** The result of eABR wave by stimulus strength. The second positive (P2) wave gradually increased in amplitude as the sound stimulus increased.

ganglion neurons were stimulated by the electrical output, and the eABR was recorded from the deafened guinea pig. The eABR recordings were acquired according to the intensity of sound stimuli (**Figure 3C**).

Evaluation of Electrical Output (*in vitro*) and eABR Recording in Animals (*in vivo*) Using a Combined Unit of the ABM and EM

In the *in vitro* test, the electrical output from ABM was applied to the EM, which produced biphasic current output. The ABM produced a maximum of 3.7 mV electrical output at 540 Hz upon vibrational input by the piezoactuator. The electrical output from ABM was amplified by approximately 40 dB (equivalent to approximately one hundred times) through the amplification part of the EM. Finally, the amplified voltage signal was converted into 8-bit digital signals by the analog-to-digital converter (ADC), and the biphasic current signal was generated by the current stimulator (**Figures 4A,B**).

In an *in vivo* animal experiment using a combined unit of the ABM and EM, the same method mentioned in the previous paragraph was used to introduce deafening, and the same surgical procedures such as postauricular incision, exposure of the bulla, bullotomy, and cochleostomy were performed in two guinea pigs.

Spiral ganglion neurons were stimulated by the biphasic current output from the combined unit of the ABM and EM. The input vibration to the ABM was produced by a piezoactuator. As the input signal to the piezoactuator amplifier increases from 1 to 10 V, the electrical output from the ABM increases and generates a higher biphasic current output through the EM. The current output signal was transmitted to the auditory nerve, and we measured it with an eABR (**Figure 4C**).

Measurement of Electrical Output From the ABM With a Tube-Type Connector and Rod-Type Connector Coupled to the Ossicles in a Cadaveric Temporal Bone

We developed a tube-type connector coupled to the umbo and a rod-type connector coupled to the malleus head. Detailed specifications of the design of each connector's length, diameter, and angle were demonstrated in **Supplementary Figure 2**. To find the optimized coupling to the umbo, we chose the suitable design (Type F-2) for the human middle ear among several designs that changed the size and shape of the umbo connection site, the length and diameter of tube, and the angle of tube (**Supplementary Figure 3**). The selection for the most suitable connector was conducted through experiments in which many preliminary connectors were directly attached to the umbo site

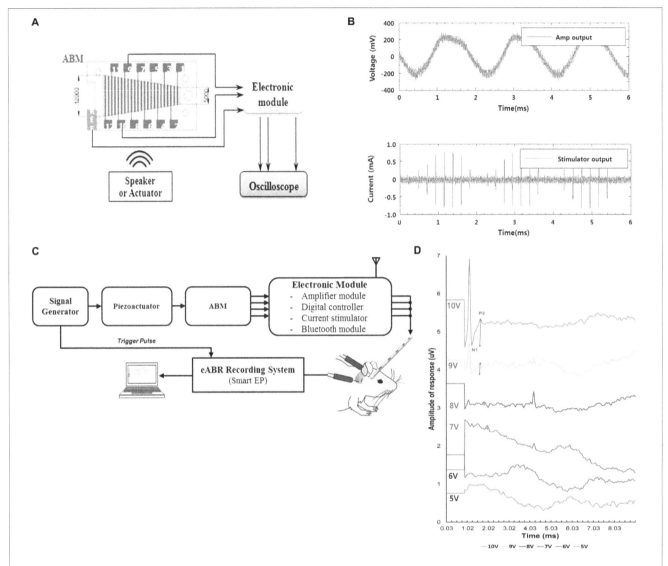

FIGURE 4 | Evaluation of Output Pulse and eABR recordings after Connection between the ABM and the Electronic Module (*in vivo* and *in vitro*). **(A)** Measurement setup of output pulse in ABM puls EM (*in vitro*). **(B)** The graph of output pulse in ABM plus EM (*in vitro*). **(C)** The experimental setup measuring the eABR in a subject. **(D)** Auditory brainstem responses of deafened guinea pigs stimulated by amplified output of electricity generated by the ABM in response to piezoactuator. The red two-way arrow indicates the N1-P2 wave. The N1-P2 wave gradually increased in amplitude as the intensity of the stimulus increased from 7V-10V.

of the human cadaveric temporal bone. The tube-type connector had a membranous part that was coupled to the umbo and a tube part that was filled with liquid and connected to the base port of the ABM packaging (**Figure 5A**). Using a fresh frozen temporal bone, the tube-type connector and the rod-type connector were connected directly to the ossicles of the cadaveric temporal bone to measure the electrical output from the ABM after applying sound stimuli. Sound stimuli were generated by a mouth simulator (B&K, 4,227, Denmark) and applied through a tube-shaped earphone to the external auditory canal. The magnitude and frequency of the applied sound stimuli on the eardrum were 70–120 dB SPL and 200 ~ 8,000 Hz (**Figure 5B**). In order to exclude the noise effect, the electrical output from the ABM was measured when the connector was coupled to the ossicle and when not coupled to the ossicle.

By subtracting the latter value from the value obtained from the former, we obtained an electrical signal that excludes the noise effect. During ossicular coupling to rod-type connectors, the maximum transfer function could be delivered to the ABM when the axis contacting the rod and the malleus head was perpendicular. In addition, to deliver movement of the natural middle ear ossicles to the sensor without energy loss, we should reduce the mechanical loading of the ABM. We had to create a free joint state with little mechanical loading between the ossicle and the rod-type connector. For this purpose, the ABM was fixed in mastoid bone with bone cement. The positioning of rod-type connector at optimistic angle with little loading to the ossicle was very difficult and time-consuming. However, in the tube-type connector, the connection between the membranous part and umbo was relatively easy.

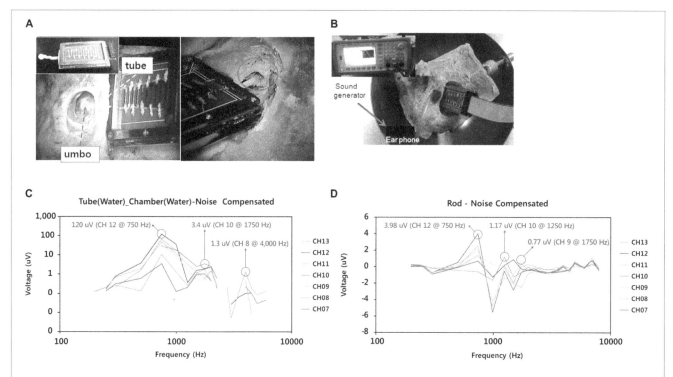

FIGURE 5 | Measurement of electrical output from the ABM with tube-type connector and rod type connector coupled to the ossicles in the cadaveric temporal bone. **(A)** Tube type connector coupled to the umbo (left); Rod type connector coupled with the malleus head (right), **(B)** The process of measuring the electrical output from the ABM package with the connector coupled with the ossicles after applying the sound pressure to the eardrum with sound generator. **(C)** Electrical output from the ABM coupled with tube type connector. **(D)** Electrical output from the ABM coupled with rod type connector.

RESULTS

Measuring Electrical Output Generated From the ABM by Vibratory Input From the Piezoactuator

The relationship between the displacement of the base port and applied voltage input to the piezoactuator demonstrated a proportional relationship of linearity (**Figure 2B**). The input voltage of the piezoactuator and the output voltage of the ABM showed a proportional relationship of linearity (**Figure 2C**). The input voltage of 6 V generated an electrical output of 6 mV from the ABM. Therefore, we assessed the relationship between the displacement of the base port and the electrical output from ABM using **Figures 2B,C**, and a linear relationship between the two was detected in the displacement range from 0 to 5 μm (**Figure 2D**). The sensitivity or efficacy (mV/μm) of the ABM was 1.82 mV/μ m.

Measurement of EM Function (*in vivo*)

Using sound stimuli (from 77 to 85 dB SPL), a conventional microphone transmits the electrical signal to the EM. The signal amplified by the EM is transmitted through the electrode to stimulate the auditory nerve. The electrical currents on the electrode ranged from 200 to 600 μA. The graph shows the varying eABR by stimulus strength (**Figure 3C**). The second peak (P2) wave appeared from the sound stimuli of 77 dB SPL. We

observed that wave patterns gradually increased in amplitude as the stimulus increased.

Measurement of Electrical Output Using the Combined Unit of ABM and EM (*in vitro*)

When the ABM and EM were connected, several mV electrical outputs were generated from the ABM when the actuator was stimulated, and the EM then amplified the electrical output one hundred times to hundreds of mV. The EM converted it into a biphasic current signal, producing a few hundred microamperes of current. This was sufficient to stimulate the subjects' auditory nerves (**Figure 4B**).

eABR Recording in Animals Using the Combined Unit of ABM and EM (*in vivo*)

Figure 4D shows the typical eABR waveforms recorded. The intensity of the stimulus voltage for the actuator was changed from approximately 1 to 10 V in 1 V steps. The first negative peak (N1) and the second positive peak (P2) were always clearly visible and were not obscured by the electrical artifact nor by the digastric muscle response (Hall, 1990). Therefore, wave N1–P2 was analyzed. The thresholds and amplitudes of the N1–P2 wave were measured. The threshold of this animal was 7 V. In **Figure 4D**, according to each stimulus intensity, the magnitude of the red two-way arrow indicates the amplitude of N1-P2 wave.

As the intensity of the stimulus increased from 7 to 10 V, the tracing waveform showed a larger N1–P2 amplitude and shorter latency in general.

Electrical Output From the ABM With Tube-Type Connector and Rod-Type Connector Coupled to the Ossicles in a Cadaveric Temporal Bone

Noise correction was obtained by subtracting the measured electrical output when the ossicle and connector were detached from the measured electrical output when the ossicle and connector were connected. In the tube-type connector coupled to the umbo, we measured 120 μV of electrical output from the ABM applying sound stimuli (110 dB SPL, 750 Hz) (**Figure 5C**). Frequency characteristics showed that ABM with the tube-type connector coupled to the umbo is reduced to three channels compared to six channels in the ABM in response to actuator stimulation. The rod-type connector also has a frequency specificity of three channels and an electrical output of up to 3.98 μV (**Figure 5D**). The positioning of rod type connector at optimistic angle with little loading to the ossicle was very difficult and time-consuming. In addition, the output of the ABM when coupled with the rod-type connector was not constant from experiment to experiment. However, in the tube connector, the connection between the membranous part and umbo was relatively easy, and constant electrical output was obtained from the ABM regardless of the connection angle or contact state. Therefore, a tube-type connector coupled to the umbo was a better option for piezoelectric acoustic sensors in transmitting the vibrational energy of ossicles compared to the rod type connector because it obtained a relatively constant electrical output regardless of the experimental conditions and a larger electrical output than the rod-type connector.

DISCUSSION

We developed a fabricated-packaged ABM with clear frequency separation characteristics within an audible frequency range (450–5,000 Hz) (Jung et al., 2015). The ABM functions as a frequency analyzer that separates vibratory inputs according to their frequency. The ABM converts them into electrical outputs without an external power source by mimicking the function of the human cochlea. The ABM is a fully implantable system using the ME microphone, which reduces the power consumption (20–40 mW) (Zeng et al., 2008) of wireless power transmissions and implements a concept called a self-power generating frequency analyzer. Since ABM serves as a frequency analyzer and our 16-channel amplifier array has reduced power consumption compared to DSP (about 5 mW) (Marsman et al., 2006) the existing CI (may be 1/25), the overall power consumption of the ABM system might be reduced. Conventional CIs require high power consumption and frequent recharging. By using the characteristics of our ABM, which functions as a frequency analyzer and self-generates electricity, the need for frequent

battery recharging can be reduced, and it is possible to develop totally implantable CIs.

However, the electrical output from the current ABM is not sufficient to stimulate auditory neurons. To acquire sufficient stimulation of auditory neurons, the electrical output should be amplified throughout the EM, and we developed an EM different from the existing speech processors. In the present study, we report the recording of eABRs in guinea pigs using a combination of the ABM and the EM. Through this experiment, we confirmed the feasibility of a totally implantable ABM system using ABM. Further, the recording of eABRs was obtained according to the frequency of the input stimuli. Low-frequency sounds or input stimuli peaked near the apex of the ABM, which transmitted its signal to the electrode placed at the apex of the cochlea. In addition, we designed various types of connectors to determine the most suitable connection method for coupling with the ossicle. Although the electrical output from the ABM decreased during coupling with the ossicles, the output of the ABM when coupled with the tube-type connector was greater than when coupled with the rod type connector. The development of connectors has opened the possibility of bioelectronics middle ear microphones obtaining acoustic energy from the ossicles and the possibility of full implantation without the need for an external microphone.

Several ABMs have been developed so far, and each ABM has advantages and disadvantages. Jang et al. (2015) demonstrated an ABM based on a piezoelectric cantilever array with frequency selectivity in the range of 2.92–12.6 kHz. Comparing this ABM with ours, our ABM is closer to a totally implantable cochlear implant because the frequency range is closer to the speech frequency range (450–5,000 Hz) and it is packaged with a liquid chamber for implantation into the body. To improve the efficacy of the ABM in the frequency band of the human speech range, our team utilized the PVDF film instead of more efficient piezoelectric materials, modified the design of ABM, and included a liquid chamber. Moreover, we explored the ossicular connection with the ABM for a totally implantable ABM system. Inaoka et al. (2011) examined whether sound stimuli applied to the stapes generated electrical output from the piezoelectric membrane after implantation into the cochlea. When sound stimuli at 100 dB SPL at frequencies of 5, 10, or 20 kHz were directly applied to the stapes using an actuator, peak-to-peak voltage outputs of 23.7, 5.7, or 29.3 μV were recorded, respectively. This piezoelectric membrane was used as small sizes for implantation into the guinea pig cochlea. Therefore, the electrical output from this device is not sufficient to stimulate auditory primary neurons. This output was approximately 50 times smaller than the electrical output of our ABM. The electrical output should be 10^5-fold higher than the output of this device for effective stimulation of auditory primary neurons when electrodes are placed in the scala tympani, similar to conventional CIs. In addition, we compared our ABM with the existing literatures on ABM development using PVDF. Saadatzi et al. (2020) developed the ABM with PVDF plates and gold electrodes mounted on the PDMS elastomer matrix. This ABM showed five channels of frequency separation characteristics within the frequency range of 3 to 8 kHz. Another ABM reported in 2018 had a novel vibration control technique of an artificial auditory cochlear epithelium that mimics the function of outer hair cells (Tsuji et al., 2018). It showed four channels of frequency separation characteristics at frequency more than 4.6 kHz. Conversely, our ABM reduced the resonant frequency to 450 Hz, had biocompatible packaging, and implemented a prototype for a totally implantable ABM system using the EM module. In this study, we obtained eABR responses in experimental animals when the ABM system (ABM + EM) is applied *in vivo* and evaluated the feasibility of the ABM system in terms of electrical power and frequency selectivity. This point is a distinction from the existing studies that studied only the characteristics of the ABM itself, and the possibility of clinical application can be evaluated through *in vivo* study of ABM systems implanted in the guinea pig. Our ABM system requires 100 times amplification for effective stimulation of auditory primary neurons compared to the output current from the conventional CI.

Despite the advantages of our ABM system, some limitations need to be improved upon for its practical use for transplants: (1) insufficient sensitivity as a sensor, (2) reduction in ABM sensitivity during coupling with the ossicle, and (3) insufficient electrical power of the whole ABM system.

ABM Sensitivity as a Sensor and Improvement of Sensitivity

The ABM efficiency was 1.82 mV/μm, as shown in **Figure 2C**. As much as the base port is pushed by the actuator in the experimental range of 0–5 μm, the electrical output was produced in proportion to the displacement of the base port. This is a new finding that was not discovered in the previous study. In addition, using the finite element (FE) model to convert the displacement of the base port to sound pressure, **Figure 6A** shows the sensitivity of ABM (mV/Pa). To calculate the equivalent sound pressures applied to the base port as a function of the displacement by the piezoactuator, finite element modeling including the ABM, liquid chamber, and base port was carried out. We aimed to measure the electrical output from the ABM based on the input sound pressure and to evaluate the sensitivity of the ABM as a sensor. We measured the electrical output generated from the ABM by the vibratory input from the piezoactuator in the same way as in the previous paper (Jung et al., 2015). The ABM sensitivity was 0.120 mV/Pa in this study. In the ABM based on piezoelectric cantilever array, the maximum sensitivity was 1.67 mV/Pa, and the sensitivity of the ABM was in the range of 0.354–1.67 mV/Pa (Jang et al., 2015). Despite the difference in material and characteristics between the membrane-type ABM and cantilever-type ABM, our ABM should increase the sensitivity as a sensor to increase the efficacy of the whole system. To improve the efficacy of the ABM, more efficient piezoelectric material with self-powered sensing capability should be developed. A comparative study on the different piezoelectric materials can be performed to determine the best candidate for sensor integration. We used film PVDF for our ABM. However, lead zirconite titanate (PZT) showed a 10 times higher piezoelectric charge/force ratio than that of PVDF film (Boukabache et al., 2014). Our team has made many attempts to find more efficient piezoelectric materials. In general, polymer type piezoelectric materials has much lower piezoelectric response in the range of 0.1 ∼ 42 pC/N, while ceramic type piezoelectric materials such as PZT has piezoelectric response of 490 pC/N (Guerin et al., 2019). However, polymer type piezoelectric materials such as PVDF has much lower Young's modulus of 1.7 GPa compared to that of PZT (∼60 GPa). The trade-off between piezoelectric response and Young's modulus should be carefully considered for developing ABM as it required high signal output in the human audible frequency range. Considering piezoelectric response and Young's modulus of PZT and PVDF, we selected PVDF as the best material to produce a larger signal output at human audible frequency range, which is biocompatible, and has no problem with its performance even after prolonged exposure to heat and moisture. In addition, our research team also attempted to develop a partially etched form of ABM to increase the efficiency of existing ABMs for next-generation ABM research (Kang et al., 2015). In an effort to improve the frequency separation performance, a partially etched-type ABM was presented by varying the thickness of ABM. By mimicking the longitudinal pattern of human basilar membrane, the partially etched-type ABM showed improved frequency separation performance and lowered the responsive frequency range. Also, the vibrational displacement was increased almost 3 times compared to non-etched ABM. To increase the power of a piezoelectric membrane, attempts to reduce the thickness of a piezoelectric membrane and to change into multilayer construction should be done (Inaoka et al., 2011). Efforts are ongoing to discover more efficient piezoelectric materials and develop more efficient ABM structures in terms of the electrical output and frequency selectivity.

The Concept of the Middle Ear Microphone

The middle ear microphone converts the vibration of the tympanic membrane or ossicles into an electrical signal (Mitchell-Innes et al., 2017). For the total implantable CI system, we used the middle ear microphone to obtain the vibration from the ossicle and connect it to the base port of the ABM. In a previous study, we measured the displacement transfer function of each part of the ossicles using laser Doppler vibrometry to determine the site of maximum ossicular motion that would be optimal for attachment of the sensor portion of the fully implantable prosthesis (Chung et al., 2013). The malleus head and the incus body turned out to be an optimal ossicular site for coupling to middle ear microphones. We used the malleus head as the site to connect to the ABM with the rod type connector. However, since the umbo is a straightforward access area and site of maximum ossicular vibration, there has been an attempt to detect the ossicular vibration for totally implantable hearing devices by attaching the piezoelectric sensor directly to the umbo (Gesing et al., 2018). In this study, the size of ABM was too large to directly contact the umbo, so we designed the most appropriate tube-type connector coupled to the umbo and conducted several trial-and-error methods, actually experimented with various designs and forms of the tube-type connectors several times. This is

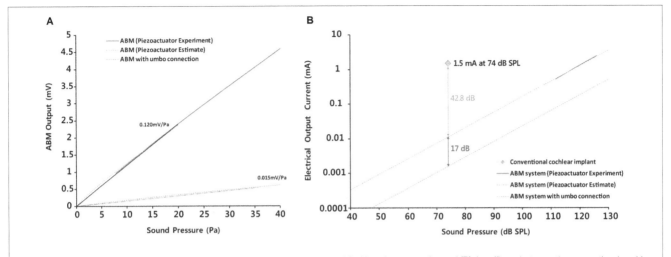

FIGURE 6 | The comparison of **(A)** the sensitivity as a sensor between ABM and ABM with umbo connection and **(B)** the efficacy between the conventional cochlear implant, ABM system, and ABM system with umbo connection.

meaningful because it is the first attempt to use the umbo as a coupling site, unlike the Carina or Esteem, which have been coupled to the malleus head or incus body.

The Causes and Solutions of Reduction in ABM Sensitivity During Coupling With the Ossicle

The efficacy of the ABM was reduced by approximately 17 dB (approximately 10 times) owing to the coupling to the umbo (**Figures 6A,B**) as the vibration energy was lost in the connection part. The electrical output of the ABM may decrease due to the decrease in the displacement of the base port during umbo connection, resulting in a decrease in overall ABM sensitivity. There were reasons for the reduction in ABM sensitivity during umbo connection and ways to improve this limitation.

The contact point between a tube-type connector and the umbo is critical because too much or too little force will result in a conductive loss and finally reduce sensitivity (Bruschini et al., 2009). Therefore, some middle ear implants use intraoperative loading devices to improve coupling efficiency and consistency (Jenkins and Uhler, 2014). Using an intraoperative loading device can control the contact point of the umbo connection and can improve the reduction in ABM sensitivity due to coupling.

The mass effect of the coupling between a tube-type connector and the umbo should also be considered as the displacement of the ossicular chain decreases with added mass, thereby decreasing sensitivity (Nishihara et al., 1993). Also, we can reduce the mass effect by fixing the connected ABM to the mastoid.

Another consideration is the ambient pressure changes, which can lead to large displacements of the ossicular chain (Mitchell-Innes et al., 2017). If the middle ear microphone is fixed to the temporal bone, then this ossicular displacement will result in a sustained increased force on the ossicles at the contact point, and there is the possibility of bone resorption and a subsequent loose fit (Mitchell-Innes et al., 2017). To solve this problem, a hydroacoustic transmission system with soft

contact to the ossicles was developed, consisting of a water-filled flexible tube covered on the ossicular side by a soft balloon-like tip with a thin wall, which was connected to a piezo-electric transducer at its other end (Hüttenbrink et al., 2001). The soft coupling of the water-filled balloon can prevent a localized pressure load and cannot restrain the free movement of the ossicle during ambient pressure changes, thus reducing the potential risk of bone resorption, which might occur with a rigid coupling (Hüttenbrink et al., 2001). The structure of the tube-type connector, which is filled with fluid inside the tube and has a flexible membrane structure to transmit vibration well to the umbo side, could be a good connector design that can be a good alternative to solving the existing coupling problem.

Results showed a decrease in frequency specificity at the umbo connection. In order to obtain the ideal ossicular coupling possible, we have experienced many trials and errors during the experiment about the rod-type and tube-type connector. Depending on the angle of connection with the ossicle, or the axis pressed by the connector, the electrical output from the ABM in the rod-type connector is inconsistent and difficult to control. In addition, the process of fixing the ABM to the temporal bone to reduce mass effect and the load on the ossicle is time-consuming. In comparison, the tube-type connector was considered a more suitable connector because it obtained a relatively constant electrical output regardless of the experimental conditions and a larger electrical output than the rod-type connector. To find the optimized coupling to the umbo, we chose the best design (Type F-2) for the human middle ear among several designs that changed the size and shape of the umbo connection site, the length and diameter of tube, and the angle of tube (**Supplementary Figure 3**). The selection for the most suitable connector was conducted through experiments in which many preliminary connectors were directly attached to the umbo site of the human cadaveric temporal bone. There is a solution to improve the shape of the junction that connect the umbo, so that the movement of the umbo can be delivered to the ABM system as much as possible. More research is needed to determine whether the loss of frequency specificity in a cadaveric temporal bone connected with the ABM is caused by a connectivity technology issue, an intrinsic characteristic of the ossicle, or a fresh frozen temporal bone problem. To improve the ossicular connection problem, an effective method for ossicular connection should be devised. Moreover, it may be possible to increase the frequency selectivity by adjusting the thickness of the ABM. Further studies are needed to improve the loss of frequency selectivity in ossicular connections.

Efficiency of the Entire ABM System and How to Improve Insufficient Efficiency

In the entire ABM system, to sufficiently stimulate the acoustic nerve, the EM was required to amplify the electrical output from the ABM by 100 times. After amplifying the electrical output from the ABM 100 times and processing it with a biphasic signal through the electrical module, we obtained an eABR waveform in guinea pigs. Inaoka et al. (2011) were the first to conduct animal testing of an ABM and showed eABRs using a membrane-type ABM applying sound stimuli at 100 dB SPL at a frequency of 5, 10, or 20 kHz. The electrical output ($5.7 \sim 29.3$ μV) should be 105-fold higher than the output of this device for effective stimulation of auditory primary neurons when electrodes are placed in the scala tympani similar to conventional CIs. We evaluated the efficiency of the entire ABM system compared to the conventional CI to assess the feasibility of our ABM system. We analyzed and compared the electrical output of the entire ABM system (ABM + EM + electrode), ABM system with umbo connection, and conventional CI according to the sound pressure (**Figure 6B**). As shown in **Figure 6B**, the efficacy of the entire ABM system is lesser by 42.8 dB (approximately 100 times) compared to generating an electrical signal of 1.5 mA at a sound pressure of 74 dB SPL on conventional CI electrodes (Maarefvand et al., 2017). Thus, the electrical output should be approximately 10^2-fold higher than the output of the present ABM system for effective stimulation of auditory primary neurons when electrodes are placed in the scala tympani compared to conventional CIs. The graph of the electrical output according to the sound pressure showed that in the case of the ABM system with umbo connection, the electrical output is lesser by 17 dB compared with that of the ABM system without coupling. In the case of the ABM system with umbo connection, the electrical output should be approximately 10^3-fold higher for effective stimulation of auditory primary neurons. Therefore, the magnitude of the electrical output from the ABM is not high enough to stimulate the acoustic nerve sufficiently without amplification, and further improvement of electrical efficiency is still required. To increase the efficiency of the whole system, there has to be an increase in the sensitivity of the ABM, increase the efficiency of the coupling to the umbo, or increase the efficiency of the EM. In order to increase the efficiency of the EM, there are solutions such as (1) increasing the amplifier gain of EM, and (2) adding amplification circuits between ABM and EM. If the amplifier array gain of the new EM is 100 times (40 dB) higher than that of the existing EM (1,000 times, 60 dB), the overall amplification is 100,000 times (100 dB). And

since the power consumption will be several hundreds of μW when an amplifier array is added, it does not significantly affect the overall system power consumption. However, designing an ultra-high gain amplifier array greater than 60 dB ($1,000\times$) is faced with many other challenges such as noise reduction and input-output non-linearity.

In addition, Our ABM had 13 electrodes and showed six channels of frequency separation characteristics (Jung et al., 2015). When connected to the ossicular chain, the frequency characteristics were reduced to three channels. A number of studies have suggested that speech recognition does not typically improve beyond 8–10 spectral channels for cochlear implant recipients (Friesen et al., 2001; Croghan et al., 2017; Schvartz-Leyzac et al., 2017; Berg et al., 2019). This performance plateau could be explained by limited independent neural populations, channel interaction, ceiling effects on some tasks, and limitations of envelope-based speech coding (Friesen et al., 2001; Croghan et al., 2017; Schvartz-Leyzac et al., 2017; Berg et al., 2019). Based on previous studies, we wanted the ABM to distinguish more than eight channels, but only six channels could be obtained due to the characteristics of the membrane type of piezoelectric material. Therefore, improvements are needed in terms of frequency selectivity and power. Improvements in frequency selectivity and power can be obtained by changing the ABM structure to cantilever form or combining multiple ABMs with different operating conditions. In addition, improvements in the material of ABM are needed, and efficient coupling methods should be devised. The method for ossicular connection is also important, but improving ABM sensitivity can improve the frequency separation characteristics because it increases the effective response from the ABM in more frequency ranges. We have already described earlier how to improve ABM sensitivity. Another option is to change the current membrane-type ABM to cantilever type ABM to improve the frequency response characteristics. The partially etched-type ABM developed by our team was presented to overcome both the limitations of cantilever types ABM that only respond to specific frequencies and the limitations of membrane-type ABM that do not clearly show frequency separation characteristics. However, it did not show definite increase in frequency separation (Kang et al., 2015). Finally, there will be a way to improve the transfer function of the junction by 3D printing the shape of the junction between umbo and the ABM to match the three-dimensional structure.

The previous papers only showed the possibilities of each ABM; however, in this study we numerically estimated how insufficient our whole ABM system is in terms of efficiency compared to the existing CI. Thus, the novelty of this study is that it evaluates the feasibility of the ABM system.

CONCLUSION

In conclusion, we developed a prototype of the totally implantable ABM system, consisting of the ABM, EM, and electrode, and evaluated its feasibility. We obtained meaningful auditory brainstem responses by implanting the output electrode of the ABM system into guinea pigs. Also, we successfully measured the electrical signal output from the ABM system through a middle ear connection from the umbo vibration with external sound stimuli. The power of the whole ABM system was 100 times lesser than that of conventional CIs and the umbo connection further deteriorate the output power, but we found a possibility of a self-powered ABM system, which might be one of the future options for a completely implantable device. Improving the intrinsic efficiency of the ABM and developing an efficient ossicular connection (coupling) technology are the challenges that lie ahead.

ETHICS STATEMENT

The animal study was reviewed and approved by all animal and experimental protocols were approved by the Seoul National University Hospital Institutional Animal Care and Use Committee (SNUH-IACUC, No. 12-0144). All animals were treated in accordance with the Guide for the Care and Use of Laboratory Animals (8th ed., 2010).

REFERENCES

1. Berg, K. A., Noble, J. H., Dawant, B. M., Dwyer, R. T., Labadie, R. F., and Gifford, R. H. (2019). Speech recognition as a function of the number of channels in perimodiolar electrode recipients. *J. Acoust. Soc. Am.* 145, 1556–1564. doi: 10.1121/1.5092350
2. Boukabache, H., Escriba, C., and Fourniols, J.-Y. (2014). Toward smart aerospace structures: design of a piezoelectric sensor and its analog interface for flaw detection. *Sensors* 14, 20543–20561. doi: 10.3390/s141120543
3. Briggs, R. J., Eder, H. C., Seligman, P. M., Cowan, R. S., Plant, K. L., Dalton, J., et al. (2008). Initial clinical experience with a totally implantable cochlear implant research device. *Otol. Neurotol.* 29, 114–119. doi: 10.1097/MAO. 0b013e31814b242f
4. Bruschini, L., Forli, F., Santoro, A., Bruschini, P., and Berrettini, S. (2009). Fully implantable Otologics MET Carina™ device for the treatment of sensorineural hearing loss. Preliminary surgical and clinical results. *Acta Otorhinolaryngol. Ital.* 29, 79–85.
5. Chung, J., Song, W. J., Sim, J. H., Kim, W., and Oh, S.-H. (2013). Optimal ossicular site for maximal vibration transmissions to coupled transducers. *Hear. Res.* 301, 137–145. doi: 10.1016/j.heares.2013.01.007
6. Croghan, N. B., Duran, S. I., and Smith, Z. M. (2017). Re-examining the relationship between number of cochlear implant channels and maximal speech intelligibility. *J. Acoust. Soc. Am.* 142, EL537–EL543. doi: 10.1121/1.5016 044
7. Friesen, L. M., Shannon, R. V., Baskent, D., and Wang, X. (2001). Speech recognition in noise as a function of the number of spectral channels: comparison of acoustic hearing and cochlear implants. *J. Acoust. Soc. Am.* 110, 1150–1163. doi: 10.1121/1.1381538
8. Gesing, A., Alves, F., Paul, S., and Cordioli, J. (2018). On the design of a MEMS piezoelectric accelerometer coupled to the middle ear as an implantable sensor for hearing devices. *Sci. Rep.* 8:3920. doi: 10.1038/s41598-018-22219-7
9. Guerin, S., Tofail, S. A., and Thompson, D. (2019). Organic piezoelectric materials: milestones and potential. *NPG Asia Mater.* 11, 1–5. doi: 10.1038/s41427-019- 0110-5
10. Hall, R. D. (1990). Estimation of surviving spiral ganglion cells in the deaf rat using the electrically evoked auditory brainstem response. *Hear. Res.* 49, 155–168. doi: 10.1016/0378-5955(90)90102-u
11. Hüttenbrink, K.-B., Zahnert, T., Bornitz, M., and Hofmann, G. (2001). Biomechanical aspects in implantable microphones and hearing aids and development of a concept with a hydroacoustical transmission. Acta Otolaryngol. 121, 185–189. doi: 10.1080/000164801300043424
12. Inaoka, T., Shintaku, H., Nakagawa, T., Kawano, S., Ogita, H., Sakamoto, T., et al. (2011). Piezoelectric materials mimic the function of the cochlear sensory epithelium. *Proc. Natl. Acad. Sci. U.S.A.* 108, 18390–18395. doi: 10.1073/pnas. 1110036108

13. Jang, J., Lee, J., Woo, S., Sly, D. J., Campbell, L. J., Cho, J.-H., et al. (2015). A microelectromechanical system artificial basilar membrane based on a piezoelectric cantilever array and its characterization using an animal model. *Sci. Rep.* 5:12447. doi: 10.1038/srep12447
14. Jenkins, H. A., and Uhler, K. (2014). Otologics active middle ear implants. *Otolaryngol. Clin. North Am.* 47, 967–978. doi: 10.1016/j.otc.2014.08.007
15. Jung, Y., Kwak, J.-H., Kang, H., Kim, W. D., and Hur, S. (2015). Mechanical and electrical characterization of piezoelectric artificial cochlear device and biocompatible packaging. *Sensors* 15, 18851–18864. doi: 10.3390/s150818851
16. Kang, H., Jung, Y., Kwak, J.-H., Song, K., Kong, S. H., and Hur, S. (2015). Fabrication and vibration characterization of a partially etched-type artificial basilar membrane. *J. Sens. Sci. Technol.* 24, 373–378. doi: 10.5369/JSST.2015.24. 6.373
17. Lee, M. Y., Kim, D. H., Park, S.-K., Jun, S. B., Lee, Y., Choi, J.-J., et al. (2017). Disappearance of contralateral dominant neural activity of auditory cortex after single-sided deafness in adult rats. *Neurosci. Lett.* 657, 171–178. doi: 10.1016/j. neulet.2017.08.001
18. Maarefvand, M., Blamey, P. J., and Marozeau, J. (2017). Pitch matching in bimodal cochlear implant patients: effects of frequency, spectral envelope, and level. *J. Acoust. Soc. Am.* 142, 2854–2865. doi: 10.1121/1.5009443
19. Maniglia, A. J., Abbass, H., Azar, T., Kane, M., Amantia, P., Garverick, S., et al. (1999). The middle bioelectronic microphone for a totally implantable cochlear hearing device for profound and total hearing loss. *Otol. Neurotol.* 20, 602–611.
20. Marsman, E. D., Senger, R. M., Carichner, G. A., Kubba, S., Mccorquodale, M. S., and Brown, R. B. (2006). "DSP architecture for cochlear implants," in *Proceedings of the 2006 IEEE International Symposium on Circuits and Systems*, (Piscataway, NJ: IEEE), 4. doi: 10.1109/ISCAS.2006.1692671
21. Mitchell-Innes, A., Morse, R., Irving, R., and Begg, P. (2017). Implantable microphones as an alternative to external microphones for cochlear implants. *Cochlear Implants Int.* 18, 304–313. doi: 10.1080/14670100.2017.1371974
22. Nishihara, S., Aritomo, H., and Goode, R. L. (1993). Effect of changes in mass on middle ear function. *Otolaryngol.Head Neck Surg.* 109, 899–910. doi: 10.1177/ 019459989310900520
23. Pulcherio, J. O. B., Bittencourt, A. G., Burke, P. R., Da Costa, Monsanto, development of a concept with a hydroacoustical transmission. Acta R., De Brito, R., et al. (2014). Carina® and Esteem®: a systematic review of fully implantable hearing devices. *PLoS One* 9:e110636. doi: 10.1371/journal. pone.0110636
24. Saadatzi, M., Saadatzi, M. N., and Banerjee, S. (2020). Modeling and fabrication of a piezoelectric artificial cochlea electrode array with longitudinal coupling. *IEEE Sens. J.* 20, 11163–11172. doi: 10.1109/JSEN.2020.2996192
25. Schvartz-Leyzac, K. C., Zwolan, T. A., and Pfingst, B. E. (2017). Effects of electrode deactivation on speech recognition in multichannel

AUTHOR CONTRIBUTIONS

S-HO and Y-HC designed the present study. JC designed and performed the experiments, analyzed data, and wrote the manuscript. YJ and JK designed and performed the experiments. SH and WK collected and analyzed the data. SK provided the statistical advice in some of the analyses and was involved in the interpretation of the data. All authors discussed the results and implications, and revised the manuscript critically for important intellectual content at all stages.

SUPPLEMENTARY MATERIAL

Supplementary Figure 1 | The photographs of surgical procedure for implantation in guinea pigs (*in vivo*). Under anesthesia, a retroauricular incision, a bullotomy, and cochleostomy was done. Then, the subjects were implanted with intracochlear stimulating electrodes into cochlea.

Supplementary Figure 2 | Detailed design diagram for the length, diameter, and angle of tube-type connector (**A**) and rod-type connector (**B**).

Supplementary Figure 3 | The diagrams for several preliminary designs that changed the size and shape of the umbo connection site, the length and diameter of tube, and the angle of tube.

cochlear implant recipients. *Cochlear Implants Int.* 18, 324–334. doi: 10.1080/14670100.2017.1359457

26. Tanaka, K., Abe, M., and Ando, S. (1998). A novel mechanical cochlea" Fishbone" with dual sensor/actuator characteristics. *IEEE/ASME Trans. Mechatron.* 3, 98–105. doi: 10.1109/3516.686677

27. Tsuji, T., Nakayama, A., Yamazaki, H., and Kawano, S. (2018). Artificial cochlear sensory epithelium with functions of outer hair cells mimicked using feedback electrical stimuli. *Micromachines* 9:273. doi: 10.3390/mi9060 273

28. Wang, Z., Mai, S., and Zhang, C. (2008). "Power issues on circuit design for cochlear implants," in *Proceedings of the 4th IEEE International Symposium on Electronic Design, Test and Applications (delta 2008)*, (Piscataway, NJ: IEEE), 163–166. doi: 10.1109/DELTA.2008.13

29. Xu, T., Bachman, M., Zeng, F.-G., and Li, G.-P. (2004). Polymeric micro-cantilever array for auditory front-end processing. *Sens. Actuators A* 114, 176–182. doi: 10.1016/j.sna.2003.11.035

30. Yip, M., Jin, R., Nakajima, H. H., Stankovic, K. M., and Chandrakasan, A. P. (2014). A fully-implantable cochlear implant SoC with piezoelectric middle-ear sensor and arbitrary waveform neural stimulation. *IEEE J. SolidState Circuits* 50, 214–229. doi: 10.1109/JSSC.2014.2355822

31. Zeng, F.-G., Rebscher, S., Harrison, W., Sun, X., and Feng, H. (2008). Cochlear implants: system design, integration, and evaluation. *IEEE Rev. Biomed. Eng.* 1, 115–142. doi: 10.1109/RBME.2008.2008250

3D Printed Patient-Specific Complex Hip Arthroplasty Models Streamline the Preoperative Surgical Workflow

Michael Jiang[1,2], Jasamine Coles-Black[1,2]*, Gordon Chen[1], Matthew Alexander[2], Jason Chuen[1,2] and Andrew Hardidge[2]

[1] 3dMedLab, Austin Health, The University of Melbourne, Parkville, VIC, Australia, [2] Department of Surgery, Austin Health, The University of Melbourne, Heidelberg, VIC, Australia

*Correspondence:
Jasamine Coles-Black
jasaminecb@gmail.com

Introduction: Surgical planning for complex total hip arthroplasty (THA) often presents a challenge. Definitive plans can be difficult to decide upon, requiring unnecessary equipment to be ordered and a long theatre list booked. We present a pilot study utilising patient-specific 3D printed models as a method of streamlining the pre-operative planning process.

Methods: Complex patients presenting for THA were referred to the research team. Patient-specific 3D models were created from routine Computed Tomography (CT) imaging. Simulated surgery was performed to guide prosthesis selection, sizing and the surgical plan.

Results: Seven patients were referred for this pilot study, presenting with complex conditions with atypical anatomy. Surgical plans provided by the 3D models were more detailed and accurate when compared to 2D CT and X ray imaging. Streamlined equipment selection was of great benefit, with augments avoided post simulation in three cases. The ability to tackle complex surgical problems outside of the operating theatre also flagged potential complications, while also providing teaching opportunities in a low risk environment.

Conclusion: This study demonstrated that 3D printed models can improve the surgical plan and streamline operative logistics. Further studies investigating the optimal 3D printing material and workflow, along with cost-benefit analyses are required before this process is ready for routine use.

Keywords: 3D printing, orthopaedic surgery, simulation, presurgical planning, healthcare systems

INTRODUCTION

Total hip arthroplasty (THA) has been a highly successful operation worldwide since its inception (1). The main indications for the procedure are pathologies which alter the biomechanics of the hip joint: most commonly osteoarthritis, fracture, and tumour infiltration. These conditions displace the centre of rotation of the joint via bony destruction. THA aims to correct these defects by restoring the centre of rotation, maintaining alignment and offset of the joint, preserving adequate bone stock and ensuring stability of the hip joint through either a cemented or uncemented prosthesis (2). Uncemented acetabular prostheses require ~50–60% surface area coverage and two thirds rim fit to provide adequate fixation for native bone to heal into and create union (3). The optimal position for an uncemented prosthesis requires both sufficient fixation and orientation, with 6 degrees of freedom in which errors can occur (4). In patients with atypical anatomy, this can be very challenging to achieve.

In routine THA, the size and position of the required implants is optimised using templating X rays (XR) (5). In patients with atypical or disrupted acetabular anatomy, more extensive investigation is necessary (6). Computed tomography (CT) is used in these cases to image the relevant anatomy in three-dimensional space; however preoperative planning based on CT alone is often insufficient to decide upon a definitive procedure. Multiple surgical plans must be prepared, leading to an increased workload for the surgical team, along with increased logistical and financial burden. 3D printed patient-specific models for preoperative planning have been suggested as an approach for these complex cases, and have demonstrated clinical benefit in this patient cohort (7).

Previous studies regarding the use of 3D models in surgical planning noted intraoperative benefits of reduced theatre time, decreased blood loss and shorter fluoroscopy time (7). Most studies shared a similar workflow, using preoperative CT imaging to create a digital render which was transferred to a 3D printer for model creation (8–12). Models were used for anatomical appraisal of relevant surgical anatomy, simulated surgery and templating of implants. Some studies also sterilised the 3D prints to be used in the intraoperative field as a reference to better orient the surgical anatomy, with this process being possible with inexpensive materials such as polylactic acid (PLA) which was able to be sterilised without deformity using high pressure steam (13–15). Consistently in the studies, surgeons felt that the 3D models were particularly useful in complex cases. Chen et al. (16) noted that visualisation of atypical anatomy alone was of benefit in planning the approach, with simulation and implant templating adding to the utility of the procedure. Bizzotto et al. (13) reported similar findings with 3D printed models being most useful for complex intra articular fractures with intra-articular steps of 2 mm or more.

While other methods such patient-specific instruments, custom 3D printed implants and computer aided preoperative planning have also been reported in the literature, the barrier to access with regards to initial investment is much greater (17, 18). In this pilot study, the authors present our initial experiences with 3D printed patient-specific models produced in-house with open source software for pre-surgical planning. We describe how models have improved surgical planning and the perioperative workflow in complex THA.

METHODS

Patient Selection

Patients included in this study were those requiring THA with challenging surgical anatomy from July 2018 to December 2019 at Austin Health, Melbourne, Australia. Inclusion criteria included complex anatomy which was difficult to appreciate through CT reconstruction alone. Conditions included complex pelvic fractures, osteoarthritis complicated by substantial bone loss and patients with Perthes disease or developmental hip dysplasia. Suitable patients were referred to the research team by the orthopaedic unit at Austin Health. This study was approved by the Austin Health Human Research Ethics Committee in accordance with its guidelines. Informed consent was obtained from all patients when consenting for their surgical procedure.

Medical Image Processing and Printing

Following routine preoperative CT, raw medical imaging data was processed using soft fines and bone fines algorithms, under guidance from the radiology department, and exported as Digital Imaging and Communications in Medicine (DICOM) files. Scans were performed using a GE Revolution CT scanner (Milwaukee, WI, USA) with 0.625 mm slice thickness, 100–120 kVp, modulated current of 300–600 mA and 30–40 cm FOV. A virtual 3D model of the patient anatomy was created using 3D Slicer (version 4.9; Harvard, US, 2019) (19), an open source medical image processing software. The workflow involved selectively including voxels above the 200–250 Hounsfield Unit (HDU) range, under advice from the radiology department at Austin Health, as this value was the lowest possible to reliably delineate bony anatomy from soft tissue while preserving cancellous bone architecture from the scan. Manual deletion of the femur was performed to define the acetabulum. Meshmixer (version 3.5; California, US, 2019), an open source computer aided design software, was used to repair mesh defects, remove extraneous surfaces and down-mesh the model to reduce file size prior to printing. Average processing time from acquiring the DICOM data to the completed Standard Triangle Language (STL) file suitable for 3D printing was 1 hour over the length of the study, with it being reduced to as little as 30 min by case 7. No difference in processing time was attributed to complexity of the case. Members of the orthopaedic team performed processing of digital images with technical input regarding printing parameters provided by the university engineering laboratory affiliated with the study. Previous studies have validated the dimensional accuracy of models created using this technique (15, 16, 20).

Completed STL files were 3D printed within 24 h, using a variety of materials as described in **Table 1**. The first three cases were created using VeroWhite resin (Stratasys, Eden Prairie, MN, USA), with the following three created from plaster. The final case utilised all three materials and was the basis for the material comparison.

Simulated Surgery

Surgical simulation was performed by the consultant and registrar responsible for each case. Each model was placed on a theatre tray, fixed in the position expected for a posterior approach, with a routine THA instrumentation set up prepared for reaming. The consultant and registrar then reamed the acetabulum in successive increments replicating the intraoperative process. Reaming was attempted to the appropriate size, with some models reamed further to test for acetabular wall integrity while aiming to maximise rim fit. Templating of the cup was based on the seating of the

TABLE 1 | A summary of the three materials trialled for 3D printed patient-specific models and cost per model.

Material	3D Printer	Average cost per model (US$)
Plaster	Projet 660 (3D Systems Corporation, Rock Hill, SC, USA)	200
VeroWhite Resin	Objet 30 (Stratasys, Eden Prairie, MN, USA)	1,500
Nylon	Jet Fusion 4200 (Hewlett-Packard, Paola Alto, CA, USA)	100

implant, rim fit and bone stock in the surrounding walls post reaming. Post reaming, a trial cup was secured and impacted where possible to assess for fixation. Finally, further implants such as plates, augments and cages were trialled to demonstrate suitability and templated where required. The femoral side was unable to be templated as all materials used in this study deformed to an unacceptable level upon impaction.

Simulation on average required 15 min for a straightforward case with one type of material. Additional time was required for contouring of plates and when complications, such as fracture, were encountered. Following simulation, the surgeons recorded a surgical plan and estimated sizing of any prostheses required in the surgery, which was then compared to the data obtained from planning using templating XRs.

RESULTS

Seven patients underwent complex THA during the study period, using 3D printed models as an adjunct to pre-surgical planning (**Table 2**). Patient-specific models were 3D printed in plaster, resin, and nylon.

Simulation with patient-specific 3D printed models conferred superior clinical, logistical and educational outcomes compared to CT and XR. Deliberate practice with the models prior to the operation streamlined equipment selection and revealed potential complications, allowing them to be accounted for intraoperatively. Ordering of equipment was able to be reduced to only the necessary trays, reducing the logistical and financial burden involved. Surgical simulation also provided a low-pressure environment for teaching without risk to the patient (21).

Material Properties

Plaster performed best when reaming the models with the most realistic haptic feedback of the three materials (**Figure 1**). Plaster models are created by fusion of layers of plaster powder, thus allowing each cycle of the reamer to scrape away a small layer and most effectively reproduced the grasp of an intraoperative ream which was not reproduced by the resin or nylon. However, these models often had deficiencies in the surrounding acetabulum due to lack of bony detail within the cancellous bone on CT imaging. This rendered them prone to shattering if reamed too far past the acetabular shell of bone. In comparison, resin provided the most realistic trial of implant impaction due to the presence of

support material which was left *in situ* in anatomical locations to approximate soft tissue. The support material in the resin models prevented this issue, and allowed impaction of the implant into the model without breakage. However, as the layers of resin and support are fused together, reaming was more strenuous. For the average hemi-pelvis printed in this study, each plaster model cost ~USD$200, while resin models were the most expensive at USD$1,500 including both the resin and the necessary support material. The costs of these models would be increased if a larger section of the pelvis was required. Nylon models were the most cost-effective at USD$100 per model, however its material properties were found to be least favourable on simulation, in accordance with findings from other studies (22). These models were prone to warping on reaming, and bony architecture quickly became distorted. Rotation of the reamer within the model resulted in rotational stretching of the layers within the model, thus losing anatomical accuracy.

DISCUSSION

Our pilot study reports encouraging findings indicating that simulation with patient-specific models narrows the definitive surgical plan, streamlines prosthesis selection and predicts potential complications prior to complex THA.

Limitations

The authors acknowledge the limitations of this pilot study, due to the small cohort size. Furthermore, comparison to a control group is extremely challenging in a cohort of unique and complex cases, where even patients with the same condition often present with vastly different anatomy. Both these limitations are inherent to the nature of the pathologies addressed with complex THA. This dilemma has been raised previously by Karlin et al. (9) who commented on the difficulty in creating a satisfactory control group for complex pathologies with clinical heterogeneity within the same disease classification. In this study, more complex patients were enrolled into the 3D print group as planning would have been extremely challenging with conventional planning methods.

Longer term outcome data is also required in order reach a definitive conclusion on the benefits to patient safety and quality of life. As 3D printing technologies continue to improve, the methods for creating models requires further streamlining to ascertain the most appropriate material and printer type as well as integration into the wider surgical system.

Clinical Benefits

Surgical simulation allowed us to trial multiple approaches to the same surgical problem. Patients recruited for this study provided unique challenges with complex atypical anatomy rendering traditional templating methods unreliable. Deliberate practice with patient specific anatomy provided the surgeon with key information including if an augment was required, whether a rim fit acetabular cup was adequate for fixation or if alternatives were required, and the size progression and orientation of the intraoperative ream achieved safely. A more confident approach into the acetabulum can also be made, with visualisation and

TABLE 2 | A summary of the cases involved in this pilot study including demographic data, causative pathology leading to THA and changes to surgical management.

Case	Age	Gender	Pathology	Templated size of acetabular cup (mm)			Changes to surgical plan	Material	Notes on image processing	Cost (USD)
				2D	3D	Intra-operative				
1	92	F	Acetabular fracture	48	48	52	On simulation, it was found that there was an undiscovered fracture of the posterior ramus which fractured on reaming. The decision was made to pre counter a plate and sterilise it for moulding on the back table to stabilise the fracture. Trialling also indicated the patient was not suitable for a cage, therefore one was not ordered. A femoral head graft was opted for to fill the posterior wall defect. On reaming the cortical edges spun dangerously, and the decision was made to cut the femur directly under the head to ream.	VeroWhite	This model provided an acceptable representation of patient anatomy. The support material provided an analogue to the soft tissue and cancellous bone. Reaming and impaction was well supported. The fracture pattern was well preserved by the support material. Processing time of the model was 1.5 hrs	1,600
2	52	M	Perthes' disease	54	52	52	When viewing the CT imaging, augments were decided upon. On simulation it was determined that augments were not necessary and that adequate fixation was able to be achieved. Augments were not ordered.	Verowhite	This model provided an accurate representation of patient anatomy, with adequate assessment of fixation. Not difficulties were encountered on reaming. Processing time for this model was 1.5 hrs	1,500
3	53	M	Perthes' disease	46	60	50	This patient was trialled with the Stryker RAS system which included an augment within the acetabular cup itself, hence the large difference in templating size. Augments were considered for this case however intraoperatively there was adequate fixation with the superior edge uncovered.	Verowhite	The resin model was able to withstand reaming using the oversized RAS system, however impaction was not satisfactory with a poor rim fit resulting in a unsatisfactory simulation of cup fit. Processing time of the model was 1 h	1,550
4	89	M	Acetabular fracture	64	60	62	The patient had a complex acetabular fracture with anterior column discontinuity. Augments and a cup/cage complex were prepared for this case. Augments were trialled on the model and sized at 50 mm. The superior bone stock was deemed adequate for screws on visualisation of the model. Intraoperatively, the superior screws provided adequate fixation and other implants were not required.	Plaster	The fracture pattern printed using the plaster was quite frail. The posterior wall segment and anterior column discontinuity required additional construction as they both fell off post print. Processing time for the model was 1 h.	250
5	84	F	Severe osteoarthritis and femoral head necrosis	48	48	48	The anterior wall of this model was shown to be deficient on reaming. The decision was made to bias reaming posteriorly to preserve anterior bone stock. A 48 mm cup press fit in the model which was reflected intraoperatively.	Plaster	The plaster model in this case provided an accurate haptic mimic to bone. The acetabular wall had solid bone stock on CT and as such reaming was very realistic with an accurate representation of rim fit which was replicated intraoperatively. Processing time for this model was 1 hr	200
6	46	F	Severe osteoarthritis and femoral head necrosis	46	52	54	Patient presented with bilateral severe OA and femoral head necrosis. 2D templating proved difficult using the affected or contralateral acetabulum. 3D simulation was much more reflective of the intraoperative conditions.	Plaster	Reaming of this model required care due to the lack of support material within the acetabulum. The anterior wall was nearly breached and almost failed. Processing time for this model was 0.5 hrs.	200
7	50	M	Severe osteoarthritis and femoral head necrosis	54	58	58	2D templating was difficult as patient had considerable bone loss and was not comparable to the contralateral side. Augment was trialled. Intraoperatively there was adequate fixation with 3 screws.	Plaster, VeroWhite, Nylon	This case provided the material comparison noted in the material properties section. Image processing was 0.5 hrs with a longer simulation time to account for all models.	Resin: 1,200 Plaster: 250 Nylon: 100

Templated size of implant on XR and CT (2D) vs. on the patient specific model (3D) is shown and compared to the size of definitive implant decided upon intraoperatively.

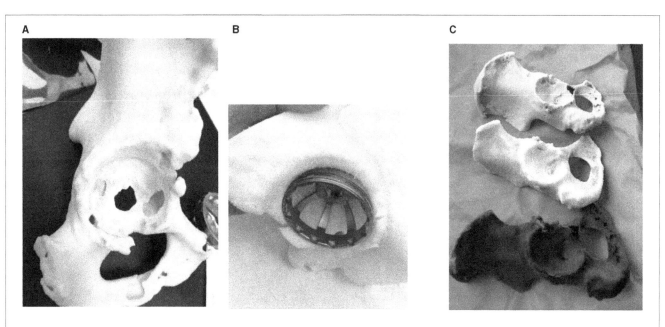

FIGURE 1 | From left to right **(A)** The plaster models possessed the most realistic haptic feedback during simulated surgery, with each revolution of the reamer removing a layer of plaster which closely reflects what occurs intraoperatively. **(B)** The resin models performed best when simulating implant fixation due to the surrounding support material which mimicked soft tissue structures absent in other models. **(C)** A comparison of all three materials with the same model created in from top down plaster, resin and nylon.

simulation informing the surgeon of any potential obstructions from osteophyte or other bony prominence along with the knowledge of which of these can be safely resected to improve access without compromising fixation later on.

In cases of pelvic fracture, the model better visualised the fracture pattern and allowed all fragments to be accounted for intraoperatively, with the additional benefit of allowing trialling and pre-contouring of plates and screws required.

For example, Case 3 involved an acetabulum with 3 plane mismatch which would have likely caused blow out of the medial wall with a cup that could secure a rim fit in the acetabulum. Due to this, a smaller cup with augments was planned. On simulation, it was shown that a smaller cup was able to be secured with adequate fixation and no augmentation despite leaving the superior edge exposed. This avoided the increased operating time, equipment cost and potential for failure associated with the augment. Templating via this method is extremely valuable in these cases, as the affected side is often too disrupted to confidently template, with the contralateral side too dissimilar to use reliably.

Pre-contouring of implants was another valuable aspect when simulating complex THA with patient-specific models. Templating of plates, cages and screw placements with 3D printed models led to significant reductions in operating time, as reflected in the study by Chana-Rodriguez et al. in which a plate was able to be implanted intra-operatively in a case of complex acetabular fracture without adjustment post templating on a 3D printed model (23). This was reflected in the first case, with the patient presenting with a complex acetabular fracture and associated protrusio acetabuli. Upon reaming of the model,

a fracture line previously thought insignificant on review in radiology meetings failed, causing a posterior ramus fracture. The decision was made to plate this prior to reaming to prevent this complication intraoperatively hence a lead plate was contoured using the 3D model. The model allowed trialling of multiple plate positions with the most optimal decided upon for the final fixation. This plate was then sterilised and used to fashion the definitive implant intraoperatively on the back table, while the fracture site was prepared. The implant was secured with minimal further adjustment.

Similarly, screw placements were able to be assessed for viable bone stock, as seen in Cases 2, 4, and 7. Future cases which require similar screw, plate, cage or augment constructs could see significant operative benefit from the use of models to prefabricate the required implants.

Our pilot study also allowed for the identification of other potential complications, allowing preparation of contingency plans. Aside from the pubic ramus fracture identified in Case 1, adjustments were made to the femoral head graft. Originally, a subcapital cut was chosen, planning for the head to be placed into the acetabulum and reamed into the posterior wall defect. However, there was significant cortical bone present which caught on reaming and started to spin dangerously. Therefore, the femoral head was cut further superiorly, allowing the graft to be safely reamed into the defect. 3D printed patient-specific models were invaluable in predicting these intraoperative difficulties ahead of time, preventing stressful situations in the operating theatre.

Replication of the intraoperative process creates an environment of known processes from a previously uncertain

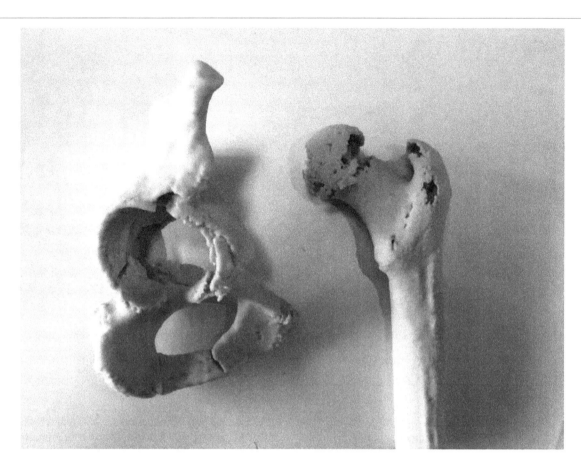

FIGURE 2 | Plaster model from Case 4 showing an acetabular fracture with anterior column discontinuity. Despite the anterior column disruption it was shown that the posterior column was intact and stable, allowing for screws to be placed in the posterior and superior aspects of the cup to stabilise the construct without need for augments or cages.

procedure. The operation becomes streamlined as the optimal alignment and positioning of the ream along with the fit and orientation of the implant is being recreated instead of discovered. Stress inducing questions such as if increasing the size of the ream will improve the fit or cause a wall blowout, which obstructing anatomy can be removed, and if a non-conventional fixation is sufficient or will cause impingement have already been answered, giving the surgeon the confidence to proceed with their predetermined plan. The reduction in stress related to operative uncertainty can also be communicated to the patient, informing them of the risks associated with their complex procedure and the steps taken to mitigate the complications. Our study found these factors positively impacted surgical preparation from both a clinician and patient perspective.

Logistical Benefits

Preparation for complex THAs involves the logistics of ordering, transport and sterilisation of all prostheses that may be required for the case. For complex cases, multiple sizes of acetabular cup, augments and cages are required in preparation for a definitive plan based on intraoperative findings. This equipment can comprise up to 14 trays for a standard THA with further equipment required for complex cases (24), conferring

a significant logistical burden on the healthcare system. In addition, reducing the number of trays required in preparation would reduce the financial and environmental impact of the hospital. In our study, 3 cases which were originally planned for augments were shown to not require them post simulation. Simulation in Case 3 demonstrated that the smaller cup was able to be repositioned and medialised adequately such that augments were not required, with similar findings in Case 2. In Case 1, the femoral head was demonstrated as being suitable as a graft to fill the acetabular defect, again avoiding the need for augments. A further two cases were less definitive, with augments subsequently ordered but not used (**Figure 2**). Similar findings have been commented on in previous studies involving 3D modelling software in complex arthroplasty (25–27).

Reducing the unpredictability of complex cases also allows for theatre time to be allocated more efficiently. Difficult cases can be highly variable in the theatre time required, resulting in more conservative theatre bookings and staffing allocations. Simulation of complex cases provides greater clarity on the approach and techniques required, giving a more precise indication of case duration and allowing theatre bookings to be allocated more efficiently.

Teaching

Although not initially a focus of our pilot study, it became apparent that simulating complex hip arthroplasty using 3D printed patient-specific models also provides a valuable teaching opportunity for trainees in a unique and low risk learning environment. Deliberate practice outside of the operating theatre allows the opportunity for trainees to plan, prepare and execute complex cases under the supervision of surgical educators while preserving patient safety. Due to this, simulated surgery using 3D models can not only provide a valuable tool in surgical planning but also a unique tool in surgical training (21).

Workflow

This study aimed to demonstrate an example of a workflow from routine preoperative CT imaging to model creation that occurs entirely within a hospital environment for the planning of complex hip arthroplasty. Image processing and model creation was performed by members of the Orthopaedic team, with a rapid improvement in processing time noted from Cases 1 to 7. Once the initial learning curve had been overcome, cases could be processed in as little as 30 min. With utilisation of an in-house 3D printer, total turnaround was 24 h from scan to model. With use of open source software, this process could be integrated into a surgical unit with minimal outlay: primarily education of staff in the image processing procedure and the cost of the prints themselves.

In our experience, the decision to print in-house compared to a third party is influenced by cost and time. Third party production of the model is more expensive due to extra labour costs and has a longer turnaround time between scan and print. However, outsourcing the process eliminates the extra time requirement for the in-house staff and eliminates the set up and maintenance costs of housing the printer. Conversely, development of an in-house process can have drastically improved turnaround times. With a 24 h turnaround it may even be possible to apply this process to emergency trauma, which has been previously reported as unfeasible due to prolonged processing times (28). An in-house process in these cases could compress the time between scan, model creation and simulated surgery to one working day, while also providing greater input from the surgeon into the modelling process (29). This study also demonstrates that the learning curve can be quickly overcome by a surgical unit with minimal disruption to clinical workflow. The volume of models printed also weighs into the cost-benefit analysis, with set up and maintenance costs being less enticing if faced with a smaller case load (30).

While many options for segmentation and CAD software exist, the software selected in the study had the lowest barrier to access. Although lacking the automation and advanced features of some proprietary software, 3D slicer (version 4.9; Harvard, US, 2019) and Meshmixer (version 3.5; California, US, 2019) were sufficient for the manual segmentation and creation of 3D models of bony anatomy. If soft tissue structures were to be involved in further research, more advanced software would need to be considered to lessen the technical and time burden that would be associated. We encountered no patients with metalware *in situ* and the resultant flare artefacts.

Regarding material selection, the ideal material would mimic the biomechanical properties of bone, while also allowing incorporation of surrounding soft tissues into the print. The haptic feedback would ideally mimic the grasp of the reamer as it removes layers of cortical and cancellous bone. However, this would need to be balanced against the brittleness of the material which would leave it prone to shattering when force was applied. In this pilot study, the plaster models reflected this best with the resin models providing additional resistance to what would be expected due to the fusion of layers of material. The material would also require sufficient viscoelasticity to allow testing for rim fit as the acetabular cups inserted are typically 1–2 mm greater in diameter than the reamer. In this aspect the resin was superior as the plaster was prone to shattering on impaction.

The current literature regarding the biomechanics of 3D printed materials mainly focuses on qualitative surgeon assessment of haptics, with quantitative studies still lacking (31). The femoral side was not investigated in this study due to material deficiencies. One femur was templated using resin however this model failed on impaction and was unable to withstand the forces necessary to hold the femoral prosthesis. While additional material could be used to reinforce the acetabular walls of the plaster models, this may confer extra strength not present within normal anatomy. As such, an ideal material combination still requires further research.

CONCLUSION

Complex acetabular surgery continues to challenge orthopaedic surgeons, with new solutions and approaches continually emerging. This pilot study suggests that in-house creation of 3D printed patient-specific models can be rapidly integrated into a surgical unit, and can provide an array of benefits to the surgeon through the trialling of multiple approaches, devices and implants for complex THA, streamlining the logistics involved. In addition, they provided a unique teaching opportunity for surgical trainees.

This pilot study has informed our next steps to further streamline our workflow with regards to case selection, model creation and pre-operative rehearsals prior to the implementation of a larger-scale prospective trial. More broadly in the orthopaedic literature, further studies into the optimal printing workflow along with quantification of the financial benefits of the models are required before it can be justified for routine use.

ETHICS STATEMENT

The studies involving human participants were reviewed and approved by Austin Health Department of Ethics. The patients/participants provided their written informed consent to participate in this study.

AUTHOR CONTRIBUTIONS

MJ, AH, and JC-B were involved in study conceptualisation and design. MJ and GC were involved in data collection. MJ, J-CB, AH, and MA were involved in manuscript writing. MA, GC, AH, and JC were involved in editing the final manuscript. All authors contributed to the article and approved the submitted version.

ACKNOWLEDGMENTS

The authors would like to acknowledge contributions from the Austin Health Departments of Orthopaedics, Radiology and Vascular surgery for their involvement in this study. The authors would also like to acknowledge advice received from the Melbourne University NExT laboratory.

REFERENCES

1. Falez F, Papalia M, Favetti F, Panegrossi G, Casella F, Mazzotta G. Total hip arthroplasty instability in Italy. *Int Orthop.* (2017) 41:635–44. doi: 10.1007/s00264-016-3345-6

2. Sheth NP, Melnic CM, Paprosky WG. Evaluation and management of chronic total hip instability. *Bone Joint J.* (2016) 98-B(1 Suppl A):44–9. doi: 10.1302/0301-620X.98B1.36516

3. Tabata T, Kaku N, Hara K, Tsumura H. Initial stability of cementless acetabular cups: press-fit and screw fixation interaction—an in vitro biomechanical study. *Eur J Orthop Surg Traumatol.* (2015) 25:497–502. doi: 10.1007/s00590-014-1571-4

4. Bou Monsef J, Parekh A, Osmani F, Gonzalez M. Failed total hip arthroplasty. *JBJS Rev.* (2018) 6:e3. doi: 10.2106/JBJS.RVW.17. 00140

5. Atesok K, Galos D, Jazrawi LM, Egol KA. Preoperative planning in orthopaedic surgery: Current practice and evolving applications. *Bull Hospital Joint Dis.* (2015) 73:257–68.

6. Kavalerskiy GM, Murylev VY, Rukin YA, Elizarov PM, Lychagin AV, Tselisheva EY. Three-dimensional models in planning of revision hip arthroplasty with complex acetabular defects. *Indian J Orthop.* (2018) 52:625–30. doi: 10.4103/ortho.IJOrtho_556_16

7. Jiang M, Chen G, Coles-Black J, Chuen J, Hardidge A. Three-dimensional printing in orthopaedic preoperative planning improves intraoperative metrics: a systematic review. *ANZ J Surg.* (2020) 90:243–520. doi: 10.1111/ans.15549

8. Cherkasskiy L, Caffrey JP, Szewczyk AF, Cory E, Bomar JD, Farnsworth C, et al. Patient specific 3D print models improve deformity correction after proximal femoral osteotomy for slipped capital femoral epiphysis. *J Investig Med.* (2016) 64:197. doi: 10.1302/1863-2548-11-1 70277

9. Karlin L, Weinstock P, Hedequist D, Prabhu SP. The surgical treatment of spinal deformity in children with myelomeningocele: the role of personalized three-dimensional printed models. *J Pediatr Orthopaed Part B.* (2017) 26:375–82. doi: 10.1097/BPB.0000000000000411

10. Li C, Yang M, Xie Y, Chen Z, Wang C, Bai Y, et al. Application of the polystyrene model made by 3-D printing rapid prototyping technology for operation planning in revision lumbar discectomy. *J Orthop Sci.* (2015) 20:475–80. doi: 10.1007/s00776-015-0706-8

11. Toyoda K, Urasaki E, Yamakawa Y. Novel approach for the efficient use of a full-scale, 3-dimensional model for cervical posterior fixation a technical case report. *Spine.* (2013) 38:E1357–E60. doi: 10.1097/BRS.0b013e3182a1f1bd

12. Yamazaki M, Okawa A, Fujiyoshi T, Kawabe J, Yamauchi T, Furuya T, et al. Simulated surgery for a patient with neurofibromatosis type-1 who had severe cervicothoracic kyphoscoliosis and an anomalous vertebral artery. *Spine.* (2010) 35:E368–E73. doi: 10.1097/BRS.0b013e3181c 42559

13. Bizzotto N, Tami I, Santucci A, Adani R, Poggi P, Romani D, et al. 3D printed replica of articular fractures for surgical planning and patient consent: a two years multi-centric experience. *3D Print Med.* (2015) 2:2. doi: 10.1186/s41205-016-0006-8

14. Jentzsch T, Vlachopoulos L, Furnstahl P, Muller DA, Fuchs B. Tumor resection at the pelvis using three-dimensional planning and patient-specific instruments: a case series. *World J Surg Oncol.* (2016) 14:249. doi: 10.1186/s12957-016-1006-2

15. Yang L, Grottkau B, He Z, Ye C. Three dimensional printing technology and materials for treatment of elbow fractures. *Int Orthop.* (2017) 41:2381–7. doi: 10.1007/s00264-017-3627-7

16. Chen C, Cai L, Zhang C, Wang J, Guo X, Zhou Y. Treatment of die-punch fractures with 3D printing technology. *J Investig Surg.* (2017) 31:1–8. doi: 10.1080/08941939.2017.1339150

17. Wang M, Li D, Shang X, Wang J. A review of computer-assisted orthopaedic surgery systems. *Int J Med Robot Comp Assist Surg.* (2020) 16:e2118. doi: 10.1002/rcs.2118

18. Moralidou M, Laura AD, Henckel J, Hothi H, Hart AJ. Three-dimensional pre-operative planning of primary hip arthroplasty: a systematic literature review. *EFORT Open Rev.* (2020) 5:845–55. doi: 10.1302/2058-5241.5.2 00046

19. Kikinis R, Pieper SD, Vosburgh KG. 3D Slicer: a platform for subject-specific image analysis, visualization, and clinical support. In: Jolesz FA, editor. *Intraoperative Imaging and Image-Guided Therapy*. New York, NY: Springer New York (2014). p. 277–89.

20. Brouwers L, Teutelink A, van Tilborg FAJB, de Jongh MAC, Lansink KWW, Bemelman M. Validation study of 3D-printed anatomical models using 2 PLA printers for preoperative planning in trauma surgery, a human cadaver study. *Eur J Trauma Emerg Surg.* (2019) 45:1013–20. doi: 10.1007/s00068-018-0970-3

21. Mulford JS, Babazadeh S, Mackay N. Three-dimensional printing in orthopaedic surgery: review of current and future applications. *ANZ J Surg.* (2016) 86:648–53. doi: 10.1111/ans. 13533

22. Haffner M, Quinn A, Hsieh T-y, Strong EB, Steele T. Optimization of 3D Print Material for the Recreation of Patient-Specific Temporal Bone Models. *Ann Otol Rhinol Laryngol.* (2018) 127:338–43. doi: 10.1177/00034894187 64987

23. Chana-Rodriguez F, Mananes RP, Rojo-Manaute J, Gil P, Martinez-Gomiz JM, Vaquero-Martin J. 3D surgical printing and pre contoured plates for acetabular fractures. *Injury.* (2016) 47:2507–11. doi: 10.1016/j.injury.2016.08.027

24. Capra R, Bini SA, Bowden DE, Etter K, Callahan M, Smith RT, et al. Implementing a perioperative efficiency initiative for orthopedic surgery instrumentation at an academic center: A comparative before-and-after study. *Medicine.* (2019) 98:e14338-e. doi: 10.1097/MD.0000000000 014338

25. Lattanzi R, Viceconti M, Zannoni C, Quadrani P, Toni A. Hip-Op: an innovative software to plan total hip replacement surgery. *Med Inform Internet Med.* (2002) 27:71–83. doi: 10.1080/146392302101 50346

26. Viceconti M, Lattanzi R, Antonietti B, Paderni S, Olmi R, Sudanese A, et al. CT-based surgical planning software improves the accuracy of total hip replacement preoperative planning. *Med Eng Phys.* (2003) 25:371–7. doi: 10.1016/S1350-4533(03)00018-3

27. Di Laura A, Henckel J, Hothi H, Hart A. Can 3D surgical planning and patient specific instrumentation reduce hip implant inventory? A prospective study. *3D Print Med.* (2020) 6:25. doi: 10.1186/s41205-020-00 077-2

28. Wong TM, Jin J, Lau TW, Fang C, Yan CH, Yeung K, et al. The use of three-dimensional printing technology in orthopaedic surgery. *J Orthop Surg.* (2017) 25. doi: 10.1177/23094990166 84077

29. Schwartz A, Money K, Spangehl M, Hattrup S, Claridge RJ, Beauchamp C. Office-based rapid prototyping in orthopedic surgery: a novel planning technique and review of the literature. *Am J Orthop.* (2015) 44:19–25.

30. Eltorai A, Nguyen E, Daniels AH. Three-dimensional printing in orthopedic surgery. *Orthopedics.* (2015) 38:684–7. doi: 10.3928/01477447-2015 1016-05

31. Meglioli M, Naveau A, Macaluso GM, Catros S. 3D printed bone models in oral and cranio-maxillofacial surgery: a systematic review. *3D Print Med.* (2020) 6:30. doi: 10.1186/s41205-020-00082-5

A World-First Surgical Instrument for Minimally Invasive Robotically-Enabled Transplantation of Heart Patches for Myocardial Regeneration

Christopher David Roche [1,2,3*†], Yiran Zhou [4†], Liang Zhao [4‡] and Carmine Gentile [1,2‡]

[1] Northern Clinical School of Medicine, University of Sydney, Sydney, NSW, Australia, [2] School of Biomedical Engineering, Faculty of Engineering and IT, University of Technology Sydney, Sydney, NSW, Australia, [3] Department of Cardiothoracic Surgery, University Hospital of Wales, Cardiff, United Kingdom, [4] School of Mechanical and Mechatronic Engineering, Faculty of Engineering and IT, University of Technology Sydney, Sydney, NSW, Australia

*Correspondence:
Christopher David Roche
croche@doctors.org.uk

[†] These authors share first authorship

[‡] These authors share last authorship

Background: Patch-based approaches to regenerating damaged myocardium include epicardial surgical transplantation of heart patches. By the time this therapy is ready for widespread clinical use, it may be important that patches can be delivered via minimally invasive and robotic surgical approaches. This brief research report describes a world-first minimally invasive patch transplantation surgical device design enabled for human operation, master-slave, and fully automated robotic control.

Method: Over a 12-month period (2019–20) in our multidisciplinary team we designed a surgical instrument to transplant heart patches to the epicardial surface. The device was designed for use via uni-portal or multi-portal Video-Assisted Thorascopic Surgery (VATS). For preliminary feasibility and sizing, we used a 3D printer to produce parts of a flexible resin model from a computer-aided design (CAD) software platform in preparation for more robust high-resolution metal manufacturing.

Results: The instrument was designed as a sheath containing foldable arms, <2 cm in diameter when infolded to fit minimally invasive thoracic ports. The total length was 35 cm. When the arms were projected from the sheath, three moveable mechanical arms at the distal end were designed to hold a patch. Features included: a rotational head allowing for the arms to be angled in real time, a surface with micro-attachment points for patches and a releasing mechanism to release the patch.

Conclusion: This brief research report represents a first step on a potential pathway towards minimally invasive robotic epicardial patch transplantation. For full feasibility testing, future proof-of-concept studies, and efficacy trials will be needed.

Keywords: instrumentation, regeneration, thorascopic surgery, myocardial patch, automation, keyhole, chest

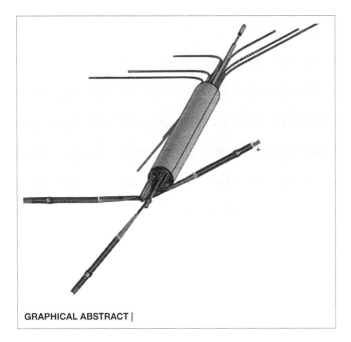

GRAPHICAL ABSTRACT |

INTRODUCTION

Since the first reports of robotic minimally invasive cardiac surgery (1), there has been increasing attention given to the role of minimally invasive robotics in cardiothoracic surgery (2–6). Meanwhile, tissue engineers have been making gains toward regenerating the myocardium (7–9). The first human trials of patches containing biomaterials/cells applied to the epicardial surface to regenerate the heart have been reported with promising results (10–14). Moreover, increasingly accessible techniques such as 3D bioprinting (one approach to generating heart tissue patches) promise scalability, reproducibility, and highly refined control over the characteristics of the patch to be grafted (7). However, many approaches to regenerate the myocardium surgically using patches applied to the epicardial surface have worked toward a model of open surgery via median sternotomy (8). There is an unanswered but pressing question whether surgical patch-based repair of the heart will need to be delivered by minimally invasive and/or robotic surgery by the time it reaches widespread clinical use (7). Additionally, for heart failure patients who may not be fit for a heart transplant or major surgery but who may tolerate a less invasive keyhole procedure (15), this solution may open up a therapeutic avenue for them.

Our team therefore conceptualised and designed a novel surgical instrument to deliver heart tissue patches to the epicardium. Our multidisciplinary team included a cardiothoracic surgeon, a bioengineer and two specialists in robotics, mechanical engineering, and mechatronics. To our knowledge, the early-stage design we present is a world-first with no similar design existing. This descriptive brief research report represents the initial step on a potentially significant pathway to pivot the field away from its focus on traditional open surgery.

METHOD
Design Process, Objectives, Reasoning

The design process was initiated with several discussions amongst the team to determine the objectives, requirements, and feasibility of the idea. An initial outline of the design was sketched with attention to the ergonomics at human surgery, the size and material requirements for thorascopic insertion and manipulation of the instrument within the chest cavity, the shape requirements to ensure suitability for human cardiothoracic anatomy, the mechanism to allow for an operator to manoeuvre the instrument using handles outside the chest cavity at the proximal (external) end of the instrument and the ability for the device to be controlled in future by both master-slave robotics and fully automated robotics.

Using SOLIDWORKS® (Dassault Systèmes SOLIDWORKS Corp, Waltham, MA, USA) computer aided design (CAD) software, the instrument blueprint was created and revised several times to ensure it was optimised. At this stage, attention was given to the points of attachment for patches onto the instrument and the details of how the patch would fold into the instrument when retracted and then be spread out for deployment when expanded (without damaging the patch). Another challenge was the releasing mechanism for the patch to release it from the instrument. It was decided that tiny attachment nodules/hooks would be placed at the distal ends of the manoeuvrable arms and at the apex of the pyramid created by the three arms converging. When the arms are expanded (outfolded) this stretches out the patch between the metal arms. This has the effect that when outstretched the patch itself would move away from the apex and fold out to form the base of a pyramid.

The patches will be made from alginate 4%/gelatin 8% in cell culture medium, which is a hydrogel that becomes fluid at temperatures over ~28°C and is more solid at lower temperatures. It can be crosslinked ionically by adding calcium chloride (2% w/v in phosphate buffered saline) which increases the strength of the material. A similar hydrogel with a modified molecular structure, gelatin methacryloyl (GelMA), can be used in a similar way to alginate/gelatin but is more robust when it is crosslinked which is done by UV light photocuring. Therefore, we created the instrument design to include areas for attachment nodules/hooks which would be attached to areas within the patch containing small rings of GelMA at the corners and the centre. These reinforced patch ring-corners would be attached to the arms distally. In the folded position, the patch centre will be similarly attached to the instrument platform where the proximal ends of the three arms converge (the apex of the pyramid formed by the arms). When opening the arms (pitch rotational movement) this will pull the patch away from the platform where the proximal ends of the arms converge as it unfolds and expands to become the outstretched base of the pyramid. Next, to release the three patch corners from the apex, the instrument arms can be moved laterally (yaw rotational movement). To ensure that release happens first at the apex/central connection the strength of the GelMA ring will be modified by using fewer layers so that this connection releases first (before the GelMA ring connection to the distal tips of the arms). In case of failure to release by

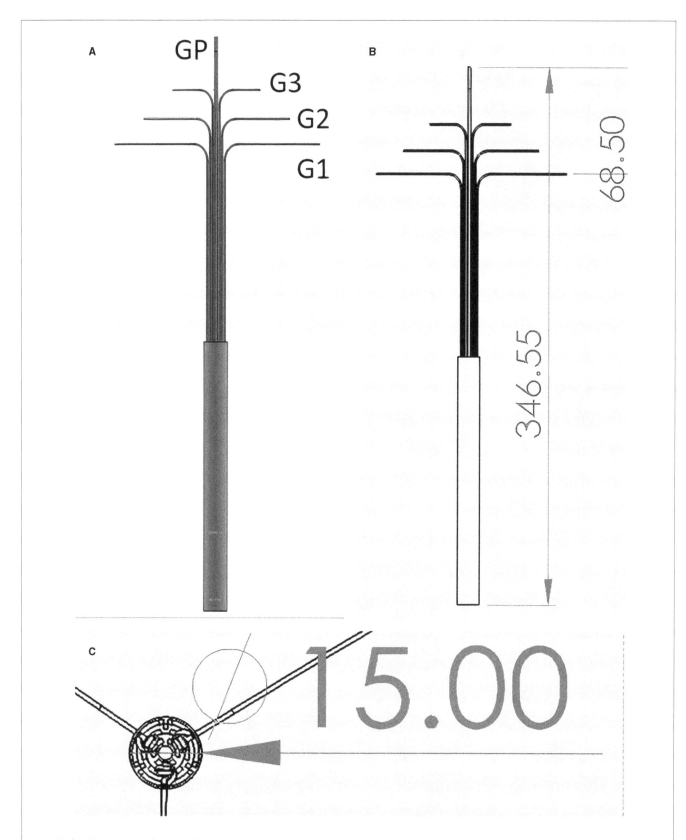

FIGURE 1 | (A,B) Lateral view. One single Grip (GP) controls forward protrusion and backwards retraction of the instrument. Grips G1–G3 are triplicate (only two of each are visible in the 2D lateral view images shown), and control each of the three distal arms to which they are attached (distal arms not visible - infolded and covered by sheath). G3 Grips control the curvature of the patch, G2 the rotation angle of the arm, and G1 the deployment angle of the arm. **(C)** "Top down" view showing triplicate arrangement of Grips when in line with each other and opened with 120 degree angles between each set of three Grips. Grips exit the cylindrical instrument body which has diameter of 15 mm. All measurements in mm. See **Supplementary Video 1** for dynamic demonstration *in silico*.

this mechanism, the platforms with the hook/nodule attachments can be moved in a sliding movement distally away from the instrument body, theoretically releasing them by breaking the GelMA rings.

The head has a rotational mechanism (role rotational movement) which allows for the rotation of the patch through 360 degrees. One arm is able to be made shorter than the other two during patch deployment. This means that by opening that arm past 90 degrees to the main instrument body whilst shortening it, the patch should be able to open and face any lateral direction (similar to the triangle that can be made with the extended index and middle finger to the thumb in opposition). This gives the instrument three degrees of rotational movement in addition to the three degrees of translational movement in the X, Y, and Z axis which are achieved by movements at the entry into the chest (similar to moving a pencil pinched lightly between the thumb and index finger). Additional to these six degrees of freedom, each arm is capable of pitch and yaw rotation individually. The shortenable arm has the additional benefit of being openable in a confined space, for example, if facing the surface of the heart when opening, so that its excursionary movement can be completed without damaging surrounding structures. Overall, these movements will allow for the patch to be expanded in the hemithorax and then rotated to face the surface of the heart at the correct angle.

One surgical approach for the operation of this instrument is via standard left-sided anterolateral multiportal video-assisted thoracoscopic surgery (VATS)—similar to a left lower lobectomy approach but with the left lung deflated via endobronchial intubation and single lung ventilation of the right lung. The pericardium would need to be partly opened to gain access to the epicardial surface. In particular, for a chronic ischaemic cardiomyopathy heart failure patient or after myocardial infarction (MI), the target area may be the anterolateral surface of the heart over the left ventricle. With the rotational head and the releasing mechanism, it should be possible to manoeuvre the patch and apply it to the epicardium on most surfaces reachable without moving the heart: a minimally invasive VATS transplantation of a regenerative cardiac patch.

Following these discussions and revisions aimed at optimising the instrument design we 3D printed a version of the instrument to assess for size and identify learning points. This "sizing and learning" print was in preparation for the full metal prototyping which will use 17-4 Ph Stainless Steel (SAE Type 630 stainless steel—hardened stainless steel containing ~15% chromium, 5% nickel, 5% copper).

RESULTS

Early-Stage Design Outcomes

The device has nine Grips plus one push-out Grip (**Figure 1**, **Supplementary Video 1**). Each arm has three Grips (**Figure 1A**, Labels G1, G2, and G3). The top Grip (G3) controls the attachment platforms and therefore the curvature of the patch (it also acts as a releasing mechanism if attachment platforms are moved beyond the maximal boundary of the outfolded patch), the middle Grip (G2) controls the rotation angle of the arm, and

the bottom Grip (G1) controls the deployment angle of the arm. The push out Grip (GP) protracts or retracts the arms from their sheath. **Supplementary Figure 1** shows a frontal and trimetric view of the mechanism with the sheath removed.

The designed length of the instrument was 35 cm and cylinder diameter was 1.5 cm (**Figures 1B,C**). Each arm was 60 mm, thus the maximum size of a triangular outfolded patch would be ~18 cm^2. The tips of each arm are 11.2 cm apart while opened at 90 degrees to the body of the instrument. The smallest parts in our instrument were the joints which are cylindrical type joins (which act like screws connecting two linked pieces) and these were 1 mm diameter and 1 mm height.

Special features of the instrument included a space between the arms when infolded where the folded patch could be stored prior to deployment (**Figure 2**). The patch could therefore be inserted into the chest within the mechanism (and covered by the outer sheath) without damaging it during insertion. Control over each of the three arms was achieved by three separate mechanisms connecting the arms to the Grips at the proximal end of the device (**Supplementary Figure 2**).

The arms were designed so that they could be individually rotated, including when the arms are folded out from their closed position. The region conveying rotationary control is shown in **Supplementary Figure 3**. In **Supplementary Figure 3B** the proximal (operator's end) region where the Grips converge is shown.

Along each arm the design includes a moveable attachment platform which can be controlled using Grip number 3 (control pathway highlighted in **Supplementary Figure 2A**). **Supplementary Video 1** shows the releasing mechanism as it moves along one of the three arms. This movement from the distal aspect of an arm to the proximal aspect allows for the attachment platforms to be moved, pulling them away from the patch connections and releasing the patch. These patch connecting platforms are shown in more detail in **Figure 3**.

The attachment platforms will have small hooks (not shown in the figure) where they will be able to attach to rings of a semi-robust crosslinked hydrogel (GelMA) at the corners of the patch. If the releasing mechanism fails to move the hook from the patch and release that corner, the arm could be rotated using the rotationary mechanism shown in **Supplementary Figure 3** to pull the connection away from the patch. To reduce the risk of injury to surrounding structures, the edges of the design are curved and smooth (**Figure 4**).

3D Printing of Sizing and Learning Resin Prototype

Some of the parameters for the 3D printer settings for the sizing and learning prototype are shown in **Supplementary Figure 4**. We used a Stratasys J750™ polyjet multi-material 3D printer (Stratasys, Eden Prairie, MN, USA). The materials used to print the test (sizing and learning) prototype parts were VeroVivid (a translucent colour material) and Agilus (an elastomeric polymer) which cost under £10 GBP ($14 USD). The total cost (excluding hardware purchase) of the sizing and learning print was <£60

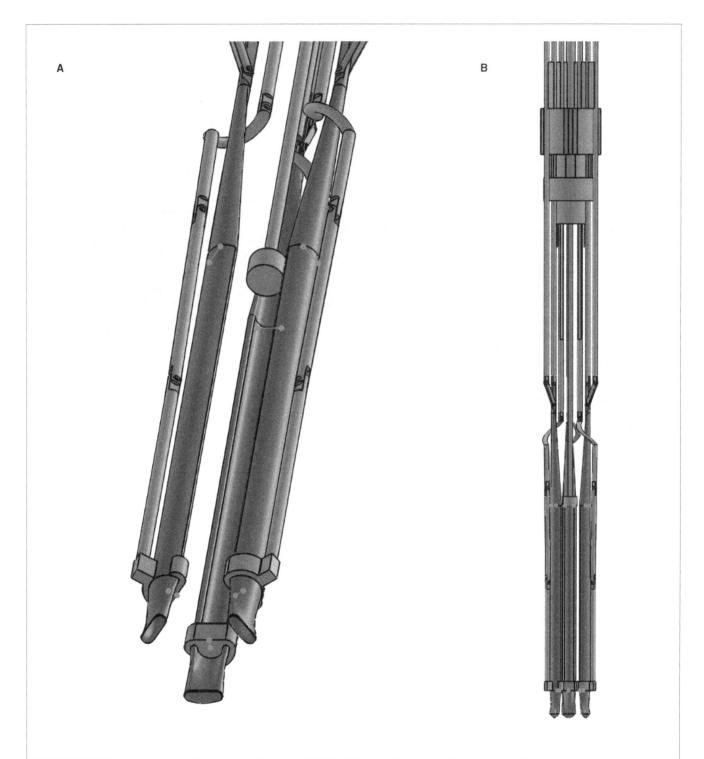

FIGURE 2 | (A,B) Close-up angled view (A) and complete lateral view (B) of the distal end of the instrument (the patient end where the patch would be enclosed). Movements of this compartment are controlled at the other (operator's) end of the instrument by the connected Grips shown in **Figure 1**.

GBP ($83 USD). A comparison of the resin size to the computer-aided design blueprint is shown in **Figure 4**. The printed product underwent a chemical bath (in a solvent named Opteon SF-79, which is used to dissolve the support material for the printed parts) and during this final phase some of the tiny cylinder joints (6 out of 13) were lost.

A World-First Surgical Instrument for Minimally Invasive Robotically-Enabled Transplantation of Heart Patches...

35

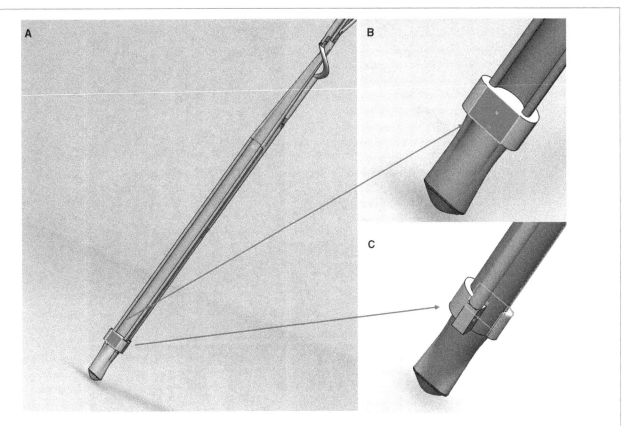

FIGURE 3 | The patch releasing mechanism in close-up. **(A)** Shows an arm patch attachment point/platform (highlighted in blue); **(B)** shows anterior view close-up of the platform where a hook/nodule (not shown) will attach patch corners; **(C)** shows a posterior view of the platform shown in **(B)**.

DISCUSSION

Brief Research Report key Considerations and Unanswered Questions

Our novel surgical instrument design is aimed at minimally invasive approaches to transplant patches for myocardial regeneration and is enabled for future robotic control of the device. Whilst it has not been designed to fit with current commercially available cardiothoracic surgical robots, it has been designed to be ready for robotic control, where the instrument itself would be attached as a forearm to a robotic arm. This was based on the capabilities in our department to build a full robotic arm and the instrument could be used for master-slave or full automation. It is important that any new instrument design is enabled for compatibility to these envisaged future robotic controls.

The sizing and learning resin 3D print gave several insights which will be invaluable for the full prototyping phase from stainless steel. Firstly, it showed us that a major challenge is going to be accounting for the manufacturing machine error with such small parts (our smallest components are 1 mm diameter × 1 mm height cylinder joints). The printer we used has a high resolution (horizontal build layers down to $14\,\mu m$) but there is also print error margin of ±150–$200\,\mu m$ (up to 1% of the diameter of our instrument and 20% of our 1 mm cylinder joints). These valuable

learning points taught us that the next phase will likely require both a slight enlarging of the instrument and also the use of a very low error manufacturing technique for the stainless steel prototype. Furthermore, each part in the design is a perfect fit and therefore allowed no space for collision volume (the distance away from the molecular centre which may come into contact with adjacent parts). The metal print in future will require micro-adjustments across every part of the design to add $\pm100\,\mu m$ space around each part so that there is room for manufacturing machine error in the generation of the stainless steel prototype.

Another consideration is that following the initial fabrication of the instrument it will have to be immersed in the same chemical bath used for the resin sizing and learning print (Opteon SF-79) during which time our tiny joints can still be lost. In fact, during the resin learning print 6 of our 13 joints were lost during the chemical bath. Therefore, we may need to include over 20, adding in extra joints in anticipation that some will be lost during the manufacturing process. Future trials by our group will determine whether these issues can be minimised by increasing the size of the instrument without removing the clinical utility.

We have envisaged the instrument being used for VATS approaches and it should be highly versatile so it can be used with multiple surgical approaches via uniportal (one large "keyhole" in the chest for all instruments) or multiportal (several keyhole incisions) VATS—for example with a left anterolateral approach.

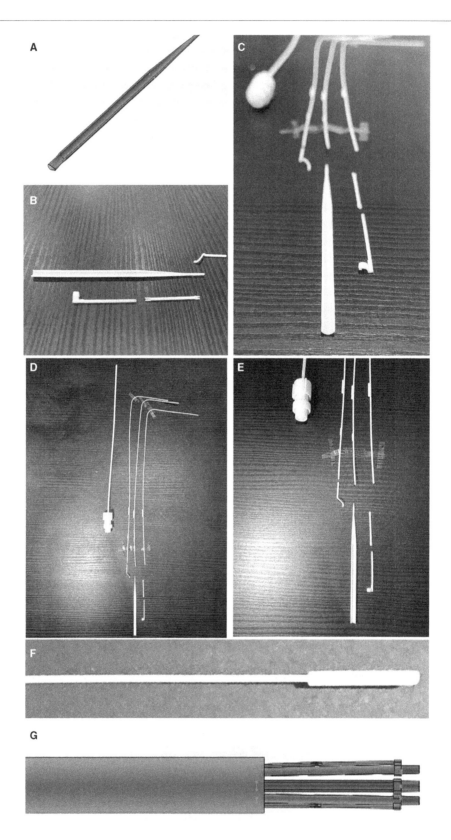

FIGURE 4 | Curved edges of the arm to reduce risk of injury to surrounding structures inside the chest. **(A)** Shows the CAD blueprint for the main component of one of the arms. The photographs in **(B,C)** show the same curved edged arm with surrounding component parts after the sizing and learning resin print (VeroVivid and Agilus). These parts were reproduced with a high degree of accuracy to the blueprint and the surrounding component parts fitted with the main body of the arm. This

(Continued)

FIGURE 4 | suggests these components will be accurately fabricated in the subsequent stainless steel prototype. Photographs in (D,E) show component parts outcome of Agilus/VeroVivid resin sizing and learning print. Despite inherent printer error margin, sizes were accurate to the CAD blueprint and appropriate for surgical use. There were limitations to the resolution printable by this method shown by the fusion of resin material at the distal tip in the photograph (F) compared to the input CAD image shown in (G). This has shown that subsequent prototyping will require a manufacturing method capable of retaining the detail of small parts within the device.

The exact approach would depend on the target area of the heart (for instance we would probably want to deploy the patch over a specific infarcted or failing area of the left ventricle). This will likely need a wide space and multiple ports to get a good view and manoeuvre into the best position.

The patch itself (see **Supplementary Video 1**) can be customised in many ways with different biomaterials to control the viscosity of the patch and also for different cell types within the patch (16). Many different cells have been tried by researchers in this field, often derived from stem cells (7). Our approach might be able to treat heart failure for patients who would otherwise not be eligible for a transplant (in a less invasive standalone procedure to patch the myocardium rather than replace the whole heart). There are many complex considerations for this, including whether one could generate a patch of patient-specific heart tissue from stem cells reprogrammed from the patient's own skin cells and transplant that (7). Importantly, all approaches to myocardial regeneration with a patch have so far have imagined an open surgical transplantation method which may actually preclude this treatment in many of the heart failure patients it is ultimately intended to benefit.

The therapeutic approach will be different for the acute vs. chronic phase of ischaemic cardiomyopathy and/or MI and initially this instrument has been designed with a view to being applicable in a non-acute situation as a standalone procedure. In the acute phase it may not even be required to transplant cells but just putting a patch as an adjunct to regular treatment which stimulates macrophages and other inflammatory responses may be beneficial for remodelling and cardiac function after MI (17). For this instrument, it is clinically most likely to be useful for chronic heart failure caused by ischaemia or MI. There are many open questions and a large amount of research is focused on regenerating the myocardium (7, 8). The unique selling point of this instrument is that no one has yet presented a solution to the question of how to transplant patches without open surgery. By the time regenerative patches for the myocardium are ready for clinical use they may need to be able to be transplanted by minimally invasive and/or robotic approaches. If patch transplant were to be used as an adjunct in a patient already undergoing another procedure, a minimally invasive method would need to exist because the primary procedure may not be via open surgery. As a standalone treatment for high-risk patients with heart failure who cannot have open surgery, it may be beneficial for them if this can be done by a less invasive approach.

This brief research report represents the first time this approach has been presented (without restriction for anyone to build upon). Whilst it has been developed for cardiac applications, it could even be co-opted for other applications (e.g. abdominopelvic) where diverse minimally invasive robotic approaches are also being developed (5' 6). Its main limitation is that the descriptive work herein is at an early stage. It is likely that future instrument designs will have to be larger, perhaps more fitting for a 5–6 cm incision rather than a 2 cm one. This would also have the potential benefit of bypassing the major challenge of how to infold a patch then outfold it like a net (without crushing it). Specifically, a 5–6 cm diameter instrument could potentially accommodate a non-folded patch large enough to be used without repeated application of small patches. Future studies will be needed to optimise designs, fully prototype them and then assess the actual performance of any prototype in proof-of-concept surgery followed by full *ex-vivo* (cadaver) and *in-vivo* trials. Efficacy will need to be evaluated in terms of transplantation success over repeated applications (with full measurement of parameters such as time to delivery, deployment accuracy in a non-beating and beating heart, patch size, covered epicardial surface area and a full range of quantitative and qualitative analyses—all compared to relevant controls). Then trials will be needed for a functional demonstration of a clinically and statistically significant improvement in cardiac function (including non-inferiority against the alternative approach of traditional open surgery). Whilst this brief report article has focused on a surgical instrument design, significant work will also be needed to show that the patch matrix we propose— alginate 4%/gelatin 8% patches ± cells based on our previous optimisation for cardiac applications (9, 16, 18)—is superior to reference patch materials. Translating these technologies is a lengthy process, which is part of the point: it should happen in parallel to the advancements currently underway in the field of myocardial regeneration, or the field risks unveiling a successful new treatment to a world that might have moved away from traditional open surgery (2, 19), limiting how to actually deliver it.

CONCLUSION

Over 12 months our multidisciplinary team has invented a design for a novel surgical instrument which is at the leading edge of innovation in this field. Findings from our sizing and learning resin print of this instrument have prepared the way for the stainless-steel prototype to be manufactured. This is a world-first achievement which may alter the direction of research for surgical transplantation of patches for myocardial regeneration. This brief research report presents the first step on this pathway, for which further trials will be needed.

AUTHOR CONTRIBUTIONS

YZ: conceptualization, data curation, formal analysis, investigation, methodology, resources, software, validation, visualization, and writing—review and editing. CR: conceptualisation, data curation, formal analysis, funding acquisition, investigation, methodology, project administration, supervision, validation, writing—original draught, and writing—review and editing. CG and LZ: conceptualisation, data curation, funding acquisition, methodology, project administration, supervision, and writing—review and editing. All authors contributed to the article and approved the submitted version.

SUPPLEMENTARY MATERIAL

Supplementary Figure 1 | The instrument with the sheath covering the distal

arms removed. Frontal **(A)** and trimetric **(B)** views show the instrument with arms in the infolded position.

Supplementary Figure 2 | Control pathways linking the operator's end to the distal arms. **(A–C)** Highlighted views of the three Grips controlling the distal arms.

Supplementary Figure 3 | Mechanism allowing for adjustment of the rotational angle of the arms. Infolded arms **(A)** can be outfolded to open position and rotated individually by the grips shown in **(B)**. View shown in **(A)** is the distal (patient's end) and **(B)** shows a "top down" view of the proximal (operator's end) of the instrument (looking down onto the Grips).

Supplementary Figure 4 | 3D printing parameters for the resin sizing and learning prototyping of individual parts.

Supplementary Video 1 | Video walkthrough of patch delivery device, including background and mechanistic demonstration from the computer-aided design (CAD).

REFERENCES

1. LaPietra A, Grossi EA, Derivaux CC, Applebaum RM, Hanjis CD, Ribakove GH, et al. Robotic-assisted instruments enhance minimally invasive mitral valve surgery. *Ann Thoracic Surg.* (2000) 70:835–8. doi: 10.1016/S0003-4975(00)01610-6
2. Torregrossa G, Balkhy HH. The role of robotic totally endoscopic coronary artery bypass in the future of coronary artery revascularization. *Eur J Cardiothorac Surg.* (2020) 58:217–20. doi: 10.1093/ejcts/ezaa104
3. Güllü AÜ, Senay S, Ersin E, Demirhisar Ö, Kocyigit M, Alhan C. Feasibility of robotic-assisted atrial septal defect repair in a 6-year-old patient. *Int J Med Robot.* (2021) 17:e2185. doi: 10.1002/rcs.2185
4. McBride K, Steffens D, Stanislaus C, Solomon M, Anderson T, Thanigasalam R, et al. Detailed cost of robotic-assisted surgery in the Australian public health sector: from implementation to a multi-specialty caseload. *BMC Health Serv Res.* (2021) 21:108. doi: 10.1186/s12913-021-06105-z
5. Bai W, Cao Q, Wang P, Chen P, Leng C, Pan T. Modular design of a teleoperated robotic control system for laparoscopic minimally invasive surgery based on ROS and RT-Middleware. *Ind Rob.* (2017) 44:596–608. doi: 10.1108/IR-12-2016-0351
6. Zhou X, Zhang H, Feng M, Zhao J, Fu Y. New remote centre of motion mechanism for robot-assisted minimally invasive surgery. *Biomed Eng Online.* (2018) 17:170. doi: 10.1186/s12938-018-0601-6
7. Roche CD, Brereton RJL, Ashton AW, Jackson C, Gentile C. Current challenges in three-dimensional bioprinting heart tissues for cardiac surgery. *Eur J Cardiothorac Surg.* (2020) 58:500–10. doi: 10.1093/ejcts/ezaa093
8. Wang H, Roche CD, Gentile C. Omentum support for cardiac regeneration in ischaemic cardiomyopathy models: a systematic scoping review. *Eur J Cardiothorac Surg.* (2020) 58:1118–29. doi: 10.1093/ejcts/ezaa205
9. Roche CD, Gentile C. Transplantation of a 3D bioprinted patch in a murine model of myocardial infarction. *J Vis Exp.* (2020) e61675. doi: 10.3791/61675
10. Menasché P, Vanneaux V, Hagege A, Bel A, Cholley B, Cacciapuoti I, et al. Human embryonic stem cell-derived cardiac progenitors for severe heart failure treatment: first clinical case report. *Eur Heart J.* (2015) 36:2011–7. doi: 10.1093/eurheartj/ehv189
11. Menasché P, Vanneaux V, Hagege A, Bel A, Cholley B, Parouchev A, et al. Transplantation of human embryonic stem cell-derived cardiovascular progenitors for severe ischemic left ventricular dysfunction. *J Am Coll Cardiol.* (2018) 71:429–38. doi: 10.1016/j.jacc.2017.11.047
12. Chachques JC, Trainini JC, Lago N, Masoli OH, Barisani JL, Cortes-Morichetti M, et al. Myocardial assistance by grafting a new bioartificial upgraded myocardium (MAGNUM clinical trial): one year follow-up. *Cell Transplant.* (2007) 16:927–34. doi: 10.3727/096368907783338217
13. Sawa Y, Miyagawa S, Sakaguchi T, Fujita T, Matsuyama A, Saito A, et al. Tissue engineered myoblast sheets improved cardiac function sufficiently to discontinue LVAS in a patient with DCM: report of a case. *Surg Today.* (2012) 42:181–4. doi: 10.1007/s00595-011-0106-4
14. Sawa Y, Yoshikawa Y, Toda K, Fukushima S, Yamazaki K, Ono M, et al. Safety and efficacy of autologous skeletal myoblast sheets (TCD-51073) for the treatment of severe chronic heart failure due to ischemic heart disease. *Circ J.* (2015) 79:991–9. doi: 10.1253/circj.CJ-15-0243
15. Moscarelli M, Lorusso R, Abdullahi Y, Varone E, Marotta M, Solinas M, et al. The effect of minimally invasive surgery and sternotomy on physical activity and quality of life. *Heart Lung Circ.* (2021) 30:882–7. doi: 10.1016/j.hlc.2020.09.936
16. Roche CD, Sharma P, Ashton AW, Jackson C, Xue M, Gentile C. Printability, durability, contractility and vascular network formation in 3D bioprinted cardiac endothelial cells using alginate-gelatin hydrogels. *Front Bioeng Biotechnol.* (2021) 9:e636257. doi: 10.31219/osf.io/ct6rk
17. Vagnozzi RJ, Maillet M, Sargent MA, Khalil H, Johansen AK, Schwanekamp JA, et al. An acute immune response underlies the benefit of cardiac stem-cell therapy. *Nature.* (2019) 577:405–9. doi: 10.1101/506626
18. Polonchuk L, Surija L, Lee MH, Sharma P, Liu Chung Ming C, Richter F, et al. Towards engineering heart tissues from bioprinted cardiac spheroids. *Biofabrication.* (2021) 13:045009. doi: 10.1088/1758-5090/ac14ca
19. Leonard JR, Rahouma M, Abouarab AA, Schwann AN, Scuderi G, Lau C, et al. Totally endoscopic coronary artery bypass surgery: a meta-analysis of the current evidence. *Int J Cardiol.* (2018) 261:42–6. doi: 10.1016/j.ijcard.2017.12.071

5

Development and *in vivo* Assessment of a Rapidly Collapsible Anastomotic Guide for Use in Anastomosis of the Small Intestine: A Pilot Study Using a Swine Model

Alisha P. Pedersen[1†], Karrer M. Alghazali[2,3*†], Rabab N. Hamzah[2], Pierre-Yves Mulon[1], Megan McCracken[4], Rebecca E. Rifkin[1], Anwer Mhannawee[2], Zeid A. Nima[2], Christopher Griffin[2], Robert L. Donnell[5], Alexandru S. Biris[2] and David E. Anderson[1]*

[1] Department of Large Animal Clinical Sciences, College of Veterinary Medicine, University of Tennessee, Knoxville, TN, United States, [2] Center for Integrative Nanotechnology Sciences, University of Arkansas at Little Rock, Little Rock, AR, United States, [3] NuShores BioSciences LLC, Little Rock, AR, United States, [4] Equine Hospital, Veterinary Health Center, University of Missouri College of Veterinary Medicine, Columbia, MO, United States, [5] Department of Biomedical and Diagnostic Sciences, College of Veterinary Medicine, University of Tennessee, Knoxville, TN, United States

Correspondence:
Alisha P. Pedersen
apotte14@vols.utk.edu
Karrer M. Alghazali
karrer@nushores.com

[†] *These authors have contributed equally to this work and share first authorship*

Various conditions in human and veterinary medicine require intestinal resection and anastomosis, and complications from these procedures are frequent. A rapidly collapsible anastomotic guide was developed for small intestinal end-to-end anastomosis and was investigated in order to assess its utility to improve the anastomotic process and to potentially reduce complication rates. A complex manufacturing method for building a polymeric device was established utilizing biocompatible and biodegradable polyvinylpyrrolidone and polyurethane. This combination of polymers would result in rapid collapse of the material. The guide was designed as a hollow cylinder composed of overlaying shingles that separate following exposure to moisture. An *in vivo* study was performed using commercial pigs, with each pig receiving one standard handsewn anastomosis and one guide-facilitated anastomosis. Pigs were sacrificed after 13 days, at which time burst pressure, maximum luminal diameter, and presence of adhesions were assessed. Burst pressures were not statistically different between treatment groups, but *in vivo* anastomoses performed with the guide withstood 10% greater luminal burst pressure and maintained 17% larger luminal diameter than those performed using the standard handsewn technique alone. Surgeons commented that the addition of a guide eased the performance of the anastomosis. Hence, a rapidly collapsible anastomotic guide may be beneficial to the performance of intestinal anastomosis.

Keywords: end-to-end anastomosis, anastomotic guide, side-to-side anastomosis, polyvinylpyrrolidone, polyurethane

INTRODUCTION

Small intestinal anastomosis is a relatively common procedure that may be performed in either emergency or elective situations and commonly involves resection of a diseased or damaged segment of the bowel (1–5). Numerous pathological conditions indicate the need for an intestinal anastomosis, including vascular compromise, bowel gangrene, obstruction, intussusception, volvulus, polyps, neoplasia, impaction, perforation due to trauma, severe inflammatory bowel disease refractory to medical therapy, chronic constipation, various congenital abnormalities, and severe inflammation due to disease. There are several techniques for performing an intestinal anastomosis. The operative technique chosen is at the discretion of the surgeon and is often based on the particular situation, personal preference, benefits or hindrances of specific techniques, cost, feasibility, availability of instruments, the diameter of the affected area of bowel, presence or lack of edema, location within the abdominal cavity, type of disease or condition, and time constraints (1, 2). Regardless of the techniques used, practices that provide the best post-operative recovery include adequate accessibility of the affected bowel segment, gentle manipulation of the bowel and surrounding abdominal structures, appropriate hemostasis and maintenance of vascularization following transection, avoidance of tension at the anastomotic site, proper surgical technique, and prevention of contamination of the abdomen with intestinal contents (2).

The most common anastomotic techniques can be divided into two broad categories, handsewn and stapled, within which are numerous sub-categories. Categories of handsewn anastomoses include simple continuous suture pattern vs. interrupted suture pattern (5–8); single-layered or double-layered closure (9–11); inverting, everting, or appositional pattern (12–15); end-to-end (EEA) or side-to-side (SSA) positioning of intestinal segments; use of absorbable vs. non-absorbable suture material and choice of a specific type of suture material; extramucosal or full-thickness suturing; and choice of spacing between suture placements (16, 17). Categories of stapled anastomoses include: end-to-end or side-to-side positioning; oversewing the stapled area or burying it; and choice of stapling device used (1). No matter the technique, several potential complications may occur during or after an intestinal anastomosis procedure, some of which are life-threatening. A complication that may present itself early in the recovery period is leakage from the anastomotic site. During the first 5–7 days of recovery, the efficacy of the anastomotic site largely relies on the integrity of the suture material or staples to holdfast in the tissues. Leakage that occurs within the first day or two after surgery is often associated with the techniques utilized to perform the anastomosis. If leakage occurs beyond the first 5–7 days in the postoperative recovery period, it is more likely to be associated with poor intestinal healing (2). Leakage may take the form of diffuse peritonitis or localized abscess formation. Peritonitis has a high morbidity and mortality rate and requires additional surgical intervention (2). Leakage has been reported to increase the expected mortality rate after bowel anastomosis from 7.2 to 22% (1, 18).

Another commonly encountered complication is excessive bleeding from the anastomotic site, either intraoperatively or postoperatively. The integrity of the anastomosis should be re-evaluated if this occurs and hemostasis achieved as needed. Postoperative bleeding can be evident as hematemesis, melena, bleeding through an intra-abdominal drain, progressive anemia, and abdominal distension, among other signs. These cases may need to be treated with medical management or, if persistent or severe, surgical intervention. Stapled anastomoses in particular have been shown to result in disruption of mesenteric blood vessels, increasing the risk of ischemia of the bowel (2). Stricture of the intestine at the anastomosis is a serious complication that has been reported to occur more frequently after stapled EEA than handsewn EEA (2, 19). Medical management of anastomotic leakage after surgery is a significant risk factor contributing to the development of a stricture, and dilatation or surgical revision may be necessary to treat this complication (2).

We hypothesized that the use of an anastomotic guide (AG), placed within the lumen of the intestine during surgery would improve the accuracy of EEA by providing a means to appose the cut ends of the intestine so that precise sutures could be placed. This precision surgery would result in increased lumen diameter and reduced potential for leakage after anastomosis. The device was designed such that it would rapidly collapse after surgery so as not to be predisposed to complications associated with other intraluminal intestinal devices. Intraluminal stents have been used to expand and maintain the lumen size of strictured bowel after colon resection and anastomosis. To date, intestinal stents used to expand the intestinal wall contain non-degradable or slowly degraded materials (20). Intestinal stents may increase morbidity rates associated with interruption of intestinal motility, impaction of the stent by digesta, stent migration, and re-obstruction (20–22). A slowly degrading (up to 3 months) intraluminal colonic stent was described for treatment of strictures of the colon after anastomotic leakage (23). A rapidly degraded or collapsed intraluminal device would eliminate post-operative morbidity associated with the use of the device. We aimed to assess the feasibility of a rapidly collapsible, intraluminal small intestinal AG to reduce the potential for post-operative complications, as well as to improve the accuracy and efficiency of the anastomotic procedure (23). A prototype AG was fabricated and underwent numerous characterization assessments prior to application in an *in vivo* swine model, which was established in order to assess post-surgical complications when compared with a standard handsewn EEA method.

MATERIALS AND METHODS

Anastomotic Guide Composition and Fabrication

Non-degradable 3D-printed models of an intraluminal guide were initially fabricated based on expected bowel size in an ~70 kg pig, as well as the length predicted to be of greatest

---

Abbreviations: EEA, End-to-end anastomosis; SSA, Side-to-side anastomosis; AG, Anastomotic guide; PVP, Polyvinylpyrrolidone; PU, Polyurethane.

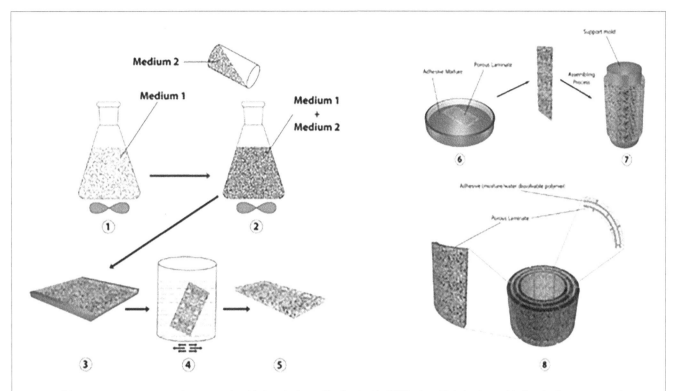

FIGURE 1 | General protocol used to fabricate the device. Medium 1 refers to PU dissolved in 90/10 ethanol/deionized water. Medium 2 refers to salt porosity agents with 75–150 pm diameter.

benefit to the technical performance of an anastomosis. A hollow cylindrical tube was determined to be the ideal shape. These prototypes were used as models for creation of a rapidly collapsible, intraluminal AG. The desired specifications were that the guide would collapse no <30 min and no longer than 3 h after implantation within the intestine.

A guide (patent pending: PCT/US2019/041550) was fabricated using a hollow cylindrical tube composed of layers of biocompatible polymer polyurethane (PU) (HydroMed:AdvanSource Biomaterials; Wilmington, MA) and moisture/fluid-degradable polymer polyvinylpyrrolidone (PVP) (polyvinylpyrrolidone: Sigma-Aldrich: Average MW 10000, St. Louis, MO). These polymers were chosen based on their water responses (water uptake and ability to dissolve in water). The polymer layers were produced using a modified salt leaching method. Briefly, the PU polymer was dissolved in 90/10 ethanol/deionized water to form medium 1, then 10 g of 75–150-μm particles (porosity agents — medium 2) for each 1 g of PU were added (**Figure 1**). The material was mixed extensively, poured over a glass mold, and transferred into a water bath to remove the salt particles. The resulting polymer film was dried and cut into a small laminate (3 × 1.5 cm). Next, the porous polymer laminate was saturated with PVP. The polymer laminates were then assembled to form multilayers over the support mold. The mold was removed, and the samples were left to dry (**Figure 2**).

The device was fabricated to serve as a temporary supportive intraluminal anastomotic guide that can rapidly lose its integrity

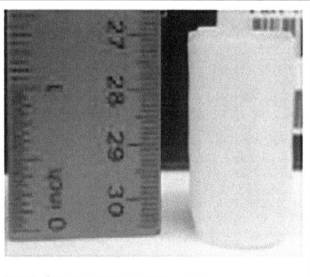

FIGURE 2 | Fabricated device measuring 3 × 1.5 cm.

after becoming wet and within the desired time. The desired specifications were that the guide would lose its integrity in no <30 min and no more than 3 h after implantation within the intestine. To test the device's ability to meet these specifications, the fabricated samples were immersed in a water bath, and the integrality was observed over time.

In vivo Investigation

In vivo studies were done after approval by the Institutional Animal Care and Use Committee (IACUC protocol #2522) at the University of Tennessee, Knoxville. Six domestic cross-bred pigs, weighing 35 to 70 kg, were housed in separate adjacent pens and acclimated to their environment for 12 days. Each pig was fasted for a minimum of 12 h prior to surgery, and water access was restricted a minimum of 2 h before surgery. Peri-operative analgesia was provided by placement of transdermal fentanyl patches (1 μg/kg) along the dorsal midline in the mid-thoracic region at least 12 h prior to surgery. Subjects were pre-medicated with xylazine (2 mg/kg, IM), induced with a combination of midazolam (0.1–0.2 mg/kg, IM) and ketamine (10 mg/kg, IM), an endotracheal tube was placed, and anesthesia maintained using isoflurane (range 1 to 5%) vaporized into oxygen (100%). Each subject was placed into dorsal recumbency, clipped, and aseptically prepared along the ventral midline. The surgical model, briefly depicted in **Figure 3**, consisted of a 10 cm ventral midline laparotomy with subsequent exteriorization of 20–40 cm of jejunum. The bowel was milked free of intraluminal contents and a 15 cm segment was isolated with Doyen intestinal clamps. A complete, transverse enterotomy was performed at a 90° angle and single interrupted sutures of #3-0 PDS (Ethicon, INC. Somerville, New Jersey) were placed at the mesenteric and anti-mesenteric margins of the cut edges for stabilization and to aid in apposition of the edges. The anastomosis was completed with an interrupted simple continuous appositional pattern (two suture segments, each placed hemi-circumferentially) using #3-0 PDS. Integrity, blood perfusion, and complete closure of the anastomosis was evaluated. Approximately 20 cm distal to the first anastomosis, a second enterotomy was performed in like manner, except after the first single interrupted suture was placed and before closing the cut edges of the bowel with the same technique, the collapsible intraluminal anastomotic guide was placed within the lumen traversing and centered on the cut edges. Following replacement of the jejunum within the abdominal cavity, the linea alba was closed using #0 PDS, the subcutaneous layer with #2-0 PDS, and finally the skin with #1 polypropylene, all utilizing a simple continuous pattern. Surgeons were consulted regarding their subjective opinion of the utility of the AG during surgery.

Pigs received intramuscular ceftiofur (Excede, Zoetis Services LLC, Parsippany, New Jersey; 5 mg/kg dose) prior to surgery. The pigs were monitored frequently for signs of pain, incision site abnormalities, vomiting, abdominal distention, diarrhea, or constipation. Peri-operative analgesia was managed using fentanyl patches (1 μg/kg, TD, 72 h) and meloxicam (0.4 mg/kg, PO, q24 h × 5 d). Pigs were monitored for activity, appetite, and clinical signs of pain through day 13 at which time the study was terminated.

All pigs were sacrificed 13 days after surgery, and necropsy examinations performed to assess the gross appearance of the bowel and anastomoses, as well as the surrounding abdominal cavity. Burst pressure withstood by the anastomotic sites was determined by instilling saline into the anastomotic region and observing for leakage. Fluid pressure was assessed using a digital pressure monitor (Surgivet® V6400 Invasive Blood Pressure Monitor, Smiths Medical PLC, Minneapolis, MN). The vicinity of the anastomotic site was occluded using surgical clamps, leaving an ~12 cm long segment centered on the anastomosis. A 16-gauge needle and IV line were used to instill saline solution into one side of this region, and a second 16-gauge needle was placed into the opposing side and attached to the pressure monitor. The lumen was gradually distended with saline while the anastomosis was observed for leaks. Once a leak occurred, the pressure reading was recorded and considered the maximum burst pressure withstood by the anastomotic site for that sample.

The external diameter of the bowel was also measured for the assessment of stricture of the anastomotic site. Diameter difference was calculated based on diameter measurements of the intestinal regions just proximally and distally adjacent to the anastomosis, as well as at the anastomotic site, utilizing calipers while saline remained infused in the segments following burst pressure measurement. Histologic evaluation included hematoxylin and eosin and trichrome stains to assess fibrosis and collagen deposition, presence and characterization of inflammation at the anastomotic sites and within the adjacent tissue, approximate width of anastomotic sites, serosal thickness, and any additional abnormalities.

RESULTS
Anastomotic Guide Characteristics
3D Keyence Laser Microscope Analysis
Three-dimensional (3D) laser microscopy (LSCM, VK-X260K, Keyence, Itasca, IL) was used to evaluate the surface morphology and topography of the samples, allowing visualization of the porous structure of the polymer laminate. The porous polymer laminate was examined using 20X and 10X lenses. The data was analyzed with Keyence's Multi-File Analyzer software. 3D microscopy confirmed that the polymer laminate has a porous structure, as shown in **Figure 4**.

Device Testing
Generally, when dry, the device is a rigid structure due to the solidification of PVP. The fabricated samples were immersed in a water bath, and the integrality was observed over time. The device lost its integrity as a function of the water/fluid response of its two polymers, causing it to collapse.

In vivo Investigation
Morbidities observed after surgery included minimal incidences of diarrhea, mild pyrexia that resolved after treatment with antibiotics, and mild swelling at the incision site. No remnants of the AGs were recovered in feces.

Following sacrifice of the pigs, gross examination of the anastomoses and surrounding abdominal cavity was performed. Adhesions were discovered at eleven out of the twelve EEA sites and at adjacent regions within the abdominal cavity in five out of the six pigs. There were no significant differences in adhesion development between the anastomotic sites that involved the AG and those that did not. A standard handsewn EEA in one pig was noted to have had minor dehiscence, and no leakage or

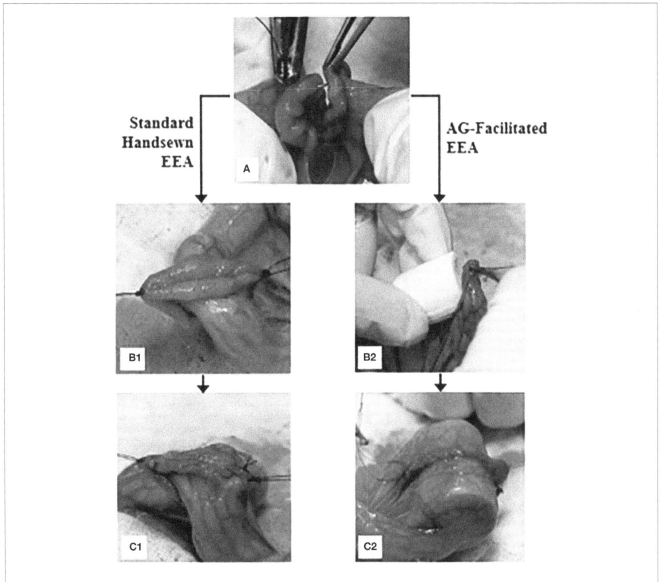

FIGURE 3 | End-to-end anastomosis procedure; **(A)** a single interrupted suture is placed on the anti-mesenteric margin of the bowel immediately following performance of a transverse enterotomy; **(B1)** single simple interrupted sutures are secured on both the anti-mesenteric and mesenteric margins, and the bowel edges are apposed for further suturing; **(C1)** a row of simple continuous sutures is placed hemi-circumferentially; **(B2)** an AG is placed into the lumen of the bowel; **(C2)** the anastomosis is performed overtop the AG after complete placement within the lumen.

dehiscence was noted in any of the EEA performed with the AG. The gross appearance of the healed margins of the bowel were similar for all EEA sites.

Burst pressure was found to be ∼10% greater at AG-facilitated anastomotic sites than those of standard handsewn EEA sites (**Table 1**); however, this difference was not statistically significant. The maximum diameter achieved at the anastomotic sites that utilized an AG was significantly greater than that achieved with the standard handsewn anastomoses (**Table 1**). Subjective evaluation by surgeons performing the anastomoses noted that the guide aided in the placement of more evenly spaced sutures and eased the performance of the EEA. The surgeons noted that there was some difficulty placing the guide within the lumen

due to its pliability (accountable to submersion in saline prior to surgery).

Histologic evaluation revealed characteristics of expected healing within all of the samples, including suture granulomas adjacent to anastomotic sites, fibrosis and collagen deposition within sites, serosal thickness at sites between 2 and 4 times that of the adjacent normal tissue, and sites ranging in width from <0.5 to 5 mm. All anastomotic sites contained a normal expected amount of mild-to-moderate inflammatory cell infiltration, typically mixed eosinophilic and lymphocytic inflammation. Two anastomotic sites (one standard and one AG) in two separate pigs appeared to have features of both jejunum and ileum, dependent on the section examined. The standard handsewn anastomosis

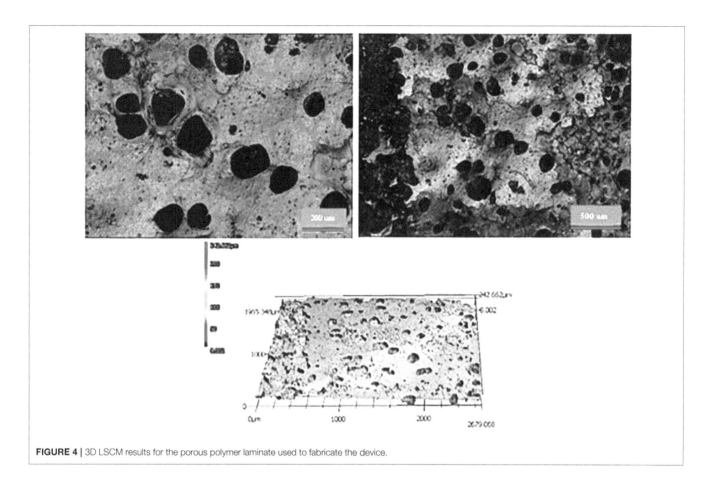

FIGURE 4 | 3D LSCM results for the porous polymer laminate used to fabricate the device.

TABLE 1 | Comparison of the average number of adhesions at the anastomotic site, burst pressure, and maximum diameter for each anastomotic technique.

	Standard handsewn EEA	Anastomotic guide EEA
Average number of adhesions at site	1	1
Average burst pressure (mmHg)[b]	150.6 ± 49.3	166.0 ± 47.5
Average maximum diameter at anastomotic site (mm)[a]	22.73 ± 2.0	26.59 ± 3.9
Diameter difference of anastomotic sites (%)[a]		+17%

Burst pressure was obtained at only five of the six anastomotic sites of each technique due to perforation of the anastomotic site or adjacent bowel in two samples. Presence of adhesions at the anastomotic sites and local regions of the abdominal cavity was assessed grossly. Burst pressure was measured by instilling saline into the anastomotic region and observing the maximum pressure withstood by the anastomosis via a digital pressure monitor. Maximum diameter at each anastomotic site was measured while saline remained infused in the segments following burst pressure measurement. Diameter difference is the difference between the average diameter of the anastomoses performed with and without the use of an AG.
[a]Statistically significant difference (p < 0.05), [b]No significant difference.

in one pig demonstrated a focal region of ulceration and marked inflammatory infiltrates, including dead or degenerate segmented eosinophils and neutrophils. This sample demonstrated an increased presence of macrophages within an area of fibrosis. Within this same pig, the bowel edges of the AG site appeared to be overlapped in one region. Another standard handsewn

anastomosis in a different pig similarly demonstrated an area of ulceration, along with the presence of hemorrhage, imbedded plant material or suture, and marked suppurative and eosinophilic inflammation. Hemorrhage was found within the serosa of this sample. Within the standard handsewn site of an additional pig, there was a focal region of pyogranulomatous inflammation, and in the AG site of this same pig, there was a mild-to-moderate amount of inflammation and hemorrhage within the serosa which was deemed likely not significant.

DISCUSSION

During post-mortem assessment, anastomotic site diameter was deemed to be improved in the sites in which an AG was used. Although small, this difference may be clinically significant, resulting in a decreased likelihood of stricture and impaction at surgical sites. A meta-analysis examining complications following sutured and stapled colorectal anastomosis in 1,233 human patients determined that strictures occurred in 2 and 8% of patients, respectively (1, 24). One limitation to evaluating the diameter difference by measuring the external diameter with calipers is that any inverted mucosa resulting in a further narrowed intraluminal diameter would not be accounted for. Two alternative methods of assessing the intraluminal diameter and anastomotic index are by instillation of a contrast agent into the delineated region of the anastomosis and subsequent

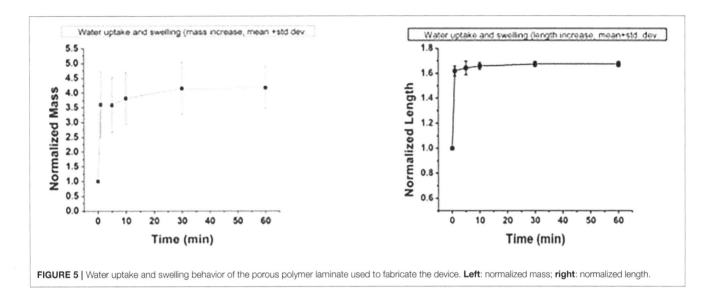

FIGURE 5 | Water uptake and swelling behavior of the porous polymer laminate used to fabricate the device. **Left**: normalized mass; **right**: normalized length.

radiographic imaging (25, 26), or by measurement of the wall thickness at the anastomotic site and proximally and distally to it utilizing calipers (26).

Differences in burst pressure between the groups were not significantly different. This suggests that the healing process in the intestine with EEA is similar regardless of the technique employed. Maximum burst pressures achieved were physiologically appropriate, and in fact were in excess to normal physiological pressures (27, 28), so it does not appear that the performance of anastomoses produced a risk of bowel disruption during motility, at least when assessed 2 weeks post-operatively.

Adhesion development occurred at nearly all anastomotic sites and within local areas of the abdominal cavity. It was difficult to differentiate which anastomotic site may have incited the additional adhesions within the abdomen, and the ~20 cm distance between the two anastomoses may ultimately have been too close in proximity to allow this determination. Intraluminal appearance of each anastomosis was not noticeably different, supporting the likelihood that the methods did not adversely affect the normal process of intestinal healing. One pig appeared to have developed a small dehiscence at the standard handsewn anastomotic site, which was sealed with an adhesion. Histologic evaluation of the samples did not reveal any substantial concerns in regards to integrity of the anastomotic sites or presence of excessive inflammation that would be expected to progress to significant disease, including within the samples that demonstrated focal regions of inflammation. All samples revealed anticipated indicators of healing, including granuloma formation at suture sites, fibrosis and collagen deposition within the anastomotic sites, and thickening of the serosa.

The EEA technique was noted by the surgeons to be easier to perform with the use of the AG. This is likely owing to the ability to place sutures more easily within the cut edges of bowel due to the edges being dilated by the guide as opposed to the natural contraction and eversion that occurs when the bowel is transected. Precision and accuracy in reconstruction of the continuity and patency of the bowel is critical to ensuring that

devastating dehiscence or stricture does not occur (2, 29). The only concern noted with the use of the AG regarded difficulty placing the guide within the lumen due to its pliability. The guides were briefly soaked in saline prior to surgery, which likely accounts for the majority of this pliability. However, sturdiness of the guide may also be addressed in modified designs by altering the thickness or polymer composition. Time to collapse of the guide was assessed in hydration studies prior to placement within the subjects and was deemed appropriate. No remnants remained within the lumen upon necropsy evaluation, which further supports that the guides broke apart.

One concern about placement of a medical device within the bowel lumen is the potential for complications associated with the device itself. Non-degradable or slowly degrading intestinal stents that have been previously available or investigated may increase morbidity rates associated with hindrance to normal peristalsis, dislodgement, blockage of the intestinal lumen with the stent, and impaction of the lumen of the stent with digesta (20–22). We designed a rapidly collapsible polymeric device to avoid these potential complications. Should the guide dislodge shortly after the surgery, it would quickly collpase with the passage of digesta within the bowel. The testing of the device by water bath immersion demonstrated that the device lost its integrity over time as a function of the water/fluid response of its two polymers, causing it to collapse. Generally, the two polymers have different responses to fluid. PU uptakes fluid into its structure, with the ability to increase in mass by about 300% of its dry weight and expand in size by about 60%, as shown in **Figure 5**. In contrast, PVP dissolves when exposed to fluid, causing the device to lose its polymer-polymer bonds.

The ability of an intraluminal anastomotic guide to aid in increasing the diameter of an intestinal anastomosis site, as well as ease the performance of the technique itself, without presenting any additional complications, supports the use of guides for this particular procedure. This could ultimately reduce complications that occur post-operatively, including dehiscence, leakage, peritonitis, stricture, and impaction. Any reduction in time of performance would also be beneficial as some patients undergoing this procedure may be physiologically and anesthetically unstable. The use of a swine model is advantageous for translation to human medicine, as swine have gastrointestinal tracts that are comparable to humans. Continued research is warranted to develop a collapsible or degradable intraluminal guide for small intestinal anastomosis for use in human and animal patients, and the data from this study will be utilized in the planning of a follow-up validation study employing a larger number of swine with assignment of animals to a single treatment group rather than the performance of both procedures within the same animal.

ETHICS STATEMENT

The animal study was reviewed and approved by Institutional Animal Care and Use Committee at the University of Tennessee, Knoxville.

REFERENCES

1. Goulder F. Bowel anastomoses: the theory, the practice and the evidence base. *World J Gastrointest Surg.* (2012) 4:208–13. doi: 10.4240/wjgs.v4.i9.208
2. Medscape. *Intestinal Anastomosis Technique.* (2016). Available online at: http://emedicine.medscape.com/article/1892319-technique (accessed June 30, 2017).
3. Tobias KM, *Intestinal resection and anastomosis. Manual of Small Animal Tissue Surgery.* Ames, IA: Wiley-Blackwell (2010). p. 175-182.
4. Ralphs SC, Jessen CR, Lipowitz AJ. Risk factors for leakage following intestinal anastomosis in dogs and cats: 115 cases (1991-2000). *J Am Vet Med Assoc.* (2003) 223:665–82. doi: 10.2460/javma.2003.223.73
5. Weisman DL, Smeak DD, Birchard SJ, Zweigart SL. Comparison of a continuous suture pattern with a simple interrupted pattern for enteric closure in dogs and cats: 83 cases (1991-1997). *J Am Vet Med Assoc.* (1999) 214:1507–10.
6. Burch JM, Franciose RJ, Moore EE, Biffl WL, Offner PJ. Single-layer continuous versus two-layer interrupted intestinal anastomosis: a prospective randomized trial. *Ann Surg.* (2000) 231:832–7. doi: 10.1097/00000658-200006000-00007
7. Ellison GW, Jokinen MP, Park RD. End-to-end approximating intestinal anastomosis in the dog: a comparative fluorescein dye, angiographic, and histopathologic evaluation. *J Am Anim Hosp Assoc.* (1982) 18:729–36.
8. Allen DA, Smeak DD, Schertel ER. Prevalence of small intestinal dehiscence and associated clinical factors: a retrospective study of 121 dogs. *J An Anim Hosp Assoc.* (1992) 28:70–6.
9. Shikata S, Yamagishi H, Taji Y, Shimada T, Noguchi Y. Single- versus two-layer intestinal anastomosis: a meta-analysis of randomized controlled trials. *BMC Surg.* (2006) 6:2. doi: 10.1186/1471-2482-6-2
10. Garude K, Tandel C, Rao S, Shah N. Single layered intestinal anastomosis: a safe and economic technique. *Indian J Surg.* (2013) 75:290–3. doi: 10.1007/s12262-012-0487-7
11. Sajid MS, Siddiqui MR, Baig MK. Single layer versus double layer suture anastomosis of the gastrointestinal tract. *Cochrane Database Syst Rev.* (2012) 1:CD005477. doi: 10.1002/14651858.CD005477.pub4
12. Getzen LC, Roe RD, Holloway CK. Comparative study of intestinal anastomotic healing in inverted and everted closures. *Surg Gynecol Obstet.* (1966) 123:1219–27.
13. Goligher JC, Morris C, McAdam WA, De Dombal FT, Johnston D. A controlled trial of inverting versus everting intestinal suture in clinical large-bowel surgery. *Br J Surg.* (1970) 57:817–22. doi: 10.1002/bjs.18005 71106
14. Holt, DE. "Large intestines". In: Slatter DH, editor. *Textbook of Small Animal Surgery*, 3rd ed. Philadelphia, PA: Saunders (2003). p. 665–82.
15. Bellenger CR. Comparison of inverting and appositional methods for anastomosis of the small intestine in cats. *Vet Rec.* (1982) 110:265–8. doi: 10.1136/vr.110.12.265
16. Deveney KE, Way LW. Effect of different absorbable sutures on healing of gastrointestinal anastomoses. *Am J Surg.* (1977) 133:86–94. doi: 10.1016/0002-9610(77)90199-4
17. Milovancev M, Weisman DL, Palmisano MP. Foreign body attachment to polypropylene suture material extruded into the small intestine lumen after enteric closure in three dogs. *J Am Vet Med Assoc.* (1982) 225:265–8.
18. Fielding LP, Stewart-Brown S, Blesovsky L, Kearney G. Anastomotic integrity after operation for large-bowel cancer: a multicentre study. *Br Med J.* (1980) 281:411–14. doi: 10.1136/bmj.281.6237.411
19. Leung TTW, MacLean AR, Buie WD, Dixon E. Comparison of stapled versus handsewn loop ileostomy closure: a meta-analysis. *J Gastrointest Surg.* (2008) 12:939–44. doi: 10.1007/s11605-007-0435-1
20. Wang Z, Li N, Li R, Li Y, Ruan L. Biodegradable intestinal stents: a review. *Nat Sci-Mater.* (2014) 24:423–32. doi: 10.1016/j.pnsc.2014.08.008
21. Brightwell NL, McFee AS, Aust JB. Bowel Obstruction and the Long Tube Stent. *Arch Surg.* (1977) 112:505–11. doi: 10.1001/archsurg.1977.01370040157024
22. Son SR, Franco RA, Bae SH, Min YK, Lee BT. Electrospun PLGA/gelatin fibrous tubes for the application of biodegradable intestinal stent in rat model. *J Biomed Mater Res Part B.* (2013) 101B:1095–105. doi: 10.1002/jbm.b.32923
23. Wang Y, Cai X, Jin R, Liang Y, Huang D, Peng S. Experimental study of primary repair of colonic leakage with a degradable stent in a porcine model. *J Gastrointest Surg.* (2011) 15:1995–2000. doi: 10.1007/s11605-011-1593-8
24. Lustosa SA, Matos D, Atallah AN, Castro AA. Stapled versus handsewn methods for colorectal anastomosis surgery. *Cochrane Database Syst Rev.* (2001) 3:CD003144. doi: 10.1002/14651858.CD003144.pub2
25. Gandini M. *In vitro* evaluation of a closed-bowel technique for one-layer hand-sewn inverting end-to-end jejunojejunostomy in the horse. *Vet Surg.* (2006) 35:683–8. doi: 10.1111/j.1532-950X.2006.00209.x
26. Zilling TL, Jansson O, Walther BS, Ottosson A. Sutureless Small bowel anastomoses: experimental study in pigs. *Eur J Surg.* (1999) 165:61–8. doi: 10.1080/110241599750007522

AUTHOR CONTRIBUTIONS

AP contributed to the design of the device and performed all of the animal studies. KA and AB contributed to the design and performed all of the fabrication, characterization, and testing of the anastomotic guide. AP and KA wrote the manuscript. RH, AM, ZN, and CG contributed to the development and testing of the anastomotic guide. DA, P-YM, MM, and RR contributed to the application of the device in the live animal model. AB and DA were mentors during the development and progression of the entire study. All authors contributed to the article and approved the submitted version.

ACKNOWLEDGMENTS

Additional thanks for technical support during these investigations is given to Dr. Madhu Dhar, Dr. Xiaocun Sun, Dr. Tom Doherty, Dr. Christopher Smith, Katie Waller, Sara Root, Paxton Parker, Richard Steiner, Austin Bow, Steven Newby, Rachel Rodriguez, Tammy Howard, Kaitlin Siegfried, Phil Snow, and Wampler's Farm Sausage.

27. Coolman BR, Ehrhart N, Pijanowski G, Ehrhart EJ, Coolman SL. Comparison of skin staples with sutures for anastomosis of the small intestine of dogs. *Vet Surg.* (2000) 29:293–302. doi: 10.1053/jvet.2000. 7539

28. Ellison, GW. End-to-end anastomosis in the dog: a comparison of techniques." *Comp Cont Ed Pract Vet.* (1981) 3:486–95.

29. Shandall A, Lowndes R, Young HL. Colonic anastomotic healing and oxygen tension. *Br J Surg.* (1985) 72:606–9. doi: 10.1002/bjs.1800720808

6

Application of Collagen I and IV in Bioengineering Transparent Ocular Tissues

Yihui Song[1†], Morgan Overmass[1†], Jiawen Fan[2], Chris Hodge[1,3,4], Gerard Sutton[1,3,4], Frank J. Lovicu[1,5] and Jingjing You[1,6]*

[1] Save Sight Institute, Faculty of Medicine and Health, The University of Sydney, Sydney, NSW, Australia, [2] Key Laboratory of Myopia of State Health Ministry, Department of Ophthalmology and Vision Sciences, Eye and Ear, Nose, and Throat (ENT) Hospital, Shanghai Medical College, Fudan University, Shanghai, China, [3] New South Wales (NSW) Tissue Bank, Sydney, NSW, Australia, [4] Vision Eye Institute, Chatswood, NSW, Australia, [5] Discipline of Anatomy and Histology, School of Medical Sciences, The University of Sydney, Sydney, NSW, Australia, [6] School of Optometry and Vision Science, University of New South Wales, Sydney, NSW, Australia

*Correspondence:
Jingjing You
jing.you@sydney.edu.au

[†] These authors have contributed equally to this work and share first authorship

Collagens represent a major group of structural proteins expressed in different tissues and display distinct and variable properties. Whilst collagens are non-transparent in the skin, they confer transparency in the cornea and crystalline lens of the eye. There are 28 types of collagen that all share a common triple helix structure yet differ in the composition of their α-chains leading to their different properties. The different organization of collagen fibers also contributes to the variable tissue morphology. The important ability of collagen to form different tissues has led to the exploration and application of collagen as a biomaterial. Collagen type I (Col-I) and collagen type IV (Col-IV) are the two primary collagens found in corneal and lens tissues. Both collagens provide structure and transparency, essential for a clear vision. This review explores the application of these two collagen types as novel biomaterials in bioengineering unique tissue that could be used to treat a variety of ocular diseases leading to blindness.

Keywords: bioengineering, collagen type IV, cornea, lens, retina, collagen type I

INTRODUCTION

The cornea and lens facilitate a pathway for light to pass through the eye to reach the retina, which then receives and transfers visual signals onto the brain for processing. These three major ocular tissues are critical for generating clear vision; therefore, any damage to the cornea, lens, and/or retina will undoubtedly impair eyesight and often lead to blindness. Tissue engineering, in particular, the development of biomaterials with specific properties, has been increasingly researched for treating ocular disease (1). Due to its abundance in the corneal stroma, collagen type I (Col-I) has been a popular and versatile biomaterial developed to replace diseased corneal layers; however, it has become evident that no singular biomaterial can be an effective substitute for the intact cornea because of the differences in composition between each of the corneal layers (2). Collagen type IV (Col-IV) is the predominant member of Descemet's membrane of the cornea, the supportive layer of the corneal endothelium (3, 4). Furthermore, it is also the main collagen type detected in the lens capsule (5), and in both Bruch's membrane and the internal limiting membrane (ILM) of the retina (6). Therefore, the application of Col-IV as a biomaterial could potentially be useful in creating a natural environment and substratum for corneal endothelial cells and the epithelial cells of the lens and retina. In this paper, previous publications on Col-I and -IV in ocular-related applications were reviewed and the insights into the future direction of development of these two collagen types in ocular bioengineering are discussed.

The Distribution of Col- I and Col-IV in the Cornea, the Lens, and the Retina

The human cornea is a transparent, avascular, highly innervated, and organized tissue that is located at the front of the eye (**Figure 1**). The cornea acts as a transparent window making up two-thirds of the refractive power of the eye and consists of five main layers from anterior to posterior sides: corneal epithelium, Bowman's layer, corneal stroma, Descemet's membrane, and corneal endothelium (2) (**Figure 1**). One major structural protein in the cornea is collagen. The human cornea consists of many types of collagen and different collagen combinations are detected within different layers (**Table 1**).

The central thickness of a normal adult human cornea approximately measures 530 μm (19). In the context of bioengineering, the stroma is critical because it constitutes the majority of the corneal volume and provides a significant contribution to both its overall transparency and strength (20). The corneal stroma is predominantly made up of Col-I fibrils organized into ~300 orthogonally arranged lamellae (2). These fibrils have a unique, smaller diameter, and regular interfibrillar spacing that supports the transparency of the tissue (21). Furthermore, when stress is applied to the cornea, these well-organized collagen fibers of the stroma are stretched to counterbalance this force, allowing the cornea to maintain its existing shape (22). In addition to the stroma, the corneal

endothelium is comprised of a monolayer of interconnected hexagonal cells sitting on the Descemet's membrane. This layer is key to maintaining relative stromal deturgescence/dehydration that is essential for corneal transparency (2). The Descemet's basement membrane is comprised primarily of Col-IV, as well as laminin, perlecan (a heparan sulfate proteoglycan), nidogen, and to a lesser degree, collagen type VIII (Col-VIII) (3, 4). While both Col-IV and Col-VIII are present in the Descemet's membrane, only Col-IV is located adjacent to endothelial cells in both the infant and adult structure (19). In comparison, Col-VIII chains initially face the endothelial cells in the infant Descemet's membrane, but lose contact as we age and shift to face the stroma (3, 4).

The lens is a transparent, biconvex orb that consists of the lens capsule, the lens epithelium, and lens fibers (**Figure 2**). Col-IV is the main type of collagen found in the lens capsule, which is a thick, uninterrupted basement membrane surrounding the lens. The lens capsule is structurally analogous to the corneal Descemet's membrane, as it consists of interlinking Col-IV and

TABLE 1 | Distribution of collagen types in the human cornea.

Layer	Collagen type
Epithelium	IV, XV, XVIII, XII (7–13)
Bowman's layer	I, III, V (14)
Stroma	I, III, V, VI, XII, XIV (15–17)
Descemet membrane	IV, VIII (15, 18)

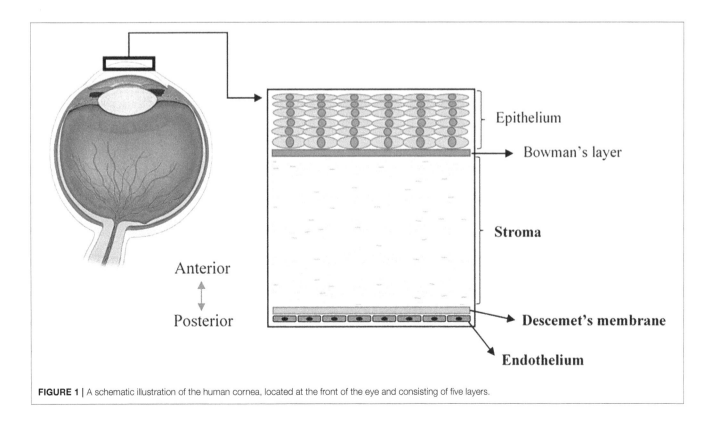

FIGURE 1 | A schematic illustration of the human cornea, located at the front of the eye and consisting of five layers.

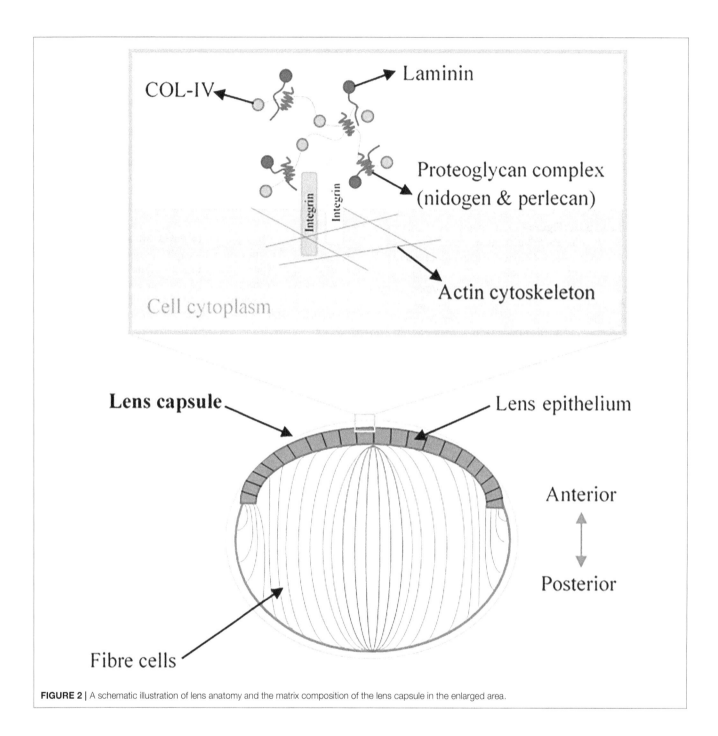

FIGURE 2 | A schematic illustration of lens anatomy and the matrix composition of the lens capsule in the enlarged area.

laminin networks bound together by nidogen and perlecan (5) (**Figure 2**). The lens capsule acts as a supporting matrix for lens epithelial cells anteriorly and fiber cells posteriorly. As a result of this structure encapsulating all lens cells, it also protects them from infection. In younger eyes, the lens capsule also has a role in determining the force required for lens accommodation, a process where the lens changes shape to alter our field of focus (23).

The human retina is the sensory tissue that lines the inner surface of the back of the eye, which senses light and sends signals to the brain to provide vision (6). It contains multiple layers with various cell types (**Figure 3**). Retinal ganglion cells (RGC) represent a type of neuron located at the inner surface of the retina. The RGCs receive visual information from the photoreceptors (rods and cones) *via* intermediate neuron types including bipolar cells, amacrine cells, and horizontal cells. Rods and cones are responsible for sensing light. Bipolar cells transfer visual information from photoreceptor cells to amacrine cells. Amacrine cells are interneurons in the retina that have short neurotic processes to connect to adjacent neurons and to

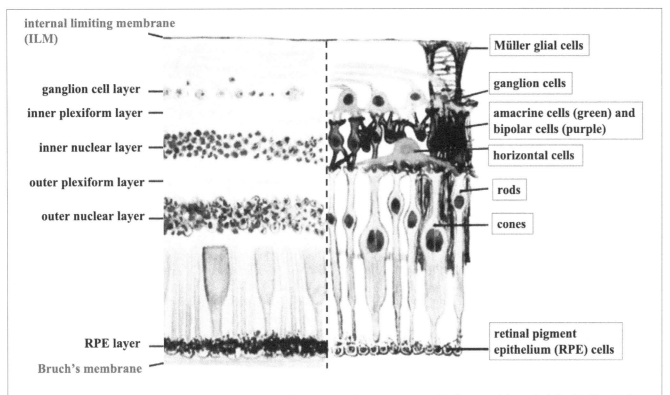

FIGURE 3 | A cross-sectional histological image of the retina, with its different layers (left) and the corresponding diagrammatic image depicting the different cell types of the retinal neural layers (right).

transfer neuronal signals. Horizontal cells, which are the laterally interconnecting neurons, have cell bodies in the inner nuclear layer of the retina. They help integrate and regulate the input from multiple photoreceptors (6). Retinal pigmented epithelial (RPE) cells make up a single layer of the postmitotic cells. This epithelia functions as a natural barrier and a regulator of the overlying photoreceptors (24). The final type of retinal-specific cells is the Müller glial cells. These cells span the entire retina and connect with all other cell types *via* cellular processes that reach out to wrap around the neurons and the synapses. They also reach out to blood vessels, so as to act as an intermediary between neurons and the circulatory system, thus regulating the flow of nutrients to the retina. Müller glia plays a critical role in maintaining neuronal health and supporting visual function (6). When light first enters the retina, it passes through the ganglion cell layer (GCL), then the inner plexiform layer (IPL), inner nuclear layer (INL), outer plexiform layer (OPL), and outer nuclear layer (ONL) (6). All these neural layers comprising eight types of retinal cells are located between the ILM and Bruch's membrane (**Figure 3**).

Basement membranes are specialized structures of the extracellular matrix that play an essential role in tissue development and maintenance. Type IV collagens are abundant components of all basement membranes (25). Bruch's membrane and ILM represent two significant basement membranes within the human retina and are located at the inner and outer retina, respectively (**Figure 3**) (6). Bruch's membrane primarily regulates

the passage of nutrients and metabolites between the RPE and underlying choriocapillaris (6). Bruch's membrane also offers a solid base and attachment site for RPE cells, acting as a part of the blood-retinal barrier (26). Bruch's membrane may also be involved in RPE differentiation (27) and wound healing (28, 29). Type IV collagen is present on both sides of Bruch's membrane in a sandwich style with the middle layer containing elastic fiber-like bands, and can also be detected in the extracellular matrix surrounding human RPE cells (30).

The ILM is not a true membrane, resulting from the fusion of the foot processes of the glia-like Müller cells. It forms a physical barrier that protects the retina from toxins and from traction from the vitreous as the eye moves. Col-IV is the predominant extracellular matrix (ECM) protein in human ILM and accounts for ∼60% of its total proteins (31). Col-IV has been detected throughout the entire thickness of ILM and is likely to be secreted by retinal Müller cells (32). Several studies have identified that Col-IV is critical not only for the structural integrity of the basement membrane but also for neuron survival and angiogenesis (33, 34). Higher expression of Col-VI has been found on the posterior side of the retina compared to its anterior side (35).

The Structure of Col-I and -IV

Collagens make up a supra-family of ECM proteins possessing a distinct triple-helical region formed from three polypeptide chains (36). Currently, 28 genetically distinct collagen types have been identified and described in the literature (37, 38). Within this group, Col-I is classified as fibril-forming, while Col-IV is defined as network-forming due to their unique supramolecular organization. Due to its predominance in body tissues, Col-I biosynthesis has been more extensively explored and will be outlined in this review; however, there is a notable lack of focus on the differences between Col-I and Col-IV biosynthesis, which can be predicted on the basis of their differing supramolecular structures.

At its most basic level, collagen biosynthesis involves the processing and aggregation of collagen monomers into functional structures. Synthesis begins within the nucleus in generating relevant mRNAs, followed by the transcription of mRNA molecules into a different α-chain (38). While Col-I only possesses two types of α-chains (α1 and α2), Col-IV has 6 α-chains (α1–6) that form different network configurations to provide basement membrane specificity (39, 40). Col-I and Col-IV are also considered heterotrimeric. This classification results from the number of α-chain genes associated with each subtype; for example, Col-I trimers are composed of two α1 chains and one α2 chain (39). Col-IV heterotrimers have greater complexity as they can organize into three different isoforms: α1α1α2, α3α4α5, and α5α5α6. The α1α1α2 Col-IV heterotrimer is predominant throughout the basement membranes of the body (40); however, the α3α4α5 network has been identified within specific tissues, including basement membranes within the eye. The adult human lens capsule contains only α3α4α5 network (41), whereas only α1α1α2 was found in the retinal ILM (42). Both α1α1α2 and α3α4α5 collagen IV networks co-exist in Bruch's membrane (43), and all of six isoforms have been detected in adult Descemet's membrane (3).

Within the primary structure of collagen is a high proportion of the repeating triplet sequence, Gly-X-Y. X, and Y in this sequence are predominantly occupied by proline (Pro) and hydroxyproline (Hyp), respectively (38). High proportions of Hyp are essential as this amino acid has a critical role in stabilizing the triple helix through the formation of intramolecular hydrogen bonds. Accordingly, Xu et al. (2019) found hydrogen bond energy within helical regions to positively correlate with greater thermal stability (44). The formation of the triple helix in the procollagen molecule is likely a shared process for Col-I and Col-IV. While uninterrupted triple helical domains are the dominant structure of Col-I and have been found to have a defined length of 300 nm (45, 46), Col-IV instead contains 21–26 interruptions within the Gly-X-Y sequence of the triple helix, leading to greater intramolecular flexibility, more suited for network formation (47, 48).

Within the extracellular space, self-assembly is initiated, and due to the significant differences in the resulting matrices, Col-I and Col-IV deviate at this stage. Released Col-I tropocollagen molecules undergo a spontaneous but organized aggregation process (38); albeit this spontaneous process has also been found to be dependent on temperature, pH, ionic strength of the solution, and the concentration of collagenous and non-collagenous components (38, 49). Molecular assembly of Col-I involves a linear alignment, with N- and C-terminal ends opposed in different tropocollagen trimers. Formed elongated fibrils can be 500 μm or more in length with a width of 500 nm (36, 38). These fibrils also have a specific 3-dimensional packing arrangement involving lateral associations between fibrils as they are staggered by about one-fourth of a molecular length. This staggering also provides Col-I fibrils with a striated organization where bands appear every 67 nm (50). Fibrillar organizations of Col-I show a degree of crystallinity; however, this organization varies throughout different tissues. Col-I aligns into straight parallel fibrillar arrangements in tendons, while in the human corneal stroma, Col-I fibrils are arranged in 300 orthogonally arranged sheets (51, 52).

Following the spontaneous molecular arrangement, additional stabilization of collagen is provided through crosslinking. Lysyl oxidase (LO) facilitates crosslink formation both in the head-to-tail alignment between adjacent telopeptide regions and in adjacent helical regions laterally (53, 54). LO initiates the formation of aldehydes from previously modified amino acid residues, lysine, and hydroxylysine (38). Aldehydes formed in each region are then able to trigger aldol reactions with lysine residues in adjacent molecules, resulting in the formation of aldimine crosslinks. Intermolecular crosslinks following spontaneous molecular organization provide the required mechanical strength and stability for collagen organization. In comparison, Col-IV supramolecular assembly aims to create a mesh-like network structure. Within its polypeptide structure, Col-IV chains have an N-terminal collagenous 7S domain, and a C-terminal non-collagenous/globular domain (NC1), in addition to the central triple helix (40). In the creation of a network, varying arrangements of Col-IV trimers are created. Two Col-IV trimers can covalently interact *via* their NC1 domain to form dimers while four 7S domains are able to crosslink into tetramers allowing for the creation of a strong and stable network (40, 47, 55). More specifically, the 7S domains bond through the formation of disulphide bridges and covalent bonding of lysine and hydroxylysine residues (47). This is a unique feature seen in the Col-IV quaternary structure as the 7S domain contains cysteine and lysine residues. LO also plays a role in Col-IV crosslink formation as it again facilitates oxidative deamination of lysine and hydroxylysine allowing for the formation of aldimine links, as seen in Col-I (56).

CURRENT DEVELOPMENT OF TISSUE ENGINEERING IN TREATING OCULAR DISEASES

The ability to manufacture bioengineered tissue that mimics existing intact tissue that can act as a means of repairing damage or to replace diseased layers presents obvious benefits in disease treatments. Using native matrix protein as the base material is a plausible direction and collagen, in particular Col-I, has been widely investigated as a suitable candidate biomaterial. The current landscape of tissue engineering in cornea, lens, and retina is detailed in Section Cornea.

Cornea

Corneal blindness is a worldwide problem that affects at least 10 million people (57–59). Corneal transplantation is an effective way to treat corneal blindness; however, there are still several significant barriers to this procedure including shortage of donor tissue and graft rejection. Currently, only one cornea is available for every 70 patients worldwide (60). The lack of fully functional eye bank facilities in third world countries, usually accompanied by other limitations, such as the lack of staff training, equipment, and public awareness of corneal donation, impact the access and ability to complete this vision rehabilitative procedure (61). High tissue graft rejection rates have also been reported potentially leading to reduced visual acuity. One study found that 10% of grafts are rejected within the 1st year, increasing in up to 50% of patients who have had multiple prior graft procedures. Each rejection episode represents a risk of total graft failure and permanent blindness (62). Donor viability may be further impacted by the presence of transmissible diseases like hepatitis A and HIV. Similarly, donor numbers may be impacted by the increasing popularity of corneal laser refractive surgery which represents a relative contraindication for use in corneal transplant procedures (58).

Corneal tissue engineering has become increasingly popular to treat severe corneal injuries and is used in two main applications: constructing a bioengineered tissue to replace donor tissue and serving as a filler/implant to fill/replace partial damaged tissue. Due to its abundance within the cornea, Col-I is one of the main natural polymers studied in this area. Researchers have developed and used plastically compressed collagen (PC) to construct bioengineered corneal grafts (63). PC refers to collagen gel from rat-tail collagen I being self-crosslinked at 37°C, and then compressed and dehydrated to provide strength and corneal shape. During this process, keratocytes (corneal cells located in the stroma) may be seeded into the structure. It is reported that minimal cell death was induced by the compression of the gel, where the collagen fibers were dense and homogeneous, similar to that of the intact corneal stroma (64). Its strength and optical properties can be further improved by introducing electrospun poly(lactic-co-glycolic acid) (PLGA) mats and using a laser to create micro-holes in the matrix resulting in increased (15 times higher) light transmittance than the previous model (65).

There are other physical methods to make collagen-based corneal implants, including centrifugal ultrafiltration and vitrification (66, 67). The process of centrifugal ultrafiltration involves the concentration of a collagen solution (from 5 to 125 mg/ml) with 30 h of centrifugation, followed by rehydration in water with an additional 10 h of centrifugation. The final collagen solution was neutralized and molded into a corneal shape. The Young's modulus of the structure was 4.83 MPa, which was between the strength of anterior corneal stroma (9.72 MPa) and posterior corneal stroma (2.04 MPa) (66). Further crosslinking including photocrosslinking or chemical crosslinking were also tested, displaying a mean light transmittance rate of over 85% and higher Young's modulus (34.89 MPa), compared to the native corneal stroma (66). This was also compatible with keratocytes and corneal epithelial cells, further representing the ability to closely mimic natural tissue (66). Collagen structures

produced by vitrification, called "Collagen vitrigel," can support re-epithelialisation on its surface, and stop epithelial cells from migrating into the cornea stroma (68). An attempt to increase its optical and mechanical properties was achieved by mixing the collagen solution with β-cyclodextrin to regulate collagen fibers to better mimic the normal corneal stromal structure (69). This resulted in comparable mechanical properties to the native cornea; however, only with moderate transparency (60–80% light transmission in visible light range), representing a relative disadvantage of this process. It was also found that the optical properties of the collagen vitrigel can be improved by replacing β-cyclodextrin with α-cyclodextrin, and inducing further chemical crosslinking with 1-ethyl-3-(3-dimethylaminopropyl)carbodiimide hydrochloride (EDC), suggesting further improvements may still be possible (70).

Chemical crosslinking is widely used in fabricating bioengineered corneal implants. The most common chemical crosslinker is EDC and N-hydroxysuccinimide (NHS). Animal collagen (porcine collagen) and recombinant human collagen (type I and type III) have been crosslinked with EDC and NHS to fabricate an artificial cornea (71–73). These collagen structures have shown good mechanical properties (with up to 260 KPa tensile strength), optical properties (with up to 92.5% light transmittance), and show compatibility with corneal cells (71, 73). Other materials, such as silk fibroin, may be added into the chemically crosslinked collagen hydrogel prior to crosslinking, to enhance certain mechanical properties, such as maximum tensile strain without affecting the biocompatibility (74).

Electro-compacted (EC) collagen gels are produced by compacting collagen using a pH gradient created by electrodes. This can improve the packing density of the collagen gel. Kishore et al. developed a collagen matrix using this method (75). The collagen matrix was further crosslinked by EDC and NHS to enhance its strength. The results show that although chemical crosslinking reduced the visible light transmission (from 79–93% to 67–89%), it dramatically increased the tensile modulus of the collagen gel (from 16 kPa to 1.8 MPa) (75). The structure is also shown to be compatible with primary keratocytes. Another bioengineered corneal stroma layer fabricated by electro-compaction and stacking collagen film has been developed by Chen et al. (76). The EC-compacted collagen solution showed a 5-fold of increase of storage modulus compared to non-EC compacted collagen and remains capable of promoting the proliferation of human keratocytes. These collagen layers, with aligned collagen fibers and human corneal stromal cells cultured on them, can be stacked and integrated by weighting down, to form a layered microstructure that closely mimics the corneal stromal structure. No further chemical crosslinking processes are introduced in the weighting down process, with the stacked structure having a much lower Young's modulus than the native cornea (0.23 kPa compared to 23.05 kPa) (76). Alternatively, magnetic fields have been used to align the collagen fibers during the self-assembling process of the collagen gel (77). The magnetic field-generated collagen gel had a similar arrangement of collagen fibers to the EC collagen gel, and it also supported keratocyte growth (77). Proteoglycans extracted from

TABLE 2 | Main advantages and disadvantages of Collagen-crosslinking method in corneal bioengineering.

Collagen-crosslinking method	Main advantages in corneal bio engineering	Main disadvantages in corneal bio engineering
Physical-crosslinking	High mechanical strength (65)	Lower optical properties (65, 70)
Chemical-crosslinking	High mechanical strength (71) High optical properties (73)	Potential cell toxicity (80)
Photo-crosslinking	Higher biocompatibility (81)	Slow crosslinking process (66)
Electro-compaction	Organized collagen fiber (76)	Lower mechanical property (76)

porcine corneal tissues (35% of decorin and 65% of lumican, keratocan, and osteoglycin) have also been incorporated during the fabrication of the collagen gel to improve the transparency; however, the details of the transmittance was not reported (77).

While there are many studies on collagen-based corneal implants in development, the development of collagen-like material-based corneal fillers/sealants are more recent. Collagen-like material-based filler can be used to seal corneal perforations and has been made and tested by Samarawickrama et al. (78). The collagen-like material-based filler was based on a modified collagen peptide conjugated to polyethylene glycol (CLP-PEG). After its application to the wound site, the filler was further crosslinked by 4-(4,6-dimethoxy-1,3,5-triazin-2-yl)-4-methylmorpholinium chloride (DMTMM) to form a structure that adheres to and seals the perforation. DMTMM was tested individually with human epithelial and endothelial cell lines and was shown to have no cell toxicity. The performance of this filler was compared to cyanoacrylate glue, a currently used treatment in clinics, with the results showing that the CLP-PEG filler glue, with an internal collagen patch, generated a much smoother surface than the cyanoacrylate glue. One disadvantage was that the bursting pressure of the CLP-PEG filler was much lower than the cyanoacrylate glue (86.6 mm Hg compared to 325.9). According to Islam et al., the CLP-PEG hydrogel is significantly weaker than normal human cornea due to its higher water content (90% compared to 78%) (79). While *in vivo* safety has been proven after 5-week long animal experiments done by implanting the gel into the cornea of guinea pigs (78), its weaker mechanical properties raise the concern of whether the CLP-PEG hydrogel may be stable under constant internal pressure for an extended period of time. The main advantages and disadvantages of the collagen-crosslinking method in corneal bioengineering are summarized in **Table 2**.

In conclusion, collagen corneal implants have already achieved good mechanical properties, optical properties, and biocompatibility; however, there are limitations. The collagen gel without additional crosslinking usually has a mechanical property weaker than the human cornea (66). Some of the chemical crosslinkers, such as EDC, while can achieve good mechanical properties, may exhibit health risks if remaining

within the implant structure. The implants mentioned above adopt traditional manufacturing processes, such as casting that lack flexibility compared to modern fabrication processes, such as 3-D printing.

Lens

Although the cornea represents the primary structure responsible for light refraction, the lens remains important for fine-tuning and precisely focusing the light that passes through it to the retina. A cloudy lens will prevent light transmission and can therefore lead to reduced visual acuity, and if significant, blindness. Cataract, a condition of irreversible clouding of the natural lens, is the leading cause of blindness affecting ~20 million individuals globally (82–84). Cataract surgery is currently the only method for treating cataract, with 28 million operations performed annually (85). Cataract surgery requires the removal of the clouded lens material and insertion of a prosthetic intraocular lens (IOL). IOLs have varied biomaterial composition and design in order to produce the best visual acuity outcomes and prevent surgical complications; the most common of which is posterior capsular opacification (PCO). PCO results from remaining LECs post-surgery that are attached to the damaged anterior lens capsule. These cells can undergo an epithelial-to-mesenchymal transition (EMT) as they migrate to the posterior capsule (86, 87). These trans-differentiated cells are contractile and deposit excessive extracellular matrix, including Col-I and Col-III that are not normally found within the normal adult lens (86, 88). These activities cause lens capsular wrinkling and opacification, correlated with loss of vision. Historically, PCO rates were as high as 20–40% of patients at 2–5 years follow-up after surgery (89), albeit more recent figures suggest a significantly decreased incidence. Neodymium: YAG (Nd:YAG) laser capsulotomy is an effective procedure used within the clinic to treat PCO. It involves the disruption of the central posterior capsule by the laser to clear the visual axis, thereby improving visual acuity (90). It uses a solid-state laser with a wavelength of 1,064 nm that can deliver high energy to ocular tissue resulting in tissue disruption without physically touching the tissue (91). Although successful, Nd:YAG laser treatment is not without risk, with damage to the IOL and retinal detachment noted in some cases (90, 92, 93).

Clinical and laboratory-based studies identified two key factors affecting associated PCO incidence: IOL material and design. Historically, most IOLs have been made up of three standard synthetic materials: polymethyl methacrylate (PMMA), silicone, and acrylic polymers. PMMA was the first IOL material; however, PMMA IOLs were rigid and inflexible requiring a larger incision in surgery for appropriate insertion (>5 mm). This has previously been correlated with an increased risk of PCO due to the disruption of the blood-aqueous barrier and lens capsule (94, 95). In comparison, foldable IOLs (silicone and acrylic polymers) requiring only small incisions (<2.5 mm) are associated with fewer complications resulting in more widespread use (96, 97). There is a strong influence of IOL material on PCO incidence. Past studies have found that PMMA IOLs are consistently associated with high rates of PCO in comparison to silicone or acrylic IOLs (98, 99); however, recent comparative studies have presented mixed results concerning PCO risk in silicone and acrylic IOLs. It has been found that instead of the material itself defining biocompatibility, the material's hydrophobicity/hydrophilicity may be the defining factor for PCO incidence. IOLs with a hydrophobic character produce significantly lower rates of PCO in comparison to hydrophilic IOLs (100). In addition, when comparing PMMA, silicone, hydrophobic acrylic, and hydrophilic acrylic IOLs, the hydrophobic acrylic IOL produced significantly less PCO compared to other materials (101). It is widely accepted that this hydrophobicity increases adhesion to the Col-IV of the lens capsule, and therefore creates closer apposition of the IOL and remaining posterior capsule following surgery (102, 103). This close adherence provides a barrier to the migrating transdifferentiating lens epithelial cells (LECs). In comparison, IOLs with hydrophilic character have PCO rates not dissimilar to PMMA IOLs, as they have been described to promote aberrant LEC proliferation and migration (102, 104).

Extracellular matrix molecules including Col-IV, fibronectin, and laminin have been evaluated as potential adhesive coatings or materials for IOLs and have been found to mimic the effects of hydrophobic IOLs, producing minimal PCO (105–107). Past studies have noted that IOLs, either made from Col-IV or with a Col-IV coating produced significantly less PCO (108). In these studies, Col-IV was found to assist in stabilizing damage to the blood-aqueous barrier and preventing EMT transformations that normally initiate fibrotic PCO. The incorporation of native lens capsules containing ECM molecules, in particular, Col-IV, therefore, appears promising but requires more development and further research.

Another significant factor determining PCO incidence is IOL edge design. This factor holds significance as these edges also have the potential to form a physical barrier to LEC movement. Studies comparing PCO outcomes between hydrophobic acrylic IOLs and silicone IOLs both made with sharp edges found no significant differences after 3 years of observation (109–111). Sharp edges in combination with other IOL design factors, like uninterrupted edges and appropriately angled haptics, have all been found to contribute to the reduction in PCO (112–114).

Presently no treatment, surgical technique, or IOL design/material arising from engineering this artificial lens replacement has been found to eliminate PCO completely. Therefore, moving forward, researchers have begun to look at options to create/regenerate natural lens structures, a process in which tissue engineering may play a significant role. Mammals have been found to possess lens regenerative abilities contingent upon the remaining LECs being relatively undisrupted and on an intact anterior and posterior lens capsule (115). This method of lens regeneration is driven by these LECs and is called "LEC-mediated regeneration." Studies in both rabbits and macaques found that upon fiber cell mass removal, a whole lens structure was able to regenerate on the remaining lens capsule within 7 weeks and 5 months, respectively (116); however, these regenerated lenses showed irregular fiber cell growth that led to the development of opacities. To address this problem, other studies have inserted tissue-engineered scaffolds following fiber mass removal. For example, Gwon and Gruber utilized a biodegradable hyaluronic acid scaffold and found lenses of greater optical clarity and normal fiber arrangement regenerated (117). It is believed these scaffolds provide the necessary mechanical support to the remaining lens capsule and LECs, mimicking the support previously provided by the natural fiber mass (118). Furthermore, this then encourages normal regeneration as opposed to aberrant proliferation and migration of LECs (i.e., PCO also linked to a sudden disruption of contact inhibition) (119, 120). With positive results for Col-IV-coated IOLs previously observed, Col-IV could also be a suitable scaffold candidate to be incorporated in future tissue engineering-based approaches to address both lens regeneration and PCO concerns. This type of approach has yet to be trialed in humans and there are limiting factors to consider. For example, older patients in whom the majority of cataract surgeries are performed (121), have hard cataracts that may require more significant intraocular surgical manipulation. This can lead to a significant loss of crucial LECs and possible damage to the supporting lens capsule, both of which are essential for LEC-mediated regeneration. Adult lenses also have larger capsules "stretched" from years of continuous lens growth (118). This impacts on the mechanical environment present and makes it unconducive to regeneration. Therefore, tissue-engineered scaffolds should consider these elements that may impact an outcome following scaffold implantation. For example, if Col-IV-based scaffolds were developed, they may require specific dimensions or design to appropriately stretch a "looser" capsule. Col-IV as a biomaterial could also be cast into a "patch" and utilized to substitute the lens capsule lost during surgery and hence minimize LEC disruption to maximize regeneration potential. The use of collagen biomaterials or scaffolds in this field is not widely seen and the previous study on the benefits of a Col-IV-based IOL is outdated (105–108). Therefore, moving forward, a tissue-engineering approach, utilizing collagen-based scaffolds to encourage lens regeneration is a potential and promising path that still requires a significant amount of work.

Retina

Tissue engineering in the retina has previously been investigated, with studies using a range of materials including decellularised natural tissues, such as amniotic membrane, lens capsule, Bruch's membrane (BM), collagen I as well as synthetic materials (122); however, to date, there are no reports of Col-IV usage in such retinal bioprinting studies. It is unclear why Col-IV was not used as a main biomaterial for retinal tissue engineering. Col-IV is an important protein for ocular health. Alport syndrome is the most typical Col-IV-related pathology in the eyes. In 1990, a role for Col-IV in an inherited genetic disease was subsequently discovered when mutations in Col-IV a5, and later Col-IV a3, and Col-IV a4, were found to underlie X-linked and autosomal recessive forms of Alportsyndrome, respectively (123). Ophthalmologic findings include anterior lenticonus characterized by a thin, fragile lens capsule (124), dot-and-fleck retinopathy (125), and temporal retinal thinning (126).

Despite no reports for collagen IV as a bioink, it has been used in retinal gluing. The aim of gluing is to achieve a strong

TABLE 3 | A summary of bioprinting methods.

Printing methods			Advantages	Disadvantages
Inkjet bioprinting	SJI		Fast, cost-friendly	Requires low viscosity material
	DOD	Thermo		
		Piezoelectric		
		Electrostatic		
Laser-assisted bioprinting			Fast, more controllable	Limited printable structure, high cell death
Stereolithography (SLA)			Good cell viability	Selective in the material of the bioink
Extrusion bioprinting			Simple, flexible, and low-cost	Requires shear-thinning material

and immediate adhesion between the retina and retinal pigment epithelium (RPE). In 1989, researchers tried to apply "Matrigel" that contained Col-IV and laminin, to study the effects of successful adhesives on retinal cells *in vitro,* and to investigate the potential biocompatibility of substrates. They found that the "Matrigel" preparation stimulates the proliferation of bovine retinal glial cells around retinal breaks. Pre-treatment with fibronectin supported the growth of retinal cells after sealing (127); however, there are little to no further studies on Col-IV as a retinal sealant, with most studies conducted prior to the 1990's. This may be due to advancements in vitreoretinal surgery to treat retinal diseases. More recently, gluing associated with retinal tissue engineering appears to represent a renewed focus in retinal surgery-related developments (122), with further potential application in clinics. Tyagi and Basu performed glue-assisted retinopexy for rhegmatogenous retinal detachments (GuARD) in patients, which allowed early visual recovery while avoiding the problems of gas or oil tamponade and obviating the need for postoperative positioning that represents a significant practical limitation for patients in the early postoperative period (128). Ophthalmologists also found fibrin glue provided a superior adhesive for sealing retinal breaks, while showing no additional adverse effects in patients (129). With the early successes reported in 1989, Col-IV may be a valuable biomaterial that is to be used in gluing applications in clinical surgery.

COLLAGEN-I AND -IV IN BIOPRINTING OCULAR TISSUES

Bioprinting belongs to 3D printing and is classified as additive manufacturing. The fundamental mechanism adopted here is by stacking materials layer by layer to form a scaffold/structure based on computational images (130). Compared to classic molding methods, bioprinting has been in the spotlight in recent years, with its advantages and capability to generate customized structures based on recorded images, as well as the reproducibility of cell printing. In recent years, publications about *in situ* printing, directly printing biomaterials/cells to injured sites using hand-held printers to reconstruct the wound and promote healing, gave us a glimpse of what future surgeries may be like (131).

Bioprinting

Unlike materials used in traditional 3D printing such as plastics, the materials used in bioprinting refer to biomaterials, usually organic materials, such as collagen, gelatine and alginate, or bioink with a cell-laden ability (130). The most frequently used methods in 3D bioprinting are inkjet bioprinting, laser-assisted bioprinting, and extrusion-based bioprinting (**Table 3**). Additional technologies like vat photopolymerisation may also be used in bioprinting.

Inkjet bioprinting, which is similar to the conventional inkjet printer, prints the structure by precisely depositing micro-drops of bioinks to a substrate. The inkjet printing technique can be divided into two categories, continuous inkjet printing (SIJ), which means continuously printing a stream of drops whilst selecting the drops that are needed to be printed to the substrate, and drop on demand inkjet printing (DOD), where the ink drop is only ejected out of the nozzle as needed (132, 133). The DOD technique can be further divided by the method used to form the micro-droplets; thermo-inkjet printing, piezoelectric inkjet printing, and electrostatic inkjet printing (134). The DOD technique has been applied to fabricating a corneal-like structure incorporated with corneal stromal cells, thus achieving good cell viability (up to 7 days) (135). Inkjet bioprinting has been investigated in its potential of fabricating other tissues, including bone and cartilage tissues (136, 137), blood vessels (138), and retinal layers (139). Inkjet printing is fast and cost-effective compared to other bioprinting methods (140) but is limited by the requirement of low-viscosity material to prevent clogging during printing (141).

Laser-assisted bioprinting during the printing process involves a pulse laser that is applied to a laser absorption layer, with bioink-containing cells covering its lower surface not directly exposed to the laser. This causes thermal expansion that ejects micro-droplets of the bioink onto the substrate (142). This method can precisely control the type and density of the cells during printing (143); hence, is often used to manufacture scaffold-free cell structures (144). A human corneal-like stroma with high cell viability has been produced with this technique, using a Col-I based bioink and human stem cells (145). Further developments have improved the strength of the laser-assisted bioprinted structure, as evidenced by this technique that is used to successfully print mesenchymal stromal cells for bone regeneration, with the aid of pre-printed nHA-collagen disks (146). Laser-assisted bioprinting does not carry the risk of blocking the printing nozzles and remains a relatively fast process. The main current limitation of this technique is the high rates of cell death during the printing process that may impact the long-term survival of the tissue (142, 147).

Photopolymerisation or photocrosslinking is a further technique used in 3D bioprinting, known as stereolithography (SLA). For this technology, a laser beam is applied directly to the printing material to initiate photopolymerisation/photocrosslinking in a selected area of bioink and the 3D structure is printed layer-by-layer. The bioink used in this printing process is usually required to be photopolymerisable or to contain a photoinitiator to be able to crosslink. As an example, methacrylate gelatine (GelMa) and eosin-Y combined with visible light are common materials and photoinitiators used for this cell printing process (148). This combination has been successfully used to print human corneal-like stroma and shows good cell compatibility post-printing (149). Lithium phenyl-2,4,6-trimethylbenzoylphosphinate (LAP) is another photoinitiator used with GelMa and UV. Other studies printing different tissue or organs, including artificial cartilage and liver using this same combination, also have good cell viability (150, 151). Stereolithography has been adopted in making artificial blood vessels with a photopolymerisable polyacrylate material (152). As the bioink used in printing is required to be photo-cross linkable, this remains a relative limitation of the technique.

Extrusion bioprinting is the most common bioprinting used in current applications (153). During extrusion printing processes, the shear-thinning bioink is extruded from a syringe by the pressure created by either air, a piston, or screw. The extrusion 3D printer can be a single syringe, a multi-syringe, or joint syringes, with coaxial printing tips to meet different needs. Extrusion printing is widely used in tissue engineering with a variety of bioinks. Multi-syringe extrusion printing has been used in printing human skin with two different layers, both dermis and epidermis (154). An example of coaxial extrusion bioprinting has been published in a study that used alginate as the shell that was immediately crosslinked by the calcium ion that was contained in the mixture of GelMa and calcium chloride during the initial mixing process, binding the GelMa together before further crosslinking (155). Extrusion bioprinting has great potential in surgery. In addition to printing the entire structure, it can also be used in *in situ* printing. O'Connell et al. developed an extrusion printing-based hand-held device called a "biopen" for treating cartilage injuries (131, 156). As a hand-held device, it increases surgical dexterity and portability. It adopts the coaxial extrusion printing mechanism and integrates a UV-curing attachment to solidify the material during, and post-printing. Another device, developed by Hakimi et al., is also a handheld 3D printer based on double syringe extrusion printing (157). Targeting a range of tissues, this dispensing method uses a cartridge that applies a crosslinker on the top of the material while printing (157). In the above-reviewed extrusion methods, a viscous bioink is usually required to maintain the shape of the printed structure during the printing process. For low viscous bioinks, a method called "freeform reversible embedding of suspended hydrogels (FRESH)" has been developed. In this method, the bioink was printed in a supporting material to obtain higher resolution and structural support for printing low-viscosity bioinks that have difficulty maintaining the printed shape during printing. This technique has already been used to print a range of human tissue including artificial human corneal stroma and heart tissues (158, 159).

Collagen-I Based Bioink

Since Col-I is the major component of the human corneal stroma, most of the bioink under current investigation for use in corneal applications contains this as its major constituent; however, this is usually combined with other materials in order to gain enough printability or postprinting mechanical properties. These bioinks can be printed with the earlier mentioned bioprinting methods.

The bioink used in 3D printing of human cornea using FRESH printing by Isaacson et al. was a combination of up to 8 mg/ml methacrylated bovine Col-I and sodium alginate (158). The authors reported that with increased concentration of collagen in the bioink, and the addition of sodium alginate, the printability and transparency were improved. A formulation of the bioink that contained 2.66 mg/ml Col-I and 2% of sodium alginate was reported as their choice of best overall properties (158). Another example of combining bovine Col-I with sodium alginate to make the collagen-based bioink for corneal bioprinting was developed by Kutlehria et al. (160). In this study, they used the SLA technique to fabricate the supporting structure and then used extrusion printing to print corneal stroma-like tissue onto the structure. The collagen in use was an acid-soluble bovine Col-I. The sodium alginate used acted to assist the solidification of the printed structure with the use of calcium chloride as a crosslinking agent. Gelatine, incorporated with the bioink, was added to enhance its printability. The optimized concentrations of the components of the bioink include 4% gelatin, 3.25% alginate, and 5 mg/ml collagen (160). A similar formulation of bioink was used by Wu et al., who also combined collagen with other natural polymers, including gelatine and sodium alginate (161); however, they used normal extrusion-based bioprinting techniques, and Col-I sourced from rat tail. As extrusion printing requires the bioink to have high printability, this bioink has high gelatine content at 10% weight per volume, to improve printability. The collagen concentration was low at 0.83 mg/ml and the bioink also contained 1% alginate. The printed structure was immersed with calcium chloride to further strengthen the structure. The printed structure was found to be transparent and cell compatible; however, the authors also reported that the alginate structure could not be degraded by cells, therefore potentially inhibiting cell proliferation (161).

Other methods to facilitate the liquid to gel transition of collagen-based bioink included using temperature-sensitive biomaterials and other natural cross-linkers. Duarte Campos et al. used low gelling temperature agarose as a component in their bovine Col-I based bioink (135). The composition included 2 mg/ml Col-I and 5 mg/ml agarose. The bioink was held in the printer with a temperature above the gelation point and the printed structure was held at room temperature for the gelling of agarose, then at 37°C for gelling the collagen. The structure printed by this bioink can show letters of text placed under it without distortion, and had good cell compatibility (over 95% cell viability); however, it had a lower mechanical strength than cornea (135). Sorkio et al. have used a bioink with 1.2 mg/ml human collagen in combination with human plasma, thrombin, and hyaluronic acid to print the cell-loaded corneal-like structure (145). Thrombin served as a crosslinker to assist bioink gelation. Stem cells were printed by laser-assisted bioprinting in parallel with the main structure, forming a corneal-like structure, with cells surrounded by collagen fibers. The structure showed good cell compatibility; however, it required non-transparent supporting material during printing, resulting in a translucent final structure, with no report of its mechanical properties (145).

A bioink primarily incorporating decellularised cornea was used to print a corneal model using an extrusion printing technique (162). The decellularised cornea was dissolved in acetic acid and pepsin with a concentration of 20 mg/ml and later neutralized by NaOH to make the bioink. The printed corneal model had over 75% light transmittance in the visible light spectrum and was compatible with human turbinate-derived mesenchymal stem cells (hTMSCs) (162). The collagen content of the decellularised cornea solution was suggested to be ~86% (163); however, the detail of the collagen types was not given (163).

In conclusion, the printing method used in published studies is FRESH (158), extrusion printing (160–162), DoD (135), and laser-assisted printing (145). For the crosslinking methods, the chemical crosslinkers that are widely used in fabricating collagen-based corneal-like structures are not popular among the 3-D cell printing projects. As all these projects incorporated cells in the bioink, more gentle crosslinking methods were used that include crosslinking using natural biomaterials, such as alginate-calcium, gelatin and thrombin, and low-temperature agarose. Most of the reported corneal bioprinting research studies used lower concentrations of Col-I (0.82 to 5 mg/ml) to maintain transparency of printed structure but required additional gentle crosslinkers. The only bioink that appears to have a higher Col-I concentration used 20 mg/ml of the decellularised cornea with 86% being collagen (162). This higher concentration of collagen has sufficient printability for extrusion printing without the need to add gelatine (162); however, it would be challenging to define the composition of the material obtained from decellularised corneas that contain many different proteins. This uncertainty could be a significant potential limitation to the broader applicability and use of the bioink. The collagen sources are either animal-based, such as bovine (135, 158, 160) and rat (161), or from human tissue (145, 162). The current studies of 3-D printing of corneal tissue remain primarily proof-of-concept studies that still have a notable period before their actual clinical use. The printed structures are mainly focused on corneal stromal layers and cells, except the study done by Wu et al. that explored the cell viability of encapsulated epithelial cells (161). Although a number of tissues represent potential alternatives to natural tissue, none of the above-mentioned printed structures have reported similar or exceeded the mechanical properties compared to the intact human cornea. It is also notable that none of the above-mentioned projects used photo-crosslinking, either during the printing process or post-printing. This may be because of the

concern that the photoinitiator and the light-curing process may be cytotoxic. Sorkio et al. suggested that photocrosslinking can be important not only to further enhance the mechanical properties of the printed structure but also expressed concern for its impact on cell viability (145). Diamantides et al., reported that the cell viability of the chondrocytein, the collagen bioink decreased to 76%, with 10 s of 1.2 W/cm^2 blue light, and 0.5 mm riboflavin photo-crosslinking (164); however, Ibusuki et al., have shown that with 40 s of photocrosslinking using 0.5 W/cm^2 blue light and 0.5 mM riboflavin, the cell viability of chondrocytesin, the collagen solution, was still over 90% (81). The cytotoxic effect of photocrosslinking could be reduced by lowering the strength of the curing light, and therefore, it is possible to introduce photocrosslinking into the development of cell encapsulating collagen-based bioinks to enhance methods on bioengineering a cornea.

Collagen-IV Based Bioink

To date, there is little to no exploration into the field of Col-IV bioprinting, and the utilization of Col-IV as a versatile bioink. Hence, the current use of collagen in bioinks is essentially limited to Col-I as previously discussed. In comparison, the current use of Col-IV emphasizes cell culturing, where it is utilized as a coating. A previous study tested a number of coatings of a polydimethylsiloxane substrate including Col-I and Col-IV (165). Substrates coated with Col-IV were found to produce the most ideal phenotypic expression in bovine corneal endothelial cells, with strong ZO-1 expression and minimal cytoskeletal α-SMA, indicating no abnormal EMT. This was a predicted result as normal corneal endothelial cells have been found to secrete Col-IV as their native collagen, but following an EMT, these cells instead produced Col-I (166, 167). A follow-up study tested cultured primary human cells on coated Col-I gels and found that only gels coated with Col-IV produced confluent monolayers of high cell density suitable for transplant (168). A similar study found that of the different ECM-coating proteins tested, only Col-IV-coated silk fibroin films allowed for the formation of confluent monolayers of primary human corneal endothelial cells that maintained apolygonal morphology (169).

For future applications of bioprinting, including the construction of a full-thickness corneal substitute, Col-IV printing, with or without cells, could hold significant promise. Col-IV bioprinting of layers extends beyond the printing of layers in a potential biomimetic corneal substitute, as this collagen is ubiquitous in the basement membranes of the body. Hence, the development of Col-IV inks and bioinks is essential for the recreation of 3D scaffolds for research, and clinical applications in which the cultured cells require a basement membrane to support their physiological function.

CONCLUSION AND FUTURE TRENDS

We have reviewed the application of tissue engineering in the cornea, the lens, and the retina with a focus on Col-I and Col-IV. Compared to the lens and the retina, tissue engineering of corneal structures is heavily studied. This may be due to its relatively simple-layered structure and a strong practical need to overcome the current global shortage of donor corneas. Despite the natural lens representing a relatively simple-structured tissue to the cornea, the success of IOLs has appeared to limit the need for tissue engineering, a lens alternative. Subsequently, most studies found emphasized coating or enhancing the compatibility of IOLs in the lens to reduce the need for secondary cataract (PCO). The more complicated structure of the retina has made it the most challenging to engineer; however, a few studies have successfully engineered retinal-like layers and structures, albeit with variable current practical application (29, 122, 139).

Collagen is a widely used biomaterial and a key structural protein in ocular tissues; however, most studies focused on the application of Col-I. Various methods have been developed to make Col-I- based structures, and all have shared one common principle, that is, to cross-link Col-I fibers. As some of the cross-linking methods, such as gentle cross-linking using alginate, or photo-crosslinking, are compatible with 3D printing, this has enabled further development of printing Col-I based structures. In the cornea, numerous studies have developed various types of Col-I bioinks and printed cell-laden corneal-like structures that have shown similar morphology and transparency to the native intact cornea, albeit with limited comparable tensile strength in many examples. Despite Col-IV being an essential component for lens and basement membranes in the cornea and the retina, it was mainly used as a coating material to support cell growth. Development of a Col-IV based scaffold or bioink remains limited. It could be that fabricating a Col-IV based structure is more challenging than Col-I, given their structural differences, but it can also be that the importance of incorporating Col-IV in tissue engineering for the lens and the retina has not yet been widely investigated. Col-IV is an essential protein for retinal and lens cell growth, and to develop a Col-IV based structure could greatly enhance cell compatibility.

The application of 3D printing was not limited to print an entire structure but also used for *in situ* printing to fill or seal injuries. *In situ* printing is novel in treating diseases, and has been used to treat cartilage injuries (131, 156). With the right biomaterial and biopen developed to fit the size of different ocular tissues, this could provide a useful tool to treat ocular injuries and diseases. Based on the published findings, it is no longer a technical barrier to produce bioengineered ocular tissues, at least not for cornea, in the laboratory; however, translating these developments to the clinic or surgery remains challenging. The complexity of bioengineered tissues, including both biomaterials and cells, and the unique manufacturing process makes these products distinct from other clinical products currently being regulated (170). Their mechanisms of action do not fall into the existing regulatory definition of potency, and long-term survival and integration of bioengineered tissues in host tissues remains unknown and requires ongoing, careful assessment (170). A whole new system that involves regulatory bodies and policymakers is likely required.

AUTHOR CONTRIBUTIONS

YS and MO conducted literature search, structured the layout, and wrote the majority part of paper. JF wrote the retina related section and conducted literature search. CH contributed in structuring and reviewing the paper. JY and GS contributed to conception of design and review of the paper. JY also contributed to literature search. FL contributed to the critical analysis of key literatures of the paper and review of the paper. All authors contributed to manuscript revision, read, and approved the submitted version.

ACKNOWLEDGMENTS

We acknowledge the support of NHMRC (APP1181415), the Sydney Eye Hospital Foundation (SEHF), and the Fudan-University of Sydney Partnership.

REFERENCES

1. Chen Z, You J, Liu X, Cooper S, Hodge C, Sutton G, et al. Biomaterials for corneal bioengineering. *Biomed Mater.* (2018) 13:032002. doi: 10.1088/1748-605X/aa92d2
2. Nishida T, Saika S, Morishige N. Chapter 1- cornea and scelar: anatomy and physiology. In: Mannis M, Holland E, editors, *Cornea Fundamentals, Diagnosis and Management.* 4th ed. Amsterdam: Elsevier. (2017) 1–22.
3. Kabosova A, Azar DT, Bannikov GA, Campbell KP, Durbeej M, Ghohestani RF, et al. Compositional differences between infant and adult human corneal basement membranes. *Invest Ophthalmol Vis Sci.* (2007) 48:4989–99. doi: 10.1167/iovs.07-0654
4. Eghrari AO, Riazuddin SA, Gottsch JD. Overview of the cornea: structure, function, and development. *Prog Mol Biol Transl Sci.* (2015) 134:7–23. doi: 10.1016/bs.pmbts.2015.04.001
5. Danysh BP, Duncan MK. The lens capsule. *Exp Eye Res.* (2009) 88:151–64. doi: 10.1016/j.exer.2008.08.002
6. Grossniklaus HE, Geisert EE, Nickerson JM. Introduction to the retina. *Prog Mol Biol Transl Sci.* (2015) 134:383–96 doi: 10.1016/bs.pmbts.2015.06.001
7. Torricelli AA, Singh V, Santhiago MR, Wilson SE. The corneal epithelial basement membrane: structure, function, and disease. *Invest Ophthalmol Vis Sci.* (2013) 54:6390–400. doi: 10.1167/iovs.13-12547

8. Sakai LY, Keene DR, Morris NP, Burgeson RE. Type VII collagen is a major structural component of anchoring fibrils. *J Cell Biol.* (1986) 103:1577--86. doi: 10.1083/jcb.103.4.1577
9. Gipson IK, Spurr-Michaud SJ, Tisdale AS. Anchoring fibrils form a complex network in human and rabbit cornea. *Invest Ophthalmol Vis Sci.* (1987) 28:212–20.
10. Ljubimov AV, Burgeson RE, Butkowski RJ, Michael AF, Sun TT, Kenney MC. Human corneal basement membrane heterogeneity: topographical differences in the expression of type IV collagen and laminin isoforms. *Lab Invest.* (1995) 72:461–73.
11. Wessel H, Anderson S, Fite D, Halvas E, Hempel J, SundarRaj N. Type XII collagen contributes to diversities in human corneal and limbal extracellular matrices. *Invest Ophthalmol Vis Sci.* (1997) 38:2408–22.
12. Maatta M, Heljasvaara R, Sormunen R, Pihlajaniemi T, Autio-Harmainen H, Tervo T. Differential expression of collagen types XVIII/endostatin and XV in normal, keratoconus, and scarred human corneas. *Cornea.* (2006) 25:341–9. doi: 10.1097/01.ico.0000178729.57435.96
13. Nakayasu K, Tanaka M, Konomi H, Hayashi T. Distribution of types I, II, III, IV and V collagen in normal and keratoconus corneas. *Ophthalmic Res.* (1986) 18:1–10. doi: 10.1159/000265406
14. Gordon MK, Foley JW, Birk DE, Fitch JM, Linsenmayer TF. Type V collagen and Bowman's membrane. Quantitation of mRNA in corneal epithelium and stroma. *J Biol Chem.* (1994) 269:24959–66. doi: 10.1016/S0021-9258(17)31483-7

15. Nishida K. Tissue engineering of the cornea. *Cornea.* (2003) 22(7Suppl.):S28–34. doi: 10.1097/00003226-200310001-00005

16. Berlau J, Becker HH, Stave J, Oriwol C, Guthoff RF. Depth and age-dependent distribution of keratocytes in healthy human corneas: a study using scanning-slit confocal microscopy *in vivo. J Cataract Refract Surg.* (2002) 28:611–6. doi: 10.1016/S0886-3350(01)01227-5

17. Young BB, Zhang G, Koch M, Birk DE. The roles of types XII and XIV collagen in fibrillogenesis and matrix assembly in the developing cornea. *J Cell Biochem.* (2002) 87:208–20. doi: 10.1002/jcb.10290

18. Sawada H, Konomi H, Hirosawa K. Characterization of the collagen in the hexagonal lattice of Descemet's membrane: its relation to type VIII collagen. *J Cell Biol.* (1990) 110:219–27. doi: 10.1083/jcb.110.1.219

19. Doughty MJ, Zaman ML. Human corneal thickness and its impact on intraocular pressure measures: a review and meta-analysis approach. *Surv Ophthalmol.* (2000) 44:367–408. doi: 10.1016/S0039-6257(00)00110-7

20. Meek KM, Knupp C. Corneal structure and transparency. *Prog Retin Eye Res.* (2015) 49:1–16. doi: 10.1016/j.preteyeres.2015.07.001

21. Hassell JR, Birk DE. The molecular basis of corneal transparency. *Exp Eye Res.* (2010) 91:326–35. doi: 10.1016/j.exer.2010.06.021

22. Boote C, Dennis S, Newton RH, Puri H, Meek KM. Collagen fibrils appear more closely packed in the prepupillary cornea: optical and biomechanical implications. *Invest Ophthalmol Vis Sci.* (2003) 44:2941–8. doi: 10.1167/iovs.03-0131

23. Ziebarth NlM, Borja D, Arrieta E, Aly M, Manns F, Dortonne I, et al. Role of the lens capsule on the mechanical accommodative response in a lens stretcher. *Investig Ophthalmol Vis Sci.* (2008) 49:4490–6. doi: 10.1167/iovs.07-1647

24. Boulton M, Dayhaw-Barker P. The role of the retinal pigment epithelium: topographical variation and aging changes. *Eye.* (2001) 15:384–9. doi: 10.1038/eye.2001.141

25. Mao M, Alavi MV, Labelle-Dumais C, Gould DB. Type IV collagens and basement membrane diseases: cell biology and pathogenic mechanisms. *Curr Top Membr.* (2015) 76:61–116. doi: 10.1016/bs.ctm.2015.09.002

26. Del Priore LV, Geng L, Tezel TH, Kaplan HJ. Extracellular matrix ligands promote RPE attachment to inner Bruch's membrane. *Curr Eye Res.* (2002) 25:79e 9. doi: 10.1076/ceyr.25.2.79.10158

27. Gong J, Sagiv O, Cai H, Tsang SH, Del Priore LV. Effects of extracellular matrix and neighboring cells on induction of human embryonic stem cells into retinal or retinal pigment epithelial progenitors. *Exp Eye Res.* (2008) 86:957–65. doi: 10.1016/j.exer.2008.03.014

28. Tezel TH, Del Priore LV. Repopulation of different layers of host human Bruch's membrane by retinal pigment epithelial cell grafts. *Invest Ophthalmol Vis Sci.* (1999) 40:767–74.

29. Tezel TH, Del Priore LV, Kaplan HJ. Reengineering of aged Bruch's membrane to enhance retinal pigment epithelium repopulation. *Invest Ophthalmol Vis Sci.* (2004) 45:3337–—48. doi: 10.1167/iovs.04-0193

30. Campochiaro PA, Jerdon JA, Glaser BM. The extracellular matrix of human retinal pigment epithelial cells *in vivo* and its synthesis *in vitro. Invest Ophthalmol Vis Sci.* (1986) 27:1615–21.

31. Candiello J, Cole GJ, Halfter W. Age-dependent changes in the structure, composition and biophysical properties of a human basement membrane. *Matrix Biol.* (2010) 29:402–10. doi: 10.1016/j.matbio.2010.03.004

32. Bu SC, Kuijer R, van der Worp RJ Li XR, Hooymans JM, Los LI. The ultrastructural localization of type II, IV, and VI collagens at the vitreoretinal interface. *PLoS ONE.* (2015) 10:e0134325. doi: 10.1371/journal.pone.0134325

33. Poschl E, Schlotzer-Schrehardt U, Brachvogel B, Saito K, Ninomiya Y, Mayer U. Collagen IV is essential for basement membrane stability but dispensable for initiation of its assembly during early development. *Development.* (2004) 131:1619–28. doi: 10.1242/dev.01037

34. Halfter W, Willem M, Mayer U. Basement membrane-dependent survival of retinal ganglion cells. *Invest Ophthalmol Vis Sci.* (2005) 46:1000–9. doi: 10.1167/iovs.04-1185

35. Lange CA, Luhmann UF, Mowat FM, Georgiadis A, West EL, Abrahams S, et al. Von Hippel-Lindau protein in the RPE is essential for normal ocular growth and vascular development. *Development.* (2012) 139:2340–50. doi: 10.1242/dev.070813

36. Gelse K, Ptl-Lindau protein in the RPE is essential for normal ocular growth

37. Gordon MK, Hahn RA. Collagens. *Cell Tissue Res.* (2010) 339:247–57. doi: 10.1007/s00441-009-0844-4

38. Sorushanova A, Delgado LM, Wu Z, Shologu N, Kshirsagar A, Raghunath R, et al. The collagen suprafamily: from biosynthesis to advanced biomaterial development. *Adv Mater.* (2019) 31:1801651. doi: 10.1002/adma.201801651

39. Henriksen K, Karsdal MA. Chapter 1 - type I collagen. In: Karsdal MA, editor, *Biochemistry of Collagens.* Laminins and Elastin: Academic Press (2016). p. 1–11. doi: 10.1016/B978-0-12-809847-9.00001-5

40. Sand JMB, Genovese F, Gudmann NS, Karsdal MA. Chapter 4 - type IV collagen. In: Karsdal MA, editor, *Biochemistry of Collagens.* 2nd ed. Laminins and Elastin: Academic Press (2019). p. 37-49. doi: 10.1016/B978-0-12-817068-7.00004-5

41. Kelley PB, Sado Y, Duncan MK. Collagen IV in the developing lens capsule. *Matrix Biol.* (2002) 21:415–23. doi: 10.1016/S0945-053X(02)00014-8

42. Bai X, Dilworth DJ, Weng YC, Gould DB. Developmental distribution of collagen IV isoforms and relevance to ocular diseases. *Matrix Biol.* (2009) 28:194–201. doi: 10.1016/j.matbio.2009.02.004

43. Chen L, Miyamura N, Ninomiya Y, Handa JT. Distribution of the collagen IV isoforms in human Bruch's membrane. *Br J Ophthalmol.* (2003) 87:212–5. doi: 10.1136/bjo.87.2.212

44. Xu S, Gu M, Wu K, Li G. Unraveling the role of hydroxyproline in maintaining the thermal stability of the collagen triple helix structure using simulation. *J Phys Chem B.* (2019) 123:7754–63. doi: 10.1021/acs.jpcb.9b05006

45. Bateman JF, Lamande SR, Ramshaw JA. Collagen superfamily. *Extracellular matrix.* (1996) 2:22–67.

46. Von der Mark K. *Components of the Organic Extracellular Matrix of Bone and Cartilage: Structure and Biosynthesis of Collagens. Dynamics of Bone and Cartilage Metabolism.* Amsterdam: Elsevier Inc. (1999). p. 3–18.

47. Khoshnoodi J, Pedchenko V, Hudson BG. Mammalian collagen IV. *Microsc Res Tech.* (2008) 71:357–70. doi: 10.1002/jemt.20564

48. Hwang ES, Brodsky B. Folding delay and structural perturbations caused by type IV collagen natural interruptions and nearby Gly missense mutations. *J Biol Chem.* (2012) 287:4368–75. doi: 10.1074/jbc.M111.269084

49. Zhu S, Yuan Q-J, Yin T, You J, Xiong S, Hu Y. Self-assembly of collagen-based biomaterials: Preparation, characterizations and biomedical applications. *J Mater Chem B.* (2018) 6:2999. doi: 10.1039/C7TB02999C

50. Lodish H, Berk A, Zipursky SL, Matsudaira P, Baltimore D, Darnell J. *Molecular Cell Biology.* 4 ed. Bookshelf: National Center for Biotechnology Information (2000). p. 9.

51. Rossert J, de Crombrugghe B. *Type I Collagen: Structure, Synthesis, and Regulation. Principles of Bone Biology.* Cambridge, MA: Elsevier (2002). p. 189-XVIII. doi: 10.1016/B978-012098652-1.50114-1

52. Nishida T, Saika S. Cornea and sclera: anatomy and physiology. *Cornea.* (2011) 8:3–24. doi: 10.1016/B978-0-323-06387-6.00008-8

53. Smith-Mungo LI, Kagan HM. Lysyl oxidase: properties, regulation and multiple functions in biology. *Matrix biology.* (1998) 16:387–98. doi: 10.1016/S0945-053X(98)90012-9

54. Yamauchi M, Taga Y, Hattori S, Shiiba M, Terajima M. Chapter 6 - analysis of collagen and elastin cross-links. In: Mecham RP, editor, *Methods in Cell Biology.* Cambridge, MA: Academic Press (2018). p. 115–32. doi: 10.1016/bs.mcb.2017.08.006

55. Hudson B, Reeders ST, Tryggvason K. Type IV collagen: structure, gene organization, and role in human diseases. Molecular basis of Goodpasture and Alport syndromes and diffuse leiomyomatosis. *J Biol Chem.* (1993) 268:26033–6 doi: 10.1016/S0021-9258(19)74270-7

56. A4270-7cal asis of Goodpasture and Alport syndromes and diffuse leiomyo, et al. Lysyl oxidase-like-2 cross-links collagen IV of glomerular basement membrane. *J Biol Chem.* (2016) 291:25999–6012. doi: 10.1074/jbc.M116.738856

57. Robaei D, Watson S. Corneal blindness: a global problem. *Clin Experiment Ophthalmol.* (2014) 42:213–4. doi: 10.1111/ceo.12330

58. Ghezzi CE, Rnjak-Kovacina J, Kaplan DL. Corneal tissue engineering: recent advances and future perspectives. *Tissue Eng B Rev.* (2015) 21:278–87. doi: 10.1089/ten.teb.2014.0397

59. Barrientez B, Nicholas SE, Whelchel A, Sharif R, Hjortdal J, Karamichos D. Corneal injury: clinical and molecular aspects. *Exp Eye Res.* (2019)

186:107709. doi: 10.1016/j.exer.2019.107709

60. Gain P, Jullienne R, He Z, Aldossary M, Acquart S, Cognasse F, et al. Global survey of corneal transplantation and eye banking. *JAMA Ophthalmol.* (2016) 134:167–73. doi: 10.1001/jamaophthalmol.2015.4776

61. Pineda R. Corneal transplantation in the developing world: lessons learned and meeting the challenge. *Cornea.* (2015) 34(Suppl.10):S35–40. doi: 10.1097/ICO.0000000000000567

62. Boisjoly HM, Tourigny R, Bazin R, Laughrea PA, Dubè I, Chamberland G, et al. Risk factors of corneal graft failure. *Ophthalmology.* (1993) 100:1728–35. doi: 10.1016/S0161-6420(93)31409-0

63. Mi S, Connon CJ. The formation of a tissue-engineered cornea using plastically compressed collagen scaffolds and limbal stem cells. In: Wright B, Connon CJ, editors, *Corneal Regenerative Medicine: Methods and Protocols.* Totowa, NJ: Humana Press (2013). p. 143–55. doi: 10.1007/978-1-62703-432-6_9

64. Mi S, Chen B, Wright B, Connon CJ. Plastic compression of a collagen gel forms a much improved scaffold for ocular surface tissue engineering over conventional collagen gels. *J Biomed Mater Res A.* (2010) 95:447–53. doi: 10.1002/jbm.a.32861

65. Kong B, Sun W, Chen G, Tang S, Li M, Shao Z, et al. Tissue-engineered cornea constructed with compressed collagen and laser-perforated electrospun mat. *Sci Rep.* (2017) 7:970. doi: 10.1038/s41598-017-01072-0

66. Zhang J, Sisley AM, Anderson AJ, Taberner AJ, McGhee CN, Patel DV. Characterization of a novel collagen scaffold for corneal tissue engineering. *Tissue Eng Part C Methods.* (2016) 22:165–72. doi: 10.1089/ten.tec.2015.0304

67. Takezawa T, Ozaki K, Nitani A, Takabayashi C, Shimo-Oka T. Collagen vitrigel: a novel scaffold that can facilitate a three-dimensional culture for reconstructing organoids. *Cell Transplant.* (2004) 13:463–73. doi: 10.3727/000000004783983882

68. Chae JJ, Ambrose WM, Espinoza FA, Mulreany DG, Ng S, Takezawa T, et al. Regeneration of corneal epithelium utilizing a collagen vitrigel membrane in rabbit models for corneal stromal wound and limbal stem cell deficiency. *Acta Ophthalmol.* (2015) 93:e57–66. doi: 10.1111/aos.12503

69. Majumdar S, Wang XK, Sommerfeld SD, Chae JJ, Athanasopoulou EN, Shores LS, et al. Cyclodextrin modulated type I collagen self-assembly to engineer biomimetic cornea implants. *Adv Funct Mater.* (2018) 28:1804076. doi: 10.1002/adfm.201804076

70. Guo Q, Shores L, Schein O, Trexler MM, Elisseeff JH. Developing biomimetic collagen-based matrix using cyclodextrin for corneal repair. In: *2014 40th Annual Northeast Bioengineering Conference (NEBEC)*, Boston, MA. (2014). p. 25–27. doi: 10.1109/NEBEC.2014.6972807

71. Liu W, Merrett K, Griffith M, Fagerholm P, Dravida S, Heyne B, et al. Recombinant human collagen for tissue engineered corneal substitutes. *Biomaterials.* (2008) 29:1147–58. doi: 10.1016/j.biomaterials.2007.11.011

72. Pasyechnikova N, Vit V, Leus M, Iakymenko S, Buznyk O, Kolomiichuk S, et al. Collagen-based bioengineered substitutes of donor corneal allograft implantation: assessment and hypotheses. *Med Hypothesis Discov Innov Ophthalmol.* (2012) 1:10–3.

73. Buznyk O, Pasyechnikova N, Islam MM, Iakymenko S, Fagerholm P, Griffith M. Bioengineered corneas grafted as alternatives to human donor corneas in three high-risk patients. *Clin Transl Sci.* (2015) 8:558–62. doi: 10.1111/cts.12293

74. Long K, Liu Y, Li W, Wang L, Liu S, Wang Y, et al. Improving the mechanical properties of collagen-based membranes using silk fibroin for corneal tissue engineering. *J Biomed Mater Res A.* (2015) 103:1159–68. doi: 10.1002/jbm.a.35268

75. Kishore V, Iyer R, Frandsen A, Nguyen TU. *In vitro* characterization of electrochemically compacted collagen matrices for corneal applications. *Biomed Mater.* (2016) 11:055008. doi: 10.1088/1748-6041/11/5/055008

76. Chen Z, Liu X, You J, Song Y, Tomaskovic-Crook E, Sutton G, et al. Biomimetic corneal stroma using electro-compacted collagen. *Acta Biomater.* (2020) 113:360–71. doi: 10.1016/j.actbio.2020.07.004

77. Torbet J, Malbouyres M, Builles N, Justin V, Roulet M, Damour O, et al. Orthogonal scaffold of magnetically aligned collagen lamellae for corneal stroma reconstruction. *Biomaterials.* (2007) 28:4268–76. doi: 10.1016/j.biomaterials.2007.05.024

78. Samarawickrama C, Samanta A, Liszka A, Fagerholm P, Buznyk O, Griffith M, et al. Collagen-based fillers as alternatives to cyanoacrylate glue for the sealing of large corneal perforations. *Cornea.* (2018) 37:609–16. doi: 10.1097/ICO.0000000000001459

79. Islam MM, Ravichandran R, Olsen D, Ljunggren MK, Fagerholm P, Lee CJ, et al. Self-assembled collagen-like-peptide implants as alternatives to human donor corneal transplantation. *RSC Adv.* (2016) 6:55745–9. doi: 10.1039/C6RA08895C

80. Nishi C, Nakajima N, Ikada Y. *In vitro* evaluation of cytotoxicity of diepoxy compounds used for biomaterial modification. *J Biomed Mater Res.* (1995) 29:829–34. doi: 10.1002/jbm.820290707

81. Ibusuki S, Halbesma GJ, Randolph MA, Redmond RW, Kochevar IE, Gill TJ. Photochemically cross-linked collagen gels as three-dimensional scaffolds for tissue engineering. *Tissue Eng.* (2007) 13:1995–2001. doi: 10.1089/ten.2006.0153

82. Foster A, Gilbert C, Johnson G. Changing patterns in global blindness: 1988–2008. *Community Eye Health.* (2008) 21:37–9.

83. Lindfield R, Vishwanath K, Ngounou F, Khanna RC. The challenges in improving outcome of cataract surgery in low and middle income countries. *Indian J Ophthalmol.* (2012) 60:464–9. doi: 10.4103/0301-4738.100552

84. Pascolini D, Mariotti SP. Global estimates of visual impairment: 2010. *Br J Ophthalmol.* (2012) 96:614–8. doi: 10.1136/bjophthalmol-2011-300539

85. McGhee CNJ, Zhang J, Patel DV, A. perspective of contemporary cataract surgery: the most common surgical procedure in the world. *J R Soc N Z.* (2020) 50:245–62. doi: 10.1080/03036758.2020.1714673

86. Wormstone IM, Wang L, Liu CS. Posterior capsule opacification. *Exp Eye Res.* (2009) 88:257–69. doi: 10.1016/j.exer.2008.10.016

87. Wernecke L, Keckeis S, Reichhart N, Strauapsule opacification. ataracmesenchymal transdifferentiation in pediatric lens epithelial cells. *Invest Ophthalmol Vis Sci.* (2018) 59:5785–94. doi: 10.1167/iovs.18-23789

88. Wormstone IM, Tamiya S, Anderson I, Duncan G. TGF-beta2-induced matrix modification and cell transdifferentiation in the human lens capsular bag. *Invest Ophthalmol Vis Sci.* (2002) 43:2301–8.

89. Awasthi N, Guo S, Wagner BJ. Posterior capsular opacification: a problem reduced but not yet eradicated. *Arch Ophthalmol.* (2009) 127:555–62. doi: 10.1001/archophthalmol.2009.3

90. Karahan E, Er D, Kaynak S. An overview of Nd:YAG laser capsulotomy. *Med Hypothesis Discov Innov Ophthalmol.* (2014) 3:45–50.

91. Mamalis N, Grossniklaus HE, Waring GO 3rd, Werner L, Brubaker J, Davis D, et al. Ablation of lens epithelial cells with a laser photolysis system: histopathology, ultrastructure, and immunochemistry. *J Cataract Refract Surg.* (2010) 36:1003—10. doi: 10.1016/j.jcrs.2009.11.021

92. Keates RH, Steinert RF, Puliafito CA, Maxwell SK. Long-term follow-up of Nd:YAG laser posterior capsulotomy. *J Am Intraocul Implant Soc.* (1984) 10:164–8. doi: 10.1016/S0146-2776(84)80101-9

93. Newland TJ, Auffarth GU, Wesendahl TA, Apple DJ. Neodymium:YAG laser damage on silicone intraocular lenses. A comparison of lesions on explanted lenses and experimentally produced lesions. *J Cataract Refract Surg.* (1994) 20:527–33. doi: 10.1016/S0886-3350(13)80233-7

94. Oshika T, Tsuboi S, Yaguchi S, Yoshitomi F, Nagamoto T, Nagahara K, et al. Comparative study of intraocular lens implantation through 32- and 55-mm incisions. *Ophthalmology.* (1994) 101:1183–90. doi: 10.1016/S0161-6420(94)31189-4

95. Ursell PG, Spalton DJ, Pande MV, Hollick EJ, Barman S, Boyce J, et al. Relationship between intraocular lens biomaterials and posterior capsule opacification. *J Cataract Refract Surg.* (1998) 24:352–60. doi: 10.1016/S0886-3350(98)80323-4

96. Chehade M, Elder MJ. Intraocular lens materials and styles: a review. *Aust N Z J Ophthalmol.* (1997) 25:255–63. doi: 10.1111/j.1442-9071.1997.tb01512.x

97. Lloyd AW, Faragher RG, Denyer SP. Ocular biomaterials and implants. *Biomaterials.* (2001) 22:769–85. doi: 10.1016/S0142-9612(00)00237-4

98. Hollick EJ, Spalton DJ, Ursell PG, Pande MV. Lens epithelial cell regression on the posterior capsule with different intraocular lens materials. *Br J Ophthalmol.* (1998) 82:1182–8. doi: 10.1136/bjo.82.10.1182

99. Coombes A, Seward H. Posterior capsular opacification prevention: IOL design and material. *Br J Ophthalmol.* (1999) 83:640–1. doi: 10.1136/bjo.83.6.640

100. Zhao Y, Yang K, Li J, Huang Y, Zhu S. Comparison of hydrophobic and hydrophilic intraocular lens in preventing posterior capsule opacification

after cataract surgery: an updated meta-analysis. *Medicine*. (2017) 96:e8301. doi: 10.1097/MD.0000000000008301

101. Hayashi K, Hayashi H. Posterior capsule opacification after implantation of a hydrogel intraocular lens. *Br J Ophthalmol*. (2004) 88:182–5. doi: 10.1136/bjo.2003.023580

102. Dorey MW, Brownstein S, Hill VE, Mathew B, Botton G, Kertes PJ, et al. Proposed pathogenesis for the delayed postoperative opacification of the hydroview hydrogel intraocular lens. *Am J Ophthalmol*. (2003) 135:591–8. doi: 10.1016/S0002-9394(02)02154-2

103. P2154-291halmolo: 10.is forinfluence on intraocular lens performance: an overview. *J Ophthalmol*. (2018) 2018:2687385.

104. Gauthier L, Lafuma A, Laurendeau C, Berdeaux G. Neodymium:YAG laser rates after bilateral implantation of hydrophobic or hydrophilic multifocal intraocular lenses: twenty-four month retrospective comparative study. *J Cataract Refract Surg*. (2010) 36:1195–200. doi: 10.1016/j.jcrs.2010.01.027

105. Linnola RJ, Sund M, Ylgive study. Berdeaux. Adhesion of soluble fibronectin, laminin, and collagen type IV to intraocular lens materials. *J Cataract Refract Surg*. (1999) 25:1486–91. doi: 10.1016/S0886-3350(99)00238-2

106. Linnola RJ, Werner L, Pandey SK, Escobar-Gomez M, Znoiko SL, Apple DJ. Adhesion of fibronectin, vitronectin, laminin, and collagen type IV to intraocular lens materials in pseudophakic human autopsy eyes. Part 1: histological sections. *J Cataract Refract Surg*. (2000) 26:1792–806. doi: 10.1016/S0886-3350(00)00748-3

107. Linnola RJ, Werner L, Pandey SK, Escobar-Gomez M, Znoiko SL, Apple DJ. Adhesion of fibronectin, vitronectin, laminin, and collagen type IV to intraocular lens materials in pseudophakic human autopsy eyes. Part 2: explanted intraocular lenses. *J Cataract Refract Surg*. (2000) 26:1807–18. doi: 10.1016/S0886-3350(00)00747-1

108. Miyake K, Maekubo K, Gravagna P, Tayot JL. Collagen IOLs: a suggestion for IOL biocompatibility. *Eur J Implant Refract Surg*. (1991) 3:99–102. doi: 10.1016/S0955-3681(13)80495-9

109. Schauersberger J, Amon M, Kruger A, Abela C, Schild G, Kolodjaschna J. Comparison of the biocompatibility of 2 foldable intraocular lenses with sharp optic edges. *J Cataract Refract Surg*. (2001) 27:1579–85. doi: 10.1016/S0886-3350(01)01019-7

110. Kohnen T, Fabian E, Gerl R, Hunold W, Hütz W, Strobel J, et al. Optic edge design as long-term factor for posterior capsular opacification rates. *Ophthalmology*. (2008) 115:1308–14e1-3. doi: 10.1016/j.ophtha.2008.01.002

111. Zemaitien.ogydesign as long-term factor for posterior capsular opacification rates. the biocompatibility of 2 intraocular lens materials. cal intraocular leMedicina. (2011) 47:595–9.

112. Vock L, Crnej A, Findl O, Neumayer T, Buehl W, Sacu S, et al. Posterior capsule opacification in silicone and hydrophobic acrylic intraocular lenses with sharp-edge optics six years after surgery. *Am J Ophthalmol*. (2009) 147:683–90.e2. doi: 10.1016/j.ajo.2008.11.006

113. Nixon DR, Woodcock MG. Pattern of posterior capsule opacification models 2 years postoperatively with 2 single-piece acrylic intraocular lenses. *J Cataract Refract Surg*. (2010) 36:929–34. doi: 10.1016/j.jcrs.2009.12.040

114. Nanu RV, Ungureanu E, Instrate SL, Vrapciu A, Cozubas R, Carstocea L, et al. An overview of the influence and design of biomaterial of the intraocular implant of the posterior capsule opacification. *Rom J Ophthalmol*. (2018) 62:188–93. doi: 10.22336/rjo.2018.29

115. Gwon A. Lens regeneration in mammals: a review. *Surv Ophthalmol*. (2006) 51:51–62. doi: 10.1016/j.survophthal.2005.11.005

116. Lin H, Ouyang H, Zhu J, Huang S, Liu Z, Chen S, et al. Lens regeneration using endogenous stem cells with gain of visual function. *Nature*. (2016) 531:323–8. doi: 10.1038/nature17181

117. Gwon A, Gruber L. Engineering the crystalline lens with a biodegradable or non-degradable scaffold. *Exp Eye Res*. (2010) 91:220–8. doi: 10.1016/j.exer.2010.05.011

118. Kumar B, Reilly MA. The development, growth, and regeneration of the crystalline lens: a review. *Curr Eye Res*. (2020) 45:313–26. doi: 10.1080/02713683.2019.1681003

119. Nagamoto T, Hara E. Lens epithelial cell migration onto the posterior capsule *in vitro*. *J Cataract Refract Surg*. (1996) 22:841–6. doi: 10.1016/S0886-3350(96)80172-6

120. Nishi O, Yamamoto N, Nishi K, Nishi Y. Contact inhibition of migrating lens epithelial cells at the capsular bend created by a sharp-edged intraocular lens after cataract surgery. *J Cataract Refract Surg*. (2007) 33:1065–70. doi: 10.1016/j.jcrs.2007.02.022

121. Cho HK, Na KS, Jun EJ, Chung SK. Cataracts among adults aged 30 to 49 years: a 10-year study from 1995 to 2004 in Korea. *Korean J Ophthalmol*. (2013) 27:345–50. doi: 10.3341/kjo.2013.27.5.345

122. Tan YSE, Shi PJ, Choo CJ, Laude A, Yeong WY. Tissue engineering of retina and Bruch's membrane: a review of cells, materials and processes. *Br J Ophthalmol*. (2018) 102:1182–7. doi: 10.1136/bjophthalmol-2017-311390

123. Barker DF, Hostikka SL, Zhou J, Chow LT, Oliphant AR, Gerken SC, et al. Identification of mutations in the COL4A5 collagen gene in Alport syndrome. *Science*. (1990) 248:1224–7. doi: 10.1126/science.2349482

124. Choi J, Na K, Bae S, Roh G. Anterior lens capsule abnormalities in Alport syndrome. *Korean J Ophthalmol*. (2005) 19:84–9. doi: 10.3341/kjo.2005.19.1.84

125. Savige J, Liu J, DeBuc DC, Handa JT, Hageman GS, Wang YY, et al. Retinal basement membrane abnormalities and the retinopathy of Alport syndrome. *Invest Ophthalmol Vis Sci*. (2010) 51:1621–7. doi: 10.1167/iovs.08-3323

126. Savige J, Sheth S, Leys A, Nicholson A, Mack HG, Colville D. Ocular features in Alport syndrome: pathogenesis and clinical significance. *Clin J Am Soc Nephrol*. (2015) 10:703–9. doi: 10.2215/CJN.10581014

127. Gilbert CE, Grierson I, McLeod D. Retinal patching: a new approach to the management of selected retinal breaks. *Eye*. (1989) 3:19–26. doi: 10.1038/eye.1989.3

128. Tyagi M, Basu S. Glue-assisted retinopexy for rhegmatogenous retinal detachments (GuARD): a novel surgical technique for closing retinal breaks. *Indian J Ophthalmol*. (2019) 67:677–80. doi: 10.4103/ijo.IJO_1943_18

129. Wang Q, Zhao J, Xu Q, Han C, Hou B. Intraocular application of fibrin glue as an adjunct to pars plana vitrectomy for rhegmatogenous retinal. *Retina*. (2020) 40:718–24. doi: 10.1097/IAE.0000000000002584

130. Ozbolat IT, Hospodiuk M. Current advances and future perspectives in extrusion-based bioprinting. *Biomaterials*. (2016) 76:321–43. doi: 10.1016/j.biomaterials.2015.10.076

131. Di Bella C, Duchi S, O'Connell CD, Blanchard R, Augustine C, Yue Z, et al. *In situ* handheld three-dimensional bioprinting for cartilage regeneration. *J Tissue Eng Regen Med*. (2018) 12:611–21. doi: 10.1002/term.2476

132. Starly B, Shirwaiker R. *3D Bioprinting Techniques. 3D Bioprinting and Nanotechnology in Tissue Engineering and Regenerative Medicine*, Cambridge, MA: Academic Press. (2015). p. 57–77. doi: 10.1016/B978-0-12-800547-7.00003-5

133. Hoath SD. *Fundamentals of Inkjet Printing: The Science of Inkjet and Droplets*. Hoboken, NJ: John Wiley & Sons (2016). doi: 10.1002/9783527684724

134. Ovsianikov A, Yoo J, Mironov V. *3D Printing and Biofabrication*. New York, NY: Springer. (2018). doi: 10.1007/978-3-319-45444-3

135. Duarte Campos DF, Rohde M, Ross M, Anvari P, Blaeser A, Vogt M, et al. Corneal bioprinting utilizing collagen-based bioinks and primary human keratocytes. *J Biomed Mater Res A*. (2019) 107:1945–53. doi: 10.1002/jbm.a.36702

136. Gao G, Schilling AF, Hubbell K, Yonezawa T, Truong D, Hong Y, et al. Improved properties of bone and cartilage tissue from 3D inkjet-bioprinted human mesenchymal stem cells by simultaneous deposition and photocrosslinking in PEG-GelMA. *Biotechnol Lett*. (2015) 37:2349–55. doi: 10.1007/s10529-015-1921-2

137. Cui X, Gao G, Yonezawa T, Dai G. Human cartilage tissue fabrication using three-dimensional inkjet printing technology. *J Vis Exp*. (2014) 2014:e51294. doi: 10.3791/51294

138. Xu C, Chai W, Huang Y, Markwald RR. Scaffold-free inkjet printing of three-dimensional zigzag cellular tubes. *Biotechnol Bioeng*. (2012) 109:3152–60. doi: 10.1002/bit.24591

139. Masaeli E, Forster V, Picaud S, Karamali F, Nasr-Esfahani MH, Marquette C. Tissue engineering of retina through high resolution 3-dimensional inkjet bioprinting. *Biofabrication*. (2020) 12:025006. doi: 10.1088/1758-5090/ab4a20

140. Bishop ES, Mostafa S, Pakvasa M, Luu HH, Lee MJ, Wolf JM, et al. 3-D bioprinting technologies in tissue engineering and regenerative medicine: current and future trends. *Genes Dis*. (2017) 4:185–95. doi: 10.1016/j.gendis.2017.10.002

141. Gudapati H, Dey M, Ozbolat I, A. comprehensive review on droplet-based bioprinting: past, present and future. *Biomaterials.* (2016) 102:20–42. doi: 10.1016/j.biomaterials.2016.06.012

142. Barron JA, Wu P, Ladouceur HD, Ringeisen BR. Biological laser printing: a novel technique for creating heterogeneous 3-dimensional cell patterns. *Biomed Microdevices.* (2004) 6:139–47. doi: 10.1023/B:BMMD.0000031751.67267.9f

143. Guillotin B, Souquet A, Catros S, Duocastella M, Pippenger B, Bellance S, et al. Laser assisted bioprinting of engineered tissue with high cell density and microscale organization. *Biomaterials.* (2010) 31:7250–6. doi: 10.1016/j.biomaterials.2010.05.055

144. Koch L, Gruene M, Unger C, Chichkov B. Laser assisted cell printing. *Curr Pharm Biotechnol.* (2013) 14:91–7. doi: 10.2174/138920113804805368

145. Sorkio A, Koch L, Koivusalo L, Deiwick A, Miettinen S, Chichkov B, et al. Human stem cell based corneal tissue mimicking structures using laser-assisted 3D bioprinting and functional bioinks. *Biomaterials.* (2018) 171:57–71. doi: 10.1016/j.biomaterials.2018.04.034

146. Keriquel V, Oliveira H, Remy M, Ziane S, Delmond S, Rousseau B, et al. *In situ* printing of mesenchymal stromal cells, by laser-assisted bioprinting, for *in vivo* bone regeneration applications. *Sci Rep.* (2017) 7:1778. doi: 10.1038/s41598-017-01914-x

147. Ferris CJ, Gilmore KG, Wallace GG, Panhuis MIH. Biofabrication: an overview of the approaches used for printing of living cells. *Appl Microbiol Biotechnol.* (2013) 97:4243–58. doi: 10.1007/s00253-013-4853-6

148. Wang Z, Kumar H, Tian Z, Jin X, Holzman JF, Menard F, et al. Visible light photoinitiation of cell-adhesive gelatin methacryloyl hydrogels for stereolithography 3D bioprinting. *ACS Appl Mater Interfaces.* (2018) 10:26859–69. doi: 10.1021/acsami.8b06607

149. Mahdavi SS, Abdekhodaie MJ, Kumar H, Mashayekhan S, Baradaran-Rafii A, Kim K. Stereolithography 3D bioprinting method for fabrication of human corneal stroma equivalent. *Ann Biomed Eng.* (2020) 48:1955–70. doi: 10.1007/s10439-020-02537-6

150. Lam T, Dehne T, Kruger JP, Hondke S, Endres M, Thomas A, et al. Photopolymerizable gelatin and hyaluronic acid for stereolithographic 3D bioprinting of tissue-engineered cartilage. *J Biomed Mater Res B Appl Biomater.* (2019) 107:2649–57. doi: 10.1002/jbm.b.34354

151. Grix T, Ruppelt A, Thomas A, Amler AK, Noichl BP, Lauster R, et al. Bioprinting perfusion-enabled liver equivalents for advanced organ-on-a-chip applications. *Genes.* (2018) 9:176. doi: 10.3390/genes9040176

152. Huber B, Engelhardt S, Meyer W, Kruger H, Wenz A, Schonhaar V, et al. Blood-vessel mimicking structures by stereolithographic fabrication of small porous tubes using cytocompatible polyacrylate elastomers, biofunctionalization and endothelialization. *J Funct Biomater.* (2016) 7:11. doi: 10.3390/jfb7020011

153. Gillispie G, Prim P, Copus J, Fisher J, Mikos AG, Yoo JJ, et al. Assessment methodologies for extrusion-based bioink printability. *Biofabrication.* (2020) 12:022003. doi: 10.1088/1758-5090/ab6f0d

154. Cubo N, Garcia M, Del Canizo JF, Velasco D, Jorcano JL. 3D bioprinting of functional human skin: production and *in vivo* analysis. *Biofabrication.* (2016) 9:015006. doi: 10.1088/1758-5090/9/1/015006

155. Liu W, Zhong Z, Hu N, Zhou Y, Maggio L, Miri AK, et al. Coaxial extrusion bioprinting of 3D microfibrous constructs with cell-favorable gelatin methacryloyl microenvironments. *Biofabrication.* (2018) 10:024102. doi: 10.1088/1758-5090/aa9d44

156. O'Connell DC, Di Bella C, Thompson F, Augustine C, Beirne S, Cornock R, et al. Development of the Biopen: a handheld device for surgical printing of adipose stem cells at a chondral wound site. *Biofabrication.* (2016) 8:15019. doi: 10.1088/1758-5090/8/1/015019

157. Hakimi N, Cheng R, Leng L, Sotoudehfar M, Ba PQ, Bakhtyar N, et al. Handheld skin printer: *in situ* formation of planar biomaterials and tissues. *Lab Chip.* (2018) 18:1440–51. doi: 10.1039/C7LC01236E

158. Isaacson A, Swioklo S, Connon CJ. 3D bioprinting of a corneal stroma equivalent. *Exp Eye Res.* (2018) 173:188–93. doi: 10.1016/j.exer.2018.05.010

159. Lee A, Hudson AR, Shiwarski DJ, Tashman JW, Hinton TJ, Yerneni S, et al. 3D bioprinting of collagen to rebuild components of the human heart. *Science.* (2019) 365:482–7. doi: 10.1126/science.aav9051

160. Kutlehria S, Dinh TC, Bagde A, Patel N, Gebeyehu A, Singh M. High-throughput 3D bioprinting of corneal stromal equivalents. *J Biomed Mater Res B Appl Biomater.* (2020) 108:2981–94. doi: 10.1002/jbm.b.34628

161. Wu Z, Su X, Xu Y, Kong B, Sun W, Mi S. Bioprinting three-dimensional cell-laden tissue constructs with controllable degradation. *Sci Rep.* (2016) 6:24474. doi: 10.1038/srep24474

162. Kim H, Jang J, Kim H, Kim KH, Cho D. 3D cell printed corneal stromal analogues for corneal tissue engineering. In: *2018 IEEE International Conference on Cyborg and Bionic Systems (CBS)*, Shenzhen. (2018). doi: 10.1109/CBS.2018.8612218

163. Hong H, Kim H, Han SJ, Jang J, Kim HK, Cho D-W, et al. Compressed collagen intermixed with cornea-derived decellularized extracellular matrix providing mechanical and biochemical niches for corneal stroma analogue. *Mater Sci Eng C.* (2019) 103:109837. doi: 10.1016/j.msec.2019.109837

164. Diamantides N, Wang L, Pruiksma T, Siemiatkoski J, Dugopolski C, Shortkroff S, et al. Correlating rheological properties and printability of collagen bioinks: the effects of riboflavin photocrosslinking and pH. *Biofabrication.* (2017) 9:034102. doi: 10.1088/1758-5090/aa780f

165. Palchesko RN, Lathrop KL, Funderburgh JL, Feinberg AW. *In vitro* expansion of corneal endothelial cells on biomimetic substrates. *Sci Rep.* (2015) 5:7955. doi: 10.1038/srep07955

166. Kay EP. Expression of types I and IV collagen genes in normal and in modulated corneal endothelial cells. *Invest Ophthalmol Vis Sci.* (1989) 30:260–8.

167. Chen S, Zhu Q, Sun H, Zhang Y, Tighe S, Xu L, et al. Advances in culture, expansion and mechanistic studies of corneal endothelial cells: a systematic review. *J Biomed Sci.* (2019) 26:2. doi: 10.1186/s12929-018-0492-7

168. Palchesko RN, Funderburgh JL, Feinberg AW. Engineered basement membranes for regenerating the corneal endothelium. *Adv Healthc Mater.* (2016) 5:2942-–50. doi: 10.1002/adhm.201600488

169. Madden PW, Lai JN, George KA, Giovenco T, Harkin DG, Chirila TV. Human corneal endothelial cell growth on a silk fibroin membrane. *Biomaterials.* (2011) 32:4076–84. doi: 10.1016/j.biomaterials.2010.12.034

170. Murphy SV, De Coppi P, Atala A. Opportunities and challenges of translational 3D bioprinting. *Nat Biomed Eng.* (2020) 4:370–80. doi: 10.1038/s41551-019-0471-7

7

Actually Seeing What is Going on – Intravital Microscopy in Tissue Engineering

Ravikumar Vaghela, Andreas Arkudas, Raymund E. Horch and Maximilian Hessenauer*

Department of Plastic and Hand Surgery, University Hospital of Erlangen, Friedrich–Alexander University Erlangen–Nürnberg (FAU), Erlangen, Germany

*Correspondence:
Maximilian Hessenauer
maximilian.hessenauer@
uk-erlangen.de;
maxhessenauer@aol.com

Intravital microscopy (IVM) study approach offers several advantages over *in vitro*, *ex vivo*, and 3D models. IVM provides real-time imaging of cellular events, which provides us a comprehensive picture of dynamic processes. Rapid improvement in microscopy techniques has permitted deep tissue imaging at a higher resolution. Advances in fluorescence tagging methods enable tracking of specific cell types. Moreover, IVM can serve as an important tool to study different stages of tissue regeneration processes. Furthermore, the compatibility of different tissue engineered constructs can be analyzed. IVM is also a promising approach to investigate host reactions on implanted biomaterials. IVM can provide instant feedback for improvising tissue engineering strategies. In this review, we aim to provide an overview of the requirements and applications of different IVM approaches. First, we will discuss the history of IVM development, and then we will provide an overview of available optical modalities including the pros and cons. Later, we will summarize different fluorescence labeling methods. In the final section, we will discuss well-established chronic and acute IVM models for different organs.

Keywords: tissue engineering, intravital microscopy, leukocyte recruitment, biomaterial, fluorescence, *in vivo*

INTRODUCTION

In vitro study models have immensely endorsed our knowledge of cellular physiology. *In vitro* study models hold many advantages over *in vivo* study models. Cells can be isolated from the particular organ, manipulated and propagated as per the requirement of the study (Kapałczyńska et al., 2018; Chen et al., 2019). Simplicity and low-cost maintenance requirements make 2D culture the first choice for researchers to understand cell biology, tissue development, disease mechanisms, and drug development. 2D culture studies are been used for better understanding of cancer biology, vascular development, cell secretomes and their influences on the immediate environment (Kapałczyńska et al., 2018; Al-Abboodi et al., 2019; Kengelbach-Weigand et al., 2019; Ahmadzadeh et al., 2020). However, *in vitro* 2D models fail to mimic the native tissue environment which is important to study tissue physiology (Weigand et al., 2016; Duval et al., 2017; Kapałczyńska et al., 2018). Therefore, 3D models were designed to propagate the cells in a more native tissue environment (Witt et al., 2017; Tong et al., 2018; Kengelbach-Weigand et al., 2019). Many researchers are shifting from traditional 3D models to biofabricated 3D models which facilitates replication of the complex tissue architecture in a more precise and controlled manner (Horch et al., 2018). Though, most 3D models lack other influencing factors of native tissue, such as the presence of other cell types as well as signal molecules from the immediate and distant environment (Weigand et al., 2016; Kapałczyńska et al., 2018). Hence, conducting *in vivo* studies is required to overcome above-mentioned limitations. A typical *in vivo* study ends with the killing of the animal followed by a collection of an organ of interest. The histological analysis provides information at one static point which fails to describe the dynamics of ongoing cellular processes (Steiner et al., 2019).

At this point, IVM studies excel *in vitro, ex vivo* and 3D models. IVM provides imaging of cellular events in its native tissue environment as well as in real-time setting. It can be used to examine proliferation, migration, differentiation of cells as well as their specific interactions and behavior (such as leukocyte–endothelial, tumor cell–cell, and bacterial-cell interaction). IVM enables acute and/or chronic as well as repetitive imaging in the same animal, which provides a comprehensive picture of the overall complex dynamic processes. IVM provides an opportunity to analyze different stages of tissue regeneration simultaneously.

Various optical modalities, ranging from wide field to multiphoton microscopy, are available for imaging of the targeted organ (Wang et al., 2005; Wang H. et al., 2018; Jonkman and Cm, 2015). The conventional wide-field microscope is adequate for semitransparent tissue structures such as cremaster muscle and skin (Lemaster et al., 2017). Confocal microscopy can further increase the resolution. Additional deep imaging of complex organs can be achieved with improved optic modalities such as multiphoton microscopy (Theer et al., 2003; Horton et al., 2013; Weigert et al., 2013; Ouzounov et al., 2017). Combination of appropriate microscopic modality and genetic tools or contrast agents can be applied to understand specific organ physiology via IVM.

Earlier IVM studies were restricted to acute duration. However, the advent of window and chamber models helped to elongate the experimental period. IVM window models provide further benefits such as elimination of repeated surgical preparation and observation of the same region for multiple times in the same animal (Hackl et al., 2013; Reichel et al., 2015; Hessenauer et al., 2018). Apart from that, biomaterials play an important role in modern tissue engineering. Tissue engineered scaffolds serve to replace, repair, and maintain structural integrity of tissue. Scaffolds should be biocompatible and promote cell growth and differentiation to support regeneration (Patel and Fisher, 2008). IVM is a promising and fast approach to study interactions of different tissue engineered constructs for tissue development. Overall, it enables tracking of the entire dynamic process. Above mentioned advantages reduce the inter-animal variation and overall requirement of the number of animals (Prunier et al., 2017).

Considering all the advantages of IVM, it is indispensable to discuss various aspects of IVM. It is a need of an hour to combine advanced optical modalities and fluorescence tagging methodologies and apply them in IVM for an in-depth analysis of the healthy and diseased state of the tissue, tissue development, repair and biocompatibility as well as host reactions on implanted biomaterials. Therefore, in this review, we aim to begin with a short history of IVM development, followed by an overview

of available optical modalities and contrast agents. In the final section of the review, we will discuss well-established IVM models for different organs.

HISTORY

In the early 19th century, Rudolf Wagner for the first time reported rolling leukocytes in the blood vessel of a grass frog. This was one of the earliest report involving real-time observation of vascular physiology in the alive animal. But the roots of IVM are even deeper. The Italian scientist Marcello Malpighi attempted IVM to observe the lung in mammals as well as amphibians for the very first time in the 16th century. In the late 19th century, Elie Metchnikoff studied phagocytosis and diapedesis using IVM in frog. The earliest IVM movies were created in the early 20th century by Ries and Vles. Before that, drawing was the only tool to describe the observation. Until then, IVM imaging was limited to vasculature observation employing bright-field microscopic setup. Moreover, observation and documentation were difficult due to the lack of contrast agents (Secklehner et al., 2017).

Intravital microscopy became a more practical tool for physiological studies after the introduction of the first fluorescence microscope by Heimstadt in 1911 (Secklehner et al., 2017) and after the development of exogenous fluorophores. In 1955, the confocal scanning microscope was developed by Minsky (1988). It was designed to eliminate out-of-focus emission light with the help of pinhole. Confocal microscopy also enhances contrast and improves Z-resolution (Wang et al., 2005; Jonkman and Cm, 2015).

Physicist Maria Göppert-Mayer in 1931 introduced the idea of multiphoton microscopy. However, the application of multiphoton microscopy became only possible after the development of the required excitation lasers in 1976. Multiphoton microscopy works on the principle of simultaneous absorption of two or more photons. Advantages of multiphoton microscopy include deeper tissue penetration and lower phototoxicity. Advanced optical modalities along with newly developed window or chamber models open the door for longitudinal deep-tissue imaging (Schießl and Castrop, 2016).

The advent of fluorescent protein and fluorescent probes has played an important role in imaging. In 1994, Green fluorescent protein (GFP) originally isolated from Aequorea victoria, was successfully introduced into *Caenorhabditis elegans* as a genetic marker. 3 years later, first strains of GFP transgenic mice was reported. Later on, different fluorescent proteins such as red, yellow, and cyan fluorescent proteins (RFP, YFP, and CFP) were discovered (Hadjantonakis et al., 2003). On the other hand, application of the first fluorescently labeled antibody was already reported in 1942 by Albert Coons (Zanacchi et al., 2014).

Transgenic reporter animals, fluorescent probes, window models and advanced microscopic modalities have emerged as essential IVM tools to study target tissues at a cellular level. The development of window models is particularly useful for chronic experiments. In 1924, Sandison first used a transparent chamber in the rabbit's ear. Currently, organs such as skin, liver, kidney, lung, cremaster muscle and brain have been studied using window models. Since the mid-20th century, researchers are actively using this tool for physiological research (Secklehner et al., 2017).

MICROSCOPY TECHNIQUES

The journey of IVM started with bright field transillumination microscopy where the image is formed by the light transmitted through the sample (Pittet and Weissleder, 2011). However, transillumination is not suitable for relatively dense and thick tissues. Therefore nowadays, IVM is largely based on the epi-fluorescence principle where the image is generated from the fluorescence emitted from the object (Weigert et al., 2013). Several microscopic modalities are available for performing IVM such as wide-field fluorescence, confocal and multiphoton microscopy (**Table 1**). When light is absorbed by the fluorophore, electrons are excited from the ground state to the excited state. While returning to the ground state, electrons emit light which has a longer wavelength. This emitted light is collected in a detection system and generates fluorescence image. In wide-field microscopy, the entire field of view is illuminated. Here, the detection of out of focus light compromises the resolution of an image (Swedlow et al., 2002; Weigert et al., 2013).

This problem is resolved in confocal microscopy (White et al., 1987; Minsky, 1988). In laser confocal scanning microscopy (LCSM), the focus light is removed by the introduction of a pinhole in front of the photomultiplier detector. The specimen is scanned point-by-point. Scanned images of each depth can be combined to form a 3D image. However, scanning of all the focal plane makes the image acquisition slower and poses a phototoxicity issue. Image acquisition speed can be increased using multiple pinholes in spinning disk confocal microscopy (SDCM). Therefore, SDCM reduces phototoxicity (Wang et al., 2005; Jonkman and Cm, 2015; Bai et al., 2020).

In multiphoton microscopy (MPM) two or more photons having near-infrared wavelength are absorbed simultaneously. Fluorophore excitation takes place only at the in-focus plane, which reduces its phototoxicity and eliminates the requirement of pinholes. MPM is preferred when the imaging area is located more than 50–100 μm deep in the tissue (Weigert et al., 2013). Two photon microscopy (2 PM) can reach up to superficial cortical layers of the rodent brain (Miller et al., 2017). Light scattering and absorption of the tissue limit the penetration depth of 2 PM. Scattering and absorption both are dependent on excitation wavelength (Miller et al., 2017). However, recent developments in Three PM (3 PM) have demonstrated substantial improvement in penetration depth. Horton et al. (2013) first used 3 PM at the long-wavelength window of 1,700 nm for mouse brain imaging. 3 PM has emerged as a powerful game-changer in high-resolution, deep tissue intravital imaging. 3 PM enables imaging of vascular and neuronal structures at the depth of approximately 1.3 mm in the mouse brain (Horton et al., 2013).

Other available MPM variations include second and third harmonic generations (SHG and THG). SHG and THG provide label-free visualization of structures, such as collagen, myosin, and lipids (Reichel et al., 2015; Vielreicher et al., 2017). The signal is generated when two or more photons combine and form single photon without energy loss. SHG and THG enable 200–400 μm of imaging depth (Weigert et al., 2013).

Reflected light oblique transillumination (RLOT) microscopy works on the principle of oblique transillumination. It was developed by installing reflector directly below the specimen. The tilted reflector allows only a specific diffracted sideband of light to reach the objective lens. It can be incorporated with a wide-field epi-fluorescence microscope. RLOT can be used for imaging fast dynamic activity in the absence of specific fluorophores (Mempel et al., 2003).

STAININGS/PROBES USED IN INTRAVITAL MICROSCOPY

Most tissues are complex structures made up of different function-specific cells. Therefore, it is very important to study all cell types discretely. Using IVM alone, it can be difficult to differentiate between different tissue-specific cell types. It is important to distinguish the target via tagging or injection of contrasting dye in the animal. This can be achieved by application of fluorescence dyes, cell-specific labeling using antibodies, nanotechnology-based probes and use of genetic reporters. Some of the dyes are already being used for clinical purpose (Dunn and Ryan, 2017; Ludolph et al., 2019).

The discovery of fluorophores in conjugation with biologically active substances (peptides, antibody fragments, and nanoparticles) led to major advancements in IVM. Depending on the requirement of the study, fluorophores such as TRITC or FITCs can be conjugated to high or low molecular weight molecules such as Dextran or Albumin. TRITC or FITCs in conjugation with high molecular weight Dextran is commonly used for contrast enhancement of intravascular blood plasma. FITC conjugated to lower molecular weight Albumin easily leaks out from the endothelium, therefore it is used in plasma extravasation studies. Injectable fluorophores have played important role in studying biological processes such as leukocyte trafficking, cell–cell interaction, including inflammation, angiogenesis, apoptosis, oxidative stress, and calcium dynamics (Dunn et al., 2002; Taqueti and Jaffer, 2013; Kawakami, 2016).

Genetically encoded fluorescent proteins (FPs) are one of the most preferred approach amongst researches for *in vivo* imaging. Genetic integration and exemption of substrates or cofactors for fluorescence make FPs an ideal tool for IVM. Available FPs enable cell tracking and *in vivo* proliferation during development, tumors metastasis and in stem cells therapy models. Far-Red fluorescent proteins (RFPs) are preferred over GFPs due to lower light absorption by hemoglobin which allows efficient photon transmission and less autofluorescence (Taqueti and Jaffer, 2013). Taqueti and Jaffer (2013) used ApoE$^{-/-}$/Lysozyme $^{EGFP/EGFP}$ mice containing encoded GFP neutrophils and monocytes to study leukocyte trafficking. Looney et al. (2011) used c-fms EGFP transgenic mice for lung immune surveillance. Lee et al. (2014) used Cxcr6gfp/+mice to study NK T cells in the liver vasculature during Borrelia burgdorferi infection. Fuhrmann et al. (2010)

TABLE 1 | Imaging techniques (Mempel et al., 2003; Masedunskas et al., 2012; Weigert et al., 2013; Marques et al., 2015b; Vielreicher et al., 2017).

Excitation	Technique	Microscopy	Light source	Detection	Advantages	Disadvantages
Single-photon	Widefield		Mercury lamp/LED	CCD	• Fast acquisition • Low cost	• Limited depth • Phototoxicity
		RLOT	Xenon lamp	CCD	• Detection of fast dynamic activity in the absence of specific fluorophores	• Limited to translucent tissue
	Confocal	LCSM	Lasers	PMT	• High spatial resolution • 3D sectioning	• Limited depth • Slow acquisition • Phototoxicity • Relatively high cost and smaller field of view
		SDCM	Lasers	CCD	• Fast acquisition • Low phototoxicity • 3D sectioning	• Limited depth • Faster acquisition • Pinhole crosstalk reduces the resolution
Two or more photon	Multiphoton	Two-photon	Lasers	PMT	• Extended depth • No off-focus emissions	• High cost • Slow acquisition
		Three-photon	Lasers	PMT	• Deep tissue imaging • Improved signal to background ratio	• High cost • Slow acquisition
		SHG and THG	Lasers	PMT	• No energy absorption • Label-free imaging of collagen, myosins, myelin, and lipids	

LED, light-emitting diode; RLOT, reflected light oblique transillumination; CCD, charge-coupled device; LCSM, laser confocal scanning microscopy; PMT, photomultiplier tube; SDCM, spinning disk confocal microscopy; SHG, second-harmonic generation; THG, third-harmonic generation.

studied Alzheimer's disease-linked neuron loss in microglial Cx3cr1 knockout mice (Kawakami, 2016). Similarly, RFP and YFP have been used to study various immune as well as organ-specific cells (**Table 2**). Genetic cell labeling enables discrimination between metastatic and non-metastatic tumors cells (Condeelis and Weissleder, 2010; Taqueti and Jaffer, 2013; Kawakami, 2016). However, the considerable size of FPs (∼25–30 kDa), can interfere with protein function. Moreover. FPs exhibit low brightness and photostability (Toseland, 2013; Yan and Mp, 2015).

Another way to detect specific cell types in IVM is by using fluorescently labeled antibody against specific cell receptor. Several types of antibody-based markers are developed to specific tagging of cells. Fluorescently labeled antibody human epidermal growth factor receptor type 2 (HER2)/*neu,* epidermal growth factor receptor (EGFR) and c-MET have been used to study tumor growth (Tanaka et al., 2014). Endothelial cells can be targeted using an anti CD31 antibody. During migration endothelial cells and leukocytes express Intracellular adhesion molecule (ICAM)-1 and endothelial cells express vascular cell adhesion molecule (VCAM)-1. Antibodies against such adhesion molecule can be used to study vascular cell migration. Apart from using full antibodies, Fluorophore-conjugated antibody fragments (Fab, Diabody, and Mini body) can also be used for IVM (Condeelis and Weissleder, 2010; Taqueti and Jaffer, 2013).

Conventional fluorescent organic dyes and FPs have limitations of photobleaching, low signal intensity, and spectral overlapping (Wang H. et al., 2018). These limitations can be overcome via the application of nanotechnology-based probes known as Quantum dots (QDs). QDs show unique properties such as size-tunable light emission, high signal brightness, extended photostability and resistance against metabolic degradation, simultaneous multi-color excitation, and spectral multiplexing (Resch-Genger et al., 2008; Jin et al., 2011; Shao et al., 2011). Megens et al. (2010) used collagen-binding protein labeled with green-fluorescent quantum dots (CNA35-QD525) to study subendothelial collagen. Wang H. et al. (2018) developed mercapto succinic acid (MSA) capped cadmium telluride/cadmium sulfide (CdTe/CdS) QDs for long-term vascular IVM. Ripplinger et al. (2012) used magnetofluorescent nanoparticles (MFNP) such as cross-linked iron oxide (CLIO) AF555, CLIO-VT680 to illuminate macrophages during inflammation. Montet et al. (2006) used cRGD-CLIO(Cy5.5) and scrRGD-CLIO(Cy3.5) for imaging tumor cells. Similarly, Mulder et al. (2009) used RGD-pQDs for targeted imaging of tumor angiogenesis. Biocompatibility and specificity of QDs can be modulated by surface coating modification. However, potential toxicity poses uncertainty for the *in vivo* application of QDs. Cytotoxicity of QDs depends on factors such as charge, size, coating ligands, oxidative, photolytic, and mechanical stability (Resch-Genger et al., 2008; Jin et al., 2011; Shao et al., 2011; Progatzky et al., 2013).

MODELS/OPERATION TECHNIQUES

Over the past decades, different window and chamber models have been developed according to the location of the organ of interest. Most models required surgical procedures to expose the organ of interest and installation of window or chamber. In this section, we will discuss various IVM models. Depending on study

TABLE 2 | Fluorescence probes for intravital microscopy (Condeelis and Weissleder, 2010; Jin et al., 2011; Taqueti and Jaffer, 2013; Toseland, 2013; Caravagna et al., 2016; Kawakami, 2016; Wang H. et al., 2018).

Class	Subtypes	Examples/target
Fluorescence dyes		
	TRITC-dextran, FITC-dextran	Vascular contrast enhancement, plasma extravasation
	Texas red-dextran	
	FITC-albumin	Plasma extravasation
	Rhodamine 6G, Acridine orange	Leukocyte trafficking
	Hoechst 33342	DNA staining
	CMTMR, Calcein-AM, CFSE, CMAC	*Ex vivo* cell labeling
Genetic tags	**GFP**	
	Lysozyme-EGFP	Neutrophils and monocytes
	c-CSF1R-GFP	Neutrophils, monocytes macrophages
	CX3CR1-GFP	Monocytes, macrophages, microglia
	CXCR6-GFP	NK T cells
	RFP	
	CX3CL1-Cherry	Macrophages
	CD2-RFP	T cells
	IL17f-RFP	Th17 cells
	NG2-RFP	Pericytes
	tdTomato	HA-CTLs
	YFP	
	CD11c-EYFP	Dendritic cells
	Thy1-YFP	Neuron
Antibodies	**IgG**	
	EGFR, Her2/neu, c-MET	Tumor cells
	CD31/PECAM-1	Endothelial junctions
	ICAM-1	Endothelial cells, leukocytes
	VCAM-1	Endothelium
	CD45	Pan-leukocyte
	CD11b	Myeloid leukocytes
	Ly-6G	Neutrophils
	F4/80	Monocytes, macrophages
	GPIbβ	Platelets
	Fragments	Fab, diabody, minibody
Nanotechnology	**Q-dot**	
	CNA35-QD525	Inflammation
	CdTe/CdS	Vascular imaging
	Magnetic nanoparticles	
	CLIO-AF555, CLIO-VT750	Macrophages
	cRGD-CLIO(Cy5.5), scrRGD-CLIO(Cy3.5)	Tumor cells

TRITC, tetramethylrhodamine; FITC, fluorescein isothiocyanate; CMTMR, 5-(and-6)-(4-chloromethyl (benzoyl)amino) tetramethylrhodamine; CFSE, carboxyfluorescein succinimidyl ester; CMAC, 7-amino-4-chloromethylcoumarin; EGFP, enhanced green fluorescent protein; GFP, green fluorescent protein; CSF1, colony-stimulating factor 1; CX3CR1, C-X3-C motif chemokine receptor 1; CX3CL1, C-X3-C motif chemokine ligand 1; CD, cluster of differentiation; RFP, red fluorescent protein; IL17f, interleukin 17f; NG2, neuron glia antigen-2; EYFP, enhanced yellow fluorescent protein; Her2/neu, human epidermal growth factor receptor 2; PECAM-1, platelet endothelial cell adhesion molecule; ICAM-1, intercellular adhesion molecule 1; Ly6G, lymphocyte antigen 6 complex locus G6D; CNA35, collagen-binding adhesion protein 35; CdS/CdTe, cadmium sulfide/cadmium telluride; CLIO, crosslinked iron oxide; AF555, AlexaFluor555; VT750, VivoTag-S 750; cRGD, cyclic arginine-glycine-aspartic acid peptide; scrRGD, scrambled RGD; Cy, cyanine.

duration, IVM models can be divided into acute imaging models and chronic models.

Acute IVM Models

In acute models, the desired organ or tissue is surgically exposed for a short period and the animal is sacrificed at the end of the study. IVM is limited to a specific time point and repeated observation is unattainable.

Cremaster Muscle

The cremaster muscle is a very thin and nearly transparent layer of smooth muscle covering both testicles. It is easily accessible in male rodents via a minimally invasive surgical procedure, which allows high-resolution imaging of local the microvasculature (**Figure 1**).

The cremaster muscle is surgically exposed by a longitudinal incision of the scrotum. After freeing from the surrounding connective tissue, the apex of the cremaster muscle is fixed on a customized stage for superfusion. A longitudinal incision is made through the ventral surface of the muscle followed by detachment from epididymis and testicle. The testicle is either pushed back into the abdominal cavity or removed by orchiectomy. The remaining cremaster muscle is spread over the customized stage and can be accessed for microscopy and interventions (Bagher and Segal, 2011; Reichel et al., 2011; Donndorf et al., 2013).

This well-standardized surgical procedure can be a useful tool for visualizing and analyzing capillary perfusion, leukocyte–endothelial interaction, microvascular response to different stimuli and endothelial permeability in a defined environment (Donndorf et al., 2013; Molski et al., 2015). It can also be used to study blood cell interactions under influence of different drugs and chemokines (Reichel et al., 2012; Rius and Sanz, 2015) as well as ischemia-reperfusion (IR) injury and local effects of systemic conditions (Molski et al., 2015). Cremaster muscle is an acute IVM model. However, Siemionow and Nanhekhan (1999) developed a chronic cremaster chamber which allows imaging up to 3 days.

Heart

The heart is the essential blood pumping machinery of the body. Therefore, it is very important to understand heart physiology.

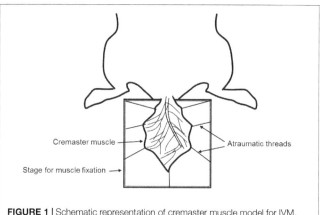

FIGURE 1 | Schematic representation of cremaster muscle model for IVM.

Application of IVM provides more accurate information compared to *in vitro* or *ex vivo* setting as it does not mimic the native physiological environment (Vinegoni et al., 2015). Similar to the lung, continuous movement is a major obstacle in heart IVM. Physical immobilization such as a using suture, a mechanical stabilizer or suction can be applied but they end up in low-resolution imaging and movement artifacts (Aguirre et al., 2014). To overcome this, a combination of approaches such as a gated acquisition algorithm, gated sequential segmented microscopy or active motion stabilization along with mechanical stabilization has been used (Lee et al., 2008).

For IVM, thoracotomy in the fourth left intercostal space is performed. Surrounding connective tissue is removed to expose the heart. Once exposed, the heart is stabilized using one of the above-mentioned technique (Lee et al., 2012; Aguirre et al., 2014; Vinegoni et al., 2015).

Heart IVM can be used to study both function of the heart muscle on single-cell level within the muscle with regard to cell metabolism as well as cell electrophysiology under physiological and pathophysiological conditions. In addition cell dynamics in pathological conditions such as ischemia-reperfusion and myocardial infarction can be closely monitored (Aguirre et al., 2014; Vinegoni et al., 2015). Most importantly microvascular events such as leukocyte trafficking as well as microvascular rearrangement under many pathological conditions such as myocardial infarction or infection can be evaluated (Ueno et al., 2016; Matsuura et al., 2018; Bajpai et al., 2019).

Ear Pinna Model

The ear pinna model is the easiest model for *in vivo* imaging as it is a non-surgical procedure (**Figure 2**). The ear contains two full-thickness layers of skin separated by a thin cartilage layer. The skin of the mouse ear contains few hair and closely resembles human skin (Chan et al., 2013). Ease of access, minimal preparation requirements, and less respiratory movement makes it an ideal site for the investigation of cell migration dynamics, cell–cell and host cell–pathogen interactions (Secklehner et al., 2017). It is very important to remove the small number of hairs present on the ear. Otherwise, it may cause autofluorescence during imaging. Shaving of the ear hair can easily lead to skin damage. Moreover, it provides only a limited area for IVM (Chan et al., 2013; Strüder et al., 2017).

The rodent ear is a suitable to model for investigating immune cells in the skin, tissue implantation, and *in vivo* tumor cell behavior (Chan et al., 2013), IR injury, and wound healing (Chan et al., 2013; Strüder et al., 2017).

Salivary Gland

Membrane traffic is a fundamental transport process that encompasses the exchange and distribution of molecules such as proteins, lipids, and polysaccharides between the cell and the extracellular space as well as among intracellular organelles (Ebrahim and Weigert, 2019). The salivary gland has emerged as a revolutionary acute IVM model to study endocytosis and regulated exocytosis. The salivary gland is situated in the neck region which makes it less susceptible to motion artifacts created by respiration and heart beating (Masedunskas et al., 2013b;

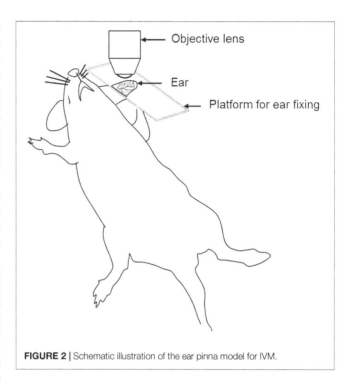

FIGURE 2 | Schematic illustration of the ear pinna model for IVM.

Ebrahim and Weigert, 2019). The salivary gland can be easily accessed by removing a small circular piece of skin from the neck (Masedunskas et al., 2013a). Relatively easy surgical access and ease of selective manipulation make it an excellent IVM model (Ebrahim and Weigert, 2019).

This model has been successfully applied to investigate mitochondrial dynamics (Porat-Shliom et al., 2019), endocytosis mediated remodeling as well as endocytosis modulation in cancer progression (Milberg et al., 2017; Ebrahim and Weigert, 2019).

Chronic IVM Models

Chronic IVM models are primarily designed for both longitudinal as well as acute studies. Chronic models involve surgical preparation along with installation of a window or chamber that enables rapid and long-term imaging.

Kidney

The kidney is a complex organ. It contains more than 20 function-specific cell types. The kidney contains several nephrons which are responsible for glomerular filtration, active tubular secretion as well as reabsorption of useful molecules (van den Berg et al., 2018). The kidney is exposed by a flank incision through the retroperitoneum. IVM is performed by placing the kidney in a coverslip-bottomed cell culture dish or immobilizing it by custom made holder (Dunn et al., 2007; Hato et al., 2018). Although, kidney IVM is primarily an acute model, Hackl et al. (2013) demonstrated the modified method involving of repeated externalization of the kidney which enables *in vivo* multiphoton imaging over several days.

Kidney IVM can be used to investigate a renal injury, IR injury, dysfunction, inflammation, cell death, microvascular blood flow, glomerular filtration and podocyte migration

(Russo et al., 2007; Devi et al., 2013; Hackl et al., 2013; Hall et al., 2013; Schießl et al., 2016b).

Lung

The lung is an essential respiratory organ situated below the rib cage. It contains a unique capillary network. Leukocytes need to undergo shape deformation for traveling through the narrow capillary segments (Wiggs et al., 1994). Pioneering work on acute imaging of lung was done by the Presson group where the dog was use as model organism. Later, this model was developed for small animals (Presson et al., 1994). Continuous movement caused by breathing and heart beating poses difficulties for *in vivo* imaging. Presson et al. (2011) for the very first time applied a customized vacuum ring imaging window with adjunctive support of gated imaging or frame registration for efficient reduction of motion artifact and maximizing clarity of the image. This organ stabilization approach revolutionized IVM in organs which are susceptible to motion artifact. Several other approaches have been used to stabilize lung for IVM which includes mechanical stabilization using Bronchus clamping, glue fixation on a coverslip and suction stabilization. However, immobilization of one area of the lung can induce shear force which can injure the lung (Looney et al., 2011; Fiole and Tournier, 2016; Rodriguez-Tirado et al., 2016).

For exposing the lung, thoracotomy is performed. The animal is placed in the right or left lateral decubitus position. An incision is made to expose the rib cage. A couple of ribs (3–4) are removed to expose the surface of a lung lobe followed by stabilization for microscopy (Looney and Bhattacharya, 2014; Rodriguez-Tirado et al., 2016). Using efficient optical tools, high-resolution lung imaging can be performed for up to 12 hours (hrs) (Rodriguez-Tirado et al., 2016). However, recently, Entenberg et al. (2018) made a ground breaking success by developing a permanently implantable and minimally invasive window that can be imagined for up to 2 weeks.

Lung IVM can be applied to study mitochondrial function in lung immunity, neutrophil as well as platelet trafficking, the gas exchange process and lung tumor biology (Eichhorn et al., 2002; Tabuchi et al., 2008; Kreisel et al., 2010; Fiole and Tournier, 2016; Rodriguez-Tirado et al., 2016; Thanabalasuriar et al., 2016; Yipp et al., 2017; Neupane et al., 2020). Apart from lung wobbling and surgical invasiveness, a major problem in the lung is penetration depth. Even highly efficient two-photon microscopy can only image superficially (up to 30–100 µm), which may not display deep tissue features of the lung (Perlman and Bhattacharya, 2007; Looney et al., 2011).

Spleen

The spleen is an important secondary lymphoid organ for IVM. It is located below the rib cage on the left-hand side within the abdominal cavity. The spleen filters pathogens and antigens from the blood. It contains the red pulp and white pulp regions, separated by the marginal zone. Red pulp macrophages recycle iron from senescent erythrocytes. The white pulp contains T cell and B cell zones which are important for antigen-specific immune responses (Martin-Jaular et al., 2011). It is relatively easy

to prepare spleen for IVM because of its superficial location in the body (Secklehner et al., 2017).

To expose the spleen, an incision is made below the ribcage on the left lateral position. Afterward, the spleen is exteriorized and placed on a customized stage and sealed with adhesive (Ferrer et al., 2012; Deniset et al., 2017). Spleen IVM is utilized in disease models such as malaria (Secklehner et al., 2017), atherosclerosis (Robbins Clinton et al., 2012) as well as cancer (Cortez-Retamozo et al., 2012). Furthermore, it can also be used for imaging of lymphocytic Calcium ion signaling (Yoshikawa et al., 2016).

Liver

The largest metabolic organ liver is located below the diaphragm. It plays an essential role in metabolism, protein synthesis and detoxification of systemic circulation (Vollmar and Menger, 2009). It receives around 80% blood supply from the portal vein and the remaining 20% oxygenated blood from the hepatic artery. Hepatocytes are the most abundant cell types inhabiting liver. Apart from that, it also contains sinusoidal Kupffer cells, endothelial cells, stellate cells and lymphocytes (Vollmar and Menger, 2009; Marques et al., 2015a).

As per the requirement of the study, liver IVM can be performed starting from a few hours to days (Ritsma et al., 2012; Park et al., 2018). The surgical procedure involves the opening of the abdominal cavity. A small part of right liver lobe is carefully exteriorized and placed on a handcraft stage (Marques et al., 2015b). Long term IVM requires installation of an observation window in the abdomen. Ritsma et al. (2012) developed a window model for long term liver IVM (up to 1 month) to study liver metastasis. The window is composed of a titanium ring along with a 1mm groove. The window is secured on an abdominal wall by a purse-string suture in the groove and a coverslip is placed on the top for imaging window (Ritsma et al., 2012).

Liver IVM has been used to investigate liver transplantation, liver regeneration, and therapeutics of liver disease or injury (Theruvath et al., 2008; Rehman et al., 2011; Czerny et al., 2012; Liu et al., 2015, 2017; Krishnasamy et al., 2019; Wimborne et al., 2020). Moreover, the liver IVM model has also been used to study hepatic transport (Dunn and Ryan, 2017; Ryan et al., 2018; Tavakoli et al., 2019), flow modulation in liver microvasculature (Clendenon et al., 2019a,b), bile dynamic and (Meyer et al., 2017) and enzyme regulation. Furthermore, this model is also utilized to investigate liver during IR injury, infections, sepsis, and endotoxemia (Vollmar et al., 1997; McAvoy et al., 2011; Lu et al., 2014; Park et al., 2018).

Dorsal Skinfold Chamber Model

The Dorsal skinfold chamber model is a widely used model for *in vivo* imaging. The chamber typically consists of two symmetrical metal frames. The frames contain a circular observation window. A double layer of depilated skin layer is sandwiched between these two frames. One of the layers of the skin along with subcutaneous tissue is removed completely in a circular area according to the diameter of the observation window. Then the circular coverslip is placed and fixed with the help of a snap ring (**Figure 3**). Titanium is the most commonly used metal to build the skinfold chamber but other varions from

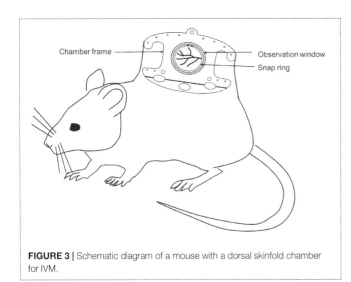

FIGURE 3 | Schematic diagram of a mouse with a dorsal skinfold chamber for IVM.

stainless steel or aluminum and non-metal materials are also used. The dorsal skinfold chamber model gives access to the striated muscle of the dorsal skin for IVM. After implanation, repetitive imaging can be performed up to 2–3 weeks (Schreiter et al., 2017; Dondossola et al., 2018; Hessenauer et al., 2018). It is suitable for both upright as well as inverted microscopes (Prunier et al., 2017).

The dorsal skinfold chamber has been extensively used in cancer biology to investigate tumor pathophysiology, tumor cell – microvasculature interaction, metastasis as well as therapy (Jain and Ward-Hartley, 1987; Jain et al., 2002; Alexander et al., 2013; Dondossola et al., 2018). It is also used to investigate the effect of chemical compounds on vascularization. Apart from that, the dorsal skinfold chamber model is also useful for studying interaction of biomaterials with surrounding host tissue, bacteria-endothelial cell interaction, organ transplantation, wound healing, fibrinolysis and thrombolysis, IR injury, inflammation, and sepsis (Laschke et al., 2011; Hillgruber et al., 2014; Miranda et al., 2015; Schreiter et al., 2017). The dorsal skinfold chamber is a widely accepted IVM model to investigate tissue angiogenesis and biocompatibility of biomaterials in tissue engineering.

Skull Cranial Window

The brain is the controlling unit of the entire body. Therefore, it is very important to understand brain physiology. *In vivo* imaging has become an important experimental tool to understand brain physiology and pathology. The brain is covered with a membrane known as the dura followed by two layers of compact cortical bone sandwiching a cancellous spongy bone layer (Yang et al., 2010; Zhao et al., 2018).

The brain can be accessed using two methods: open-skull or thinned-skull cranial window. As suggested by the name the thinned-skull cranial window is prepared by thinning of the skull bone layers with a drill. Controlled thinning is performed until the transparency for imaging is achieved without exposing the brain. On the other hand, in the open-skull window procedure, drilling is continued until all three bone layers are removed.

A coverslip is positioned on the dura and sealed with adhesive (**Figure 4**) (Dorand et al., 2014; Isshiki and Okabe, 2014).

Both methods have their merits and demerits. Thinned-skull window approach causes minimal perturbation and allows immediate imaging after surgery whereas in open-skull model a resting period of approximately 2 weeks is required before imaging. Moreover, the open-skull method is prone to cause higher inflammation, astrogliosis, and higher dendritic spine turnover due to a higher degree of perturbation. Thinned-skull window approaches require re-thinning for repeated imaging, which is not necessary for open-skull approaches. Furthermore, image quality in the thin-skull window is compromised at points deeper than 50 μm. Therefore, the open-skull window is preferred for deep high resolution imaging. Depending on the requirement both models can be used for chronic as well as acute studies (Yang et al., 2010; Dorand et al., 2014). Both models require highly skilled surgeons and the selection of the model can be done based on the aim and the duration of the study.

Transcranial imaging can be used to study Alzheimer's disease and potential treatments, brain injury, leukocyte-pathogen interaction and tumor dynamics in brain vasculature (Yang et al., 2010; Dorand et al., 2014; Isshiki and Okabe, 2014; Secklehner et al., 2017; Alieva et al., 2019).

DISCUSSION

Over the past decades, tissue engineering has made considerable progress in the field of tissue regeneration. Researchers are constantly applying novel approaches to understand tissue physiology in the normal and diseased state as well as regeneration or repair. 3D models closely resemble the native tissue environment. However, they cannot exactly mimic *in vivo* conditions where factors from the immediate and distant environment play an important role in maintaining tissue homeostasis (Kapałczyńska et al., 2018; Chen et al., 2019). Therefore, it is inevitable to perform *in vivo* studies. On the other hand, tissue repair or regeneration is a dynamic cellular process. Conventional *in vivo* studies are incapable to explain it thoroughly. Hence, performing IVM studies is the most appropriate approach for in depth understanding of tissue repair, regeneration, and cell interactions.

Researchers have developed different IVM models, which require surgical procedures to expose the area of interest and install a window or chamber. Cremaster muscle and skinfold chamber models are the most preferable models in terms of simplicity and reproducibility to visualize capillary perfusion and leukocyte–endothelial interaction under native condition and under treatment as well as during IR injury (**Figure 5**). Cremaster muscle IVM model imaging is limited from few hrs up to 3 days (Siemionow and Nanhekhan, 1999). Therefore, the dorsal skinfold chamber model is widely preferred for the long-term *in vivo* imaging.

The dorsal skinfold chamber is a key model to analyze different tissue engineering strategies for improving the vascularization of implanted biomaterials. Long term, repetitive evaluation of the same ROI, evaluation of complex immunological

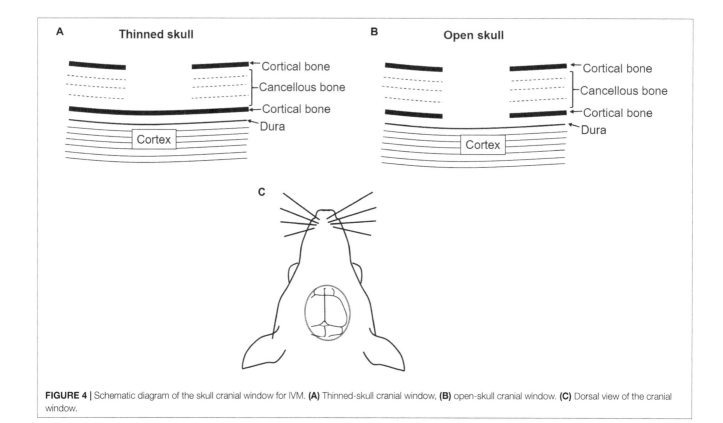

FIGURE 4 | Schematic diagram of the skull cranial window for IVM. **(A)** Thinned-skull cranial window, **(B)** open-skull cranial window. **(C)** Dorsal view of the cranial window.

phenomena is easily achieved. Kampmann et al. (2013) observed enhancement of PLGA scaffold vascularization upon application of Bone marrow-derived mesenchymal stem cells (bmMSCs) and VEGF. Reichel et al. (2015) investigated the effect of components of the Plasminogen Activation System on vascularization of porous polyethylene (PPE) implants. They observed accelerated vascularization in implants coated with urokinase-type plasminogen activator (uPA) and tissue plasminogen activator (tPA), plasminogen activator inhibitor-1 (PAI-1) (Reichel et al., 2015). Recently, improved vascularization of PPE implant coated with Vitronectin in skinfold chamber model was reported (Hessenauer et al., 2018). Adipose tissue-derived microvascular fragments (ad-MVF) contain high vascularization capacity that can be easily harvested from fat tissue. Frueh et al. (2017) seeded GFP$^+$ ad-MVF on collagen-glycosaminoglycan matrices and implanted them into full-thickness skin defects in the mice skinfold chamber. They observed significantly accelerated vascularization of the implants (Frueh et al., 2017). This strategy can be used for full-thickness skin defect treatment. In another experiment, Laschke et al. (2019) cultivated ad-MVF at 20°C and implanted it into dorsal skinfold chambers. They observed enhanced vascularization in sub normothermically cultivated ad-MVFs compared to normothermically cultivated ad-MVFs (Laschke et al., 2019).

The skinfold chamber can also be adapted to investigate the regeneration of transplanted tissue material. Lushaj et al. (2012) implanted neonatal atrial and ventricular tissues in the skinfolds chamber. This was the first successful attempt of ectopic engraftment of differentiated myocardium in the skinfold

chamber (Lushaj et al., 2012). In another experiment, Walser et al. (2013) implanted *in vitro* co-cultivated primary human osteoblasts and human dermal microvascular endothelial cells spheroids (HOB-HDMEC) into the skinfold chamber. They observed noticeable interconnection to the host microvasculature via the inosculation process. This strategy can be a very useful treatment of large bone tissue defects (Walser et al., 2013).

The dorsal skinfold chamber model is the most preferable model for investigation of biocompatibility and host reaction to different biomaterials. Jehn et al. (2020) compared the effects of mesenchymal stem cells (MSC) in combination with Poly-L-lactide-co-glycolide (PLGA) and beta-tricalcium phosphate (β-TCP) scaffold. They reported significant improvement in angiogenesis for β-TCP scaffolds compared with PLGA scaffolds (Jehn et al., 2020). Laschke et al. (2009) investigated *in vivo* biocompatibility and vascularization of porous polyurethane scaffolds. The scaffolds stimulated a weak angiogenic response after 14 days of implantation with low inflammatory reaction (Laschke et al., 2009). Gniesmer et al. (2020) studied chitosan-graft- polycaprolactone (CS-g-PCL) fiber mats for rotator cuff tear repair. Intravital investigation revealed significant increase in vascularisation in CS-g-PCL fiber mats compared to the porous polymer patch and uncoated PCL fiber mats on day 14 (Gniesmer et al., 2020). Dondossola et al. (2016) applied this model to examine foreign body response to 3D porous calcium phosphate-coated medical grade poly (ε-caprolactone) (mPCL-CaP) scaffolds. They observed a connection between giant cells and vascular endothelial growth factor (VEGF) induced neovessels as key factor stimulating the foreign body response

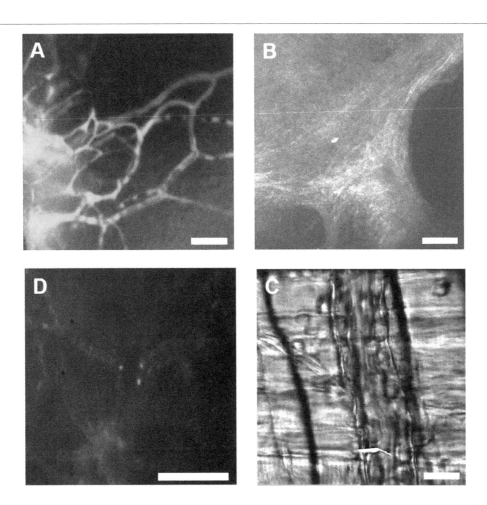

FIGURE 5 | Illustration of IVM images using different microscopy methods. **(A)** IVM image of FITC-Dextran labeled microvasculature in the skinfold chamber, scale bar: 100 μm. **(B)** 2 PM THG image of collagen in the skinfold chamber, scale bar: 100 μm. **(C)** IVM image showing leukocytes labeled with Rhodamine 6G in the skinfold chamber, scale bar: 100 μm. **(D)** RLOT image of the cremaster muscle, scale bar: 50 μm.

and late-stage fibrosis (Dondossola et al., 2016). The same group also used a skinfold chamber model to study tumor-bone interactions and therapeutic response. They implanted tissue-engineered bone constructs in prostate cancer lesions. They observed tumor growth inside the bone cavity and along the cortical bone interface. They also reported reduction in osteoclast kinetics and osteolysis on application of bisphosphonate therapy without perturbing tumor growth (Dondossola et al., 2018).

Moreover, Polstein et al. (2017) used optogenetics for controlling cell differentiation and tissue formation in the skinfold chamber. They used a light-inducible switch to control the expression of angiopoietin-1 and VEGF for stimulation of vascular sprouting in a mouse dorsal skinfold chamber (Polstein et al., 2017).

In the aforementioned studies, repetitive evolution of the same ROI (region of interest) was performed to examine a comprehensive picture of the dynamic process starting from recruitment of cells to formation of a vasculature network or inosculation of host vasculature in scaffolds within the very same alive animal. This is only possible in IVM. Moreover, IVM enables observation of the immediate and long-term response of

the native *in vivo* environment on the implantation of biomaterial in a live animal. The conventional approach for making similar observation requires termination of the experiment, extraction of the implant, and complex evaluation processes such as micro sectioning and staining. The harvesting and handling in this process itself can temper with final results. Imaging of dynamic cellular processes at multiple time points also reduces the requirement of total animals numbers for a particular study.

Skinfold chambers have also played an important role in cancer research and identification of key anti-tumor therapies. Yuan et al. (1995) used the skin fold chamber model to determine microvascular permeability in human tumor xenografts. Molecular size is one of the important determining factors for transvascular transportation of therapeutic agents in tumors. They concluded that liposomes of up to the diameter of 400 nm were permeable in human colon adenocarcinoma LS174T tumor vessels (Yuan et al., 1995). Vascular targeted therapies are showing promising results for cancer treatment. Several preclinical and clinical studies are reported which focus on blocking vasculature growth of the tumor. Savarin et al. (2018) monitored antiangiogenic or vascular disruptive effects of targeted gene and irradiation therapy from dorsal skin window. They observed a significant reduction in the tumor vessel area in animals receiving targeted gene treatment (Savarin et al., 2018). Haeger et al. (2019) determined that invading tumor cells survive DNA damage and radiotherapy via β1/αVβ3/β5 integrin crosstalk. Noticeably, effective radiosensitization can be accomplished by targeting multiple integrins (Haeger et al., 2019). Although, skin fold chamber is an excellent model for the cancer research, skin is not orthotopic location for all tumor types (Prunier et al., 2017).

The ability of reparative imaging provides an excellent opportunity to observe tumor cell metastasis and the effect of therapeutic treatment at several time points in real-time and in the same animal which is not possible in conventional cancer study designs (Condeelis and Segall, 2003).

Apart from the skinfold chamber, the skull cranial window is another important model for *in vivo* brain imaging. The skull cranial window model is more complex than the skinfold chamber. This model is very use full to study brain disease, injury and possible treatments (Yang et al., 2010; Dorand et al., 2014; Isshiki and Okabe, 2014; Secklehner et al., 2017; Alieva et al., 2019). Khosravi et al. (2018) used a cranial window chamber model to study angiogenesis and cellular events around surgical bone implants. Both cranial window and skinfold chamber models are widely used to study tumor development, cell–cell interaction, specific disease or injury and therapeutics (Upreti et al., 2011; Pai et al., 2014; Miranda et al., 2015; Reeves et al., 2015; Zhang et al., 2016; Ampofo et al., 2017; Tarantini et al., 2017; Alieva et al., 2019).

Intravital microscopy can be applied to study dynamic activities such as membrane trafficking. Endocytosis is a vital cellular process that plays an important role in the regulation of cell signaling, metabolism and motility. Moreover, the deregulation of the endocytic pathway is connected to infection, immunodeficiencies, neurodegeneration, and cancer (Ebrahim and Weigert, 2019). Molitoris group initiated an investigation of endosomal system dynamics in the kidney model. They applied multiphoton microscopy for *in vivo* imaging of uptake of systemically injected molecules such as fluorescent dextrans, folate receptors and albumin in the kidneys' proximal tubuli (Dunn et al., 2002; Sandoval et al., 2004). Recently, Kuwahara et al. (2016) revealed Megalin as a potential therapeutic target for metabolic syndrome-related chronic kidney disease. The kidney IVM model is used to understand the function of different receptors present in the renal system. Schießl et al. (2016a) used intravital microscopy to investigate the effects of the angiotensin II (Ang II) receptor on podocyte function. They demonstrated that Ang II enhances the endocytosis of albumin by podocytes that can result in impaired podocyte function (Schießl et al., 2016a). The higher amount of albumin in urine or Albuminuria is an indication of the kidney disease. The salivary glands IVM model evolved as a relatively simple model for membrane trafficking studies (Ebrahim and Weigert, 2019). Secretory cells contain secretory granules, which transport a variety of proteins. Shitara et al. (2020) demonstrated the role of Cdc42 GTPase in the biogenesis and/or maturation of these secretory granules. Membrane remodeling

is important for the regulation of different processes such as cell division, migration, and membrane trafficking that requires continuous modifications of the composition as well as the property of the lipid bilayer. Milberg et al. (2017) applied the salivary gland model to investigate the role of the actomyosin cytoskeleton in membrane remodeling. They reported that the actomyosin cytoskeleton serves as a scaffold for the recruitment of regulatory molecules and also provides necessary mechanical forces for remodeling the lipid bilayer (Milberg et al., 2017).

Hackl et al. (2013) used repeated MPM of the same glomeruli for imagining the motility of podocytes in the multi-color Pod-Confetti mouse model. They observed the appearance of a new podocyte within 24 h of the previous imaging session (Hackl et al., 2013). In a recent study, Schiessl et al. (2018) used MPM for evaluation of the cellular and molecular activities involved in renal proximal tubular regeneration. They observed proliferating tubular cells at the site of injury (Schiessl et al., 2018).

These above-mentioned dynamic portrayals of processes such as membrane trafficking and cellular motility are otherwise not possible in conventional study design without terminating the study at several timepoints.

The lung and heart are the most difficult organs for *in vivo* imaging because of continuous movement. Different methods for stabilization and software-based video editing methods are established (Presson et al., 2011; Matsuura et al., 2018). Lung IVM models are extensively used for imaging of immune cell trafficking, alveolar perfusion, and gaseous exchange. Oxygen uptake and carbon dioxide disposal is the primary function of the lung. Tabuchi et al. (2013) combined mice lung IVM along with two-dimensional oxygen saturation mapping to study pulmonary oxygen uptake. They demonstrated that 50% of total oxygen uptake takes place in precapillary arterioles of less than 30 μm in diameter before the blood enters the alveolar-capillary network (Tabuchi et al., 2013). In another similar study, they used the same methodology to study alveolar dynamics and local gas exchange in the healthy and diseased lung (Tabuchi et al., 2016). In a recent study, the role of neutrophils in a sepsis-induced lung injury model was investigated using combinations of fluorescent dyes and antibodies to differentiate leukocyte subsets. The acute lung injury decreased the functional capillary ratio due to the generation of dead space by prolonged neutrophil entrapment within lung capillaries (Park et al., 2019). Initial *in vivo* heart studies for leukocyte trafficking used heterotopic heart tissue transplantation due to inherent technical difficulties in imaging moving tissue (Li et al., 2012). Later Lee et al. (2012), introduced a two-photon method for intravital visualization of murine heart at subcellular resolution. Recently, novel cardiac stabilizers were established for imaging the beating native heart within the intrathoracic position in rats (Matsuura et al., 2018). They successfully managed real-time *in vivo* imaging of cardiac tissue dynamics under normal and IR conditions at subcellular resolution. They observed the subcellular dynamics of the myocardium and mitochondrial distribution in cardiac myocytes. They also observed IR injury induced suppression of the contraction/relaxation cycle and the resulting increase in cell permeability and leukocyte accumulation in cardiac tissue. Dynamics of immune cell trafficking immediately after events such as myocardial infarction is only possible in an IVM study design.

Liver IVM models have been used for the investigation of liver injury such as IR, and bacterial (*Mycobacterium bovis*, *Borrelia burgdorferi*, *acillus cereus*, and methicillin-resistant *Staphylococcus aureus*) and parasitic (*Plasmodium berghei*, *Leishmania donovani*, and *Schistosome granulomas*) infections and their treatment (Marques et al., 2015b). Acetaminophen is an antipyretic and analgesic drug. Recently, Hu et al. (2016) revealed that lower dosage of Acetaminophen induces reversible mitochondrial permeability resulting in mitochondrial dysfunction and steatosis in hepatocytes in the murine liver (Hu et al., 2016). Inhibition of the bile salt export pump (BSEP) is strongly connected to drug-mediated liver injury that commonly goes undetected during clinical testing. Ryan et al. (2018) used quantitative intravital microscopy to identify the dose-dependent effects of BSEP inhibitors. They used fluorescent bile salts as a biomarker for hepatobiliary transport inhibition. This model can provide valuable information on the toxic effects of the drug on human liver (Ryan et al., 2018). Dynamic processes such as cell–cell, cell–pathogen interaction, fluctuation in mitochondrial function, and bile transport can only be visualized in realtime using the IVM approach.

Imaging duration was one of the major limitations of IVM studies. Earlier models for abdominal organs were mainly acute. Ritsma et al. (2012) made a breakthrough in the area of the abdominal imaging window (AIW). They developed a window model for long-term liver IVM (up to 1 month) (Ritsma et al., 2012). Most of the current AIWs are designed and installed as described by Ritsma et al. (2012). Moreover, this window design can also be used to visualize internal organs such as the spleen, kidney, small intestine, pancreas, and liver. Perry et al. (2019) observed enhanced neovascularization and integration of pre-vascularized tissue-engineered muscle graft into abdominal wall defects compared to non-prevascularized grafts. Recently, Entenberg et al. (2018) developed a permanently implantable lung window that can be imagined for up to 2 weeks. Also, tissue regeneration is a dynamic and lengthy process that starts with the recruitment of immune cells following injury. Another imaging strategy for extension of the imaging period is the repeated externalization of organs or tissue (Hackl et al., 2013). However, surgical processes involved in repeated externalization of an organ can damage the organ of interest and delay the regeneration process or can lead to false results. Moreover, it is also prerequisite to keep organ or tissue wet and maintain the normal temperature during the surgical process. A precise experimental design is required for imaging of the entire regeneration process.

In most chamber or window models a glass coverslip is placed on the top of the tissue which can induce an inflammatory or immune response. Biocompatibility of the glass coverslip can be improved with PLL-g-PEG(poly-L-lysine-graft-poly(ethylene glycol)) coating (Ritsma et al., 2013). It is questionable if data collected from a small field can be extrapolated to the entire organ. Intravital microscopy provides high-resolution imaging of one small region that provides dynamic information of that spot only. For repeated analysis, it is important to identify the very same spot for the next microscopy. Hackl et al. (2013) used serial MPM imaging of the same glomerulus over time in the intact Pod-GFP mouse kidney. They identified Glomeruli based on a laser-induced mark placed close to the glomerulus (Hackl et al., 2013). For a better understanding of the dynamic process, imaging of more than 2 or 3 fields from a single animal is important. However, it can be difficult to fully correlate information because each field image contains small temporal heterogeneity. Here, it would be interesting to include a system that can collect data from multiple fields at the same time. However, imaging at lower magnification objectives such as 2.5× could be helpful because smaller magnification objectives provide a larger field of view than higher magnification objectives such as 25×. Though, lower magnification objectives can compromise the resolution (Dunn and Ryan, 2017).

The IVM studies are designed for imaging *in vivo* cellular dynamics. However, the surgical procedure involved during the experiment itself can interfere with the dynamics of cellular activity. Continuous exposure to light in different microscopic modalities is reported as phototoxic. Organs and tissues are a multicellular structural system. It is difficult to discriminate each cell type in one region. Here, *in vivo* imaging can be strengthened using different labeling strategies. Various approaches such as fluorescence dyes, fluorescence proteins and QDs are available. The specificity of these fluorescent probes can be increased using specific antibodies or antibody fragments. Discrimination of different cell types in one particular region can be achieved by combining one or more of the aforementioned strategies. For instance, GFP-positive animals can be injected with different cell marking dyes and marker antibodies at the same time (Dunn et al., 2002; Sandoval et al., 2004). Residual cell debris containing fluorescent proteins can result in unwanted background. Administration of all these substances can cause a toxic effect on the animal. Therefore, it is important to determine the optimal amount which exhibits minimum toxicity without interfering with the image quality. Moreover, some studies are designed for repeated *in vivo* imaging. Here, it is important to perform a preliminary study to determine the effect of long-term and repeated administration of these fluorescent probes.

From our own experience of animal studies and for both ethical and scientific reasons, it is very important to pay special attention to animal health. Animals need to be checked regularly for the overall health and healing of surgical areas. Many long-term windows or chamber installation requires placement of glass coverslips which are prone to break occasionally. Animals often tend to remove sutures placed to fix the chamber or window. Therefore, a regular check-up is necessary to prevent incidents that might affect the experiment outcome.

Penetration of depth is one of the major concerns for IVM studies. Conventional single-photon optical modalities such as epifluorescence and confocal microscopy can reach up to around $100\,\mu m$ of depth only. Compared to conventional to one-photon confocal microscopy, 2 PM can improve the depth of penetration by a factor of 2 to 3 (Kobat et al., 2011). Theer et al. (2003) used a 800 nm excitation source by using a Ti: Sapphire regenerative amplifier. They could achieve 1 mm imaging depth in the mouse brain. Later, Kobat et al. (2011) used 1,280-nm excitation to achieve a remarkable penetration depth of approximately 1.6 mm in the cortex of a mouse brain. However, in 2 PM light scattering and absorption of tissue limit the penetration depth and both of these are dependent on excitation wavelength (Miller et al., 2017). In 2 PM microscopy, the highest imaging depth is determined by the ability of excitation light to hit the focus point unscattered as well as the released fluorescence to reach the detector (Kobat et al., 2011). Horton et al. (2013) developed a revolutionary system in the field of 3 PM. They used 3 PM to imaging of subcortical structures within an intact mouse brain. In 3 PM, 1,700 nm excitation source was used. Application of longer excitation wavelength reduces the attenuation of excitation light by the tissue. Moreover, 3PE significantly reduces the out-of-focus background and improves the signal to background ratio. In the preliminary 3PM experiments, vascular and neuronal structures in the mouse brain at ∼1.3 mm depth were imagined (Horton et al., 2013). Certainly, 3 PM has the potential to play a game-changing role in the field of IVM. Current 3 PM applications are largely limited to brain IVM (Horton et al., 2013; Wang T. et al., 2018). Application of innovative microscopic methods on other organs such as heart, lung, and kidney can achieve previously unmet penetration depth. Though, the establishment of an advanced imagining system requires more money and optimization initially, once established it can uncover dynamic activities deep inside the tissue that was hidden so far.

Overall, suitable selection and application of advanced optical modalities with fluorescence tagging methodologies in IVM can enable in-depth analysis of the tissue in healthy and diseased state, tissue development, repair and biomaterial compatibility as well as host reactions on implantation. It can also provide essential information at the level of cell–cell interactions and facilitate the development of potential treatments for complex diseases such as cancer and Alzheimer.

SUMMARY/CONCLUSION

Intravital microscopy provides information at the cellular and molecular level in different dynamic complex processes. It can be performed in both acute as well as chronic settings using windows or chambers. Advancement in microscopy and fluorescent markers have changed the direction of IVM. IVM provides useful information to understand physiology and cellular interaction. It can be applied to disease models for exploring new therapeutic approaches. Selection of the right model and suitable microscopic methods are very important points to be considered. Respiration and heart beating pose problems in imaging of upper extremity organs such as heart and lung. Deep tissue imaging is possible via multiphoton microscopy. However, there is still scope for development in further deep tissue imaging and application of advanced microscopic tool such as 3 PM for deep *in vivo* imaging of organs such as lung, liver, heart, kidney, and spleen.

Intravital microscopy is a promising approach to investigate host reactions on implanted biomaterials (Dondossola et al., 2016; Gniesmer et al., 2020; Jehn et al., 2020). IVM models for different organs have already been developed but most models are currently used to analyze organ specific dynamic processes during the healthy or diseased state. The majority of current IVM experiments can be adapted to improve tissue engineering strategies. IVM has great potential to improve and expand the boundaries of regenerative medicine. Considering all the advantages of IVM, it would be beneficial to keep developing and applying IVM models compatible with tissue engineering experiments in order to gain deeper insight in angiogenesis, inflammation and immunologic processes in tissue engineering.

AUTHOR CONTRIBUTIONS

RV, AA, RH, and MH wrote the manuscript. All authors contributed to the article and approved the submitted version.

REFERENCES

1. Aguirre, A. D., Vinegoni, C., Sebas, M., and Weissleder, R. (2014). Intravital imaging of cardiac function at the single-cell level. *PNAS* 111, 11257–11262. doi: 10.1073/pnas.1401316111

2. Ahmadzadeh, N., Robering, J. W., Kengelbach-Weigand, A., Al-Abboodi, M., Beier, J. P., Horch, R. E., et al. (2020). Human adipose-derived stem cells support lymphangiogenesis in vitro by secretion of lymphangiogenic factors. *Exp. Cell Res.* 388:111816. doi: 10.1016/j.yexcr.2020.111816

3. Al-Abboodi, M., An, R., Weber, M., Schmid, R., Klausing, A., Horch, R. E., et al. (2019). Tumor-type-dependent effects on the angiogenic abilities of endothelial cells in an in vitro rat cell model. *Oncol. Rep.* 42, 350–360. doi: 10.3892/or.2019.7143

4. Alexander, S., Weigelin, B., Winkler, F., and Friedl, P. (2013). Preclinical intravital microscopy of the tumour-stroma interface: invasion, metastasis, and therapy response. *Curr. Opin. Cell Biol.* 25, 659–671. doi: 10.1016/j.ceb.2013.07.001

5. Alieva, M., Leidgens, V., Riemenschneider, M. J., Klein, C. A., Hau, P., and van Rheenen, J. (2019). Intravital imaging of glioma border morphology reveals distinctive cellular dynamics and contribution to tumor cell invasion. *Sci. Rep.* 9:2054. doi: 10.1038/s41598-019-38625-4

6. Ampofo, E., Lachnitt, N., Rudzitis-Auth, J., Schmitt, B. M., Menger, M. D., and Laschke, M. W. (2017). Indole-3-carbinol is a potent inhibitor of ischemia-reperfusion–induced inflammation. *J. Surg. Res.* 215, 34–46. doi: 10.1016/j.jss.2017.03.019

7. Bagher, P., and Segal, S. S. (2011). The mouse cremaster muscle preparation for intravital imaging of the microcirculation. *J. Vis. Exp.* 52:e2874. doi: 10.3791/ 2874

8. Bai, C., Yu, X., Peng, T., Liu, C., Min, J., Dan, D., et al. (2020). 3D imaging restoration of spinning-disk confocal microscopy via deep learning. *IEEE Photon. Technol. Lett.* 32, 1131–1134. doi: 10.1109/LPT.2020.3014317

9. Bajpai, G., Bredemeyer, A., Li, W., Zaitsev, K., Koenig, A. L., Lokshina, I., et al. (2019). Tissue resident CCR2- and CCR2+ cardiac macrophages differentially orchestrate monocyte recruitment and fate specification following myocardial injury. *Circ. Res.* 124, 263–278. doi: 10.1161/CIRCRESAHA.118. 314028

10. Caravagna, C., Jaouën, A., Debarbieux, F., and Rougon, G. (2016). Overview of innovative mouse models for imaging neuroinflammation. *Curr. Protoc. Mouse Biol.* 6, 131–147. doi: 10.1002/cpmo.5

11. Chan, K. T., Jones, S. W., Brighton, H. E., Bo, T., Cochran, S. D., Sharpless, N. E., et al. (2013). Intravital imaging of a spheroid-based orthotopic model of melanoma in the mouse ear skin. *Intravital* 2:e25805. doi: 10.4161/intv.25805

12. Chen, L., Mou, S., Li, F., Zeng, Y., Sun, Y., Horch, R. E., et al. (2019). Self-assembled human adipose-derived stem cell-derived extracellular vesicle-functionalized biotin-doped polypyrrole titanium with long-term stability and potential osteoinductive ability. *ACS Appl. Mater. Interfaces* 11, 46183–46196. doi: 10. 1021/acsami.9b17015

13. Clendenon, S. G., Fu, X., Von Hoene, R. A., Clendenon, J. L., Sluka, J. P., Winfree, S., et al. (2019a). A simple automated method for continuous fieldwise measurement of microvascular hemodynamics. *Microvasc. Res.* 123, 7–13. doi: 10.1016/j.mvr.2018.11.010

14. Clendenon, S. G., Fu, X., Von Hoene, R. A., Clendenon, J. L., Sluka, J. P., Winfree, S., et al. (2019b). Spatial temporal analysis of fieldwise flow in microvasculature. *J. Vis. Exp.* 183. doi: 10.3791/60493

15. Condeelis, J., and Segall, J. E. (2003). Intravital imaging of cell movement in tumours. *Nat. Revi. Cancer* 3, 921–930. doi: 10.1038/nrc1231

16. Condeelis, J., and Weissleder, R. (2010). In vivo imaging in cancer. *Cold Spring Harb. Perspect. Biol.* 2:a003848. doi: 10.1101/cshperspect.a003848

17. Cortez-Retamozo, V., Etzrodt, M., Newton, A., Rauch, P. J., Chudnovskiy, A., Berger, C., et al. (2012). Origins of tumor-associated macrophages and neutrophils. *PNAS* 109, 2491–2496. doi: 10.1073/pnas.1113744109

18. Czerny, C., Kholmukhamedov, A., Theruvath, T. P., Maldonado, E. N., Ramshesh, V. K., Lehnert, M., et al. (2012). Minocycline decreases liver injury after hemorrhagic shock and resuscitation in mice. *HPB Surg.* 2012:259512. doi: 10.1155/2012/259512

19. Deniset, J. F., Surewaard, B. G., Lee, W.-Y., and Kubes, P. (2017). Splenic Ly6Ghigh mature and Ly6Gint immature neutrophils contribute to eradication of S. pneumoniae. *J. Exp. Med.* 214, 1333–1350. doi: 10.1084/jem.20161621

20. Devi, S., Li, A., Westhorpe, C. L. V., Lo, C. Y., Abeynaike, L. D., Snelgrove, S. L., et al. (2013). Multiphoton imaging reveals a new leukocyte recruitment paradigm in the glomerulus. *Nat. Med.* 19, 107–112. doi: 10.1038/nm.3024

21. Dondossola, E., Holzapfel, B. M., Alexander, S., Filippini, S., Hutmacher, D. W., and Friedl, P. (2016). Examination of the foreign body response to biomaterials by nonlinear intravital microscopy. *Nat. Biomed. Eng.* 1:0007. doi: 10.1038/s41551- 016-0007

22. Dondossola, E., Alexander, S., Holzapfel, B. M., Filippini, S., Starbuck, M. W., Hoffman, R. M., et al. (2018). Intravital microscopy of osteolytic progression and therapy response of cancer lesions in the bone. *Sci. Transl. Med.* 10:eaao572. doi: 10.1126/scitranslmed.aao5726

23. Donndorf, P., Ludwig, M., Wildschütz, F., Useini, D., Kaminski, A., Vollmar, B., et al. (2013). Intravital microscopy of the microcirculation in the mouse cremaster muscle for the analysis of peripheral stem cell migration. *J. Vis. Exp.* 81:50485. doi: 10.3791/50485

24. Dorand, R. D., Barkauskas, D. S., Evans, T. A., Petrosiute, A., and Huang, A. Y. (2014). Comparison of intravital thinned skull and cranial window approaches to study CNS immunobiology in the mouse cortex. *Intravital* 3:e29728. doi: 10.4161/intv.29728

25. Dunn, K. W., and Ryan, J. C. (2017). Using quantitative intravital multiphoton microscopy to dissect hepatic transport in rats. *Methods* 128, 40–51. doi: 10.1016/j.ymeth.2017.04.015

26. Dunn, K. W., Sandoval, R. M., Kelly, K. J., Dagher, P. C., Tanner, G. A., Atkinson, S. J., et al. (2002). Functional studies of the kidney of living animals using multicolor two-photon microscopy. *Am. J. Physiol. Cell Physiol.* 283, C905–C916. doi: 10.1152/ajpcell.00159.2002

27. Dunn, K. W., Sutton, T. A., and Sandoval, R. M. (2007). Live-animal imaging of renal function by multiphoton microscopy. *Curr. Protoc. Cytom.* Chapter 12:Unit12.9. doi: 10.1002/0471142956.cy1209s41

28. Duval, K., Grover, H., Han, L.-H., Mou, Y., Pegoraro, A. F., Fredberg, J., et al. (2017). Modeling physiological events in 2D vs. 3D cell culture. *Physiology* 32, 266–277. doi: 10.1152/physiol.00036.2016

29. Ebrahim, S., and Weigert, R. (2019). Intravital microscopy in mammalian multicellular organisms. *Curr. Opin. Cell Biol.* 59, 97–103. doi: 10.1016/j. ceb. 2019.03.015

30. Eichhorn, M. E., Ney, L., Massberg, S., and Goetz, A. E. (2002). Platelet kinetics in the pulmonary microcirculation in vivo assessed by intravital microscopy. *J. Vasc. Res.* 39, 330–339. doi: 10.1159/000065545

31. Entenberg, D., Voiculescu, S., Guo, P., Borriello, L., Wang, Y., Karagiannis, G. S., et al. (2018). A permanent window for the murine lung enables high-resolution imaging of cancer metastasis. *Nat. Methods* 15, 73–80. doi: 10.1038/nmeth.4511

32. Ferrer, M., Martin-Jaular, L., Calvo, M., and del Portillo, H. A. (2012). Intravital microscopy of the spleen: quantitative analysis of parasite mobility and blood flow. *J. Vis. Exp.* 59:3609. doi: 10.3791/3609

33. Fiole, D., and Tournier, J.-N. (2016). Intravital microscopy of the lung: minimizing invasiveness. *J. Biophotonics* 9, 868–878. doi: 10.1002/jbio.201500246

34. Frueh, F. S., Später, T., Lindenblatt, N., Calcagni, M., Giovanoli, P., Scheuer, C., et al. (2017). Adipose tissue-derived microvascular fragments improve vascularization, lymphangiogenesis, and integration of dermal skin substitutes. *J. Invest. Dermatol.* 137, 217–227. doi: 10.1016/j.jid.2016.08.010

35. Fuhrmann, M., Bittner, T., Jung, C. K. E., Burgold, S., Page, R. M., Mitteregger, G., et al. (2010). Microglial Cx3cr1 knockout prevents neuron loss in a mouse model of alzheimer's disease. *Nat. Neurosci.* 13, 411–413. doi: 10.1038/nn.2511

36. Gniesmer, S., Brehm, R., Hoffmann, A., de Cassan, D., Menzel, H., Hoheisel, A. L., et al. (2020). Vascularization and biocompatibility of poly(ε-caprolactone) fiber mats for rotator cuff tear repair. *PLoS One* 15:e0227563. doi: 10.1371/journal.pone.0227563

37. Hackl, M. J., Burford, J. L., Villanueva, K., Lam, L., Suszták, K., Schermer, B., et al. (2013). Tracking the fate of glomerular epithelial cells in vivo using serial multiphoton imaging in new mouse models with fluorescent lineage tags. *Nat. Med.* 19, 1661–1666. doi: 10.1038/nm.3405

38. Hadjantonakis, A.-K., Dickinson, M. E., Fraser, S. E., and Papaioannou, V. E. (2003). Technicolour transgenics: imaging tools for functional genomics in the mouse. *Nat. Rev. Genet.* 4, 613–625. doi: 10.1038/nrg1126

39. Haeger, A., Alexander, S., Vullings, M., Kaiser, F. M. P., Veelken, C., Flucke, U., et al. (2019). Collective cancer invasion forms an integrin-dependent radioresistant niche. *J. Exp. Med.* 217:e20181184. doi: 10.1084/jem.20181184

40. Hall, A. M., Rhodes, G. J., Sandoval, R. M., Corridon, P. R., and Molitoris, B. A. (2013). In vivo multiphoton imaging of mitochondrial structure and function during acute kidney injury. *Kidney Int.* 83, 72–83. doi: 10.1038/ki.2012.328

41. Hato, T., Winfree, S., and Dagher, P. C. (2018). Kidney Imaging: – Intravital Microscopy. *Methods Mol. Biol.* 1763, 129–136. doi: 10.1007/978-1-4939-7762-8_12

42. Hessenauer, M. E. T., Lauber, K., Zuchtriegel, G., Uhl, B., Hussain, T., Canis, M., et al. (2018). Vitronectin promotes the vascularization of porous polyethylene biomaterials. *Acta Biomater.* 82, 24–33. doi: 10.1016/j.actbio.2018.10.004

43. Hillgruber, C., Steingräber, A. K., Pöppelmann, B., Denis, C. V., Ware, J., Vestweber, D., et al. (2014). Blocking von willebrand factor for treatment of cutaneous inflammation. *J. Invest. Dermatol.* 134, 77–86. doi: 10.1038/jid.2013. 292

44. Horch, R. E., Weigand, A., Wajant, H., Groll, J., Boccaccini, A. R., and Arkudas, A. (2018). [Biofabrication: new approaches for tissue regeneration]. *Handchir Mikrochir Plast Chir.* 50, 93–100. doi: 10.1055/s-0043-124674

45. Horton, N. G., Wang, K., Kobat, D., Clark, C. G., Wise, F. W., Schaffer, C. B., et al. (2013). In vivo three-photon microscopy of subcortical structures within an intact mouse brain. *Nat. Photonics* 7, 205–209. doi: 10.1038/nphoton.2012.336

46. Hu, J., Ramshesh, V. K., McGill, M. R., Jaeschke, H., and Lemasters, J. J. (2016). Low dose acetaminophen induces reversible mitochondrial dysfunction associated with transient c-Jun N-Terminal kinase activation in mouse liver. *Toxicol. Sci.* 150, 204–215. doi: 10.1093/toxsci/kfv319

47. Isshiki, M., and Okabe, S. (2014). Evaluation of cranial window types for in vivo two-photon imaging of brain microstructures. *Microscopy* 63, 53–63. doi: 10. 1093/jmicro/dft043

48. Jain, R. K., Munn, L. L., and Fukumura, D. (2002). Dissecting tumour pathophysiology using intravital microscopy. *Nat. Rev. Cancer* 2, 266–276. doi: 10.1038/nrc778

49. Jain, R. K., and Ward-Hartley, K. A. (1987). Dynamics of cancer cell interactions with microvasculature and interstitium. *Biorheology* 24, 117–125. doi: 10.3233/ bir-1987-24205

50. Jehn, P., Winterboer, J., Kampmann, A., Zimmerer, R., Spalthoff, S., Dittmann, J., et al. (2020). Angiogenic effects of mesenchymal stem cells in combination with different scaffold materials. *Microvasc. Res.* 127:103925. doi: 10.1016/j.mvr. 2019.103925

51. Jin, S., Hu, Y., Gu, Z., Liu, L., and Wu, H.-C. (2011). Application of quantum dots in biological imaging. *J. Nanomater.* 2011:e834139. doi: 10.1155/2011/834139

52. Jonkman, J. E., and Cm, B. (2015). Any way you slice it-a comparison of confocal microscopy techniques. *J. Biomol. Tech.* 26, 54–65. doi: 10.7171/jbt.15-26 02-003

53. Kampmann, A., Lindhorst, D., Schumann, P., Zimmerer, R., Kokemüller, H., Rücker, M., et al. (2013). Additive effect of mesenchymal stem cells and VEGF to vascularization of PLGA scaffolds. *Microvasc. Res.* 90, 71–79. doi: 10.1016/j. mvr.2013.07.006

54. Kapałczyńska, M., Kolenda, T., Przybyła, W., Zajączkowska, M., Teresiak, A., Filas, V., et al. (2018). 2D and 3D cell cultures – a comparison of different types of cancer cell cultures. *Arch. Med. Sci.* 14, 910–919. doi: 10.5114/ aoms.2016.63743

55. Kawakami, N. (2016). In vivo imaging in autoimmune diseases in the central nervous system. *Allergol. Int.* 65, 235–242. doi: 10.1016/j.alit.2016.02.001

56. Kengelbach-Weigand, A., Tasbihi, K., Strissel, P. L., Schmid, R., Marques, J. M., Beier, J. P., et al. (2019). Plasticity of patient-matched normal mammary epithelial cells is dependent on autologous adipose-derived stem cells. *Sci. Rep.* 9:10722. doi: 10.1038/s41598-019-47224-2

57. Khosravi, N., Mendes, V. C., Nirmal, G., Majeed, S., DaCosta, R. S., and Davies, J. E. (2018). Intravital imaging for tracking of angiogenesis and cellular events around surgical bone implants. *Tissue Eng. Part C Methods* 24, 617–627. doi: 10.1089/ten.tec.2018.0252

58. Kobat, D., Horton, N., and Xu, C. (2011). In vivo two-photon microscopy to 1.6- mm depth in mouse cortex. *J. Biomed.Opt.* 16:106014. doi: 10.1117/1.3646209

59. Kreisel, D., Nava, R. G., Li, W., Zinselmeyer, B. H., Wang, B., Lai, J., et al. (2010). In vivo two-photon imaging reveals monocyte-dependent neutrophil extravasation during pulmonary inflammation. *PNAS* 107, 18073–18078. doi: 10.1073/pnas.1008737107

60. Krishnasamy, Y., Gooz, M., Li, L., Lemasters, J. J., and Zhong, Z. (2019). Role of mitochondrial depolarization and disrupted mitochondrial homeostasis in non-alcoholic steatohepatitis and fibrosis in mice. *Int. J. Physiol. Pathophysiol. Pharmacol.* 11, 190–204.

61. Kuwahara, S., Hosojima, M., Kaneko, R., Aoki, H., Nakano, D., Sasagawa, T., et al. (2016). Megalin-mediated tubuloglomerular alterations in high-fat diet– induced kidney disease. *J. Am. Soc. Nephrol.* 27, 1996–2008. doi: 10.1681/ASN. 2015020190

62. Laschke, M. W., Heß, A., Scheuer, C., Karschnia, P., and Menger, M. D. (2019). Subnormothermic short-term cultivation improves the vascularization capacity of adipose tissue-derived microvascular fragments. *J. Tissue Eng. Regen. Med.* 13, 131–142. doi: 10.1002/term.2774

63. Laschke, M. W., Strohe, A., Scheuer, C., Eglin, D., Verrier, S., Alini, M., et al. (2009). In vivo biocompatibility and vascularization of biodegradable porous polyurethane scaffolds for tissue engineering. *Acta Biomater.* 5, 1991–2001. doi: 10.1016/j.actbio.2009.02.006

64. Laschke, M. W., Vollmar, B., and Menger, M. D. (2011). The dorsal skinfold chamber: window into the dynamic interaction of biomaterials with their surrounding host tissue. *Eur. Cell Mater.* 22, 147–164. discussion 164-167.

65. Lee, S., Nakamura, Y., Yamane, K., Toujo, T., Takahashi, S., Tanikawa, Y., et al. (2008). Image stabilization for in vivo microscopy by high-speed visual feedback control. *IEEE Trans. Rob.* 24, 45–54. doi: 10.1109/TRO.2007.914847

66. Lee, S., Vinegoni, C., Feruglio, P. F., Fexon, L., Gorbatov, R., Pivoravov, M., et al. (2012). Real-time in vivo imaging of the beating mouse heart at microscopic resolution. *Nat. Commun.* 3:1054. doi: 10.1038/ncomms2060

67. Lee, W. -Y., Sanz, M. -J., Wong, C. H. Y., Hardy, P. -O., Salman-Dilgimen, A., Moriarty, T. J., et al. (2014). Invariant natural killer T cells act as an extravascular cytotoxic barrier for joint-invading lyme borrelia. *Proc. Natl. Acad. Sci. U. S. A.* 111, 13936–13941. doi: 10.1073/pnas.1404769111

68. Lemaster, K. A., Farid, Z., Brock, R. W., Shrader, C. D., Goldman, D., Jackson, D. N., et al. (2017). Altered post-capillary and collecting venular reactivity in skeletal muscle with metabolic syndrome. *J. Physiol.* 595, 5159–5174. doi: 10.1113/JP274291

69. Li, W., Nava, R. G., Bribriesco, A. C., Zinselmeyer, B. H., Spahn, J. H., Gelman, A. E., et al. (2012). Intravital 2-photon imaging of leukocyte trafficking in beating heart. *J. Clin. Invest.* 122, 2499–2508. doi: 10.1172/JCI62970

70. Liu, Q., Rehman, H., Krishnasamy, Y., Lemasters, J. J., and Zhong, Z. (2017). 8-pCPT-cGMP prevents mitochondrial depolarization and improves the outcome of steatotic partial liver transplantation. *Int. J. Physiol. Pathophysiol. Pharmacol.* 9, 69–83.

71. Liu, Q., Rehman, H., Krishnasamy, Y., Schnellmann, R. G., Lemasters, J. J., and Zhong, Z. (2015). Improvement of liver injury and survival by JNK2 and iNOS deficiency in liver transplants from cardiac death mice. *J. Hepatol.* 63, 68–74. doi: 10.1016/j.jhep.2015.02.017

72. Looney, M. R., and Bhattacharya, J. (2014). Live imaging of the lung. *Annu. Rev. Physiol.* 76, 431–445. doi: 10.1146/annurev-physiol-021113-170331

73. Looney, M. R., Thornton, E. E., Sen, D., Lamm, W. J., Glenny, R. W., and Krummel, M. F. (2011). Stabilized imaging of immune surveillance in the mouse lung. *Nat/ Methods* 8, 91–96. doi: 10.1038/nmeth.1543

74. Lu, H.-H., Wu, Y.-M., Chang, W.-T., Luo, T., Yang, Y.-C., Cho, H.-D., et al. (2014). Molecular imaging of ischemia and reperfusion in vivo with mitochondrial autofluorescence. *Anal. Chem.* 86, 5024–5031. doi: 10.1021/ac5006469

75. Ludolph, I., Cai, A., Arkudas, A., Lang, W., Rother, U., and Horch, R. E. (2019). Indocyanine green angiography and the old question of vascular autonomy - Long term changes of microcirculation in microsurgically transplanted free flaps. *Clin. Hemorheol. Microcirc.* 72, 421–430. doi: 10.3233/CH-180544

76. Lushaj, E. B., Hu, J., Haworth, R., and Lozonschi, L. (2012). Intravital microscopy to study myocardial engraftment. *Interact. Cardiovasc. Thorac. Surg.* 15, 5–9. doi: 10.1093/icvts/ivs093

77. Marques, P. E., Antunes, M. M., David, B. A., Pereira, R. V., Teixeira, M. M., and Menezes, G. B. (2015a). Imaging liver biology *in vivo* using conventional confocal microscopy. *Nat. Protoc.* 10, 258–268. doi: 10.1038/ nprot.2015.006

78. Marques, P. E., Oliveira, A. G., Chang, L., Paula-Neto, H. A., and Menezes, G. B. (2015b). Understanding liver immunology using intravital microscopy. *J. Hepatol.* 63, 733–742. doi: 10.1016/j.jhep.2015.05.027

79. Martin-Jaular, L., Ferrer, M., Calvo, M., Rosanas-Urgell, A., Kalko, S., Graewe, S., et al. (2011). Strain-specific spleen remodelling in Plasmodium yoelii infections in Balb/c mice facilitates adherence and spleen macrophage-clearance escape. *Cell. Microbiol.* 13, 109–122. doi: 10.1111/j.1462-5822.2010.01523.x

80. Masedunskas, A., Milberg, O., Porat-Shliom, N., Sramkova, M., Wigand, T., Amornphimoltham, P., et al. (2012). Intravital microscopy: a practical guide on imaging intracellular structures in live animals. *Bioarchitecture* 2, 143–157. doi: 10.4161/bioa.21758

81. Masedunskas, A., Porat-Shliom, N., Tora, M., Milberg, O., and Weigert, R. (2013a). Intravital microscopy for imaging subcellular structures in live mice expressing fluorescent proteins. *J. Vis. Exp.* 1:50558. doi: 10.3791/50558

82. Masedunskas, A., Sramkova, M., Parente, L., and Weigert, R. (2013b). Intravital microscopy to image membrane trafficking in live rats. *Methods Mol. Biol.* 931, 153–167. doi: 10.1007/978-1-62703-056-4_9

83. Matsuura, R., Miyagawa, S., Fukushima, S., Goto, T., Harada, A., Shimozaki, Y., et al. (2018). Intravital imaging with two-photon microscopy reveals cellular dynamics in the ischeamia-reperfused rat heart. *Sci. Rep.* 8:15991. doi: 10.1038/ s41598-018-34295-w

84. McAvoy, E. F., McDonald, B., Parsons, S. A., Wong, C. H., Landmann, R., and Kubes, P. (2011). The role of CD14 in neutrophil recruitment within the liver microcirculation during endotoxemia. *J. Immunol.* 186, 2592–2601. doi: 10. 4049/jimmunol.1002248

85. Megens, R. T. A., Reitsma, S., Prinzen, L., Egbrink, M. G. A. O., Engels, W., Leenders, P. J. A., et al. (2010). In vivo high-resolution structural imaging of large arteries in small rodents using two-photon laser scanning microscopy. *JBO* 15:011108. doi: 10.1117/1.3281672

86. Mempel, T. R., Moser, C., Hutter, J., Kuebler, W. M., and Krombach, F. (2003). Visualization of leukocyte transendothelial and interstitial migration using reflected light oblique transillumination in intravital video microscopy. *JVR* 40, 435–441. doi: 10.1159/000073902

87. Meyer, K., Ostrenko, O., Bourantas, G., Morales-Navarrete, H., Porat-Shliom, N., Segovia-Miranda, F., et al. (2017). A predictive 3D multi-scale model of biliary fluid dynamics in the liver lobule. *Cell Syst.* 4, 277.e9–290.e9. doi: 10.1016/j.cels. 2017.02.008

88. Milberg, O., Shitara, A., Ebrahim, S., Masedunskas, A., Tora, M., Tran, D. T., et al. (2017). Concerted actions of distinct nonmuscle myosin II isoforms drive intracellular membrane remodeling in live animals. *J. Cell Biol.* 216, 1925–1936. doi: 10.1083/jcb.201612126

89. Miller, D. R., Jarrett, J. W., Hassan, A. M., and Dunn, A. K. (2017). Deep tissue imaging with multiphoton fluorescence microscopy. *Curr. Opin. Biomed. Eng.* 4, 32–39. doi: 10.1016/j.cobme.2017.09.004

90. Minsky, M. (1988). Memoir on inventing the confocal scanning microscope. *Scanning* 10, 128–138. doi: 10.1002/sca.4950100403

91. Miranda, M. L., Balarini, M. M., and Bouskela, E. (2015). Dexmedetomidine attenuates the microcirculatory derangements evoked by experimental sepsis. *Anesthes* 122, 619–630. doi: 10.1097/ALN.0000000000000491

92. Molski, M., Yazici, I., and Siemionow, M. Z. (2015). "Standard cremaster muscle model for ischemia reperfusion," in *Plastic and Reconstructive Surgery: Experimental Models and Research Designs*, ed. M. Z. Siemionow (London: Springer London), 83–88. doi: 10.1007/978-1-4471-6335-0_9

93. Montet, X., Montet-Abou, K., Reynolds, F., Weissleder, R., and Josephson, L. (2006). Nanoparticle imaging of integrins on tumor cells. *Neoplasia* 8, 214–222. doi: 10.1593/neo.05769

94. Mulder, W. J. M., Castermans, K., van Beijnum, J. R., Egbrink, M. G. A. O., Chin, P. T. K., Fayad, Z. A., et al. (2009). Molecular imaging of tumor angiogenesis using αvβ3-integrin targeted multimodal quantum dots. *Angiogenesis* 12, 17– 24. doi: 10.1007/s10456-008-9124-2

95. Neupane, A. S., Willson, M., Chojnacki, A. K., Vargas, E., Silva Castanheira, F., Morehouse, C., et al. (2020). Patrolling alveolar macrophages conceal bacteria from the immune system to maintain homeostasis. *Cell* 183, 110. e11–125.e11. doi: 10.1016/j.cell.2020.08.020

96. Ouzounov, D. G., Wang, T., Wang, M., Feng, D. D., Horton, N. G., Cruz-Hernández, J. C., et al. (2017). In vivo three-photon imaging of activity of GCaMP6-labeled neurons deep in intact mouse brain. *Nat. Methods* 14, 388– 390. doi: 10.1038/nmeth.4183

97. Pai, S., Qin, J., Cavanagh, L., Mitchell, A., El-Assaad, F., Jain, R., et al. (2014). Real- time imaging reveals the dynamics of leukocyte behaviour during experimental cerebral malaria pathogenesis. *PLoS Pathog.* 10:e1004236. doi: 10.1371/journal. ppat.1004236

98. Park, I., Kim, M., Choe, K., Song, E., Seo, H., Hwang, Y., et al. (2019). Neutrophils disturb pulmonary microcirculation in sepsis-induced acute lung injury. *Eur. Respir. J.* 53:1800786. doi: 10.1183/13993003.00786-2018

99. Park, S. A., Choe, Y. H., Lee, S. H., and Hyun, Y.-M. (2018). Two-photon Intravital imaging of leukocytes during the immune response in lipopolysaccharide-treated mouse liver. *J. Vis. Exp.* 132:e57191. doi: 10.3791/57191

100. Patel, M., and Fisher, J. P. (2008). Biomaterial scaffolds in pediatric tissue engineering. *Pediatr. Res.* 63, 497–501. doi: 10.1203/01. PDR.0b013e318165eb3e

101. Perlman, C. E., and Bhattacharya, J. (2007). Alveolar expansion imaged by optical sectioning microscopy. *J. Appl. Physiol.* 103, 1037–1044. doi: 10.1152 japplphysiol.00160.2007

102. Perry, L., Merdler, U., Elishaev, M., and Levenberg, S. (2019). Enhanced host neovascularization of prevascularized engineered muscle following transplantation into immunocompetent versus immunocompromised mice. *Cells* 8:1472. doi: 10.3390/cells8121472

103. Pittet, M. J., and Weissleder, R. (2011). Intravital imaging. *Cell* 147, 983–991. doi: 10.1016/j.cell.2011.11.004

104. Polstein, L. R., Juhas, M., Hanna, G., Bursac, N., and Gersbach, C. A. (2017). An engineered optogenetic switch for spatiotemporal control of gene expression. Cell differentiation. And tissue morphogenesis. *ACS Synth. Biol.* 6, 2003–2013. doi: 10.1021/acssynbio.7b00147

105. Porat-Shliom, N., Harding, O. J., Malec, L., Narayan, K., and Weigert, R. (2019). Mitochondrial populations exhibit differential dynamic responses to increased energy demand during exocytosis in vivo. *iScience* 11, 440–449. doi: 10.1016/j. isci.2018.12.036

106. Presson, R. G., Brown, M. B., Fisher, A. J., Sandoval, R. M., Dunn, K. W., Lorenz, K. S., et al. (2011). Two-photon imaging within the murine thorax without respiratory and cardiac motion artifact. *Am. J. Pathol.* 179, 75–82. doi: 10.1016/ j.ajpath.2011.03.048

107. Presson, R. G., Okada, O., Hanger, C. C., Godbey, P. S., Graham, J. A., Glenny, R. W., et al. (1994). Stability of alveolar capillary opening pressures. *J. Appl. Physiol.* 77, 1630–1637. doi: 10.1152/jappl.1994.77.4.1630

108. Progatzky, F., Dallman, M. J., and Lo Celso, C. (2013). From seeing to believing: labelling strategies for in vivo cell-tracking experiments. *Interface Focus* 3:20130001. doi: 10.1098/rsfs.2013.0001

109. Prunier, C., Chen, N., Ritsma, L., and Vrisekoop, N. (2017). Procedures and applications of long-term intravital microscopy. *Methods* 128, 52–64. doi: 10. 1016/j.ymeth.2017.06.029

110. Reeves, K. J., Hurrell, J. E., Cecchini, M., van der Pluijm, G., Down, J. M., Eaton, C. L., et al. (2015). Prostate cancer cells home to bone using a novel in vivo model: modulation by the integrin antagonist GLPG0187. *Int. J. Cancer* 136, 1731–1740. doi: 10.1002/ijc.29165

111. Rehman, H., Sun, J., Shi, Y., Ramshesh, V. K., Liu, Q., Currin, R. T., et al. (2011). NIM811 prevents mitochondrial dysfunction, attenuates liver injury, and stimulates liver regeneration after massive hepatectomy. *Transplantation* 91, 406–412. doi: 10.1097/TP.0b013e318204bdb2

112. Reichel, C. A., Hessenauer, M. E. T., Pflieger, K., Rehberg, M., Kanse, S. M., Zahler, S., et al. (2015). Components of the plasminogen activation system promote engraftment of porous polyethylene biomaterial via common and distinct effects. *PLoS One* 10:e0116883. doi: 10.1371/journal.pone.0116883

113. Reichel, C. A., Lerchenberger, M., Uhl, B., Rehberg, M., Berberich, N., Zahler, S., et al. (2011). Plasmin inhibitors prevent leukocyte accumulation and remodeling events in the postischemic microvasculature. *PLoS One* 6:e0017229. doi: 10.1371/journal.pone.0017229

114. Reichel, C. A., Puhr-Westerheide, D., Zuchtriegel, G., Uhl, B., Berberich, N., Zahler, S., et al. (2012). C-C motif chemokine CCL3 and canonical neutrophil attractants promote neutrophil extravasation through common and distinct mechanisms. *Blood* 120, 880–890. doi: 10.1182/blood-2012-01-402164

115. Resch-Genger, U., Grabolle, M., Cavaliere-Jaricot, S., Nitschke, R., and Nann, T. (2008). Quantum dots versus organic dyes as fluorescent labels. *Nat. Methods* 5, 763–775. doi: 10.1038/nmeth.1248

116. Ripplinger, C. M., Kessinger, C. W., Li, C., Kim, J. W., McCarthy, J. R., Weissleder, R., et al. (2012). Inflammation modulates murine venous thrombosis resolution in vivo: assessment by multimodal fluorescence molecular imaging. *Arterioscler Thromb. Vasc. Biol.* 32, 2616–2624. doi: 10.1161/ATVBAHA.112.251983

117. Ritsma, L., Steller, E. J. A., Beerling, E., Loomans, C. J. M., Zomer, A., Gerlach, C., et al. (2012). Intravital microscopy through an abdominal imaging window reveals a pre-micrometastasis stage during liver metastasis. *Sci. Transl. Med.* 4:158ra145. doi: 10.1126/scitranslmed.3004394

118. Ritsma, L., Steller, E. J. A., Ellenbroek, S. I. J., Kranenburg, O., Rinkes, I. H. M. B., and van Rheenen, J. (2013). Surgical implantation of an abdominal imaging window for intravital microscopy. *Nat. Protoc.* 8, 583–594. doi: 10.1038/nprot. 2013.026

119. Rius, C., and Sanz, M. J. (2015). Intravital microscopy in the cremaster muscle microcirculation for endothelial dysfunction studies. *Methods Mol. Biol.* 1339, 357–366. doi: 10.1007/978-1-4939-2929-0_26

120. Robbins Clinton, S., Chudnovskiy, A., Rauch, P. J., Figueiredo, J. L., Iwamoto, Y., Gorbatov, R., et al. (2012). Extramedullary hematopoiesis generates ly-6chigh monocytes that infiltrate atherosclerotic lesions. *Circulation* 125, 364–374. doi: 10.1161/CIRCULATIONAHA.111.061986

121. Rodriguez-Tirado, C., Kitamura, T., Kato, Y., Pollard, J. W., Condeelis, J. S., and Entenberg, D. (2016). Long-term high-resolution intravital microscopy in the lung with a vacuum stabilized imaging window. *J. Vis. Exp.* 116:54603. doi: 10.3791/54603

122. Russo, L. M., Sandoval, R. M., McKee, M., Osicka, T. M., Collins, A. B., Brown, D., et al. (2007). The normal kidney filters nephrotic levels of albumin retrieved by proximal tubule cells: retrieval is disrupted in nephrotic states. *Kidney Int.* 71, 504–513. doi: 10.1038/sj.ki.5002041

123. Ryan, J., Morgan, R. E., Chen, Y., Volak, L. P., Dunn, R. T., and Dunn, K. W. (2018). Intravital multiphoton microscopy with fluorescent bile salts in

rats as an in vivo biomarker for hepatobiliary transport inhibition. *Drug. Metab. Dispos.* 46, 704–718. doi: 10.1124/dmd.117.079277

124. Sandoval, R. M., Kennedy, M. D., Low, P. S., and Molitoris, B. A. (2004). Uptake and trafficking of fluorescent conjugates of folic acid in intact kidney determined using intravital two-photon microscopy. *Am. J. Physiol. Cell Physiol.* 287, C517–C526. doi: 10.1152/ajpcell.00006.2004

125. Savarin, M., Prevc, A., Rzek, M., Bosnjak, M., Vojvodic, I., Cemazar, M., et al. (2018). Intravital monitoring of vasculature after targeted gene therapy alone or combined with tumor irradiation. *Technol. Cancer Res. Treat* 17:1533033818784208. doi: 10.1177/1533033818784208

126. Schiessl, I. M., Grill, A., Fremter, K., Steppan, D., Hellmuth, M.-K., and Castrop, H. (2018). Renal interstitial platelet-derived growth factor receptor-β cells support proximal tubular regeneration. *J. Am. Soc. Nephrol.* 29, 1383–1396. doi: 10. 1681/ASN.2017101069

127. Schießl, I. M., and Castrop, H. (2016). Deep insights: intravital imaging with two- photon microscopy. *Pflugers Arch.* 468, 1505–1516. doi: 10.1007/s00424-016- 1832-7

128. Schießl, I. M., Hammer, A., Kattler, V., Gess, B., Theilig, F., Witzgall, R., et al. (2016a). Intravital imaging reveals angiotensin ii–induced transcytosis of albumin by podocytes. *J. Am. Soc. Nephrol.* 27, 731–744. doi: 10.1681/ASN. 2014111125

129. Schießl, I. M., Hammer, A., Riquier-Brison, A., and Peti-Peterdi, J. (2016b). Just Look! intravital microscopy as the best means to study kidney cell death dynamics. *Semin. Nephrol.* 36, 220–236. doi: 10.1016/j.semnephrol.2016. 03.009

130. Schreiter, J., Meyer, S., Schmidt, C., Schulz, R. M., and Langer, S. (2017). Dorsal skinfold chamber models in mice. *GMS Interdiscip Plast Reconstr. Surg. DGPW* 6:Doc10. doi: 10.3205/iprs000112

131. Secklehner, J., Lo Celso, C., and Carlin, L. M. (2017). Intravital microscopy in historic and contemporary immunology. *Immunol. Cell Biol.* 95, 506–513. doi: 10.1038/icb.2017.25

132. Shao, L., Gao, Y., and Yan, F. (2011). Semiconductor quantum dots for biomedicial applications. *Sensors* 11, 11736–11751. doi: 10.3390/s111211736

133. Shitara, A., Bleck, C. K. E., and Weigert, R. (2020). Cdc42 controls secretory granules morphology in rodent salivary glands in vivo. *Commun. Integr. Biol.* 13, 22–26. doi: 10.1080/19420889.2020.1724605

134. Siemionow, M., and Nanhekhan, L. V. (1999). Introduction of cremaster muscle chamber technique for long-term intravital microscopy. *Ann. Plast Surg.* 43, 161–166.

135. Steiner, D., Lang, G., Fischer, L., Winkler, S., Fey, T., Greil, P., et al. (2019). Intrinsic vascularization of recombinant eADF4(C16) spider silk matrices in the arteriovenous loop model. *Tissue Eng. Part A* 25, 1504–1513. doi: 10.1089/ten.tea.2018.0360

136. Strüder, D., Grambow, E., Klar, E., Mlynski, R., and Vollmar, B. (2017). Intravital microscopy and thrombus induction in the earlobe of a hairless mouse. *J. Vis. Exp.* 122:55174. doi: 10.3791/55174

137. Swedlow, J. R., Hu, K., Andrews, P. D., Roos, D. S., and Murray, J. M. (2002). Measuring tubulin content in *Toxoplasma gondii*: a comparison of laser- scanning confocal and wide-field fluorescence microscopy. *PNAS* 99, 2014– 2019. doi: 10.1073/pnas.022554999

138. Tabuchi, A., Mertens, M., Kuppe, H., Pries, A. R., and Kuebler, W. M. (2008). Intravital microscopy of the murine pulmonary microcirculation. *J. Appl. Physiol.* 104, 338–346. doi: 10.1152/japplphysiol.00348.2007

139. Tabuchi, A., Nickles, H. T., Kim, M., Semple, J. W., Koch, E., Brochard, L., et al. (2016). Acute lung injury causes asynchronous alveolar ventilation that can be corrected by individual sighs. *Am. J. Respir. Crit. Care Med.* 193, 396–406. doi: 10.1164/rccm.201505-0901OC

140. Tabuchi, A., Styp-Rekowska, B., Slutsky, A. S., Wagner, P. D., Pries, A. R., and Kuebler, W. M. (2013). Precapillary oxygenation contributes relevantly to gas exchange in the intact lung. *Am. J. Respir. Crit. Care Med.* 188, 474–481. doi: 10.1164/rccm.201212-2177OC

141. Tanaka, K., Ide, S., Shimura, T., Okigami, M., Toiyama, Y., Kitajima, T., et al. (2014). Intravital imaging of fluorescently labeled therapeutic monoclonal antibody on the surface of tumor cells in metastatic tumor xenografts using a multiphoton microscopy. *JCO* 32:e22062. doi: 10.1200/jco.2014.32.15_suppl. e22062

142. Taqueti, V. R., and Jaffer, F. A. (2013). High-resolution molecular imaging via intravital microscopy: illuminating vascular biology in vivo. *Integr. Biol.* 5, 278–290. doi: 10.1039/c2ib20194a

143. Tarantini, S., Fulop, G. A., Kiss, T., Farkas, E., Zölei-Szénási, D., Galvan, V., et al. (2017). Demonstration of impaired neurovascular coupling responses in TG2576 mouse model of Alzheimer's disease using functional laser speckle contrast imaging. *GeroScience* 39, 465–473. doi: 10.1007/s11357-017-9980-z

144. Tavakoli, M., Tsekouras, K., Day, R., Dunn, K. W., and Pressé, S. (2019). Quantitative kinetic models from intravital microscopy: a case study using hepatic transport. *J. Phys. Chem. B* 123, 7302–7312. doi: 10.1021/acs.jpcb. 9b04729

145. Thanabalasuriar, A., Neupane, A. S., Wang, J., Krummel, M. F., and Kubes, P. (2016). iNKT cell emigration out of the lung vasculature requires neutrophils and monocyte-derived dendritic cells in inflammation. *Cell Rep.* 16, 3260–3272. doi: 10.1016/j.celrep.2016.07.052

146. Theer, P., Hasan, M. T., and Denk, W. (2003). Two-photon imaging to a depth of 1000 μm in living brains by use of a Ti:Al$_2$O$_3$ regenerative amplifier. *Opt. Lett., OL* 28, 1022–1024. doi: 10.1364/OL.28.001022

147. Theruvath, T. P., Zhong, Z., Pediaditakis, P., Ramshesh, V. K., Currin, R. T., Tikunov, A., et al. (2008). Minocycline and N-methyl-4-isoleucine cyclosporin (NIM811) mitigate storage/reperfusion injury after rat liver transplantation through suppression of the mitochondrial permeability transition. *Hepatology* 47, 236–246. doi: 10.1002/hep.21912

148. Tong, J., Mou, S., Xiong, L., Wang, Z., Wang, R., Weigand, A., et al. (2018). Adipose-derived mesenchymal stem cells formed acinar-like structure when stimulated with breast epithelial cells in three-dimensional culture. *PLoS One* 13:e0204077. doi: 10.1371/journal.pone.0204077

149. Toseland, C. P. (2013). Fluorescent labeling and modification of proteins. *J. Chem. Biol.* 6, 85–95. doi: 10.1007/s12154-013-0094-5

150. Ueno, T., Kim, P., McGrath, M. M., Yeung, M. Y., Shimizu, T., Jung, K., et al. (2016). Live images of donor dendritic cells trafficking via CX3CR1 pathway. *Front. Immunol.* 7:412. doi: 10.3389/fimmu.2016.00412

151. Upreti, M., Jamshidi-Parsian, A., Koonce, N. A., Webber, J. S., Sharma, S. K., Asea, A. A., et al. (2011). Tumor-endothelial cell three-dimensional spheroids: new aspects to enhance radiation and drug therapeutics. *Transl. Oncol.* 4, 365–376.

152. van den Berg, C. W., Ritsma, L., Avramut, M. C., Wiersma, L. E., van den Berg, B. M., Leuning, D. G., et al. (2018). Renal subcapsular transplantation of PSC-derived kidney organoids induces neo-vasculogenesis and significant glomerular and tubular maturation in vivo. *Stem Cell Rep.* 10, 751–765. doi: 10.1016/j.stemcr.2018.01.041

153. Vielreicher, M., Gellner, M., Rottensteiner, U., Horch, R. E., Arkudas, A., and Friedrich, O. (2017). Multiphoton microscopy analysis of extracellular collagen I network formation by mesenchymal stem cells. *J. Tissue Eng. Regen. Med.* 11, 2104–2115. doi: 10.1002/term.2107

154. Vinegoni, C., Aguirre, A. D., Lee, S., and Weissleder, R. (2015). Imaging the beating heart in the mouse using intravital microscopy techniques. *Nat. Protoc.* 10, 1802–1819. doi: 10.1038/nprot.2015.119

155. Vollmar, B., Burkhardt, M., Minor, T., Klauke, H., and Menger, M. D. (1997). High-resolution microscopic determination of hepatic nadh fluorescence forin vivomonitoring of tissue oxygenation during hemorrhagic shock and resuscitation. *Microvas. Res.* 54, 164–173. doi: 10.1006/mvre.1997.2028

156. Vollmar, B., and Menger, M. D. (2009). The hepatic microcirculation: mechanistic contributions and therapeutic targets in liver injury and repair. *Physiol. Rev.* 89, 1269–1339. doi: 10.1152/physrev.00027.2008

157. Walser, R., Metzger, W., Görg, A., Pohlemann, T., Menger, M. D., and Laschke, M. W. (2013). Generation of co-culture spheroids as vascularisation units for bone tissue engineering. *Eur. Cell Mater.* 26, 222–233. doi: 10.22203/ecm. v026a16

158. Wang, E., Babbey, C. M., and Dunn, K. W. (2005). Performance comparison between the high-speed Yokogawa spinning disc confocal system and single-point scanning confocal systems. *J. Microsc.* 218, 148–159. doi: 10.1111/j.1365-2818.2005.01473.x

159. Wang, H., Yang, H., Xu, Z. P., Liu, X., Roberts, M. S., and Liang, X. (2018). Anionic long-circulating quantum dots for long-term intravital vascular imaging. *Pharmaceutics* 10:244. doi: 10.3390/pharmaceutics10040244

160. Wang, T., Ouzounov, D. G., Wu, C., Horton, N. G., Zhang, B., Wu, C.-H., et al. (2018). Three-photon imaging of mouse brain structure and function through the intact skull. *Nat. Methods* 15, 789–792. doi: 10.1038/s41592-018-0115-y

161. Weigand, A., Beier, J. P., Arkudas, A., Al-Abboodi, M., Polykandriotis, E., Horch, R. E., et al. (2016). The arteriovenous (AV) loop in a small animal model to study angiogenesis and vascularized tissue engineering. *J. Vis. Exp.* 117:54676. doi: 10.3791/54676

162. Weigert, R., Porat-Shliom, N., and Amornphimoltham, P. (2013). Imaging cell biology in live animals: ready for prime time. *J. Cell Biol.* 201, 969–979. doi: 10.1083/jcb.201212130

163. White, J. G., Amos, W. B., and Fordham, M. (1987). An evaluation of confocal versus conventional imaging of biological structures by fluorescence light microscopy. *J. Cell Biol.* 105, 41–48. doi: 10.1083/jcb.105.1.41

164. Wiggs, B. R., English, D., Quinlan, W. M., Doyle, N. A., Hogg, J. C., and Doerschuk, C. M. (1994). Contributions of capillary pathway size and neutrophil deformability to neutrophil transit through rabbit lungs. *J. Appl. Physiol.* 77, 463–470. doi: 10.1152/jappl.1994.77.1.463

165. Wimborne, H. J., Hu, J., Takemoto, K., Nguyen, N. T., Jaeschke, H., Lemasters, J. J., et al. (2020). Aldehyde dehydrogenase-2 activation decreases acetaminophen hepatotoxicity by prevention of mitochondrial depolarization. *Toxicol. Appl. Pharmacol.* 396:114982. doi: 10.1016/j.taap.2020.114982

166. Witt, R., Weigand, A., Boos, A. M., Cai, A., Dippold, D., Boccaccini, A. R., et al. (2017). Mesenchymal stem cells and myoblast differentiation under HGF and IGF-1 stimulation for 3D skeletal muscle tissue engineering. *BMC Cell Biol.* 18:15. doi: 10.1186/s12860-017-0131-2

167. Yan, Q., and Mp, B. (2015). Advances in chemical labeling of proteins in living cells. *Cell Tissue Res.* 360, 179–194. doi: 10.1007/s00441-015-2145-4

168. Yang, G., Pan, F., Parkhurst, C. N., Grutzendler, J., and Gan, W.-B. (2010). Thinned-skull cranial window technique for long-term imaging of the cortex in live mice. *Nat. Protoc.* 5, 201–208. doi: 10.1038/nprot.2009.222

169. Yipp, B. G., Kim, J. H., Lima, R., Zbytnuik, L. D., Petri, B., Swanlund, N., et al. (2017). The lung is a host defense niche for immediate neutrophil-mediated vascular protection. *Sci. Immunol.* 2:eaam8929. doi: 10.1126/sciimmunol.aam8929

170. Yoshikawa, S., Usami, T., Kikuta, J., Ishii, M., Sasano, T., Sugiyama, K., et al. (2016). Intravital imaging of Ca^{2+} signals in lymphocytes of Ca^{2+} biosensor transgenic mice: indication of autoimmune diseases before the pathological onset. *Sci. Rep.* 6:18738. doi: 10.1038/srep18738

171. Yuan, F., Dellian, M., Fukumura, D., Leunig, M., Berk, D. A., Torchilin, V. P., et al. (1995). Vascular permeability in a human tumor xenograft: molecular size dependence and cutoff size. *Cancer Res.* 55, 3752–3756.

172. Zanacchi, F. C., Bianchini, P., and Vicidomini, G. (2014). Fluorescence microscopy in the spotlight. *Microsc. Res. Tech.* 77, 479–482. doi: 10.1002/jemt.22393

173. Zhang, M., Sun, D., Liu, G., Wu, H., Zhou, H., and Shi, M. (2016). Real-time in vivo imaging reveals the ability of neutrophils to remove Cryptococcus neoformans directly from the brain vasculature. *J. Leukoc. Biol.* 99, 467–473. doi: 10.1189/jlb.4AB0715-281R

174. Zhao, Y.-J., Yu, T.-T., Zhang, C., Li, Z., Luo, Q.-M., Xu, T.-H., et al. (2018). Skull optical clearing window for *in vivo* imaging of the mouse cortex at synaptic resolution. *Light Sci. Appl.* 7:17153. doi: 10.1038/lsa.2017.153

8

Accessing 3D Printed Vascular Phantoms for Procedural Simulation

Jasamine Coles-Black[1,2]*, Damien Bolton[2] and Jason Chuen[1,2]

[1] 3dMedLab, Austin Health, The University of Melbourne, Parkville, VIC, Australia, [2] Department of Surgery, Austin Health, The University of Melbourne, Melbourne, VIC, Australia

*Correspondence:
Jasamine Coles-Black
JasamineCB@gmail.com

Introduction: 3D printed patient-specific vascular phantoms provide superior anatomical insights for simulating complex endovascular procedures. Currently, lack of exposure to the technology poses a barrier for adoption. We offer an accessible, low-cost guide to producing vascular anatomical models using routine CT angiography, open source software packages and a variety of 3D printing technologies.

Methods: Although applicable to all vascular territories, we illustrate our methodology using Abdominal Aortic Aneurysms (AAAs) due to the strong interest in this area. CT aortograms acquired as part of routine care were converted to representative patient-specific 3D models, and then printed using a variety of 3D printing technologies to assess their material suitability as aortic phantoms. Depending on the technology, phantoms cost $20–$1,000 and were produced in 12–48 h. This technique was used to generate hollow 3D printed thoracoabdominal aortas visible under fluoroscopy.

Results: 3D printed AAA phantoms were a valuable addition to standard CT angiogram reconstructions in the simulation of complex cases, such as short or very angulated necks, or for positioning fenestrations in juxtarenal aneurysms. Hollow flexible models were particularly useful for device selection and in planning of fenestrated EVAR. In addition, these models have demonstrated utility other settings, such as patient education and engagement, and trainee and anatomical education. Further study is required to establish a material with optimal cost, haptic and fluoroscopic fidelity.

Conclusion: We share our experiences and methodology for developing inexpensive 3D printed vascular phantoms which despite material limitations, successfully mimic the procedural challenges encountered during live endovascular surgery. As the technology continues to improve, 3D printed vascular phantoms have the potential to disrupt how endovascular procedures are planned and taught.

Keywords: 3D printing, vascular phantom, simulation, fluoroscopy, angiography, AAA (abdominal aortic aneurysm), EVAR, FEVAR

INTRODUCTION
3D Printed Vascular Phantoms

3D printing is a manufacturing technique which has gained attention in surgery recently as a means of rapidly producing patient-specific anatomical models for the purposes of procedural simulation and training. This accessible technology allows imaging to be converted into physical, patient-specific models within the hospital setting, enabling surgeons and other proceduralists to rapidly access true-to-scale representations of patient anatomy for superior visualization and planning.

3D printing is anticipated to represent the next step in personalized medicine. Despite the nascence of the technology, its utility as a tool in presurgical planning and intraoperative visualization is currently being examined via clinical trials (1). In addition, its potential in other settings is being explored, such as for patient education and engagement and trainee education. Due to the expiry of patents leading to the democratization of 3D printing technology, desktop 3D printers are now in the price range of office paper printers, well within reach of all surgical departments seeking to produce of patient-specific 3D printed anatomical models in-house. In the field of vascular intervention, 3D printed models have been used as presurgical simulation tools in the planning of Endovascular Aneurysm Repair (EVAR) (2), and complex endovascular aortic techniques such as fenestrated or branched EVAR (3, 4). 3D printed vascular models have also been explored in procedural simulation involving other vascular territories, such as coil embolisation of cerebral aneurysms (5) or splenic artery aneurysms (6).

Our frontier experiences with the technology mirror those of other groups, with 3D printed patient-specific vascular models providing superior anatomical insights for simulating complex procedures (**Figure** 1). This has clear advantages regarding patient safety with reduced time under anesthesia, reduction in operation time (7), shorter recovery times, and a reduction in blood loss intraoperatively (8), resulting in cost savings to health services. However, despite the promise of 3D printed patient-specific phantoms for simulation, lack of exposure to the technology amongst vascular proceduralists poses a barrier for adoption (9).

We offer an accessible, low-cost guide to producing vascular anatomical models using routine CT angiography, open source software packages and a variety of 3D printing technologies, with a focus on Abdominal Aortic Aneurysms (AAAs) to showcase its utility. However, the techniques described are equally applicable to any vascular territory imaged using Computed Tomographic (CT) angiography.

Abdominal Aortic Aneurysms

An Abdominal Aortic Aneurysm is a dilatation of the abdominal aorta to at least 1.5 times its usual size, or an outer diameter of 3 cm (10). As a true aneurysm, the dilatation affects all three layers of the aortic wall, namely the intima, media, and adventitia. AAAs cause a substantial burden on the healthcare system. Rupture results in death in 65% of cases, with a perioperative mortality of 32% (11). In addition, ruptured AAAs are responsible for 1.3% of total deaths in 65–85 year old males in developed countries (10).

The infrarenal aorta is the most common site of AAA formation, and the most favorable anatomical morphology for repair, either via an endovascular approach with EVAR or open surgical repair via infrarenal aortic clamping. Contemporary endovascular technology has made great strides, with EVAR seen as standard care in patients with appropriate anatomy (12).

However, when faced with patient anatomy beyond the standard infrarenal AAA, the endovascular surgeon must modify

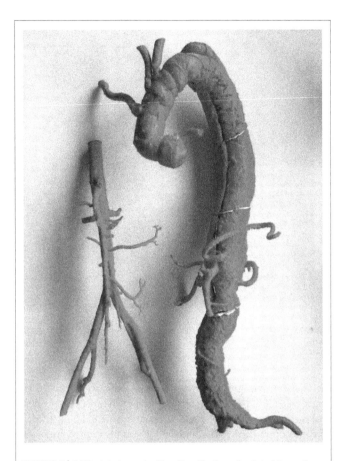

FIGURE 1 | A 3D printed complex Type B aortic dissection for reintervention (right) compared to normal aorta (left). Both models were 3D printed using FDM technology and ABS filament. Note that due to limitations in the size of the print bed, the Type B aortic dissection was printed in four pieces.

his or her approach to these complex cases. If the aneurysm extends to but does not involve the renal artery ostia, it is considered a juxtarenal AAA. If the aneurysm extends further superiorly involving the renal arteries and visceral arteries, it is termed a pararenal or paravisceral AAA. Endovascular repair of these complex anatomies is challenging, requiring branched or fenestrated stent grafts, or may be technically unfeasible with current levels of technology.

Utility of 3D Printed Phantoms in AAA Simulation

As Vascular Surgery experiences a fundamental shift with increasing endovascular and decreasing open repairs, the reach of EVAR increasingly extends to patients with complex anatomy outside of the standard infrarenal AAA, adding to the complexity of contemporary AAA repair.

Well-known potential complications of EVAR include endoleak, graft occlusion, migration or infection (13, 14), requiring further endovascular or open surgical revision and further costs incurred to the healthcare system. As such, adequate visualization of the patient's unique anatomy, appropriate graft selection, the ability to predict intraoperative difficulties and

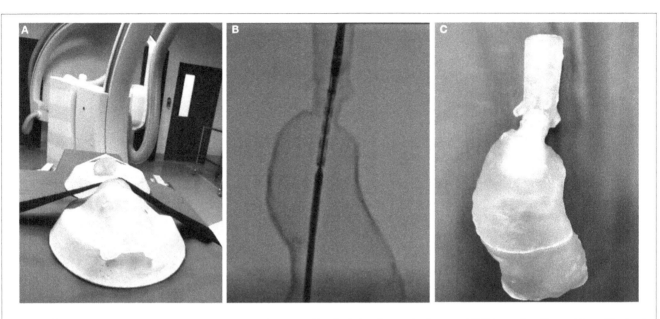

FIGURE 2 | (A) A transparent complex juxtarenal AAA phantom being prepared for simulation of a complex fenestrated EVAR procedure. The model was 3D printed with SLA technology using a transparent resin. **(B)** The AAA phantom under fluoroscopy. **(C)** The AAA phantom after deployment of a fenestrated stent graft.

the shape of the graft after deployment are paramount to the improvement of this young technique, and the cost to the public health system. Many of these complications would be mitigated with the opportunity to simulate the proposed procedure and select devices using patient-specific AAA phantoms.

In addition, there is a growing role for 3D printed EVAR simulators in training the next generation of Vascular Surgeons (7). The benefits of simulation in procedural training have been well-described in the Vascular Surgery literature (15, 16). Simulation allows for a "dry run," improving trainee confidence in procedures. It provides an opportunity for participants to apply theory into practice, and to gain experience that would otherwise potentially put patients at risk, particularly in emergency situations. In addition, simulation provides an environment where all members of the team can learn with and from one another, with the opportunity for debriefing and reflection.

Duran et al. reported an improvement in self-reported confidence levels amongst Vascular trainees afforded access to simulation, with 86% of trainees surveyed supportive of simulation training (17). Simulation accelerates the acquisition of psychomotor skills, procedural understanding, and facilitates assessment of proficiency (18, 19). Specific to EVAR, Vento et al. confirmed that simulation objectively improved the competence of trainees in performing EVAR, with reductions in total procedure time, total fluoroscopy time, time for contralateral gate cannulation, and volume contrast used when compared to the control group (20).

Endovascular techniques are evolving at a remarkable rate. Combined with decreased training hours and the unstructured nature of opportunistic on-the-job training via the traditional Halstedian apprenticeship model, simulation-based procedural training is a promising avenue. The contemporary challenge

of lack of procedural exposure is further compounded by improvements in non-invasive vascular imaging techniques, reducing the opportunities for trainees to perform diagnostic angiograms in order to gain essential wire and catheter handling skills (18). Simulation provides a solution by offering an avenue to learn the key steps required in common as well as more advanced procedures under the supervision of a surgical educator.

Study Aims

3D printed vascular phantoms have a growing role in the pre-surgical simulation and training of complex endovascular procedures. While there is growing interest in the topic, lack of familiarity with 3D printing technology has resulted in slow uptake.

In developing this methodology, our aim was to create inexpensive vascular phantoms with optimal anatomical, haptic and fluoroscopic fidelity. Through iterative prototyping, we have improved upon the workflow, particularly with regards to speed and cost to ensure that initial investment would not pose a barrier to interested departments.

We demonstrate this workflow using AAA phantoms as an example of how CT angiograms acquired as part of standard care can be converted into patient-specific 3D models. Our work has occurred at 3D Med Lab, Australia's first 3D printing laboratory in a public hospital setting. This work has resulted in hollow 3D printed thoracoabdominal aortas with branches which allow for realistic simulation under fluoroscopy.

These models, despite current material limitations, successfully mimic the cannulation and deployment challenges encountered during live endovascular surgery (**Figure 2**). As dimensional and representational material validity is improved, these AAA phantoms have the potential to serve as a powerful

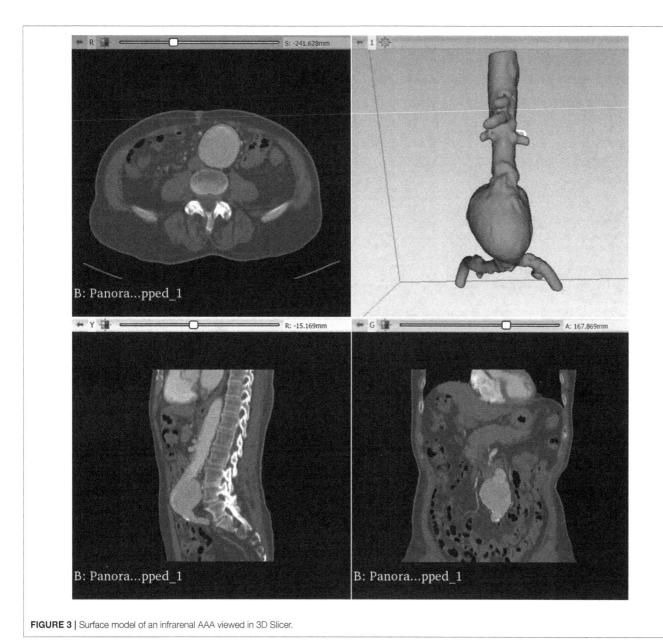

FIGURE 3 | Surface model of an infrarenal AAA viewed in 3D Slicer.

adjunct to how complex EVAR cases are planned. In addition, as these models do not degrade, they serve as a valuable tool to simulate EVAR for vascular trainees, as well as to counsel patients as part of the therapeutic relationship.

We seek to inform on the readiness of current levels of 3D printing technologies for the vascular proceduralist, and the feasibility of implementing 3D printing in the hospital setting. A readily reproducible, descriptive methodology for the creation of vascular phantoms has yet to be described in the literature, leading many groups to rely on commercial third parties to create and 3D print their vascular models. Not only would 3D printed vascular phantoms be more economical to produce within the health service setting, it allows for translation to the angiography suite with the efficiency that surgeons are accustomed to.

In summary, our aim was to develop a low cost, low complexity, CT angiogram to 3D printed vascular phantom workflow that could be easily adopted by other groups using open source segmentation packages and inexpensive, commercially available 3D printers.

MATERIALS AND EQUIPMENT

Segmentation Software

There is an ever-expanding selection of medical image processing software available, both commercial and open source. Commercial software utilized by groups in the literature include Mimics (version 23.0; Materialize NV, Leuven, Belgium, 2020), InVivoDental (version 6.0; Anatomage, San Jose, CA, 2020), OnDemand3D (APP version 1.0; CyberMed Inc, Seoul,

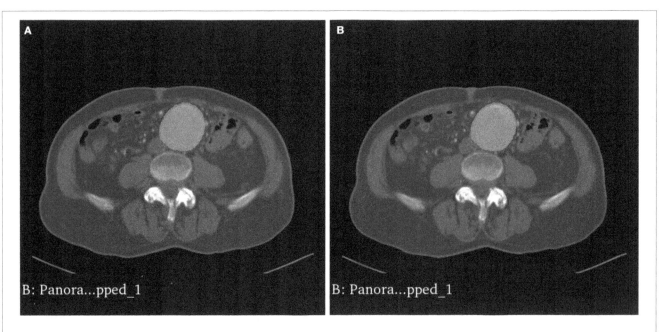

FIGURE 4 | (A) The intraluminal contrast within the AAA is highlighted. **(B)** The model is dilated outwards to approximate the external surface of the AAA, resulting in a hollow phantom.

Korea, 2020), and OsiriX Imaging Software (version 11.0; Pixmeo, Geneva, Switzerland, 2020). However, licensing fees commence at thousands of dollars, which can be challenging for surgical units to justify at the outset.

Open source software such as 3D Slicer (version 4.11; Harvard, US, 2020), and ITKsnap (version 3.6; Pennsylvania, US, 2020) present accessible alternatives. Most of our group's experience has been with the open source software 3D Slicer (21), a platform for the analysis and visualization of medical images, available for download at https://www.slicer.org/ (**Figure 3**). The user interface of 3D Slicer is modular in nature, with powerful plug-in capabilities for additional algorithms and applications.

3D Printing Technology

The most readily available 3D printing technologies for the vascular proceduralist include those accessible via university links, or those sufficiently affordable and compact to be located within the hospital setting. The most common 3D printing modalities include Fused Deposition Modeling (FDM), Stereolithography (SLA) and Inkjet techniques.

FDM is the most accessible 3D printing technique for those interested in experimenting with the technology, retailing for as little as a few hundred dollars. The technology involves the building of layers via the extrusion of heat-softened polymers. Common materials include the rigid thermoplastics Acrylonitrile Butadiene Styrene (ABS), Polylactic Acid (PLA), as well as flexible thermoplastics such as Thermoplastic Polyurethane (TPU) and Thermoplastic Elastomer (TPE), soft, rubber-like filaments. FDM has been used to 3D print surgical guides (22),

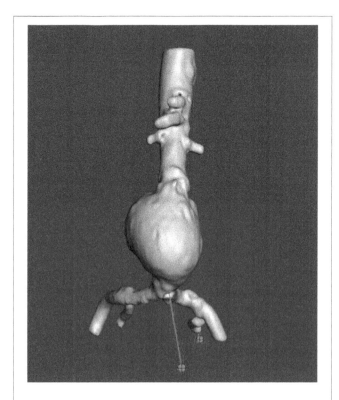

FIGURE 5 | Using Meshmixer, mesh defects in the AAA phantom are identified for repair prior to finalizing the model for 3D printing.

patient-specific anatomical models for presurgical simulation (23), and even patient-tailored pharmacotherapeutics at individualized doses (24).

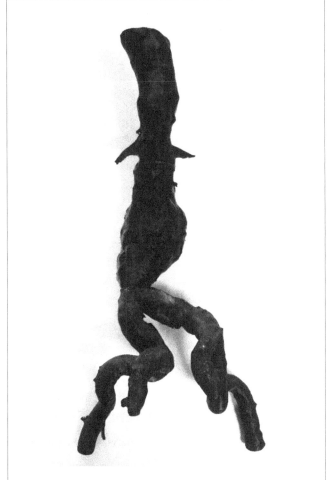

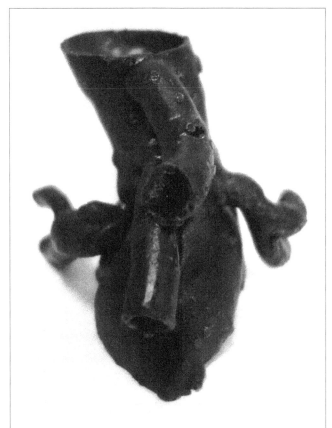

FIGURE 7 | The visceral segment of a complex juxtarenal AAA 3D printed in flexible resin using SLA technology for presurgical planning.

FIGURE 6 | A complex juxtarenal abdominal aortic aneurysm 3D printed for presurgical planning using FDM technology. In addition, the 3D printed model was used to plan the fenestrations of a commercially produced endograft.

SLA utilizes an ultraviolet laser, which is selectively scanned over a vat of photo-active photopolymer, curing and solidifying specified areas on the surface of the liquid. As the process continues, the final object is built up layer by layer. Thus far, SLA has been used for anatomical modeling in presurgical simulation (25) and training (26), and in the creation of scaffolds for tissue engineering (27).

Inkjet 3D printing is an extension of the conventional two-dimensional paper printing technique. Hundreds of microscopic nozzles selectively deposit droplets of photopolymer one layer at a time, which are flash cured using a UV lamp. Retailing for hundreds of thousands of dollars, inkjet printing is the most expensive of the 3D printing techniques described, requiring collaboration with academic centers at the outset until its expense can be justified. This technique allows for multiple anatomical structures to be 3D printed in one piece, allowing for basic discrimination between tissues for the purposes of simulation (28, 29).

We provide interested vascular proceduralists with examples of aortic phantoms 3D printed with each of these technologies, as well as our experiences regarding their suitability for common applications (**Figures 6–8**).

METHODOLOGY

We describe our methodology for isolating regions of patient vasculature to generate surface models for 3D printing, however the vascular models generated can equally be viewed on a tablet, through a Virtual Reality headset, or projected onto a screen for viewing.

Using 3D Slicer, CT aortograms were converted to representative patient-specific AAA models. The models were then prepared for printing using another open source computer aided design (CAD) software, Meshmixer (version 3.5, Autodesk, California, US, 2020), and 3D printed using a variety of 3D printing techniques in order to assess their suitability as aortic phantoms (**Figures 4, 5**). Depending on the 3D printing technology used, these models cost AUD$20–1,000 and were produced in 12–48 h.

Image Acquisition

CT aortograms acquired as part of AAA surveillance or preoperative workup are an ideal starting point for this workflow, with intraluminal contrast greatly facilitating the isolation of

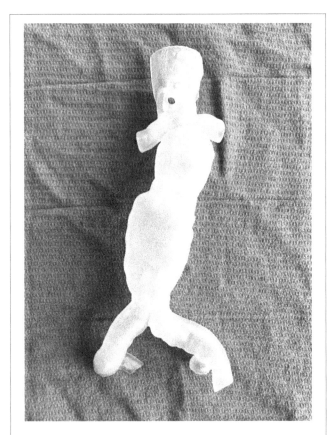

FIGURE 8 | A flexible, hollow, translucent AAA phantom 3D printed using Inkjet technology.

vascular anatomy. Due to its increasing availability and ever-improving speed and quality, non-invasive CT angiography has become the conventional imaging modality for visualizing vascular anatomy and pathology (30). The accuracy of image processing is highly dependent upon the quality and resolution of the original CT imaging, with slice thicknesses <1 mm yielding superior results.

Although not the modality of choice at our center, Magnetic Resonance Angiography (MRA) presents an ideal alternative, likewise due to the presence of intraluminal contrast. B-mode ultrasound has also been utilized with success in the literature in 3D printing arteriovenous fistulas (31), however ultrasound as a modality is more heavily operator dependent, less readily available in the clinical setting due to staffing demands, and cannot be applied to all vascular territories. A key concept is that the imaging protocol which best visualizes the vascular anatomy for surgical planning will similarly result in the best imaging for 3D printing.

Generating 3D Models From CT Angiograms

Generating 3D models from patient CT angiography is performed via the process of image segmentation, which involves partitioning an image into multiple segments for

meaningful analysis. In the context of CT aortograms, a contrast-enhanced AAA and its branches are efficiently isolated from the surrounding soft tissue by leveraging the concept of Hounsfield Units.

Using the *Segment Editor* module, CT aortogram datasets were automatically segmented using the *Threshold* function. The *Threshold* tool divides the CT angiography dataset into two segments, based on the Hounsfield Unit range selected. This labels the voxels, or three-dimensional pixels, as either colored or uncoloured, covering areas of the selected intensity values throughout all slices of the CT angiogram.

Segmentation via thresholding is performed based on intensity values alone. Hence the process, whilst automated, may result in artifact, or unwanted areas that have been highlighted due to their similar density to the region of interest. These can be removed using the *Save Island* function. *Save Island* retains the selected anatomy and removes disconnected voxels with the same intensity.

Creating a 3D Model

In 3D Slicer, a preview of the segmented AAA can be visualized in the 3D viewing screen by toggling *View 3D*. For the purposes of EVAR planning, the AAA can be cropped superior to the visceral segment of the aorta, and inferior to the bifurcation of the common iliac arteries by using the *Scissors* function. The *Hollow* function converts the external surface of the intra-luminal contrast into the internal surface, growing a wall of the specified thickness around it, preserving the diameter of the lumen. Once the process is complete, the AAA model is *Exported* to be prepared for 3D printing. The AAA model is by default saved in Visualization ToolKit (VTK) format. This is best converted to Standard Triangle Language (STL) format which is compatible with 3D printers and Computer Aided Design (CAD) software.

Preparing the AAA Phantom for 3D Printing

Depending on the presurgical simulation intended, or the lesson plan in mind, the model can be further modified using CAD software prior to 3D printing. The vascular phantom can be made modular to introduce increasing levels of complexity, or the inflow and outflow modified to allow compatibility with a fluid circuit. For these purposes, Meshmixer (version 3.5, Autodesk, California, US, 2020) is the open source CAD software favored by many groups in the literature, due to a useful feature in the *Analysis* menu. The *Inspector* tool allows the user-friendly *Auto Repair* of defects in the model prior to 3D printing.

3D Printing the AAA Phantom

Once the STL file is ready for 3D printing, it is loaded into the proprietary 3D printing software associated with the 3D printing machine and printed. Phantoms produced using the three main 3D printing modalities, Fused Deposition Modeling (FDM), Stereolithography (SLA) and Inkjet are described below in our *Results*.

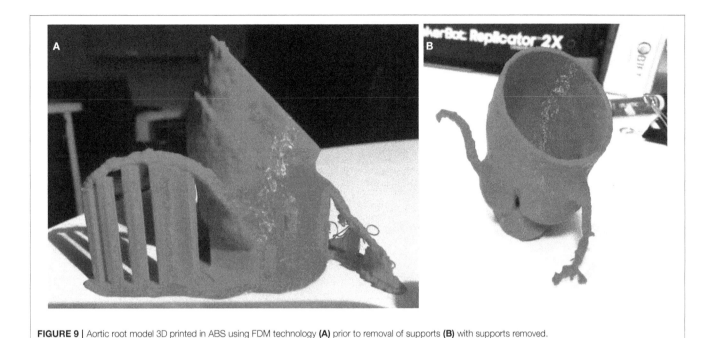

FIGURE 9 | Aortic root model 3D printed in ABS using FDM technology **(A)** prior to removal of supports **(B)** with supports removed.

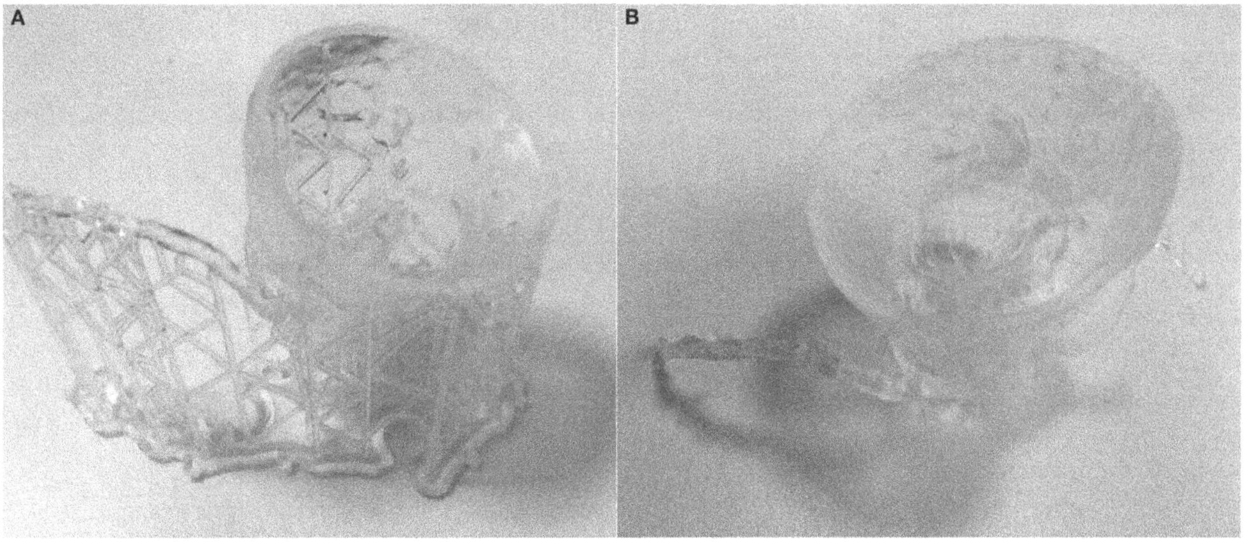

FIGURE 10 | Same aortic root model as previous 3D printed in transparent resin using SLA technology **(A)** prior to removal of supports **(B)** with supports removed.

RESULTS

In our experience, 3D printed AAA phantoms are of limited utility in the presurgical planning of standard infrarenal AAA cases. However, they have influenced surgical decision making and device selection in complex cases. In addition, these models have been 3D printed and demonstrated to be useful in a variety of settings, including patient education and engagement, surgical and anatomical education, as well as intraoperative visualization.

There remains room for improvement in the manufacturing of these models, in particular for greater cost efficiency and

material properties mimicking those of a diseased aorta as we seek to create a AAA phantom with optimal anatomical, haptic and fluoroscopic fidelity.

Fused Deposition Modeling (FDM)

FDM is an accessible avenue to begin 3D printing vascular phantoms. There is a large variety of makes and models available on the market, with our group having experience with the Makerbot Replicator 2X (Stratasys, Minnesota, USA), Flashforge Creator Pro (Zhejiang, China), Prusa I3 MK3S (Prague, Czech Republic), and Ultimaker S5 (Utrecht, Netherlands). These

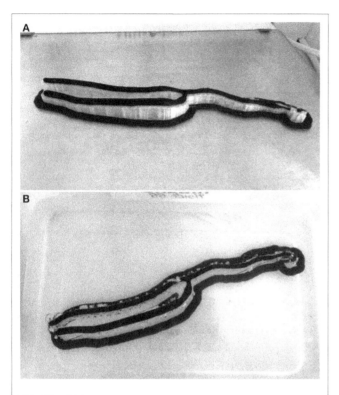

FIGURE 11 | (A) A 3D printed brachial artery model prior to removal from the print bed, with supports *in situ*. **(B)** The same model in a water bath to dissolve the PVA supports.

early work in the literature of 3D printed AAA visceral segment models for the planning of fenestrated physician modified stent grafts on the sterile back table (33).

Inkjet

Inkjet printers produce multicolored, multi-material models with variable shore hardness. Our group have used the Object500 Connex3 Polyjet (Stratasys, Minneapolis, USA), the Stratasys J750 (Stratasys, Minneapolis, USA), and the Projet 3500 3D printers (3D Systems Corporation, Rock Hill, USA) to produce flexible, translucent aortic phantoms. Due to the greater size of the print bed on these commercial 3D printers, even most large AAAs can be 3D printed in a single piece, costing $700–1,000 in materials.

At the outset, Inkjet printers require a significant financial investment or collaboration with an academic center when building a hospital-based 3D printing service. For example, the Stratasys J750 retails for $600,000, and a 1 kg cartridge of the resin required for 3D printing costs $2,000.

Postprocessing

Regardless of the 3D printing technique, FDM, SLA, and Inkjet 3D printed phantoms require postprocessing prior to use, and the removal of support material required to support the weight of the object during the 3D printing process. Disposal metal scissors and forceps allow for the removal of support material with accuracy and control. This process typically requires a few minutes of manual removal, and up to 20 min for more intricate models (**Figures 9–10**).

Dissolvable support material is an alternative, with Polyvinyl Acetate (PVA) support material available for dual-extrusion FDM machines, which is readily dissolved in water. Chemical solvents are required to dissolve the large amount of supports present on Inkjet 3D printed models (**Figure 11**). This is preferable to water jetting the support material, which risks damaging intricate anatomy, particularly when producing flexible models. A disadvantage of soluble support material is the overnight wait for supports to dissolve, adding to the production time of the workflow.

Depending on the 3D printer used, the AAA may need to be sectioned into several parts to fit the available volume for printing. In particular, conventional hobbyist FDM and SLA 3D printers are limited by small print beds, with larger thoracoabdominal aneurysms required to be 3D printed in pieces and joined together with epoxy resin.

hobbyist 3D printers retail in the range of hundreds to thousands of dollars, making them an inexpensive option to begin exploring the technology. Professional tier FDM 3D printers are more reliable and require less maintenance.

The machines consume inexpensive thermoplastics, retailing from $30–80 for a kilogram, which equates to $10–20 per AAA model. Although transparent thermoplastics exist, the resolution of FDM technology and the layered deposition results in at best a translucent end product, as reported by Chung et al. (32). Depending on the size of the AAA being printed, FDM machines require 24–48 h to 3D print the final product, with additional time required for support structures to be manually removed.

Stereolithography (SLA)

SLA printers retail in the range of thousands of dollars. Most of our experience has been with the Formlabs Form 2 (Somerville, Massachusetts, USA) SLA printer. The benefit of the SLA printer over FDM technology is in its greater resolution, allowing for the creation of transparent 3D printed AAA models which allow the trajectory of devices to be visualized during simulation. 1 L of clear or opaque resin retails for $150, equating to roughly $50–100 per model. Despite the slightly higher cost, we have come to rely on the SLA printer due to its lower print failure rate and ability to create transparent models.

In addition, Formlabs carry an autoclavable dental resin which has received FDA approval to be autoclaved. This has resulted in

Performance Under Fluoroscopy

FDM, SLA and Inkjet 3D printed AAA phantoms are equally visible under fluoroscopy, allowing for another level of realism to be added to the simulation task. Despite the fact that all three 3D printing techniques performed equally from a visual perspective, due to the resolution of FDM technology which features building melted layers of plastic to create the final product, the grooves between layers were haptically perceptible when traversed by wires (**Figure 12**). While superior to conventional CT angiography or workstation 3D reconstructions, uneven ridges have the potential to affect the trajectory of guidewires

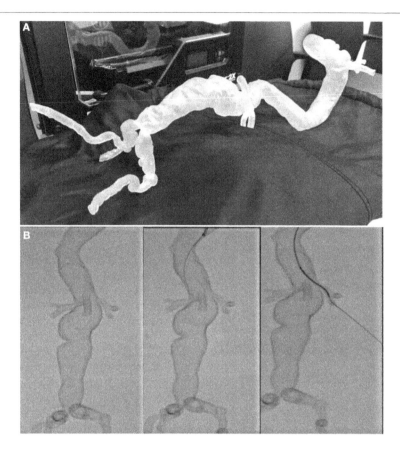

FIGURE 12 | (A) A hollow transparent complex thoracoabdominal aneurysm phantom 3D printed using SLA technology. **(B)** Stages of the phantom being cannulated under fluoroscopy for interventional planning. This "pre-flight" simulation was invaluable in predicting navigational difficulties, with the trajectory of guidewires and devices matching what was encountered during live surgery.

and devices during preoperative simulation. In addition, we have found that the lack of compliance in rigid 3D printed materials adds an additional level of difficulty when traversing tortuous iliac arteries.

DISCUSSION

AAA phantoms 3D printed using a variety of 3D printing technologies, despite material limitations, successfully mimic the cannulation and deployment challenges encountered during live endovascular surgery. As dimensional and representational material validity improves, they have the potential to serve as a powerful adjunct to how complex EVAR cases are planned.

Comparison of 3D Printed AAA Phantoms to Other Vascular Territories

3D printed AAAs, and other large vascular phantoms involving the aorta, result in greater challenges with regard to efficient production. Unless access to commercial 3D printers are readily accessible, 3D printed AAAs must often be produced in pieces and joined together prior to use, due to limitations on the size of the print bed on hobbyist machines.

In the case of simulating procedures in smaller vascular territories such as the Circle of Willis or Internal Carotid Artery it may be wiser to create a negative of the anatomy of the interest contained within a solid 3D printed block. From our experience in these smaller vascular territories this creates a more durable result in these small diameter vessels which are more prone to moving or breaking during simulation.

Anatomical Accuracy of 3D Printed Phantoms

We have outlined the workflow required to produce 3D printed vascular phantoms, with each step introducing a potential avenue for error during the imaging, segmentation, or 3D printing phases. It is evident that further work validating the accuracy of 3D printed models for surgical simulation is warranted. As with all new devices and techniques, surgeons are accustomed to the circumspect application of new technologies to meet the needs of each individual patient.

Image Acquisition

Patient-specific anatomical models are as accurate as the imaging from which they originate. A useful principle is that the imaging modality that best visualizes the anatomy for conventional

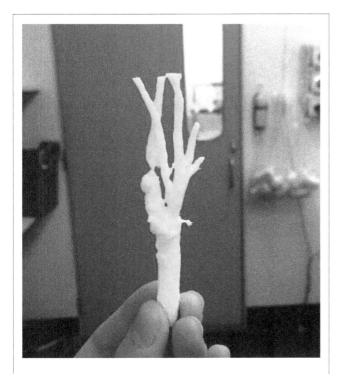

FIGURE 13 | A solid 3D printed internal carotid artery used to plan carotid endarterectomy.

surgical planning will produce the most detailed anatomical model. Imaging modalities are ever improving, with these improvements benefiting patients regardless of whether an anatomical model is 3D printed (**Figure 13**). In the vascular territories, optimizing vascular imaging requires the mitigation of motion artifact, and sufficient contrast discrimination and resolution.

For example, dual-energy CT angiography would allow for better contrast discrimination of intravascular calcium from contrast, as well as improving temporal resolution in both peripheral and aortic vascular territories (34, 35). Similarly, electrocardiographic-gated CT coronary angiography allows for the reduction of motion artifacts in valvular heart disease (36), leading to a superior 3D printed anatomical model.

It is evident that as 3D printing becomes more grounded in conventional surgical practice, improving current imaging protocols in order to optimize the final 3D printed product is a necessary area of further study.

3D Modeling

Medical image processing software is the next step in the workflow that has a potential to introduce error. Kang et al. compared four of the most readily available commercial software options, InVivoDental (version 5.0; Anatomage, San Jose, CA, 2015), Mimics (version 14.0; Materialize NV, Leuven, Belgium, 2015), OnDemand3D (APP version 1.0; CyberMed Inc, Seoul, Korea, 2015), and OsiriX Imaging Software (version 3.7; Pixmeo, Geneva, Switzerland, 2015) in the creation of craniofacial models (37), determining that InVivoDental was most accurate in producing 3D models from CT imaging.

All four segmentation software packages were accurate at the voxel or subvoxel level; however, there were statistically significant differences in all anatomical regions between the four software packages tested. Kang et al. were not able to access the proprietary coding of these commercial software packages, hence the study was unable to apply the same standardized parameters across the board, limiting direct comparison. Despite this, the fact that all models were accurate to the level of individual voxels was a reassuring finding.

3D Printing

There is currently no gold standard for validating the accuracy of patient-specific anatomical models produced by 3D printing. However, early work from multiple groups suggests the accuracy of 3D printed models are within acceptable limits for presurgical planning (38–41).

Hazeveld et al. compared the accuracy of different 3D printing technologies (42). Given what is known about the accuracy of each 3D printing technology, the study confirmed that dimensional error was lowest for Inkjet 3D printing, followed by SLA, and finally FDM. Specific to 3D printed vasculature, Takao et al. determined splenic artery aneurysms 3D printed using FDM printers to be highly precise and accurate, with the cross-sectional areas amongst the 3D printed models within SD <0.05 cm^2 (range 0.00–0.05) (6).

Determining Validity

The ideal AAA phantom is one that is not only anatomically accurate but boasts high haptic and fluoroscopic fidelity. In developing this workflow, we have sought to produce 3D printed AAAs with the highest possible representational validity within the constraints of a bench to bedside approach, accessible to the hospital vascular proceduralist.

The necessity of each measure of fidelity depends upon its intended application. For example, for the purposes of presurgical simulation and the education of trainees, high haptic and fluoroscopic fidelity are much more important than when a 3D printed AAA model is used to educate patients. As previously discussed by our group, the validity of a simulation tool can be evaluated in several ways, with a current lack of objective evidence as to how the different measures of validity can be assessed (43). Face validity involves comparing the anatomical and haptic fidelity of a simulator to the current "gold standard" trainers or to performing the procedure *in vivo* (44). It is a highly subjective, but most common measure used in the medical simulation literature. Predictive validity is a much more objective and desirable goal, and involves an assessment of patient outcomes (44) as a result of the simulation. As previously discussed, there are clinical trials underway exploring if 3D printed anatomical models for presurgical planning do indeed improve patient outcomes (1), but none on the topic of endovascular intervention.

A Hospital-Based 3D Printing Service

3D printed anatomical models present a promising new frontier in the planning and simulation of complex surgical procedures. The American Medical Association has recognized the potential

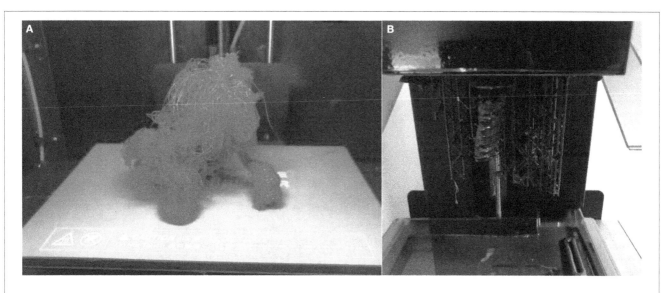

FIGURE 14 | Failed prints on **(A)** FDM. **(B)** SLA 3D printers.

of 3D printed anatomical models in presurgical planning and in producing surgical guides, introducing two reimbursement codes last year (45).

The strength of 3D printing anatomical models when compared to other technologies is its unprecedented accessibility to the vascular specialist, allowing for just-in-time manufacturing. When compared to commissioning an external commercial provider, 3D printed vascular phantoms can be translated from bench to bedside in a matter of hours, lowering costs to surgical units and the time required for the model to be shipped to the hospital. In addition, the current COVID-19 pandemic has emphasized the importance of local health services to be self-sufficient with regard to supplies.

However, the centralized manufacturing approach requires local hospitals to invest in the medical image processing, CAD and 3D printing hardware and skills outlined in this manuscript in order to access this technology. While this would result in significant cost savings for the anatomical models themselves, with flow-on effects of reduced theater time and blood loss resulting in cost savings to the hospital system, it represents a more substantial initial investment.

Limitations of Current Technology

3D printing remains a rapidly evolving technology which is becoming increasingly accessible to vascular proceduralists and the general public. With current levels of technology, inexpensive hobbyist 3D printers are less reliable than their commercial counterparts, particularly when first experimenting with the print orientation of objects. Despite this, they remain an accessible starting point for vascular specialists seeking to begin their foray into the technology (**Figure 14**). The print failure rate is lessened when printing smaller models, when compared to large vascular phantoms such as thoracoabdominal aneurysms, and when 3D printers are adequately maintained.

CONCLUSION

Once the challenges in developing this workflow were overcome, 3D printed anatomical models have become commonplace in the planning of complex procedures in our Vascular Unit and the broader Department of Surgery. Physical patient-specific models have proven to be a valuable addition to standard imaging, and in the rehearsal and modification of devices prior to surgery. When planning the approach to complex AAAs, hollow flexible models are particularly useful for the rehearsal of endograft insertion and positioning via iliac artery access, and in predicting the trajectory of guidewires and devices.

As 3D printing technologies become more common, reliable, and cost effective, their use in preprocedural simulation will flourish. In sharing this methodology, we warmly invite comments from others with an interest in 3D printing in vascular interventional planning in how we can further explore its uses.

AUTHOR CONTRIBUTIONS

JC-B contributed to the write up, study design, and experiments performed in this manuscript. DB contributed to the write up and design of this manuscript. JC contributed to the write up, design, and supervision of this manuscript. All authors contributed to the article and approved the submitted version.

REFERENCES

1. Witowski J, Sitkowski M, Zuzak T, Coles-Black J, Chuen J, Major P, et al. From ideas to long-term studies: 3D printing clinical trials review. *Int J Comput Assist Radiol Surg.* (2018) 13:1473–8. doi: 10.1007/s11548-018-1793-8

2. Marone EM, Auricchio F, Marconi S, Conti M, Rinaldi LF, Pietrabissa A, et al. Effectiveness of 3D printed models in the treatment of complex aortic diseases. *J Cardiovasc Surg (Torino).* (2018) 59:699–706. doi: 10.23736/S0021-9509.18.10324-7

3. Taher F, Falkensammer J, McCarte J, Strassegger J, Uhlmann M, Schuch P, et al. The influence of prototype testing in three-dimensional aortic models on fenestrated endograft design. *J Vasc Surg.* (2017) 65:1591–7. doi: 10.1016/j.jvs.2016.10.108

4. Leotta DF, Starnes BW. Custom fenestration templates for endovascular repair of juxtarenal aortic aneurysms. *J Vasc Surg.* (2015) 61:1637–41. doi: 10.1016/j.jvs.2015.02.016

5. Kono K, Shintani A, Okada H, Terada T. Preoperative simulations of endovascular treatment for a cerebral aneurysm using a patient-specific vascular silicone model. *Neurol Med Chir (Tokyo).* (2013) 53:347–51. doi: 10.2176/nmc.53.347

6. Takao H, Amemiya S, Shibata E, Ohtomo K. 3D printing of preoperative simulation models of a splenic artery aneurysm: precision and accuracy. *Acad Radiol.* (2017) 24:650–3. doi: 10.1016/j.acra.2016.12.015

7. Torres IO, De Luccia N. A simulator for training in endovascular aneurysm repair: The use of three dimensional printers. *Eur J Vasc Endovasc Surg.* (2017) 54:247–53. doi: 10.1016/j.ejvs.2017.05.011

8. Qiao F, Li D, Jin Z, Hao D, Liao Y, Gong S. A novel combination of computer-assisted reduction technique and three dimensional printed patient-specific external fixator for treatment of tibial fractures. *Int Orthop.* (2016) 40:835–41. doi: 10.1007/s00264-015-2943-z

9. Coles-Black J, Chao I, Chuen J. Three-dimensional printing in medicine. *Med J Aust.* (2017) 207:102–3. doi: 10.5694/mja16.01073

10. Sakalihasan N, Limet R, Defawe OD. Abdominal aortic aneurysm. *Lancet.* (2005) 365:1577–89. doi: 10.1016/S0140-6736(05)66459-8

11. Kniemeyer HW, Kessler T, Reber PU, Ris HB, Hakki H, Widmer MK. Treatment of ruptured abdominal aortic aneurysm, a permanent challenge or a waste of resources? Prediction of outcome using a multi-organ-dysfunction score. *Eur J Vasc Endovasc Surg.* (2000) 19:190–6. doi: 10.1053/ejvs.1999.0980

12. Calero A, Illig KA. Overview of aortic aneurysm management in the endovascular era. *Semin Vasc Surg.* (2016) 29:3–17. doi: 10.1053/j.semvascsurg.2016.07.003

13. Greenhalgh RM, Brown LC, Kwong GP, Powell JT, Thompson SG. Comparison of endovascular aneurysm repair with open repair in patients with abdominal aortic aneurysm (EVAR trial 1), 30-day operative mortality results: randomised controlled trial. *Lancet.* (2004) 364:843–8. doi: 10.1016/S0140-6736(04)16979-1

14. Prinssen M, Verhoeven EL, Buth J, Cuypers PW, van Sambeek MR, Balm R, et al. A randomized trial comparing conventional and endovascular repair of abdominal aortic aneurysms. *N Engl J Med.* (2004) 351:1607–18. doi: 10.1056/NEJMoa042002

15. Bismuth J, Donovan MA, O'Malley MK, El Sayed HF, Naoum JJ, Peden EK, et al. Incorporating simulation in vascular surgery education. *J Vasc Surg.* (2010) 52:1072–80. doi: 10.1016/j.jvs.2010.05.093

16. Widmer LW, Schmidli J, Widmer MK, Wyss TR. Simulation in vascular access surgery training. *J Vasc Access.* (2015) 16(Suppl. 9):S121–5. doi: 10.5301/jva.5000372

17. Duran C, Bismuth J, Mitchell E. A nationwide survey of vascular surgery trainees reveals trends in operative experience, confidence, and attitudes about simulation. *J Vasc Surg.* (2013) 58:524–8. doi: 10.1016/j.jvs.2012.12.072

18. Neequaye SK, Aggarwal R, Van Herzeele I, Darzi A, Cheshire NJ. Endovascular skills training and assessment. *J Vasc Surg.* (2007) 46:1055–64. doi: 10.1016/j.jvs.2007.05.041

19. Aggarwal R, Black SA, Hance JR, Darzi A, Cheshire NJ. Virtual reality simulation training can improve inexperienced surgeons' endovascular skills. *Eur J Vasc Endovasc Surg.* (2006) 31:588–93. doi: 10.1016/j.ejvs.2005.11.009

20. Vento V, Cercenelli L, Mascoli C, Gallitto E, Ancetti S, Faggioli G, et al. The role of simulation in boosting the learning curve in EVAR procedures. *J Surg Educ.* (2018) 75:534–40. doi: 10.1016/j.jsurg.2017.08.013

21. Fedorov A, Beichel R, Kalpathy-Cramer J, Finet J, Fillion-Robin JC, Pujol S, et al. 3D Slicer as an image computing platform for the Quantitative Imaging Network. *Magn Reson Imaging.* (2012) 30:1323–41. doi: 10.1016/j.mri.2012.05.001

22. Chana-Rodriguez F, Mananes RP, Rojo-Manaute J, Gil P, Martinez-Gomiz JM, Vaquero-Martin J. 3D surgical printing and pre contoured plates for acetabular fractures. *Injury.* (2016) 47:2507–11.

23. Scawn RL, Foster A, Lee BW, Kikkawa DO, Korn BS. Customised 3D printing: an innovative training tool for the next generation of orbital surgeons. *Orbit.* (2015) 34:216–9. doi: 10.3109/01676830.2015.1049367

24. Skowyra J, Pietrzak K, Alhnan MA. Fabrication of extended-release patient-tailored prednisolone tablets via fused deposition modelling (FDM) 3D printing. *Eur J Pharm Sci.* (2015) 68:11–7. doi: 10.1016/j.ejps.2014.11.009

25. Man QW, Jia J, Liu K, Chen G, Liu B. Secondary reconstruction for mandibular osteoradionecrosis defect with fibula osteomyocutaneous flap flowthrough from radial forearm flap using stereolithographic 3-dimensional printing modeling technology. *J Craniofac Surg.* (2015) 26:e190–3. doi: 10.1097/SCS.0000000000001456

26. Dhir V, Itoi T, Fockens P, Perez-Miranda M, Khashab MA, Seo DW, et al. Novel *ex vivo* model for hands-on teaching of and training in EUS-guided biliary drainage: creation of "Mumbai EUS" stereolithography/3D printing bile duct prototype (with videos). *Gastrointest Endosc.* (2015) 81:440–6. doi: 10.1016/j.gie.2014.09.011

27. Skoog SA, Goering PL, Narayan RJ. Stereolithography in tissue engineering. *J Mater Sci Mater Med.* (2014) 25:845–56. doi: 10.1007/s10856-013-5107-y

28. Barbosa MZ, Zylbersztejn DS, de Mattos LA, Carvalho LF. Three-dimensionally-printed models in reproductive surgery: systematic review and clinical applications. *Minerva Ginecol.* (2019) 71:235–44. doi: 10.23736/S0026-4784.19.04319-3

29. Maddox MM, Feibus A, Liu J, Wang J, Thomas R, Silberstein JL. 3D-printed soft-tissue physical models of renal malignancies for individualized surgical simulation: a feasibility study. *J Robot Surg.* (2018) 12:27–33. doi: 10.1007/s11701-017-0680-6

30. Yu T, Zhu X, Tang L, Wang D, Saad N. Review of CT angiography of aorta. *Radiol Clin North Am.* (2007) 45:461–83. doi: 10.1016/j.rcl.2007.04.010

31. Carroll JE, Colley ES, Thomas SD, Varcoe RL, Simmons A, Barber TJ. Tracking geometric and hemodynamic alterations of an arteriovenous fistula through patient-specific modelling. *Comput Methods Programs Biomed.* (2020) 186:105203. doi: 10.1016/j.cmpb.2019.105203

32. Chung M, Radacsi N, Robert C, McCarthy ED, Callanan A, Conlisk N, et al. On the optimization of low-cost FDM 3D printers for accurate replication of patient-specific abdominal aortic aneurysm geometry. *3D Print Med.* (2018) 4:2. doi: 10.1186/s41205-017-0023-2

33. Branzan D, Winkler D, Schmidt A, Scheinert D, Grunert R. 3-Dimensional aortic model to create a fenestrated stent graft for the urgent treatment of a paravisceral penetrating aortic ulcer. *JACC Cardiovasc Interv.* (2019) 12:793–5. doi: 10.1016/j.jcin.2018.10.024

34. Brockmann C, Jochum S, Sadick M, Huck K, Ziegler P, Fink C, et al. Dual-energy CT angiography in peripheral arterial occlusive disease. *Cardiovasc Intervent Radiol.* (2009) 32:630–7. doi: 10.1007/s00270-008-9491-5

35. Shaqdan KW, Parakh A, Kambadakone AR, Sahani DV. Role of dual energy CT to improve diagnosis of non-traumatic abdominal vascular emergencies. *Abdom Radiol (NY).* (2019) 44:406–21. doi: 10.1007/s00261-018-1741-7

36. Manghat NE, Rachapalli V, Van Lingen R, Veitch AM, Roobottom CA, Morgan-Hughes GJ. Imaging the heart valves using ECG-gated 64-detector row cardiac CT. *Br J Radiol.* (2008) 81:275–90. doi: 10.1259/bjr/16301537

37. Kang SH, Kim MK, Kim HJ, Zhengguo P, Lee SH. Accuracy assessment of image-based surface meshing for volumetric computed tomography images in the craniofacial region. *J Craniofac Surg.* (2014) 25:2051–5. doi: 10.1097/SCS.0000000000001139

38. Ye N, Long H, Zhu S, Yang Y, Lai W, Hu J. The accuracy of computer image-guided template for mandibular angle ostectomy. *Aesthetic Plast Surg.* (2015) 39:117–23. doi: 10.1007/s00266-014-0424-1

39. Sun Y, Luebbers HT, Agbaje JO, Schepers S, Vrielinck L, Lambrichts I, et al. Accuracy of upper jaw positioning with intermediate splint fabrication after virtual planning in bimaxillary orthognathic surgery. *J Craniofac Surg.* (2013) 24:1871–6. doi: 10.1097/SCS.0b013e31829a80d9

40. Ono I, Abe K, Shiotani S, Hirayama Y. Producing a full-scale model from computed tomographic data with the rapid prototyping technique using the binder jet method: a comparison with the laser lithography method using a dry skull. *J Craniofac Surg.* (2000) 11:527–37. doi: 10.1097/00001665-200011060-00004

41. Otawa N, Sumida T, Kitagaki H, Sasaki K, Fujibayashi S, Takemoto M, et al. Custom-made titanium devices as membranes for bone augmentation in implant treatment: Modeling accuracy of titanium products constructed with selective laser melting. *J Craniomaxillofac Surg.* (2015) 43:1289–95. doi: 10.1016/j.jcms.2015.05.006

42. Hazeveld A, Huddleston Slater JJ, Ren Y. Accuracy and reproducibility of dental replica models reconstructed by different rapid prototyping techniques. *Am J Orthod Dentofacial Orthop.* (2014) 145:108–15. doi: 10.1016/j.ajodo.2013.05.011

43. Chen G, Jiang M, Coles-Black J, Mansour K, Chuen J, Amott D. Three-dimensional printing as a tool in otolaryngology training: a systematic review. *J Laryngol Otol.* (2020) 134:14–9. doi: 10.1017/S0022215119002585

44. Gallagher AG, Ritter EM, Satava RM. Fundamental principles of validation, and reliability: rigorous science for the assessment of surgical education and training. *Surg Endosc.* (2003) 17:1525–9. doi: 10.1007/s00464-003-0035-4

45. Kemp S, Coles-Black J, Walker MJ, Wallace G, Chuen J, Mukherjee P. Ethical and regulatory considerations for surgeons as consumers and creators of three-dimensional printed medical devices. *ANZ J Surg.* (2020) 90:1477–81. doi: 10.1111/ans.15871

9

3D Printing Improved Testicular Prostheses: Using Lattice Infill Structure to Modify Mechanical Properties

Jacob Skewes[1], Michael Y. Chen[1,2,3], David Forrestal[1,2], Nicholas J. Rukin[2,3,4] and Maria A. Woodruff[1]*

[1] Engineering Faculty, Queensland University of Technology, Brisbane, QLD, Australia, [2] Herston Biofabrication Institute, Metro North Hospital and Health Service, Brisbane, QLD, Australia, [3] Redcliffe Hospital, Metro North Hospital and Health Service, Brisbane, QLD, Australia, [4] School of Medicine, University of Queensland, Brisbane, QLD, Australia

Correspondence:
Maria A. Woodruff
mia.woodruff@@qut.edu.au

Patients often opt for implantation of testicular prostheses following orchidectomy for cancer or torsion. Recipients of testicular prostheses report issues regarding firmness, shape, size, and position, aspects of which relate to current limitations of silicone materials used and manufacturing methods for soft prostheses. We aim to create a 3D printable testicular prosthesis which mimics the natural shape and stiffness of a human testicle using a lattice infill structure. Porous testicular prostheses were engineered with relative densities from 0.1 to 0.9 using a repeating cubic unit cell lattice inside an anatomically accurate testicle 3D model. These models were printed using a multi-jetting process with an elastomeric material and compared with current market prostheses using shore hardness tests. Additionally, standard sized porous specimens were printed for compression testing to verify and match the stiffness to human testicle elastic modulus (E-modulus) values from literature. The resulting 3D printed testicular prosthesis of relative density between 0.3 and 0.4 successfully achieved a reduction of its bulk compressive E-modulus from 360 KPa to a human testicle at 28 Kpa. Additionally, this is the first study to quantitatively show that current commercial testicular prostheses are too firm compared to native tissue. 3D printing allows us to create metamaterials that match the properties of human tissue to create customisable patient specific prostheses. This method expands the use cases for existing biomaterials by tuning their properties and could be applied to other implants mimicking native tissues.

Keywords: 3D printing, testicular prosthesis, meta-materials, bio-fabrication, implants, soft prostheses, bio-materials

INTRODUCTION

Testicle prostheses are offered to patients following orchidectomy for testicular tumors, loss after torsion, atrophy, and undescended testicles. These prostheses are made from silicone, like breast implants, either being fully solid, saline-filled, or silicone gel-filled. There are theoretical risks associated with silicone and liquid-filled implants, including connective tissue diseases, auto-immune disorders, and implant failure due to rupture. While these risks remain very low, there is a market push toward an alternative for silicone use in soft prosthetic implant design (1–3).

The main issues regarding testicular implants are related to the use and limitations of current materials and manufacturing methods. Recipients of testicle prostheses often describe them as being too firm, not the right size or shape, or positioned too high. These aspects can adversely affect physical exercise, sexual activity and confidence, leading to dissatisfaction and regretting the decision for accepting an implant. Sizes for testicular prostheses offered on the market are limited to small, medium, and large despite the individual nature of the human body (4–7). Additionally, they are designed to be sutured in place only in one position at the top of the prosthesis allowing them to freely rotate around that point inside the scrotum (8). The solution to these problems may lie with adopting new approaches to customized implant design using 3D scanning, modeling, and printing. Size, shape, and suture positioning could be adapted to an individual's needs using these technologies. However, a significant challenge for improving the firmness or "feel" of prosthetic testicles is the lack of medically approved bio-materials with appropriate properties.

To the best of our knowledge there is currently no study which quantifies and compares current market testicular prostheses regarding firmness, size and shape to verify patient complaints or provide a benchmark for creating an improved prosthesis. The use of 3D printing in individual testicle prosthesis design is limited and does not focus on developing prostheses with the intention to solve issues regarding firmness, soft tissue applications or using 3D printing to directly print an implant (9).

Consequently, it would be highly beneficial to create a system where already approved, well-established materials could be manufactured using innovative techniques to alter material properties. Doing so would allow a testicular prosthesis or other soft prostheses to have controllable properties that match natural tissue.

3D printing processes typically create components layer by layer from 3D computer models. Currently, 3D printing is the only method which can produce precisely controlled lattice filled structures. Research with lattice filled structures to create bio-mimetic properties has been extensively used with metals and primarily focused on mimicking bone and hard tissue properties (10–12). By creating a soft prosthesis using this method, we can overcome common problems described by patients, while avoiding the need for silicone gels or liquid infills to develop a safer, more natural-feeling product. In this study, we aim to prototype a 3D printed testicular prosthesis by engineering a lattice structure that exhibits the natural feel, size and shape of a real testicle.

A meta-material is a material engineered to have particular mechanical properties based on its sub-structure and not material composition. For example, two foams made from the same material can be either stiff or soft depending on their relative densities. However, while foam is made with randomized sub-structures, a meta-material is populated with a repeating shape called a unit cell. Properties such as the E-modulus (stiffness) and hardness can be finely tuned by manipulating the physical parameters of the unit cell. This approach was used to design a 3D printed testicular prosthesis with anatomical shape, size, and tuneable stiffness. **Figure 1** outlines the method for designing the testicular prostheses.

MATERIALS AND METHODS
Testicular Prosthesis Design
Testicle prostheses and standard sized samples were 3D printed using Visijet M2 ENT UV Curable Elastomeric material with a Projet MJP 2500 3D printer (3D Systems, Rock Hill, United States). The reported E-modulus (E_s), strength (σ_s), and density (ρ_s) of this material was 0.27–0.43 MPa, 0.2–0.4 MPa, and 1.12g/cm^3, respectively (13). The unit cell chosen to adjust the mechanical properties of the base material is the cubic lattice structure made of circular cross-sectional beams with a length (l) and radius (r). This unit cell was chosen because of its simplicity and known analytical relationships. The relative density can be adjusted using Equation (1) and the E-modulus (related to firmness, hardness and feel) can be adjusted using Equation (2).

$$\frac{\rho}{\rho_s} = 3\pi \left(\frac{r}{l}\right)^2 - 8\sqrt{2}\left(\frac{r}{l}\right)^3 \tag{1}$$

$$\frac{E}{E_S} = \frac{\pi r^2}{l^2} \tag{2}$$

These equations are based on the applied mechanics Euler-Bernoulli beam theory which suggest that a minimum of six unit cells in the X, Y, and Z dimensions of a sample is needed for the analytical solutions to begin to converge to real world expectations (14, 15).

Testicles with relative densities 0.2, 0.3, 0.4, 0.5, 0.6, 0.7, 0.8, 0.9, and 1.0 (fully solid) using the cubic lattice structure were designed. The testicular prosthesis model and shape was adapted from the BodyParts3D database (16), a collection of anatomical 3D models of an adult human male. The dimensions of the testicle model used were 29, 31, and 38 mm in the X, Y, and Z directions, respectively. Considering the size of the model and to achieve the relative densities, the length of the unit cells were held constant at 3.5 mm while the radius of the beams were adjusted as depicted in **Figure 1C**. A wall thickness of 2 mm was chosen to provide the unit cells with a protective skin while minimizing any additional stiffness contribution to the prosthesis.

Compression tests with different shaped objects cannot be compared since the shape and cross-sectional area affects how much force is needed to displace a material. Additionally, shapes with non-uniform cross-sections cannot yield E-modulus values. Standard sized test samples with a uniform cross-section provide a way for determining the E-modulus of the lattice structures independent of its final shape. Thus, to verify the analytical models through compression testing, cube-shaped samples of uniform cross-sectional area (25 × 25 mm) using the same design parameters (unit cell size, shape, and top and bottom wall thickness) as the testicular prostheses were created using 3D printing (**Figure 1E**).

All 3D models were designed in 3D Sprint software package (3D Systems, Rock Hill, United States), a tool for manipulating parameters such as wall thickness, unit cell type, model size, and preparing the final models for 3D printing.

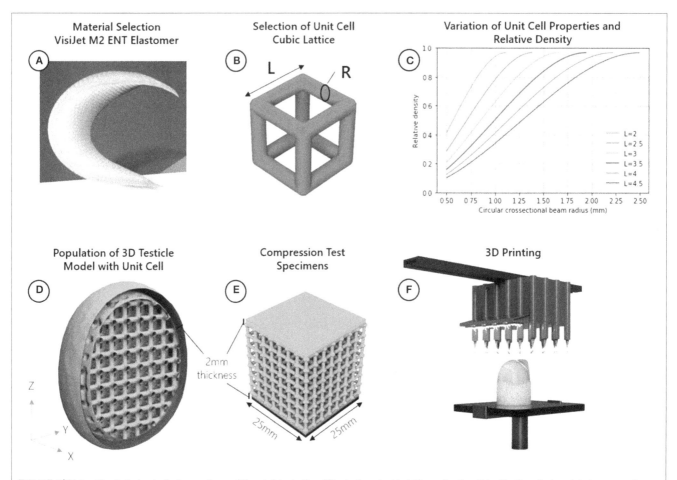

FIGURE 1 | Method for designing testicular prostheses; **(A)** material selection, **(B)** selection of cubic lattice unit cell and identification of relevant design parameters related to relative density length (L) and radius (R), **(C)** Plot showing how the radius and length of the cubic unit cell beams can be adjusted to achieve a range of relative densities, choosing a radius, or length which is too small may not be manufacturable, while choosing values too large narrows the range of achievable relative densities, **(D)** populate 3D model of testicle with cubic unit cell, **(E)** create compression test specimens with uniform cross-sectional area (25 mm²), **(F)** 3D print the testicles and compression specimens using a Multi-Jet process.

Testicular Prosthesis Manufacturing and Post-processing

The Projet MJP 2500 3D printer uses an inkjet printing head which dispenses droplets of a liquid photopolymer onto a build surface. The droplets are subsequently hardened by Ultra-Violet (UV) light. A wax support structure is simultaneously printed to fill any voids in the 3D model which requires removal post process in a hot water bath followed by an oil bath. This process is outlined in **Figure 2**. Using the 3D printer detailed here, the achievable X, Y, Z resolution is $1,600 \times 900 \times 90$ DPI, with a recommended minimum feature size of 25 μm. Based on the DPI, the resulting layer thickness in the Z direction was 32 μm. The printer parameters used regarding speed, curing time, temperature, and layer thickness were set at factory default settings by 3D Systems and cannot be changed since these parameters are optimized specifically to the MJF 2500 print head and Visijet M2 ENT UV material.

Compression Testing

Compression testing was conducted using an Instron Universal Testing System (Norwood, United States) with a 2 kN load cell compressing at 10 mm per min at a temperature of 25°C to 50% strain, along the Z axis of print direction for all samples. Cubic shaped samples of uniform cross-sectional area (**Figure 1E**) were compressed to verify the analytical model and determine the E-modulus (stiffness) of the bulk material and the relative densities. Values obtained from previously published studies using Real-Time Shear Wave Elastography to measure the E-modulus of male testicles were used to verify that the designed prostheses fell within the range of real testicular stiffness (28 ± 6 KPa) (17–19). For each relative density three samples were tested for statistical analysis.

Shore Hardness Testing

Shore hardness is a measure of a materials resistance to indentation using a device with a spring-loaded indenter. Using a

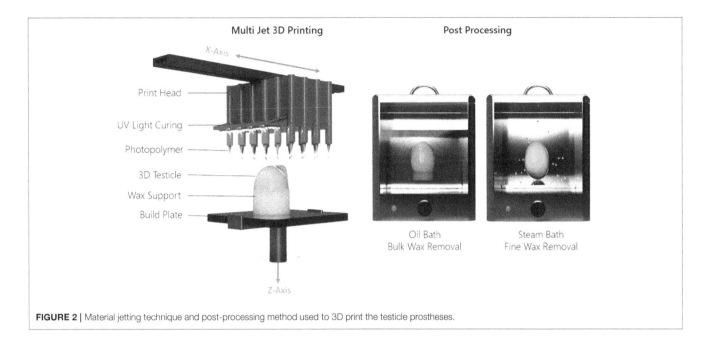

FIGURE 2 | Material jetting technique and post-processing method used to 3D print the testicle prostheses.

Shore OO Durometer device (Hildebrand, Zürich, Switzerland) we measured the hardness of the 3D printed prostheses and medical testicle prostheses, the gold standard comparison; Promedon© (Endotherapeutics, Epping, Australia), Kiwee© (Coloplast, Humlebaek, Denmark), and the Torosa© (Coloplast, Humlebaek, Denmark). These prostheses were categorized into four areas (top, bottom, left and right) to assess any change in hardness due to features or shape differences of the prostheses. The hardness was measured in the center of those areas at room temperature following the method of the ASTM D2240 standards.

RESULTS

3D Printed Testicular Prostheses and Cubic Lattice Samples

All 27 testicular prostheses and 27 cubic lattice samples, 9 of which are illustrated in **Figure 3A**, were printed together in 11.5 h. The average weight and material cost per prosthesis was 17 g and $16 AUD, respectively. A visual comparison of the market prostheses and a 3D printed testicular prosthesis with a relative density of 0.4 is shown in **Figure 3B**. The resulting testicular prostheses and samples appeared to have a smooth surface finish and layer lines often seen with 3D printed parts were not visible. **Figure 3C** captures the deformation of a 0.4 relative density cubic lattice sample under compression.

Compression Testing Results

Compression test results indicated that a 100% dense material with an E-modulus of 360 KPa is modifiable to a minimum of 10 KPa at 20% relative density. **Figure 4B** displays a comparison between the experimental and analytical results [from Equation (2)]. The averaged experimental results followed a similar trend; however, they are consistently lower than the analytical

prediction apart from relative density 0.9. At this relative density, the pore sizes are too small to allow the wax support structure to be fully removed post printing, leaving excess solid wax behind and contributing to an increase in stiffness (**Figure 4**).

Comparison with human testicle E-modulus values demonstrated that the relative densities using this model required to match the feel of a testicle were between 0.3 and 0.4 as shown in **Figure 4C**. For each specimen, a boxplot in **Figure 4D** shows the repeatability of the cubic lattice E-modulus results for a sample size of 3.

Hardness Testing Results

The results shown in **Figure 5** show how the hardness of the 3D printed testicles correlates to its relative density while revealing the hardness of the market prostheses exceeded the hardness of samples with relative densities 0.3 and 0.4 which is the range we would expect the hardness of a human testicle to be (5–15). The top side of each market prosthesis was much harder than the left, right, and bottom positions because the suture holes located there were made from a harder material. Relative density of 0.2 was omitted from the results as these prostheses were too soft to obtain reliable values.

DISCUSSION

Using 3D printing we have demonstrated with a meta-material approach and a cubic lattice unit cell that we can manufacture a novel testicular prosthesis where the shape, size, and stiffness can be finely tuned to match a human testicle. With this approach, the need for silicone or liquid infills and thus risk of rupture is eliminated. Importantly, this approach expands the potential use cases of existing medically approved materials. This provides opportunity for a single base material to be used for a range of prosthetic implant products that vary in

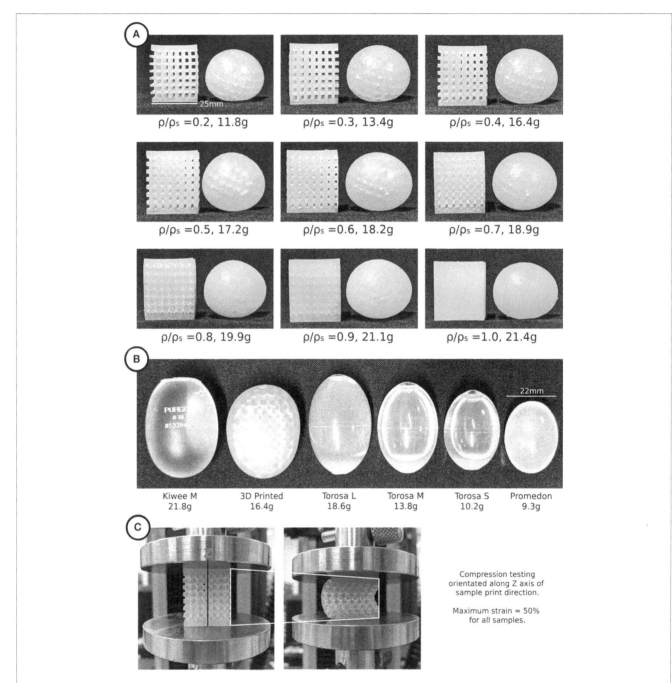

ρ/ρs =0.2, 11.8g   ρ/ρs =0.3, 13.4g   ρ/ρs =0.4, 16.4g

ρ/ρs =0.5, 17.2g   ρ/ρs =0.6, 18.2g   ρ/ρs =0.7, 18.9g

ρ/ρs =0.8, 19.9g   ρ/ρs =0.9, 21.1g   ρ/ρs =1.0, 21.4g

Kiwee M   3D Printed   Torosa L   Torosa M   Torosa S   Promedon
21.8g   16.4g   18.6g   13.8g   10.2g   9.3g

Compression testing
orientated along Z axis of
sample print direction.

Maximum strain = 50%
for all samples.

FIGURE 3 | (A) 3D printed testicular prostheses and cubic lattice compression samples of relative density 0.2–1.0, **(B)** Medical prostheses Kiwee, Torosa, and Promedon (L, large; M, medium; S, small) next to a 3D printed testicular prosthesis, **(C)** Compression testing of cubic lattice samples showing deformation.

stiffness or other mechanical properties, with cost savings from economies of scale and reduced regulatory approval or material certification processes. These advantages and benefits are directly translatable to other areas of prostheses or silicone implant designs and to patients or clinicians looking for an improved individualized product.

To our knowledge, this is the first study to quantify and compare medical testicular prosthesis characteristics using a shore hardness test. The results shown here clearly indicate that the existing medical prostheses are relatively too firm. Particularly the top section where the suture position is located, consistent with patient complaints of products being too hard (4–6).

The best performing medical prostheses regarding hardness was the Kiwee, with results in-between relative densities 0.3 and 0.4 (the ideal case). However, in October 2017 Coloplast withdrew the Kiwee prosthesis from the market due to "particles found on the surface of some implants" (20). Being the

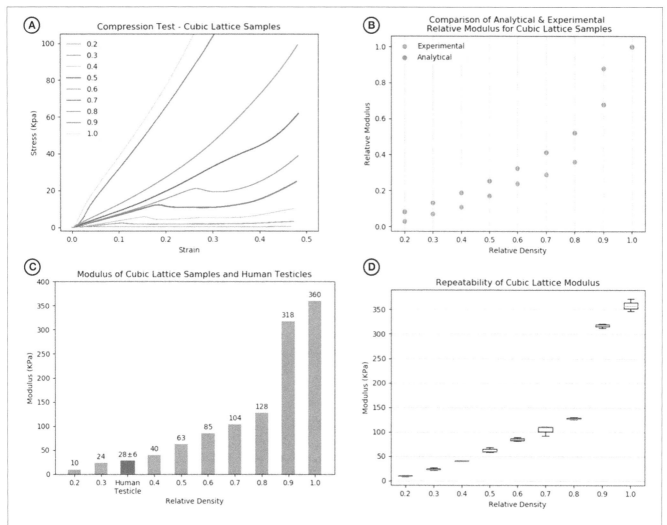

FIGURE 4 | (A) Compression test results of cubic lattice specimens showing increase in stiffness with relative density. **(B)** Comparison of analytical [Equation (1) and (2)] and experimental relative modulus for cubic lattice specimens. **(C)** Relative densities of 0.3–0.4 match with human testicle stiffness values. **(D)** The repeatability of the modulus values across a sample size of 3 for each relative density.

only silicone gel filled testicle prostheses, the removal of the Kiwee from the market leaves only two options for patients at our hospital; the Torosa (saline filled) and Promedon (solid silicone).

Hardness tests provide a useful way to determine the basic feel of a prostheses. For 3D printing prostheses, hardness can be theoretically tuneable as there is a direct correlation between the hardness results and E-modulus values; as the relative densities increase, so does the hardness value.

The cubic unit cell used in this paper was a good starting point for prototyping a 3D printed testicular prosthesis with tuneable stiffness. However, the benefits of 3D printing can allow for more complex unit cell geometries, gradients of relative density, and wall thicknesses without compromising cost or the manufacturing process. A human testicle is made of several substructures, each with unique mechanical properties. These substructures could be mimicked in a more complex prosthesis design. For example, the epididymis could also be modeled

into the prosthesis with its own firmness, as well as surgically functional aspects such as suture positions.

Such graded designed metamaterial approaches and 3D printing are beginning to be used to solve problems with or improve upon other medical device products. This includes applications for orthopedic implants where bone substructures including cortical and trabecular bone have been 3D printed with titanium in a graded lattice structure to match the anisotropic mechanical properties of bone (11, 21). These concepts could be further applied here to improve upon the testicle prosthesis design.

This technology could potentially have applications in other implants that seek to mimic the feeling of native tissue. For example, silicone breast implants have rupture rates as high as 10% at 10 years after implantation (22). Our method could create realistic feeling implants that have lower risk of rupture or shrinkage due to the lattice infill. Additionally, nose and ear prostheses or functional medical devices and training models

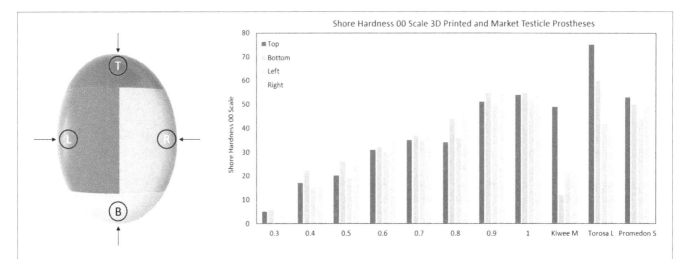

FIGURE 5 | Shore Hardness OO scale results for 3D printed testicles and medical prostheses. Notably the Kiwee which is a silicone coated silicone gel filled prostheses shows appropriate hardness results (within ranges of relative density 0.3–0.4); however, Torosa and Promedon prostheses are relatively hard compared to natural tissue. Note that the Hardness results for Torosa small and medium sized prostheses are the same as the large size, as the hardness value is dominated by the material and not minor changes in size.

which require hardness in some areas and softness in others could be achieved, owing to the versatility of printing differing structures in one print.

Different unit cells such as Triply Periodic Minimal Surfaces like the Gyroid, or Schwarz P surfaces, or other beam-based unit cells like the diamond can achieve different ranges of E-modulus for the same relative densities as the cubic unit cell (23). For example, the diamond structure can theoretically achieve a relative modulus of 0.05 with a relative density of 50%. Compared with the cubic which can achieve a relative modulus of 0.25 at relative density 50%. This means that by selecting the appropriate unit cell shape, a material which has a higher E-modulus could be used to achieve the same result, further expanding the use of existing materials.

Limitations of Current Design

A limitation of this study is that the 3D printing material used is not approved for implantation. There is a lack of available and directly 3D printable soft polymer materials on the market that can be utilized to make patient specific and life-like implants, which provides a great opportunity for the 3D printing industry to develop compatible materials. Additionally, no fatigue tests have been conducted to determine if the cubic lattice structures withstand repeated loading. This is recommended for future work on implantable materials prior to clinical trials.

Although this study was not performed with an implantable material, the concept could be applied to an implantable material with a similar bulk E-modulus range and a variety of 3D printing methods including Selective Laser Sintering (SLS) or Fused Deposition Modeling (FDM). For example, materials

such as Thermoplastic Polyurethane (TPU) which are approved for implantation such as Lubrizol Carbothane™ TPU (24) or Biomerics Quadrathane™ TPU (25) could be 3D printed using selective laser sintering (SLS) or fused deposition modeling (FDM) processes. These materials are used with injection molding systems and come in pelletised form. Therefore, they would need to be further processed into a powder or filament to be 3D printed. There are many of these TPU materials with stiffness ranges between 2.2 and 5.5 MPa. While stiffer than the material used here, using the concept in this paper with a diamond unit cell and a TPU with 2.4 MPa, a relative density of 0.25–0.35 would be recommended to match the feel of a human testicle.

CONCLUSIONS

We have demonstrated how 3D printing can be used to create a meta-material lattice structure for realistic feeling testicular prosthesis prototypes. These prototypes address the most common complaints of patients including unnatural size and shape and discomfort. This same technology could be used with various elastomeric materials and simulate the characteristics of a variety of native tissues. These developments will contribute to a future of individualized patient implants and prostheses through complete customization of shape, size and mechanical properties matching of human tissue.

AUTHOR CONTRIBUTIONS

All authors listed have made a substantial, direct and intellectual contribution to the work, and approved it for publication.

REFERENCES

1. Turek PJ, Master VA, Group TPS. Safety and effectiveness of a new saline filled testicular prosthesis. *J Urol.* (2004) 172:1427–30. doi: 10.1097/01.ju.0000139718.09510.a4
2. Bodiwala D, Summerton DJ, Terry TR. Testicular prostheses: development and modern usage. *Ann R Coll Surg Engl.* (2007) 89:349–53. doi: 10.1308/003588407X183463
3. Hillard C, Fowler JD, Barta R, Cunningham B. Silicone breast implant rupture: a review. *Gland Surg.* (2017) 6:163–8. doi: 10.21037/gs.2016.09.12
4. Dieckmann K-P, Anheuser P, Schmidt S, Soyka-Hundt B, Pichlmeier U, Schriefer P, et al. Testicular prostheses in patients with testicular cancer - acceptance rate and patient satisfaction. *BMC Urol.* (2015) 15:16. doi: 10.1186/s12894-015-0010-0
5. Yossepowitch O, Aviv D, Wainchwaig L, Baniel J. Testicular prostheses for testis cancer survivors: patient perspectives and predictors of long-term satisfaction. *J Urol.* (2011) 186:2249–52. doi: 10.1016/j.juro.2011.07.075
6. Lucas JW, Lester KM, Chen A, Simhan J. Scrotal reconstruction and testicular prosthetics. *Transl Androl Urol.* (2017) 6:710–21. doi: 10.21037/tau.2017.07.06
7. Nichols PE, Harris KT, Brant A, Manka MG, Haney N, Johnson MH, et al. Patient decision-making and predictors of genital satisfaction associated with testicular prostheses after radical orchiectomy: a questionnaire-based study of men with germ cell tumors of the testicle. *Urology.* (2019) 124:276–81. doi: 10.1016/j.urology.2018.09.021
8. Hayon S, Michael J, Coward RM. The modern testicular prosthesis: patient selection and counseling, surgical technique, and outcomes. *Asian J Androl.* (2020) 22:64–9. doi: 10.4103/aja.aja_93_19
9. Park, H-J, Kim, D-K, Lee, B-W, Kim, S-H, Wang J-P. Development of device for patient-specific artificial testicle using 3D printing. *Int J Eng Res Technol.* (2019) 12:2863–6. Available online at: https://www.scopus.com/record/display.uri?eid=2-s2.0-85078865858&origin=resultslist
10. Nazir A, Abate KM, Kumar A, Jeng J-Y. A state-of-the-art review on types, design, optimization, and additive manufacturing of cellular structures. *Int J Adv Manuf Technol.* (2019) 104:3489–510. doi: 10.1007/s00170-019-04085-3
11. du Plessis A, Broeckhoven C, Yadroitsava I, Yadroitsev I, Hands CH, Kunju R, et al. Beautiful and functional: a review of biomimetic design in additive manufacturing. *Addit Manuf.* (2019) 27:408–27. doi: 10.1016/j.addma.2019.03.033
12. Fan H, Fu J, Li X, Pei Y, Li X, Pei G, et al. Implantation of customized 3-D printed titanium prosthesis in limb salvage surgery: a case series and review of the literature. *World J Surg Oncol.* (2015) 13:1–10. doi: 10.1186/s12957-015-0723-2
13. D Systems. *Material Selection Guide for ProJet MJP 2500 and 2500 Plus - VisiJet M2 MultiJet Printing Materials for functional precision plastic and elastomeric parts 2020.* Available online at: https://www.3dsystems.com/sites/default/files/2020-08/3d-systems-visiJet-m2-material-selection-guide-usen-2020-08-20-web.pdf.
14. Ashby MF. *Materials Selection in Mechanical Design.* Fifth edit. Oxford, United Kingdom: Butterworth-Heinemann (2017).
15. Zadpoor AA, Hedayati R. Analytical relationships for prediction of the mechanical properties of additively manufactured porous biomaterials. *J Biomed Mater Res Part A.* (2016) 104:3164–74. doi: 10.1002/jbm.a.35855
16. Mitsuhashi N, Fujieda K, Tamura T, Kawamoto S, Takagi T, Okubo K. BodyParts3D: 3D structure database for anatomical concepts. *Nucleic Acids Res.* (2009) 37:D782–5. doi: 10.1093/nar/gkn613
17. Sun Z, Xie M, Xiang F, Song Y, Yu C, Zhang Y, et al. Utility of real-time shear wave elastography in the assessment of testicular torsion. *PLoS ONE.* (2015) 10:e0138523. doi: 10.1371/journal.pone.0138523
18. Pedersen MR, Møller H, Osther PJS, Vedsted P, Holst R, Rafaelsen SR. Comparison of tissue stiffness using shear wave elastography in men with normal testicular tissue, testicular microlithiasis and testicular cancer. *Ultrasound Int Open.* (2017) 3:E150–5. doi: 10.1055/s-0043-116660
19. Falanga V, Bucalo B. Use of a durometer to assess skin hardness. *J Am Acad Dermatol.* (1993) 29:47–51. doi: 10.1016/0190-9622(93)70150-R
20. Coloplast. Urgent Field Safety Notice FRMML-2015-1006-PR30xx & VS30xx 2017. Available online at: http://www.bfarm.de/SharedDocs/Kundeninfos/EN/11/2017/7295-15_kundeninfo_en.pdf;jsessionid=7CD47A0669AB724E53BF10CCE5E13111.2_cid344?__blob=publicationFile&v=1.
21. Zadpoor AA. Current trends in metallic orthopedic biomaterials: from additive manufacturing to bio-functionalization, infection prevention, and beyond. *Int J Mol Sci.* (2018) 19:E2684. doi: 10.3390/ijms19092684
22. Baek WY, Lew DH, Lee DW. A retrospective analysis of ruptured breast implants. *Arch Plast Surg.* (2014) 41:734–9. doi: 10.5999/aps.2014.41.6.734
23. Bobbert FSL, Lietaert K, Eftekhari AA, Pouran B, Ahmadi SM, Weinans H, et al. Additively manufactured metallic porous biomaterials based on minimal surfaces: a unique combination of topological, mechanical, and mass transport properties. *Acta Biomater.* (2017) 53:572–84. doi: 10.1016/j.actbio.2017.02.024
24. Lubrizol. *Carbothane TPU 2021.* Available online at: https://www.lubrizol.com/Health/Medical/Polymers/Carbothane-TPU.
25. Biomerics. *Medical Polymers 2021.* Available online at: https://biomerics.com/products/medical-polymers/.

10

Advances in Skin Tissue Bioengineering and the Challenges of Clinical Translation

Bronwyn L. Dearman[1,2,3]*, Steven T. Boyce[4] and John E. Greenwood[1,2]

[1] Skin Engineering Laboratory, Adult Burns Centre, Royal Adelaide Hospital, Adelaide, SA, Australia, [2] Adult Burns Centre, Royal Adelaide Hospital, Adelaide, SA, Australia, [3] Faculty of Health and Medical Science, The University of Adelaide, Adelaide, SA, Australia, [4] Department of Surgery, University of Cincinnati, Cincinnati, OH, United States

*Correspondence:
Bronwyn L. Dearman
bronwyn.dearman@sa.gov.au

Skin tissue bioengineering is an emerging field that brings together interdisciplinary teams to promote successful translation to clinical care. Extensive deep tissue injuries, such as large burns and other major skin loss conditions, are medical indications where bioengineered skin substitutes (that restore both dermal and epidermal tissues) are being studied as alternatives. These may not only reduce mortality but also lessen morbidity to improve quality of life and functional outcome compared with the current standards of care. A common objective of dermal-epidermal therapies is to reduce the time required to accomplish stable closure of wounds with minimal scar in patients with insufficient donor sites for autologous split-thickness skin grafts. However, no commercially-available product has yet fully satisfied this objective. Tissue engineered skin may include cells, biopolymer scaffolds and drugs, and requires regulatory review to demonstrate safety and efficacy. They must be scalable for manufacturing and distribution. The advancement of technology and the introduction of bioreactors and bio-printing for skin tissue engineering may facilitate clinical products' availability. This mini-review elucidates the reasons for the few available commercial skin substitutes. In addition, it provides insights into the challenges faced by surgeons and scientists to develop new therapies and deliver the results of translational research to improve patient care.

Keywords: skin, bioengineering, burns, wound closure, skin substitutes, clinical translation, tissue engineering, biopolymers

INTRODUCTION

The challenges of translational medicine are becoming more prevalent with developing new technologies as novel therapies for personalised medicine. One therapy where translational research is at the forefront is reducing the use of skin autografts for extensive full-thickness burns with laboratory-generated skin (1–7). The split-thickness meshed and expanded skin autograft has been the prevailing standard of care for burns surgeons for decades and remains the preferred method of wound closure due to its relatively high efficacy of stable wound closure (3, 8, 9). However, if the burn area massively exceeds the area of available donor site for skin autografts, the advantages of autologous engineered skin substitutes is compelling. To regenerate a substitute of uninjured human skin that definitively provides wound closure both anatomically and physiologically (6) is a common challenge for tissue engineers, and may involve polymer chemists, cellular and molecular biologists, surgeons, nurses, and therapists. A systematic review of clinical studies investigating autologous bilayered skin substitutes as epithelial stem cell niches after grafting, identified 16 potential studies and nine types of autologous skin substitutes over a 25-year period (10). Currently, only a small number of these are still available for therapeutic use, with no ideal substitute in the market. The current models have distinct attributes, for the majority, the scaffold type is a source or derivation of collagen (biologic) with autologous fibroblasts and keratinocytes. Another novel synthetic scaffold utilising a polyurethane (PUR) has also been used to generate a skin composite (composite cultured skin, CCS) and has reported its use for the treatment of a 95% total body surface area burn patient (11). However, these all remain deficient in pigmentation, hair, and other dermal appendages. The authors draw on combined experiences from taking the research bench to bedside. This review will describe the distinct models of bilayered tissue engineered products that have been used therapeutically, which there are few, but all address the same clinical challenges.

The Need for an Alternative to Skin Autografts for Extensive Full-Thickness Burns

Burns are a global health concern, especially for low to middle-income countries, accounting for over 95% of burn deaths (12). Burn injuries of all depths make up only a small proportion (1%) of trauma hospitalisations in Australia (13), but are one of the most costly, due to long hospital and rehabilitation stays (14, 15). In the United States, hospitalised burns cost over $1billion per year (16) and in high income countries the mean cost per 1% TBSA is US$4159.00 (17). These costs are significant, but the major indirect cost is the patient's lifelong scars and disfigurements. As the percentage of total body surface area (TBSA) burn and burn depth increases, the costs increase exponentially (14). Extensive, full-thickness burn injuries (>50% TBSA) usually require intensive care, multiple surgical procedures, physical and occupational therapy and psycho-social interventions to recover. Patients with these degrees of burn often die which obviates skin graft paucity (18). However, advances in burn care have led to increased survival rates due to early excision of eschar, temporary wound closure, advanced nutritional support, infection prevention, and improvements in critical care medicine (19–22). Although, burns in the elderly and those with coincident trauma such as inhalation injury, remain challenging.

In this patient population, temporary wound coverage provides time for utilisation of donor sites from superficially burned skin and re-harvesting to allow multiple procedures of skin autografting (23). Maximising wound coverage with available donor site involves thin, widely-meshed, or expanded (Meek-Wall technique) (24) skin autografts, resulting in poor functional and aesthetic outcomes. In addition, donor sites generated by split-thickness skin graft harvesting are extremely painful, may require opiate analgesia, limit mobilisation, and discourage compliance with physical therapy (25). Skin autografts, however, have properties that promote their continued widespread use for the closure of large, deep skin wounds (no rejection, vascular inosculation, high efficacy, long-term stability), but their correlation with increased morbidity, especially in the elderly, is a significant disadvantage, which motivates the search for alternatives (26, 27).

An ideal skin substitute should adhere, vascularise, and integrate quickly, contain both epidermal and dermal components, provide permanent and definitive wound closure, be autologous, resist infection, be easy to prepare, handle well, easy to apply, cost-effective, and resist mechanical shear forces (28). They should demonstrate high engraftment rates, restore natural pigmentation, and provide all skin appendages and sensory networks in uninjured skin. This list of qualities is comprehensive, and to simultaneously replicate these features *in vivo* requires complex engineering in the laboratory. Engineered skin fabrication is a specialised professional field with many aspects still to be elucidated and reduced to practise. A standardised universal classification system for "skin substitutes" was published by Davison-Kotler et al. in 2018 to encapsulate all adaptations (research and clinical) using a factorial design (29). Primary categories include acellular dermal substitutes, temporary skin substitutes, and permanent skin substitutes, further expanding into sub-categories (2). The many variations have been tabulated in former reviews and will not be detailed here (6, 7, 29–38). This review focuses on permanent, cellular, and mainly autologous products with dermal and epidermal components. It will explore a few commercially available products and some clinically used in extensive wounds (**Table 1**).

Large, Excised Wounds—Temporising the Wound Bed for Definitive Closure

The loss of the epidermis, and sufficient dermis to ensure loss of all the epidermal adnexa, requires rapid wound closure. The primary focus is on reducing inflammation and granulation, preventing infection and limiting contraction. The associated mortality and morbidity rates decrease with the successful implementation of the above and achieved by staged closure (69). Acellular dermal substitutes comprising a dermal and a pseudo-epidermal component have been widely used to achieve physiological closure. Their implementation has produced a paradigm shift in burn care (21, 70, 71). The dermal components may originate from decellularised human skin, biological polymers, or synthetic polymers. Their function is to temporarily close the excised wound to decrease fluid loss, allow integration and controlled granulation tissue invasion inducing a vascularised wound bed. Commercial examples include Integra® Dermal Regeneration Template, Pelnac, Terudermis, Hyalomatrix, and RenoSkin (69). These products and similar ones have limitations, including a risk of transmissible disease, loss from infection and high costs (5, 72). Despite regulatory approval for specific medical indications, most dermal substitutes have not achieved worldwide consensus as market leaders for large, deep dermal wounds. However, establishing a neo-dermis enhances structural stability and provides the time required for definitive epithelial wound closure, whether by serial grafting or by generating and applying autologous engineered skin.

TABLE 1 | Examples of clinically-available or investigative skin substitutes [adapted from Vig et al. (7), Boyce et al. (31)].

	Product-country of origin	Classification/components	Proposed clinical indication	Product limitations
Dermal-epidermal substitutes	TISSUEtech Autograft system (Hylomatrix + Laserskin)—Italy (39, 40)	Cellular, autologous Ks, Fbs with HA	Diabetic ulcers	Small wounds, difficult to use clinically
	Tissue-cultured skin autograft (TCSA's)—Germany (41)	Cellular, autologous Ks, Fbs with Matriderm^{TM}	Chronic ulcerations	Small wounds
	Engineered skin substitute (ESS)—USA (42–50)	Cellular, autologous Ks, Fbs, bovine collagen-GAG	Large burns and other skin loss conditions	Xenogeneic scaffold, small pieces, shrinkage of product, cost
	Composite cultured skin (CCS)—Australia (51–57)	Cellular, autologous Ks, Fbs, synthetic polymer	Full- thickness burns	Scaffold porosity, complex
	Self-assembled skin substitute (SASSs)—Canada (58)	Cellular, autologous Ks and Fbs	Burns	Labour intensive
	Autologous homologous skin construct (AHSC)—USA (59–61)	Cellular, autologous skin cells	Burns, acute trauma chronic wounds	Cell suspension/aggregate
	MyDerm—Malaysia (62–65)	Cellular, autologous Ks and Fbs, Fibrin	Burns, skin trauma and chronic wounds	Clinical efficiency
	StrataGraft^{TM}—USA (66, 67)	Cellular, allogeneic Ks and Fbs, non-bovine collagen	Burns and skin conditions	Allogeneic, temporary, size
	denovoSkin—Switzerland (68)	Cellular, autologous Ks and Fbs, bovine collagen	Burns	Xenogeneic scaffold

HA, Hyaluronic acid; Ks, Keratinocytes, Fbs, Fibroblasts.

The NovoSorb^{TM} Biodegradable Temporising Matrix (BTM) is a synthetic scaffold that is currently in routine use for burns and complex wound repair (73–79). It is a scaffold that temporises the wound and biodegrades after integration and establishment of dermal elements (80). Furthermore, it resists infection, can be made in large sheets, is inexpensive to produce, easy to handle, and provides integration time (76–82). With the optimisation of a dermal replacement template and a major limitation addressed, i.e., acquisition of time for cellular growth, the prospective next step is the specification of a definitive wound closure alternative.

The Current State of Bioengineered Dermal-Epidermal Substitutes

Bioengineered skin substitutes involving dermal and epidermal components are the focus of this paper; however, epidermal replacements (cellular) require brief reference to appreciate the desirability of both components. A skin substitute is yet to be achieved that replaces the anatomy and physiology of uninjured skin or completely replaces all skin autograft properties- implying why an epidermal replacement alone will not replicate a meshed, or sheet, autograft. Cultured Epithelial Autografts (CEA's) have been used since 1986 (83), and other adaptations or iterations of keratinocyte suspensions [e.g., Epicel (84, 85), Cell Spray, RECELL$^®$ (86), BioSeed (87), Laserskin (39, 40)] have evolved. These are clinical adjuncts to therapies with traditional treatments of burn care to expedite reepithelialisation rate. Clinically applicable for small wounds (88), ulcers (87, 89–92), superficial burns (93) and skin graft donor sites; they have not been universally accepted by burns surgeons independently for deep large burns due to their limited expansion rate, mechanical fragility on handling, tendency to blister *in vivo* and

vulnerability to shear after application (partly to deficiencies in basement membrane formation) (94). In addition, they are costly to produce, can take weeks to manufacture, and are epidermal derived replacements (95–100). Incorporating a substitute containing epidermal and dermal components is a logical progression toward regenerating a tissue more like uninjured skin (101).

A critical paracrine dialogue between fibroblasts and keratinocytes is essential for basement membrane synthesis, a beneficial feature for engineered skin substitutes (102–104). The basement membrane protects against shear by establishing a molecular bond that anchors the cellular epidermis to the extracellular matrix of the dermis. The most analogous to skin, and the most successful clinically to date, is an Engineered Skin Substitute (ESS) developed in Cincinnati, Ohio (105). Developed over the past 30 years, the ESS comprises autologous keratinocytes and fibroblasts in a bovine collagen-glycosaminoglycan (GAG) scaffold (42–50). The ESS model was the first to demonstrate stable closure of full-thickness burns by combination with Integra$^®$ Dermal Regeneration Template (106). In 2017, a report was published of ESS' clinical results in 16 subjects treated from 2007 to 2010. For patients with >50%, TBSA full-thickness burns, ESS's were able to reduce the need for harvesting donor skin grafts and reduce the mortality rate compared with data from similar patient populations reported in the National Burn Repository of the American Burn Association (107). The ESS results in a closed wound that has structural and functional similarities to native skin. However, this model also has limitations (lack of other cell types and adnexal structures, contraction of the collagen scaffold during ESS fabrication, relatively high cost and regulatory complexity); and is not commercially available. Pre-clinical studies have recently demonstrated the successful incorporation of melanocytes (108, 109), microvascular endothelial cells (110), and hair follicles (111) into the ESS model.

Bovine collagen is also used in denovoSkin™ (Cutiss AG, Zurich), which consists of a collagen hydrogel and human dermal fibroblasts and keratinocytes. It has been classified as an Advanced Therapy Medical Product (ATMP) and has received FDA and EMA Orphan status to treat burns in the US and EU (112, 113). It is currently undergoing clinical trial recruitment for adult and children burns, with an estimated completion date of 2023. However, the production of a dermal-epidermal equivalent with xenogeneic (non-human)-derived biologicals, such as bovine, rat, or porcine collagens or glycosaminoglycans (42) raises the potential for immune recognition and rejection and risk of prion transmission. A synthetic scaffold and autologous cell approach may reduce these risks.

Several matrices using fibroblasts alone to provide the biological extracellular matrix environment (114–117) have shown the generated skin's long-term stability *in vitro* (118). Through the Special Access Program in Canada, a Self-Assembled Skin Substitute (SASS) has shown clinical effectiveness, reporting a case series of 14 severely burned subjects (58). This substitute contains autologous fibroblasts and keratinocytes, forming a human biopolymer fibroblast scaffold with subsequent keratinocyte seeding. The constraining factor for this type of substitute, like some others, is the production time, with an average of 9 weeks from the initial biopsy (58). In addition, the SASSs post-transplantation displayed visible junctions between applications, re-iterating the need for a sizeable sheet that can be generated and transplanted with fewer anaesthetics.

Improved scalability has now been reported using a biodegradable polyurethane (PUR) as the scaffold for a dermal-epidermal alternative, known as a composite cultured skin (CCS) (51–57). The attributes for an "ideal engineered skin," as mentioned previously (119), formulated the premise of combining an engineered-epidermis to a modified BTM dermal substitute. Compared to bovine collagen (a biologic), a synthetic biodegradable PUR showed lower toxicity and cytotoxicity, reduced immunogenic reaction, and minimal inflammatory response (51, 52, 120). The BTM-CCS provided a two-stage strategy, with the CCS as a definitive second stage wound closure material. The application of NovoSorb™ BTM, a temporising matrix, addresses one of the major limitations of available skin substitutes [i.e., time required for autologous cell expansion 3–5 weeks (38)]. The integration period enables the time required for cell isolation, expansion and bilayered construction (up to 7-weeks if needed) (11, 69). The CCS is a 1 mm thick PUR porous scaffold, populated with autologous fibroblasts in a fibrin network and layered with autologous keratinocytes (53, 54). Pre-clinical studies in a porcine model initially demonstrated the efficacy of small CCS, and later large pieces, generated in an automated bioreactor (54, 57). This custom-made novel bioreactor device has taken this from research to clinic (11, 57). The two-stage strategy of BTM-CCS has been used clinically in a 95% TBSA burn injury (covering 40% TBSA of original burn) (11). The patient not only survived but, at 1.5 years post-injury, required minimal contracture release in areas where autografts were applied and none to the CCS-applied areas. The result for CCS was a smooth, supple aesthetic appearance with varying pigmentation from primary epithelial engraftment. No delineation between junctions of CCSs can be observed. ROM and SOSS scores were comparable to sheet graft, but favourable over 1:3 meshed STSG and Meek.

The subcutaneous layer (the deepest layer of skin) is absent in many investigational and clinical substitutes. Polarity TE, a US company, produces an Autologous Homologous Skin Construct (AHSC). They claim that functional full-thickness skin can be regenerated by obtaining a full-thickness biopsy with immediate application (59). A retrospective, 15-patient post-AHSC application review case series was reported (60) for various wound types (burns, acute/traumatic injuries, and chronic wounds). It differs from the conventional dermal-epidermal substitute, in that it seems not to necessitate culture and is returned to the patient within days. These wounds were closed at 3 months post application; however, further studies are required to investigate and substantiate the claims of efficacy, especially in full-thickness, excised burns (61).

Several other dermal-epidermal constructs have been used clinically or gone to clinical trial pending commercialisation (**Table 1**). Some examples include, tissue cultured skin autograft (TCSAs using Matriderm™, Germany) (41), TISSUEtech Autograft system™ (using Hylomatrix, Anika Therapeutics Inc., Bedford) (121), and others using Allodermis (122, 123), Human plasma (124, 125), and Fibrin (MyDerm, Japan) (62–65). Another bi-layered product recently receiving (2021) FDA approval for adult deep partial-thickness burns is StrataGraft® (Mallinckrodt, USA) (66, 67). Although it is not autologous, this bilayered allogeneic product comprises murine collagen and allogeneic fibroblasts and keratinocytes, this acts indirectly on the autologous cells to assist with wound closure (66). This type of treatment is limited for deep full-thickness burns as it needs another source of autologous cells e.g., meshed graft or other skin appendages, to close the wound. However, it is readily available and "off-the-shelf" ready for immediate use, whereas typical bilayered autologous substitutes can take weeks to fabricate. As with any graft, there is potential for loss if there is no neovascularization. The majority of clinically available engineered skins are avascular; however, this is under investigation by researchers (126). The loss of graft can be due to an accumulation of blood (haematoma), fluid (seroma), contamination, or mechanical shear. The different skin models mentioned have varying pore sizes and can contribute to the success of the engraftment. The density of the dermal component (i.e., too small or large pores) can inhibit or promote vascularisation (57, 127). Shear of a substitute graft or blistering will also occur if there is loss or no basement membrane and reiterates the importance of cell-cell contact of the epidermal-dermal component *in vitro* culture. When this loss occurs, the wound heals by secondary reepithelialisation and healing is delayed. Although, a systematic review of bilayered skin substitutes showed wound healing rates for leg ulcers were comparable with the standard of care (RR 1.51, 95%

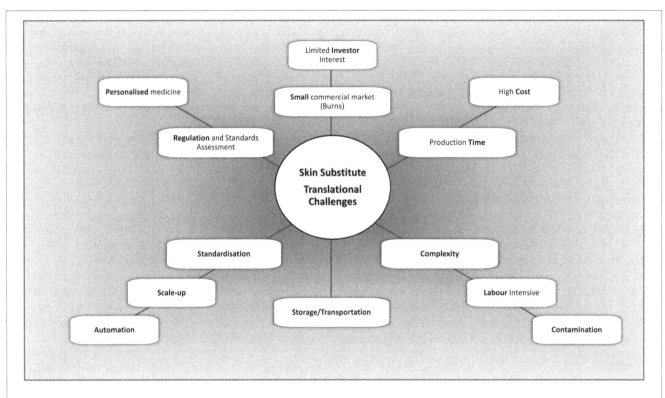

FIGURE 1 | Challenges and considerations in bioengineering of bilayered skin substitutes. Adapted from Al-Himdani et al. (133).

1.22–1.88) (128). A widely meshed STSG used for extensive wound coverage results in a weave-like pattern, producing a poor aesthetic result. In contrast, autologous engineered skin provides immediate coverage with a stratified epidermis that suppresses granulation tissue and arrests the scarring process. Producing a favourable smooth, pliable, even skin, with a reduction in pain and itch (55, 68, 107). Another major strength and benefit over skin autografts is the reduction of autologous donor skin and its associated morbidities. The diverse bilayered approaches mentioned all have their strengths and weaknesses, and in review, the ideal model may likely be combinations of biopolymer scaffolds and stem cells that can produce a functional, clinically safe and effective alternative (129, 130). Any of these tissue engineered products will face regulatory reviews and reimbursement requirements.

Clinical Challenges for Skin Substitutes

As cell-based therapeutic inventions, these products require approval by regulatory authorities to ensure high quality, safety and proven efficacy (131) (Therapeutic Goods Administration, TGA in Australia; Food and Drug Administration, FDA in the United States; European Medicines Agency (EMA), in the European Union, etc.). Several pre-clinical substitutes are being used through Special Access Programs (SAP) in designated countries. This scheme is a way of using non-licenced products to treat life-threatening injuries where other methods are not suitable, or non-existent. In the United States, the passage of the 21st Century Cures Act, in 2016 (31) and new agency programs

will facilitate the clinical use of novel products and devices to treat patients at severe medical risk.

The generation of highly manipulated tissue-engineered products follows the standards for current Good Manufacturing Practices (cGMP) (132). They should ideally be free of any xenogeneic product (131) and include mandatory testing for microbiological assessment [sterility assurance level (SAL) of 10^{-6}] and transportation validation to ensure that product integrity is maintained. Generating a clinically viable, and ethical, product suitable for market is a lengthy and labour intensive process, with high initial capital costs. These infrastructure costs, process complexity, and stringent quality control result in expensive products, making commercialisation less practical (133, 134) and are translational challenges a therapeutic product may encounter (**Figure 1**). The cost of such substitutes, however, should not be assessed directly by the cost per unit of production only (31, 135), but also indirectly by assessing overall hospital cost reductions concerning length of stay, the number of reconstructive surgeries post-major burn, patient outcome and aesthetics. Although, an experienced highly trained medical team, including specialised nurses and therapy protocols are required during the intense early stages of treatment until they become the prevailing standard of care.

The Future Opportunities of Skin Substitutes

The generation of laboratory-generated "skin substitutes," irrespective of classification, have to date only partially addressed the requirements for achieving stable wound closure. They currently produce inadequate pigmentation (hypo- or hyperpigmentation), they lack vasculature, hair, glands, and none have replicated the results of unmeshed autograft or duplicated the anatomy and physiology of uninjured skin. Due to cost, regulatory restraints, and the significant scientific challenge to incorporate all skin features simultaneously (136–139). Approaches to the refinement of fabrication systems for skin substitutes will facilitate advanced models of engineered skin to reach their markets with a consequent decrease in costs. The requirement for scalability is a compelling demand for large burn injuries and can be met by incorporating automated bioreactors (57, 140). These may assist production and provide complete automation and standardisation to improve product quality. The robotic systems are engineering advances that will move forward in parallel with medical advances. The 3D and 4D bioprinting fields coupled with the latest compatible bioinks are novel techniques that may rapidly advance the tissue engineering field (141–145).

In time, these technologies and advances in tissue engineering will at least reduce, and possibly replace, the need for skin autografts and enable easier clinical translation of an acceptable autologous engineered skin, suitable for patient use. The significance of this is that patients with life-threatening burns will no longer suffer the painful acute morbidity and later scarring that donor sites generate. Time in ICU and total hospitalisation will be reduced, the need for reconstructive surgery will decrease, with overall costs reduced. The success will also have implications for other dermatologic conditions, including but not limited to giant congenital naevi excision and engraftment, epidermolysis bullosa treatment, certain surgical reconstructions, and vitiligo. It can also contribute to the investigation and requirement for epidermal appendages, naturally matched skin pigmentation, vascular plexus, and sensory nerves (2, 139, 146, 147). As each of these advances is currently under investigation, there can be high degrees of confidence that many, if not most of these skin components (uniform skin colour, sweat glands, and hair follicles) will be incorporated into future models of skin substitutes and available clinically for the treatment of full-thickness skin wounds, including burns.

AUTHOR CONTRIBUTIONS

BD developed the outline with contributions from both JG and SB. BD wrote the manuscript with editing by JG and SB.

REFERENCES

1. Supp DM, Boyce ST. Engineered skin substitutes: practices and potentials. *Clin Dermatol.* (2005) 23:403–12. doi: 10.1016/j.clindermatol.2004.07.023
2. Boyce S, Supp D. Chapter 11 - biologic skin substitutes. in *Skin Tissue Engineering and Regenerative Medicine*, eds M. Z. Albanna and J. H. Holmes Iv (New York, NY: Academic Press/Elsevier), (2016). p. 211–38. doi: 10.1016/B978-0-12-801654-1.00011-5
3. MacNeil S. Progress and opportunities for tissue-engineered skin. *Nature.* (2007) 445:874–80. doi: 10.1038/nature05664
4. Chua AW, Khoo YC, Tan BK, Tan KC, Foo CL, Chong SJ. Skin tissue engineering advances in severe burns: review and therapeutic applications. *Burns Trauma.* (2016) 4:3. doi: 10.1186/s41038-016-0027-y
5. Nicholas MN, Yeung J. Current status and future of skin substitutes for chronic wound healing. *J Cutan Med Surg.* (2017) 21:23–30. doi: 10.1177/1203475416664037
6. Shevchenko RV, James SL, James SE. A review of tissue-engineered skin bioconstructs available for skin reconstruction. *J R Soc Interface.* (2010) 7:229–58. doi: 10.1098/rsif.2009.0403
7. Vig K, Chaudhari A, Tripathi S, Dixit S, Sahu R, Pillai S, et al. Advances in skin regeneration using tissue engineering. *Int J Mol Sci.* (2017) 18:789–807. doi: 10.3390/ijms18040789
8. Ong YS, Samuel M, Song C. Meta-analysis of early excision of burns. *Burns.* (2006) 32:145–50. doi: 10.1016/j.burns.2005.09.005
9. Ben-Bassat H, Chaouat M, Segal N, Zumai E, Wexler MR, Eldad A. How long can cryopreserved skin be stored to maintain adequate graft performance? *Burns.* (2001) 27:425–31. doi: 10.1016/S0305-4179(00)00162-5
10. Cortez Ghio S, Larouche D, Doucet EJ, Germain L. The role of cultured autologous bilayered skin substitutes as epithelial stem cell niches after grafting: a systematic review of clinical studies. *Burns Open.* (2021) 5:56–66. doi: 10.1016/j.burnso.2021.02.002
11. Greenwood JE, Damkat-Thomas L, Schmitt B, Dearman B. Successful proof of the 'two-stage strategy' for major burn wound repair. *Burns Open.* (2020) 4:121–31. doi: 10.1016/j.burnso.2020.06.003
12. World Health Organization. *A WHO Plan for Burn Prevention and Care.* World Health Organization (?2008). Available online at: https://apps.WHO.Int/iris/handle/10665/97852

13. Pointer S, Tovell A. *Hospitalised Burn Injuries, Australia, 2013–14 Injury Research and Statistics Series no 102 Cat no INJCAT 178.* Canberra, ACT: AIHW (2016).
14. Ahn CS, Maitz PK. The true cost of burn. *Burns.* (2012) 38:967–74. doi: 10.1016/j.burns.2012.05.016
15. Cleland H, Greenwood JE, Wood FM, Read DJ, Wong She R, Maitz P, et al. The burns registry of Australia and New Zealand: progressing the evidence base for burn care. *Med J Austral.* (2016) 204:195 1e. doi: 10.5694/mja15.00989
16. Finkelstein EA, Corso PS, Miller TR. *The Incidence and Economic Burden of Injuries in the United States.* New York, NY: Oxford University Press (2006).
17. Hop MJ, Polinder S, van der Vlies CH, Middelkoop E, van Baar ME. Costs of burn care: a systematic review: costs of burn care. *Wound Repair Regener.* (2014) 22:436–50. doi: 10.1111/wrr.12189
18. Chua A, Song C, Chai A, Kong S, Tan KC. Use of skin allograft and its donation rate in Singapore: an 11-year retrospective review for burns treatment. *Transplant Proc.* (2007) 39:1314–6. doi: 10.1016/j.transproceed.2006.11.028
19. Herndon DN, Barrow RE, Rutan RL, Rutan TC, Desai MH, Abston S. A comparison of conservative versus early excision. Therapies in severely burned patients. *Annal Surg.* (1989) 209:547. doi: 10.1097/00000658-198905000-00006
20. Rose J, Herndon D. Advances in the treatment of burn patients. *Burns.* (1997) 23:S19–26. doi: 10.1016/S0305-4179(97)90096-6
21. Price LA, Milner SM. The totality of burn care. *Trauma.* (2012) 15:16–28. doi: 10.1177/1460408612462311
22. Fratianne RB, Brandt CP. Improved survival of adults with extensive burns. *J Burn Care Rehab.* (1997) 18:347. doi: 10.1097/00004630-199707000-00013
23. Wurzer P, Keil H, Branski LK, Parvizi D, Clayton RP, Finnerty CC, et al. The use of skin substitutes and burn care-a survey. *J Surg Res.* (2016) 201:293–8. doi: 10.1016/j.jss.2015.10.048
24. Meek CP. Successful microdermagrafting using the meek-wall microdermatome. *Am J Surg.* (1958) 96:557–8. doi: 10.1016/0002-9610(58)90975-9
25. Huang G, Ji S, Luo P, Zhang Y, Wang G, Zhu S, et al. Evaluation of dermal substitute in a novel co-transplantation model with autologous epidermal sheet. *PLoS ONE.* (2012) 7:e49448. doi: 10.1371/journal.pone.0049448
26. Ashcroft GS, Mills SJ, Ashworth JJ. Ageing and wound healing. *Biogerontology.* (2002) 3:337. doi: 10.1023/A:1021399228395

27. Gore DC. Utility of acellular allograft dermis in the care of elderly burn patients. *J Surg Res.* (2005) 125:37–41. doi: 10.1016/j.jss.2004.11.032

28. Shores JT, Gabriel A, Gupta S. Skin substitutes and alternatives: a review. *Adv Skin Wound Care.* (2007) 20:493. doi: 10.1097/01.ASW.0000288217.83128.f3

29. Davison-Kotler E, Sharma V, Kang NV, García-Gareta E. A new and universal classification system of skin substitutes inspired by factorial design. *Tissue Eng Part B Rev.* (2018) 24:279–88. doi: 10.1089/ten.teb.2017.0477

30. Boyce ST, Lalley AL. Tissue engineering of skin and regenerative medicine for wound care. *Burns Trauma.* (2018) 6:4. doi: 10.1186/s41038-017-0103-y

31. Boyce S, Cheng P, Warner P. Chapter 2.5.8 - burn dressings and skin substitutes. In: Wagner W, Sakiyama-Elbert SE, Zhang G, Yaszemski MJ, editors. *Biomaterials Science, An Introduction to Materials in Medicine.* 4th ed. (San Diego: CA, Academic Press/Elsevier) (2020). p. 1169–80.

32. Sun BK, Siprashvili Z, Khavari PA. Advances in skin grafting and treatment of cutaneous wounds. *Science.* (2014) 346:941–5. doi: 10.1126/science.1253836

33. Metcalfe AD, Ferguson MW. Tissue engineering of replacement skin: the crossroads of biomaterials, wound healing, embryonic development, stem cells and regeneration. *J R Soc Interface.* (2007) 4:413–37. doi: 10.1098/rsif.2006.0179

34. Chocarro-Wrona C, Lopez-Ruiz E, Peran M, Galvez-Martin P, Marchal JA. Therapeutic strategies for skin regeneration based on biomedical substitutes. *J Eur Acad Dermatol Venereol.* (2019) 33:484–96. doi: 10.1111/jdv.15391

35. Zeng Q, Macri LK, Prasad A, Clark RAF, Zeugolis DI, Hanley C, et al. *5.534 - Skin Tissue Engineering,* (Amsterdam, NL: Elsevier Ltd) (2011). p. 467–99. doi: 10.1016/B978-0-08-055294-1.00186-0

36. Zeng R, Lin C, Lin Z, Chen H, Lu W, Li H. Approaches to cutaneous wound healing: basics and future directions. *Cell Tissue Res.* (2018) 374:217–32. doi: 10.1007/s00441-018-2830-1

37. Moiemen NS, Lee KC. The role of alternative wound substitutes in major burn wounds and burn scar resurfacing. In: Herndon D, editor. *Total Burn Care,* 5th edn. Edinburgh, UK: Elsevier Ltd (2018). p. 633–9.e1.

38. Stojic M, López V, Montero A, Quílez C, de Aranda Izuquiza G, Vojtova L, et al. Skin tissue engineering. In: *Biomaterials for Skin Repair and Regeneration,* ed. E. García-Gareta (Duxford, UK: Woodhead Publishing) (2019). p. 59–99.

39. Price RD, Das-Gupta V, Leigh IM, Navsaria HA. A comparison of tissue-engineered hyaluronic acid dermal matrices in a human wound model. *Tissue Eng.* (2006) 12:2985. doi: 10.1089/ten.2006.12.2985

40. Chan ES, Lam PK, Liew CT, Lau HC, Yen RS, King WW. A new technique to resurface wounds with composite biocompatible epidermal graft and artificial skin. *J Trauma.* (2001) 50:358–62. doi: 10.1097/00005373-200102000-00028

41. Golinski P, Menke H, Hofmann M, Valesky E, Butting M, Kippenberger S, et al. Development and characterization of an engraftable tissue-cultured skin autograft: alternative treatment for severe electrical injuries? *Cells Tissues Organs.* (2015) 200:227–39. doi: 10.1159/000433519

42. Boyce ST, Christianson DJ, Hansbrough JF. Structure of a collagen-GAG dermal skin substitute optimized for cultured human epidermal keratinocytes. *J Biomed Mater Res.* (1988) 22:939–57. doi: 10.1002/jbm.820221008

43. Powell HM, Boyce ST. EDC cross-linking improves skin substitute strength and stability. *Biomaterials.* (2006) 27:5821–7. doi: 10.1016/j.biomaterials.2006.07.030

44. Smiley AK, Klingenberg JM, Boyce ST, Supp DM. Keratin expression in cultured skin substitutes suggests that the hyperproliferative phenotype observed *in vitro* is normalized after grafting. *Burns.* (2006) 32:135–8. doi: 10.1016/j.burns.2005.08.017

45. Barai ND, Boyce ST, Hoath SB, Visscher MO, Kasting GB. Improved barrier function observed in cultured skin substitutes developed under anchored conditions. *Skin Res Technol.* (2008) 14:418–24. doi: 10.1111/j.1600-0846.2008.00225.x

46. Kalyanaraman B, Supp DM, Boyce ST. Medium flow rate regulates viability and barrier function of engineered skin substitutes in perfusion culture. *Tissue Eng Part A.* (2008) 14:583–93. doi: 10.1089/tea.2007.0237

47. Kalyanaraman B, Boyce ST. Wound healing on athymic mice with engineered skin substitutes fabricated with keratinocytes harvested from an automated bioreactor. *J Surg Res.* (2009) 152:296–302. doi: 10.1016/j.jss.2008.04.001

48. Klingenberg JM, McFarland KL, Friedman AJ, Boyce ST, Aronow BJ, Supp DM. Engineered human skin substitutes undergo large-scale genomic reprogramming and normal skin-like maturation after transplantation to athymic mice. *J Invest Dermatol.* (2010) 130:587–601. doi: 10.1038/jid.2009.295

49. Lander JM, Supp DM, He H, Martin LJ, Chen X, Weirauch MT, et al. Analysis of chromatin accessibility in human epidermis identifies putative barrier dysfunction-sensing enhancers. *PLoS ONE.* (2017) 12:e0184500. doi: 10.1371/journal.pone.0184500

50. Lloyd C, Besse J, Boyce S. Controlled-rate freezing to regulate the structure of collagen-glycosaminoglycan scaffolds in engineered skin substitutes. *J Biomed Mater Res B Appl Biomater.* (2015) 103:832–40. doi: 10.1002/jbm.b.33253

51. Greenwood JE, Li A, Dearman BL, Moore TG. Evaluation of novosorb novel biodegradable polymer for the generation of a dermal matrix part 2: *in-vivo* studies. *Wound Prac Res.* (2010) 18:24–34.

52. Greenwood JE, Li A, Dearman BL, Moore TG. Evaluation of novosorb novel biodegradable polymer for the generation of a dermal matrix part 1: *in-vitro* studies. *Wound Prac Res.* (2010) 18:14–22.

53. Dearman BL, Stefani K, Li A, Greenwood JE. "Take" of a polymer-based autologous cultured composite "skin" on an integrated temporizing dermal matrix: proof of concept. *J Burn Care Res.* (2013) 34:151–60. doi: 10.1097/BCR.0b013e31828089f9

54. Dearman BL, Li A, Greenwood JE. Optimization of a polyurethane dermal matrix and experience with a polymer-based cultured composite skin. *J Burn Care Res.* (2014) 35:437–48. doi: 10.1097/BCR.0000000000000061

55. Dearman B, Greenwood J. Treatment of a 95% total body surface burns patient with a novel polyurethane-based composite cultured skin. *eCM Periodical.* (2020) Collection 1(TERMIS EU Abstracts):187.

56. Dearman B, Greenwood J. A novel polyurethane-based composite cultured skin and a bespoke bioreactor in a porcine wound. *eCM Periodical.* (2020) Collection 1(TERMIS EU Abstracts):315.

57. Dearman BL, Greenwood JE. Scale-up of a composite cultured skin using a novel bioreactor device in a porcine wound model. *J Burn Care Res.* (2021). doi: 10.1093/jbcr/irab034

58. Germain L, Larouche D, Nedelec B, Perreault I, Duranceau L, Bortoluzzi P, et al. Autologous bilayered self-assembled skin substitutes (SASSs) as permanent grafts: a case series of 14 severely burned patients indicating clinical effectiveness. *Eur Cell Mater.* (2018) 36:128–41. doi: 10.22203/eCM.v036a10

59. Isbester K, Wee C, Boas S, Sopko N, Kumar A. Regeneration of functional, full-thickness skin with minimal donor site contribution using autologous homologous skin construct. *Plastic Surg Case Stud.* (2020) 6:2513826X1989881. doi: 10.1177/2513826X19898810

60. Mundinger GS, Armstrong DG, Smith DJ, Sailon AM, Chatterjee A, Tamagnini G, et al. Autologous homologous skin constructs allow safe closure of wounds: a retrospective, noncontrolled, multicentered case series. *Plast Reconstr Surg Glob Open.* (2020) 8:e2840. doi: 10.1097/GOX.0000000000002840

61. Granick MS, Baetz NW, Labroo P, Milner S, Li WW, Sopko NA. *In vivo* expansion and regeneration of full-thickness functional skin with an autologous homologous skin construct: clinical proof of concept for chronic wound healing. *Int Wound J.* (2019) 16:841–46. doi: 10.1111/iwj.13109

62. Mazlyzam AL, Aminuddin BS, Fuzina NH, Norhayati MM, Fauziah O, Isa MR, et al. Reconstruction of living bilayer human skin equivalent utilizing human fibrin as a scaffold. *Burns.* (2007) 33:355–63. doi: 10.1016/j.burns.2006.08.022

63. Seet WT, Manira M, Khairul Anuar K, Chua KH, Ahmad Irfan AW, Ng MH, et al. Shelf-life evaluation of bilayered human skin equivalent, Myderm. *PLoS ONE.* (2012) 7:e40978. doi: 10.1371/journal.pone.0040978

64. Bt Hj Idrus R, Abas A, Ab Rahim F, Saim AB. Clinical translation of cell therapy, tissue engineering, and regenerative medicine product in Malaysia and its regulatory policy. *Tissue Eng Part A.* (2015) 21:2812–6. doi: 10.1089/ten.tea.2014.0521

65. Mohamed Haflah NH, Ng MH, Mohd Yunus MH, Naicker AS, Htwe O, Abdul Razak KA, et al. Massive traumatic skin defect successfully treated with autologous, bilayered, tissue-engineered myderm skin substitute: a case

report. *JBJS Case Connect.* (2018) 8:e38. doi: 10.2106/JBJS.CC.17.00250

66. Centanni JM, Straseski JA, Wicks A, Hank JA, Rasmussen CA, Lokuta MA, et al. Stratagraft skin substitute is well-tolerated and is not acutely immunogenic in patients with traumatic wounds: results from a prospective, randomized, controlled dose escalation trial. *Ann Surg.* (2011) 253:672–83. doi: 10.1097/SLA.0b013e318210f3bd

67. Sheryl R. *Stratatech Corporation Biologics License Application (Approval Letter).* (2021). Available online at: https://www.FDA.Gov/media/150131/download

68. Schiestl C, Meuli M, Vojvodic M, Pontiggia L, Neuhaus D, Brotschi B, et al. Expanding into the future: combining a novel dermal template with distinct variants of autologous cultured skin substitutes in massive burns. *Burns Open.* (2021) 5:145–53. doi: 10.1016/j.burnso.2021.06.002

69. Greenwood JE. Chapter 10 - hybrid biomaterials for skin tissue engineering. in *Skin Tissue Engineering and Regenerative Medicine*, eds M. Z. Albanna and J. H. Holmes Iv (Amsterdam, NL: Academic Press) (2016). p. 185–210.

70. Yannas IV, Burke JF, Huang C, Gordon PL. Correlation of *in vivo* collagen degradation rate with *in vitro* measurements. *J Biomed Mater Res.* (1975) 9:623–28. doi: 10.1002/jbm.820090608

71. Yannas IV, Burke JF. Design of an artificial skin. I. Basic design principles. *Biomed Mater Res.* (1980) 14:65–81. doi: 10.1002/jbm.820140108

72. MacNeil S. Biomaterials for tissue engineering of skin. *Mater Today.* (2008) 11:26–35. doi: 10.1016/S1369-7021(08)70087-7

73. Wagstaff MJD, Schmitt BJ, Coghlan P, Finkemeyer JP, Caplash Y, Greenwood JE. A biodegradable polyurethane dermal matrix in reconstruction of free flap donor sites: a pilot study. *Eplasty.* (Springfield, IL: Open Science Co.) (2015) 15:e13.

74. Cheshire PA, Herson MR, Cleland H, Akbarzadeh S. Artificial dermal templates: a comparative study of novosorb biodegradable temporising matrix (btm) and integra((r)) dermal regeneration template (drt). *Burns.* (2016) 42:1088–96. doi: 10.1016/j.burns.2016.01.028

75. Lodescar RJ, Gibson CJ, Gallagher J. 722 an experience with a biodegradable temporizing matrix in a metropolitan burn center. *J Burn Care Res.* (2020) 41:S192. doi: 10.1093/jbcr/iraa024.306

76. Wagstaff MJ, Caplash Y, Greenwood JE. Reconstruction of an anterior cervical necrotizing fasciitis defect using a biodegradable polyurethane dermal substitute. *Eplasty.* (2017) 17:e3.

77. Greenwood JE, Schmitt BJ, Wagstaff MJ. Experience with a synthetic bilayer biodegradable temporising matrix in significant burn injury. *Burns Open.* (2018) 2:17–34. doi: 10.1016/j.burnso.2017.08.001

78. Damkat-Thomas L, Greenwood JE, Wagstaff MJD. A synthetic biodegradable temporising matrix in degloving lower extremity trauma reconstruction: a case report. *Plast Reconstr Surg Glob Open.* (2019) 7:e2110. doi: 10.1097/GOX.0000000000002110

79. Sreedharan S, Morrison E, Cleland H, Ricketts S, Bruscino-Raiola F. Biodegradable temporising matrix for necrotising soft tissue infections: a case report. *Austral J Plastic Surg.* (2019) 2:106–9. doi: 10.34239/ajops.v2i1.72

80. Greenwood JE, Dearman BL. Comparison of a sealed, polymer foam biodegradable temporizing matrix against integra(r) dermal regeneration template in a porcine wound model. *J Burn Care Res.* (2012) 33:163–73. doi: 10.1097/BCR.0b013e318233facl

81. Greenwood JE, Wagstaff MJD, Rooke M, Caplash Y. Reconstruction of extensive calvarial exposure after major burn injury in 2 stages using a biodegradable polyurethane matrix. *Eplasty.* (2016) 16:e17.

82. Solanki NS, York B, Gao Y, Baker P, Wong She RB. A consecutive case series of defects reconstructed using novosorb® biodegradable temporising matrix: initial experience and early results. *J Plastic Reconstruc Aesthetic Surg.* (2020) 73:1845. doi: 10.1016/j.bjps.2020.05.067

83. Cuono C, Langdon R, McGuire J. Use of cultured epidermal autografts and dermal allografts as skin replacement after burn injury. *Lancet.* (1986) 1:1123. doi: 10.1016/S0140-6736(86)91838-6

84. Compton CC, Hickerson W, Nadire K, Press W. Acceleration of skin regeneration from cultured epithelial autografts by transplantation to homograft dermis. *J Burn Care Rehabil.* (1993) 14:653. doi: 10.1097/00004630-199311000-00010

85. Carsin H, Ainaud P, Le Bever H, Rives J-M, Lakhel A, Stephanazzi J, et al. Cultured epithelial autografts in extensive burn coverage of severely traumatized patients: a five year single-center experience with 30 patients. *Burns.* (2000) 26:379–87. doi: 10.1016/S0305-4179(99)00143-6

86. Holmes JH, Molnar JA, Shupp JW, Hickerson WL, King BT, Foster KN, et al. Demonstration of the safety and effectiveness of the recell® system combined with split-thickness meshed autografts for the reduction of donor skin to treat mixed-depth burn injuries. *Burns.* (2019) 45:772–82. doi: 10.1016/j.burns.2018.11.002

87. Vanscheidt W, Ukat A, Horak V, Bruning H, Hunyadi J, Pavlicek R, et al. Treatment of recalcitrant venous leg ulcers with autologous keratinocytes in fibrin sealant: a multinational randomized controlled clinical trial. *Wound Repair Regen.* (2007) 15:308–15. doi: 10.1111/j.1524-475X.2007.00231.x

88. Ortega-Zilic N, Hunziker T, Lauchli S, Mayer DO, Huber C, Baumann Conzett K, et al. Epidex® Swiss field trial 2004-2008. *Dermatology.* (2010) 221:365–72. doi: 10.1159/000321333

89. Tausche AK, Skaria M, Böhlen L, Liebold K, Hafner J, Friedlein H, et al. An autologous epidermal equivalent tissue-engineered from follicular outer root sheath keratinocytes is as effective as split-thickness skin autograft in recalcitrant vascular leg ulcers. *Wound Repair Regener.* (2003) 11:248–52. doi: 10.1046/j.1524-475X.2003.11403.x

90. Limat A, Mauri D, Hunziker T. Successful treatment of chronic leg ulcers with epidermal equivalents generated from cultured autologous outer root sheath cells. *J Investigative Dermatol.* (1996) 107:128–35. doi: 10.1111/1523-1747.ep12298415

91. Moustafa M. Randomized, controlled, single-blind study on use of autologous keratinocytes on a transfer dressing to treat nonhealing diabetic ulcers. *Regen Med.* (2007) 2:887–902. doi: 10.2217/17460751.2.6.887

92. Moustafa M, Simpson C, Glover M, Dawson RA, Tesfaye S, Creagh FM, et al. A new autologous keratinocyte dressing treatment for non-healing diabetic neuropathic foot ulcers. *Diabet Med.* (2004) 21:786–9. doi: 10.1111/j.1464-5491.2004.01166.x

93. Zhu N, Warner RM, Simpson C, Glover M, Hernon CA, Kelly J, et al. Treatment of burns and chronic wounds using a new cell transfer dressing for delivery of autologous keratinocytes. *Euro J Plastic Surg.* (2005) 28:319–30. doi: 10.1007/s00238-005-0777-4

94. Middelkoop E, Sheridan RL. 15 - skin substitutes and the next level'. in: *Total Burn Care*, ed. D. Herndon, 5th edn. Edinburgh: Elsevier Ltd (2018). p. 167–73.e2.

95. Blight A, Mountford EM, Cheshire IM, Clancy JMP, Levick PL. Treatment of full skin thickness burn injury using cultured epithelial grafts. *Burns.* (1991) 17:495–98. doi: 10.1016/0305-4179(91)90079-V

96. Donati L, Magliacani G, Bormioli M, Signorini M, Baruffaldi Preis FW. Clinical experiences with keratinocyte grafts. *Burns.* (1992) 18:S19–26. doi: 10.1016/0305-4179(92)90106-5

97. Munster AM. Cultured skin for massive burns: a prospective, controlled trial. *Ann Surg.* (1996) 224:372–7. doi: 10.1097/00000658-199609000-00013

98. Raghunath M, Meuli M. Cultured epithelial autografts: diving from surgery into matrix biology. *Pediatric Surg Int.* (1997) 12:478–83. doi: 10.1007/s003830050188

99. Paddle-Ledinek JE, Cruickshank DG, Masterton JP. Skin replacement by cultured keratinocyte grafts: an Australian experience. *Burns.* (1997) 23:204–11. doi: 10.1016/S0305-4179(96)00123-4

100. Atiyeh BS, Costagliola M. Cultured epithelial autograft (CEA) in burn treatment: three decades later. *Burns.* (2007) 33:405–13. doi: 10.1016/j.burns.2006.11.002

101. Greaves NS, Iqbal SA, Baguneid M, Bayat A. The role of skin substitutes in the management of chronic cutaneous wounds. *Wound Repair Regen.* (2013) 21:194–210. doi: 10.1111/wrr.12029

102. Boyce ST, Supp AP, Swope VB, Warden GD. Vitamin C regulates keratinocyte viability, epidermal barrier, and basement membrane *in vitro*, and reduces wound contraction after grafting of cultured skin substitutes. *J Invest Dermatol.* (2002) 118:565–72. doi: 10.1046/j.1523-1747.2002.01717.x

103. Boyce ST, Warden GD. Principles and practices for treatment of cutaneous wounds with cultured skin substitutes. *Am J Surg.* (2002) 183:445–56. doi: 10.1016/S0002-9610(02)00813-9

104. Harriger MD, Warden GD, Greenhalgh DG, Kagan RJ, Boyce ST. Pigmentation and microanatomy of skin regenerated from composite grafts of cultured cells and biopolymers applied to full-thickness burn wounds. *Transplantation.* (1995) 59:702–7. doi: 10.1097/00007890-199503150-00011

105. Boyce ST, Kagan RJ, Yakuboff KP, Meyer NA, Rieman MT, Greenhalgh DG, et al. Cultured skin substitutes reduce donor skin harvesting for closure of excised, full-thickness burns. *Ann Surg.* (2002) 235:269. doi: 10.1097/00000658-200202000-00016

106. Boyce ST, Kagan RJ, Meyer NA, Yakuboff KP, Warden GD. The 1999 clinical research award. Cultured skin substitutes combined with Integra artificial skin to replace native skin autograft and allograft for the closure of excised full–thickness burns. *J Burn Care Rehabil.* (1999) 20:453–61. doi: 10.1097/00004630-199920060-00006

107. Boyce ST, Simpson PS, Rieman MT, Warner PM, Yakuboff KP, Bailey JK, et al. Randomized, paired-site comparison of autologous engineered skin substitutes and split-thickness skin graft for closure of extensive, full-thickness burns. *J Burn Care Res.* (2017) 38:61–70. doi: 10.1097/BCR.0000000000000401

108. Boyce ST, Zimmerman RL, Supp DM. Tumorigenicity testing in athymic mice of cultured human melanocytes for transplantation in engineered skin substitutes. *Cell Transplant.* (2015) 24:1423–9. doi: 10.3727/096368914X683052

109. Boyce ST, Lloyd CM, Kleiner MC, Swope VB, Abdel-Malek Z, Supp DM. Restoration of cutaneous pigmentation by transplantation to mice of isogeneic human melanocytes in dermal-epidermal engineered skin substitutes. *Pigment Cell Melanoma Res.* (2017) 30:531–40. doi: 10.1111/pcmr.12609

110. Supp DM, Wilson-Landy K, Boyce ST. Human dermal microvascular endothelial cells form vascular analogs in cultured skin substitutes after grafting to athymic mice. *FASEB J.* (2002) 16:797–804. doi: 10.1096/fj.01-0868com

111. Sriwiriyanont P, Lynch KA, McFarland KL, Supp DM, Boyce ST. Characterization of hair follicle development in engineered skin substitutes. *PLoS ONE.* (2013) 8:e65664. doi: 10.1371/journal.pone.0065664

112. Oostendorp C, Meyer S, Sobrio M, van Arendonk J, Reichmann E, Daamen WF, et al. Evaluation of cultured human dermal- and dermo-epidermal substitutes focusing on extracellular matrix components: comparison of protein and rna analysis. *Burns.* (2017) 43:520–30. doi: 10.1016/j.burns.2016.10.002

113. Pontiggia L, Klar A, Bottcher-Haberzeth S, Biedermann T, Meuli M, Reichmann E. Optimizing *in vitro* culture conditions leads to a significantly shorter production time of human dermo-epidermal skin substitutes. *Pediatr Surg Int.* (2013) 29:249–56. doi: 10.1007/s00383-013-3268-x

114. Grinnell F, Fukamizu H, Pawelek P, Nakagawa S. Collagen processing, crosslinking, and fibril bundle assembly in matrix produced by fibroblasts in long-term cultures supplemented with ascorbic acid. *Exp Cell Res.* (1989) 181:483–91. doi: 10.1016/0014-4827(89)90105-5

115. Ishikawa O, Kondo A, Okada K, Miyachi Y, Furumura M. Morphological and biochemical analyses on fibroblasts and self-produced collagens in a novel three-dimensional culture. *Br J Dermatol.* (1997) 136:6–11. doi: 10.1046/j.1365-2133.1997.d01-1134.x

116. El Ghalbzouri A, Lamme E, Ponec M. Crucial role of fibroblasts in regulating epidermal morphogenesis. *Cell Tissue Res.* (2002) 310:189–99. doi: 10.1007/s00441-002-0621-0

117. Ahlfors JE, Billiar KL. Biomechanical and biochemical characteristics of a human fibroblast-produced and remodeled matrix. *Biomaterials.* (2007) 28:2183–91. doi: 10.1016/j.biomaterials.2006.12.030

118. El Ghalbzouri A, Commandeur S, Rietveld MH, Mulder AA, Willemze R. Replacement of animal-derived collagen matrix by human fibroblast-derived dermal matrix for human skin equivalent products. *Biomaterials.* (2009) 30:71–8. doi: 10.1016/j.biomaterials.2008.09.002

119. Kailani MH, Jafar H, Awidi A. Chapter 9 - synthetic biomaterials for skin tissue engineering. in *Skin Tissue Engineering and Regenerative Medicine,* eds M. Z. Albanna and J. H. Holmes Iv (Amsterdam, NL: Academic Press/Elsevier Inc) (2016). p. 163–83.

120. Li A, Dearman BL, Crompton KE, Moore TG, Greenwood JE. Evaluation of a novel biodegradable polymer for the generation of a dermal matrix. *J Burn Care Res.* (2009) 30:717. doi: 10.1097/BCR.0b013e3181abffca

121. Uccioli L, TissueTech Autograph System Italian Study G. A clinical investigation on the characteristics and outcomes of treating chronic lower extremity wounds using the tissuetech autograft system. *Int J Low Extrem Wounds.* (2003) 2:140–51. doi: 10.1177/1534734603258480

122. Sheridan RL, Morgan JR, Cusick JL, Petras LM, Lydon MM, Tompkins RG. Initial experience with a composite autologous skin substitute. *Burns.* (2001) 27:421–24. doi: 10.1016/S0305-4179(00)00156-X

123. Takami Y, Yamaguchi R, Ono S, Hyakusoku H. Clinical application and histological properties of autologous tissue-engineered skin equivalents using an acellular dermal matrix. *J Nippon Med School.* (2014) 81:356–63. doi: 10.1272/jnms.81.356

124. Gomez C, Galan JM, Torrero V, Ferreiro I, Perez D, Palao R, et al. Use of an autologous bioengineered composite skin in extensive burns: clinical and functional outcomes. A multicentric study. *Burns.* (2011) 37:580–9. doi: 10.1016/j.burns.2010.10.005

125. Llames S, Garcia E, Garcia V, del Rio M, Larcher F, Jorcano JL, et al. Clinical results of an autologous engineered skin. *Cell Tissue Bank.* (2006) 7:47–53. doi: 10.1007/s10561-004-7253-4

126. Baltazar T, Merola J, Catarino C, Xie CB, Kirkiles-Smith NC, Lee V, et al. Three dimensional bioprinting of a vascularized and perfusable skin graft using human keratinocytes, fibroblasts, pericytes, and endothelial cells. *Tissue Eng Part A.* (2020) 26:227–38. doi: 10.1089/ten.tea.2019.0201

127. Dehghani F, Annabi N. Engineering porous scaffolds using gas-based techniques. *Curr Opin Biotechnol.* (2011) 22:661–6. doi: 10.1016/j.copbio.2011.04.005

128. Jones JE, Nelson EA, Al-Hity A, Jones JE. Skin grafting for venous leg ulcers. *Cochrane Libr.* (2013) 2013:CD001737-CD37. doi: 10.1002/14651858.CD001737.pub4

129. Sheikholeslam M, Wright MEE, Jeschke MG, Amini-Nik S. Biomaterials for skin substitutes. *Adv Healthc Mater.* (2018) 7:1700897. doi: 10.1002/adhm.201700897

130. Augustine R, Kalarikkal N, Thomas S. Advancement of wound care from grafts to bioengineered smart skin substitutes. *Progress Biomater.* (2014) 3:103–13. doi: 10.1007/s40204-014-0030-y

131. Zheng MH, Pembrey R, Niutta S, Stewart-Richardson P, Farrugia A. Challenges in the evaluation of safety and efficacy of human tissue and cell based products. *ANZ J Surg.* (2006) 76:843–9. doi: 10.1111/j.1445-2197.2006.03880.x

132. Rajab T, Rivard AL, Wasiluk KR, Gallegos RP, Bianco RW. Chapter III.2.7 - Ethical issues in biomaterials and medical devices. in *Biomaterials Science,* eds B. D. Ratner, A. S. Hoffman, F. J. Schoen and J. E. Lemons 3rd ed. (Amsterdam: NL, Academic Press/Elsevier) (2013). p. 1425–31.

133. Al-Himdani S, Jessop ZM, Al-Sabah A, Combellack E, Ibrahim A, Doak SH, et al. Tissue-engineered solutions in plastic and reconstructive surgery: principles and practice. *Front Surg.* (2017) 4:4. doi: 10.3389/fsurg.2017.00004

134. Tolkoff J, Anders R. Chapter III.2.2 - commercialization: what it takes to get a product to market. In: *Biomaterials Science.* eds B. D. Ratner, A. S. Hoffman, F. J. Schoen and J. E. Lemons. 3rd edn. (Amsterdam NL: Academic Press/Elsevier) (2013). p. 1389–99.

135. Dhasmana A SS, Kadian S, Singh L. Skin tissue engineering: principles and advances. *J Dermatol Res.* (2018) 1:101.

136. Hendrickx B, Vranckx JJ, Luttun A. Cell-based vascularization strategies for skin tissue engineering. *Tissue Eng Part B Rev.* (2011) 17:13–24. doi: 10.1089/ten.teb.2010.0315

137. Huang S, Xu Y, Wu C, Sha D, Fu X. *in vitro* constitution and *in vivo* implantation of engineered skin constructs with sweat glands. *Biomaterials.* (2010) 31:5520–25. doi: 10.1016/j.biomaterials.2010.03.060

138. Brandenburger M, Kruse C. Fabrication of a co-culture system with human sweat gland-derived cells and peripheral nerve cells. *Methods Mol Biol.* (2019) 1993:139–48. doi: 10.1007/978-1-4939-9473-1_11

139. Lalley AL, Boyce ST. Fabrication of chimeric hair follicles for skin tissue engineering. *Methods Mol Biol.* (2019) 1993:159–79. doi: 10.1007/978-1-4939-9473-1_13

140. Kalyanaraman B, Boyce S. Assessment of an automated bioreactor to propagate and harvest keratinocytes for fabrication of engineered skin substitutes. *Tissue Eng.* (2007) 13:983–93. doi: 10.1089/ten.2006.0338

141. Cubo N, Garcia M, Del Canizo JF, Velasco D, Jorcano JL. 3D bioprinting

of functional human skin: production and *in vivo* analysis. *Biofabrication.* (2016) 9:015006. doi: 10.1088/1758-5090/9/1/015006

142. Pourchet LJ, Thepot A, Albouy M, Courtial EJ, Boher A, Blum LJ, et al. Human skin 3D bioprinting using scaffold-free approach. *Adv Healthc Mater.* (2017) 6:1601101–8. doi: 10.1002/adhm.201601101

143. Koch L, Michael S, Reimers K, Vogt PM, Chichkov B. Chapter 13 - bioprinting for skin. In: Zhang LG, Fisher JP and Leong KW, editors. *3D Bioprinting and Nanotechnology in Tissue Engineering and Regenerative Medicine.* London, UK: Elsevier Inc., Academic Press (2015). p. 281–306.

144. Albanna M, Binder KW, Murphy SV, Kim J, Qasem SA, Zhao W, et al. *In situ* bioprinting of autologous skin cells accelerates wound healing of extensive excisional full-thickness wounds. *Sci Rep.* (2019) 9:1856. doi: 10.1038/s41598-018-38366-w

145. Smandri A, Nordin A, Hwei NM, Chin KY, Abd Aziz I, Fauzi MB. Natural 3D-printed bioinks for skin regeneration and wound healing: a systematic review. *Polymers.* (2020) 12:1782–1800. doi: 10.3390/polym12081782

146. Supp DM, Hahn JM, McFarland KL, Combs KA, Lee KS, Inceoglu B, et al. Soluble epoxide hydrolase inhibition and epoxyeicosatrienoic acid treatment improve vascularization of engineered skin substitutes. *Plast Reconstr Surg Glob Open.* (2016) 4:e1151. doi: 10.1097/GOX.0000000000001151

147. Supp DM, Hahn JM, Lloyd CM, Combs KA, Swope VK, Abdel-Malek Z, et al. Light or dark pigmentation of engineered skin substitutes containing melanocytes protects against ultraviolet light-induced DNA damage *in vivo*. *J Burn Care Res.* (2020) 41:751–60. doi: 10.1093/jbcr/iraa029

11

Possible Implications for Improved Osteogenesis? The Combination of Platelet-Rich Fibrin with Different Bone Substitute Materials

Sebastian Blatt[1,2]*, Daniel G. E. Thiem[1], Solomiya Kyyak[1], Andreas Pabst[3], Bilal Al-Nawas[1] and Peer W. Kämmerer[1]

[1] Department of Oral and Maxillofacial Surgery, University Medical Center, Johannes Gutenberg University Mainz, Mainz, Germany, [2] Platform for Biomaterial Research, BiomaTiCS Group, University Medical Center, Johannes Gutenberg University Mainz, Mainz, Germany, [3] Department of Oral and Maxillofacial Surgery, Federal Armed Forces Hospital, Koblenz, Germany

*Correspondence:
Sebastian Blatt
sebastian.blatt@unimedizin-mainz.de

Bone substitute materials (BSM) are widely used in oral regeneration, but sufficient angiogenesis is crucial for osteogenesis. The combination of BSM with autologous thrombocyte concentrations such as platelet-rich fibrin (PRF) may represent a clinical approach to overcome this limitation. This study analyzes the early influence on osteoblast (HOB) *in vitro*. Here, four different BSM (allogeneic, alloplastic, and two of xenogeneic origin) were combined with PRF. After the incubation with osteoblasts for 24 h, cell viability, migration, and proliferation were assessed. Next, marker of proliferation, migration, and differentiation were evaluated on gene and protein levels in comparison to the native BSM and osteoblast alone. Addition of PRF increased viability for both the xenogeneic BSM ($p = 0.0008$, $p = 0.032$, respectively) in comparison to HOB and vs. native BSM ($p = 0.008$), and led to a tendency for increased cell proliferation and migration for all BSM (each $p > 0.05$). On gene basis, allogeneic and alloplastic BSM displayed a significantly increased RUNX2 expression (each $p = 0.050$). Expression of alkaline phosphatase for alloplastic ($p = 0.050$) and collagen-1 for xenogeneic BSM ($p = 0.05$) were significantly increased in combination with PRF. In addition, bone morphogenic protein was expressed significantly higher when xenogeneic material was combined with PRF in comparison to HOB alone (each $p = 0.05$). In summary, the combination of PRF with different BSM increases initial viability and may influence early proliferation and migration potential of osteoblast via RUNX2, alkaline phosphatase, collagen, and BMP2 especially in combination with alloplastic and xenogeneic BSM. Biofunctionalization of BSM using PRF might improve osteogenesis and extend the range of indications.

Keywords: bone substitute, oral regeneration, platelet-rich fibrin, tissue engineering, osteoblast, allograft, xenograft

INTRODUCTION

Autologous bone augmentation remains the treatment therapy of choice for regenerative craniomaxillofacial surgery in case of facial bone loss due to trauma, cancer, or other pathologies (Tatullo et al., 2012). However, disadvantages may be seen in the limited offer and enhanced morbidity with respect to the donor site especially in multimorbid patients (von Arx et al., 2001).

Here, bone substitute materials (BSM) of allogeneic, xenogeneic, or alloplastic origins represent a suitable and promising therapy option with specific indications: in opposite to the osteoinductive capacity of autologous bone, BSM shows functional deficits due to their osteoconductive properties (Khosropanah et al., 2018). Only for allogeneic BSM, an osteoinductive potential could be demonstrated (Miron et al., 2016). Therefore, allogeneic materials in particular are frequently used for "bone engineering" where, e.g., via co-culture experiments, stem cell therapy or the addition of growth factors BSM were edited in order to improve bone regeneration procedures (Hinze et al., 2010).

As a key role in initial osteogenesis, a sufficient blood vessel supply and angiogenesis, the formation of new blood vessels from existing lumina, is mandatory (Rather et al., 2019). On the one hand, capillary structures supply the regenerated bony defect area with nutrients and minerals for homeostasis. In addition, they support and regulate diverse functions of the bone marrow and bone in osteogenesis processes, structurally and via paracrine pathways on different cellular levels (Grosso et al., 2017). Here, new engineering strategies may overcome the current limitations of an insufficient initial blood supply of BSM that, with an increased angiogenic potential, may lead the way to an optimized osseous regeneration.

Autologous platelet concentrate (PC) such as platelet-rich fibrin (PRF) are now broadly used in dental and craniomaxillofacial regenerative medicine (Dohan et al., 2006). Via the complex interplay of different cytokines and growth factors, the proliferation and differentiation of different cell lines is thrived (Miron et al., 2017). So far, a significant pro-angiogenic effect of the PRF could be shown especially for soft tissue regeneration procedures (Ghanaati et al., 2018; Blatt et al., 2020). Up to date, there is inconsistent data if PRF may also support bony regeneration (Miron et al., 2017). Still, raising evidence emerges that PRF may also support differentiation and proliferation of osteoblasts (Dohle et al., 2018). Lately, our working group demonstrated a positive effect after 3–10 days of co-incubation, especially in combination with an allograft in comparison to BSM alone or in combination with xenogeneic materials (Kyyak et al., 2020). However, data for a possible initial and early interaction remain spares.

Controversially, some studies and case reports report conflicting data if PRF may influence osteogenesis (Pripatnanont et al., 2013; Yoon et al., 2014). A possible explanation for the ambivalent data may be seen in the diversity of the analyzed BSM and their different biophysical properties. Furthermore, different time points of evaluation were chosen that counteract time points of the physiological wound healing phase. Therefore, the aim of this study was to investigate the early effect on viability, migration, proliferation, and differentiation of osteoblasts of the PRF when combined with BSM *in vitro* after 24 h. This way, a comprehensive understanding of the possible initial mechanism of PRF in comparison to the well-studied later time points in osteogenesis should be provided to detect intercellular implications and provide basic scientific evidence for potential clinical translation.

MATERIALS AND METHODS

Bone Substitute Materials
Four commercially available BSM were tested: allogeneic (AKM: maxgràft®, botiss biomaterials GmbH, Zossen, Germany, granularity <2 mm), alloplastic (APKM: maxresob®, botiss biomaterials GmbH, Zossen, Germany, granularity 0.8–1.5 mm), and xenogeneic BSM (XKM1: cerabone®, botiss biomaterials GmbH, Zossen, Germany, granularity 1.0–2.0 mm, XKM2: BioOss®, Geistlich Pharma AG, Wolhusen, Switzerland, granularity 1–2 mm) were used for the further experiments.

PRF Protocol
For the PRF protocol, blood was collected from three healthy volunteers who gave their informed consent to this study in accordance with the ethical standards of the National Research Committee (Ärztekammer Rheinland-Pfalz, no. "2019-14705_1") and the 1964 Helsinki declaration and its later amendments or comparable ethical standards. Ten milliliters of peripheral venous blood per sample were collected after puncturing the cephalic or the median cubital vein with the vacutainer system and specific sterile plain vacuum tubes with additional silicone within their coating surface for solid (A-PRF+, Mectron, Carasco, Italy) and liquid PRF, respectively (iPRF, Mectron, Carasco, Italy). Next, PRF was directly manufactured (1,200 rpm for 8 min, relative centrifugal force 177 g at a fixed angle rotor with a radius of 110 mm, Duo centrifuge, Mectron, Carasco, Italy), as previously described (Blatt et al., 2020).

Cell Culture
Before the incubation with osteoblast, PRF was pressed to a stable membrane with the "PRF Box" (Mectron, Carasco, Italy) as indicated by the manufacturer. Next, PRF was cut into small pieces of 10–20 mm^2, 0.3–0.5 ml of liquid PRF was added and mixed manually with an equal quantity of the respective BSM (100 mg) to obtain a sticky clot. Next, a commercially available human osteoblast cell line (HOB, PromoCell, Heidelberg, Germany) was used and cultivated with a standard HOB medium with an additive fetal calf serum (FCS, Gibco Invitrogen, Karlsruhe, Germany), Dulbecco's modified Eagle's medium (DMEM, Gibco Invitrogen), dexamethasone (100 nmol/l, Serva Bioproducts, Heidelberg, Germany), L-glutamine (Gibco Invitrogen), and streptomycin (100 mg/ml, Gibco Invitrogen). Cultivation was done at 37°C in a constant, humidified atmosphere with 95% room air and 5% CO$_2$ until a confluence of approximately 70% was reached. Next, HOB were passaged using 0.25% trypsin (Seromed Biochrom KG, Berlin, Germany). HOB at passage five were used and seeded in a 24 well plate (Merck, Darmstadt, Germany) in a density of 5 × 10^4 cells per well. Now, 100 mg of the respective BSM were added in combination with (prepared as mentioned above) or without PRF and further incubated for 24 h at 37°C with 95% room air and 5% CO$_2$. HOB alone served as control.

Cell Viability Analysis
Next, cell viability was analyzed after 24 h by 3-(4,5-dimethylthiazol-2-yl)-2,5-diphenyltetrazolium bromide (MTT) assay, as previously described (Pabst et al., 2015). In brief, MTT

(200 μL, 2 mg/mL) was added to the wells and incubated for 4 h at 37°C before the culture medium was discarded, and 10 ml of lysis buffer was added per well. Finally, a fluorescence microplate reader (Versamax, Molecular Devices, San Jose, CA, United States) was used at 570 nm to detect metabolic activity that reflects viability.

Cell Proliferation Analysis

Fluorescence red was applied after 24 h with CellTracker (Life Technologies, Thermo Fisher Scientific, Darmstadt, Germany) according to the manufacturer's instructions to track cell number and therefore, proliferation rate. After the removal of the culture media, warmed Red dye was added and incubated for 30 min. Afterward, the dye was removed, washed with serum-free medium, and incubated for 30 min. Finally, Red fluorescence was analyzed with a fluorescence microscope (BZ-9000, Keyence, Osaka, Japan). Automatic thresholding was applied to extract cell structures and the area fraction (%) was calculated as previously described (Kyyak et al., 2020).

Cell Migration Assay

A scratch test was used to detect migration ability, as previously described (Kyyak et al., 2020). HOB were incubated with BSM in combination with and without PRF in a special scratch assay plate (ibidi GmbH, Gräfelfing, Germany) for 24 h at the above mentioned conditions. Here, red cell tracker was applied as mentioned above. Quantification of the migrated cells and visualization of cell viability was done with the ImageJ software (ACTREC, Navi Mumbai, India), as previously described (Kyyak et al., 2020). In brief, images at a $10\times$ fold magnification were first converted to grayscale before image subtraction was used to correct background staining. Next, automatic thresholding was applied to extract cell structures, and cells migrated in the gap were evaluated and the area fraction (%) was calculated.

ELISA Quantification

Growth factor release on protein basis was analyzed after co-incubation with 1.4 ml of the cell supernatant, which was extracted after incubation for 24 h with HOB and the respective native and bio-activated BSM samples, as previously described (Blatt et al., 2020). Antibodies for alkaline phosphatase (AP), collagen (COL), bone morphogenic protein 2 (BMP), osteocalcin (OCN), and Runt-related transcription factor-2 (RUNX, all R&D Systems, Minneapolis, MN, United States) were evaluated according to the manufacturer's protocol and analyzed via an ELISA plate reader and the specific software (SoftMax Pro 5.4, Molecular Devices, San Jose, CA, United States). In brief, after diluting the capture antibody in a coating buffer according to the manufacturer's dilution protocol, a 96-well-plate was coated with 100 μL per well of coating solution and incubated overnight at 2–8°C. Afterward, wells were washed with a wash buffer and the excess liquid was removed. Two hundred microliters of blocking buffer was added and incubated for 1 h at room temperature and then removed. Next, 100 μl of standards and samples were added into the designated wells and incubated for 1 h at room temperature. The sample was then aspirated, the plate was then washed three times, and the excess liquid was

removed. According to the manufacturer's instructions, detection body was diluted in the blocking buffer and 100 μl was added to each well. After incubating for 2 h at room temperature, the plate was washed and the excess liquid was removed. Next, 100 μl of streptavidin-HRP diluted in the blocking buffer was added and incubated for 30 min at room temperature. After washing and removing the excess liquid, 100 μl of TMB substrate solution was added to each well and incubated for 30 min, then, 100 μl of stop solution was added and absorbance at 450 nm was measured with the ELISA plate reader and the specific software.

PCR Quantification

The evaluation of proliferation and migration marker on gene basis were done with real-time quantitative PCR (qRT-PCR, CFX Connect Real-Time PCR Detection System, Bio-Rad, Germany) using SYBR Green Supermix (BioRad, Hercules, CA, United States), as previously described (Kyyak et al., 2020), for the following genes: alkaline phosphatase (*ALPL*), bone morphogenic protein 2 (*BMP2*), collagen type 1 alpha 1 chain (*COL1A1*), bone gamma-carboxyglutamate protein (alias: osteocalcin, *OCN*), and RUNX family transcription factor 2 (*RUNX2*). For internal control, housekeeping genes actin alpha 1, skeletal muscle (*ACTA1*), and glyceraldehyde-3-phosphate dehydrogenase (*GAPDH*) were ran (primer sequences: **Table 1**). Briefly, the total RNA was extracted after 24 h of co-incubation using a commercial kit (Qiagen, Hilden, Germany) before RNA was converted to cDNA by the iScript cDNA synthesis kit (BioRad, Hercules, CA, United States) according to the manufacturers' instructions. Eleven microliters of SYBR, 1 μl of primer sense, 1 μl of primer antisense, and 5 μl of RNA-free water were used with the thermal cycler at the first step $-95°C$ for 3 min; second Step (repeated 39 times) $-95°C$ for 10 s, then 58°C for 30 s, and finally 72°C for 20 s; final step $-65°C$ for 0.5 s and then 95°C for 5 s. Quantification of gene expression was evaluated via the $\Delta\Delta$ CT method.

Statistical Analysis

The results were interpreted in mean values with its standard error and rounded to the first decimal place. For normal

TABLE 1 | Primer sequences for PCR protocol.

Primer	Sequence
ACTA1	Sense-GGAGCAATGATCTTGATCTT, antisense-CTTCCTGGGCATGGAGTCCT
GAPDH	Sense-AAAACCCTGCCAATTATGAT, antisense-CAGTGAGGGTCTCTCTCTTC
ALPL	Sense-ACTGCAGACATTCTCAAAGC, antisense-GAGTGAGTGAGTGAGCAAGG
BMP2	Sense-CCTGAAACAGAGACCCACCC; antisense-TCTGGTCACGGGGAATTTCG
COL1A1	Sense-AGAACTGGTGCAAG; antisense-GAGTTTACAAGACA
OCN	Sense-GSAAAGGTGCAGCCTTTGGT; antisense-GGCTCCCAGCCATTGATACAG
RUNX2	Sense-CCCACGAATGCACTATTCC; antisense-GGACATACCGAGGGACAT

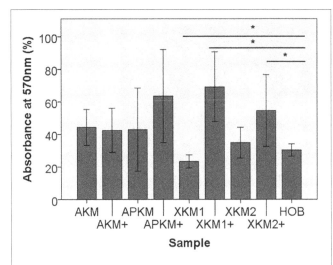

FIGURE 1 | MTT assay to evaluate viability at absorbance of 570 nm of HOB after co-incubation with the respective samples with (+)/without PRF ($^*p < 0.05$ Mann–Whitney U testing vs. HOB, XKM1: $p = 0.016$, XKM1+: $p = 0.008$, XKM2+: $p = 0.032$).

TABLE 2 | (A) MTT assay: Mean absorbances found at 570 nm for the respective samples with (+)/without PRF and respective p-values vs. HOB alone and native BSM, (B) Cell proliferation assessed with cell tracker red: Mean number of cells with its standard error and respective p-values vs. HOB alone and native BSM, (C) Scratch assay: Mean number of cells migrated into the gap for the respective samples with (+)/without PRF and respective p-values vs. HOB alone and native BSM.

(A)

Sample	Mean absorbance at 570 nm	p-Value (respective sample vs. HOB, Mann–Whitney U test)	p-Value (respective sample with PRF vs. native control, Mann–Whitney U test)
HOB	0.303 ± 0.03	–	–
AKM	0.443 ± 0.11	0.095	0.690
AKM+	0.425 ± 0.13	0.151	
APKM	0.429 ± 0.25	0.310	0.412
APKM+	0.635 ± 0.28	0.151	
XKM1	0.232 ± 0.04	0.016	0.008
XKM1+	0.698 ± 0.21	0.008	
XKM2	0.348 ± 0.09	0.222	0.222
XKM2+	0.545 ± 0.22	0.032	

(B)

Sample	Mean number of cells	p-Value (respective sample vs. HOB, Mann–Whitney U-test)	p-Value (respective sample with PRF vs. native control, Mann–Whitney U Test)
HOB	4.843 ± 8.906	–	–
AKM	5.627 ± 12.963	0.439	0.121
AKM+	5.291 ± 6.771	0.121	
APKM	4.228 ± 10.464	0.439	0.439
APKM+	5.403 ± 6.893	1.00	
XKM1	4.970 ± 11.287	0.439	0.121
XKM1+	5.239 ± 5.694	0.121	
XKM2	2.197 ± 6.181	0.121	1.00
XKM2+	4.175 ± 5.746	0.121	

(C)

Sample	Mean number of cells migrated into the gap	p-Value (respective sample vs. HOB, Mann–Whitney U test)	p-Value (respective sample with PRF vs. native control, Mann–Whitney U test)
HOB	3.584 ± 5.40	–	–
AKM	3.834 ± 5.688	0.439	1.00
AKM+	6.878 ± 7.634	0.439	
APKM	6.230 ± 6.33	1.00	0.121
APKM+	5.236 ± 9.12	0.439	
XKM1	5.813 ± 6.757	0.439	0.439
XKM1+	6.769 ± 9.368	0.439	
XKM2	3.116 ± 4.537	1.00	0.439
XKM2+	4.872 ± 5.94	1.00	

distribution, the Shapiro–Wilk test was used. In case of normally distributed values, the Student's t-test for paired samples was applied. For non-normal distributions, the Mann–Whitney test was used. In order to compare all the groups, the Kruskal–Wallis rank sum test was applied. A p-value of ≤ 0.05 was considered to be statistically significant. Finally, bar charts with error bars were used for data illustration.

RESULTS

Combination of PRF With BSM Increases Initial Viability and Tent to Improve Early Proliferation and Migration Potential of Osteoblast

First, viability of HOB after 24 h of incubation with the respective BSM with or without PRF was analyzed via 3-(4,5-dimethyl-2-yl)-2,5-diphenyltetrazolium bromide (MTT) assay (five samples in triplets each, $n = 60$, **Table 2A**). Here, all samples leveled over the negative control of HOB except for XKM1. There was no statistical significance between the groups ($p = 0.467$). In comparison to HOB alone, xenogeneic BSM did reveal a statistically significant increased viability (XKM1: $p = 0.016$, XKM1+: $p = 0.008$, XKM2+: $p = 0.032$ all other tested samples: $p > 0.05$). Metabolic activity was significantly higher for xenogeneic material 1 only when combined with PRF vs. the native material ($^*p = 0.008$, all other tested samples: $p > 0.05$, **Figure 1**). The differences between the groups were statistically significant ($p = 0.007$, **Figure 1**).

Next, cell proliferation was investigated via cell tracker (**Table 2B**, three samples in duplets for each, $n = 54$). After 24 h of incubation, no significant differences between the groups could be revealed ($p = 0.098$). However, the addition of PRF led to a tendency for increased viability for APKM in comparison to

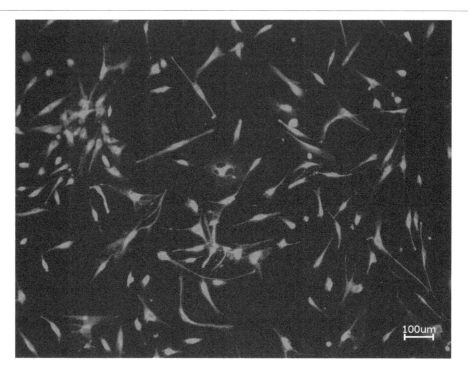

FIGURE 2 | Exemplary micrograph of cell tracker red for allogeneic BSM without the addition of PRF (10× magnification).

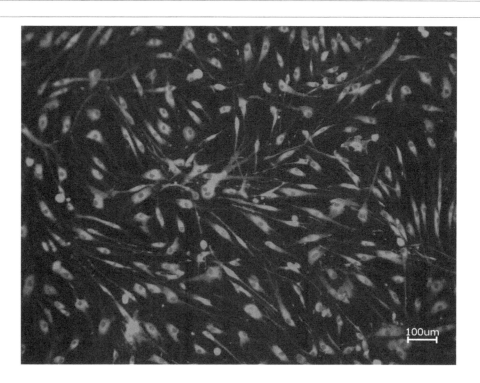

FIGURE 3 | Exemplary micrograph of cell tracker red for allogeneic BSM with the addition of PRF (10× magnification).

HOB (all tested samples: $p > 0.05$). Viability was increased when alloplastic and xenogeneic materials where combined with PRF in comparison to their native control, however without reaching statistical significance (all tested samples: $p > 0.05$, **Figures 2–4**).

To assess the differences between the groups concerning cell migration, the scratch assay was assessed (three samples in duplets for each, $n = 54$, **Figures 5–7**). Here, comparisons between all samples did not reveal any statistically significant

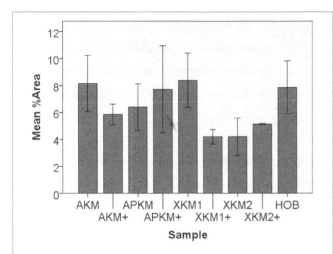

FIGURE 4 | Mean percentage of cells assessed via cell tracker assay of HOB after co-incubation with the respective samples with (+)/without PRF to detect proliferation potential (each $p > 0.05$, Mann–Whitney U testing in comparison to HOB and native BSM).

PRF in Combination With Different BSM Triggers Early Release of Marker for Osteoblast Proliferation and Differentiation

To further characterize the early interaction of PRF with the respective BSM and their influence on osteoblasts, the evident marker of proliferation and differentiation on gene and protein level via PCR and ELISA quantification, respectively, were analyzed.

Gene Expression

The PCR results (three samples in triplets each per gene, $n = 36$, **Figures 8**, **9**) showed no significant differences between the groups ($p = 0.069$, **Tables 3A–E**).

The *ALPL* expression was highest for HOB alone in comparison to other samples (all tested samples: $p > 0.05$). In comparison to the native BSM, the mean expression for *ALPL* was higher for each BSM when PRF was added with a significant increase for alloplastic material (APKM vs. APKM+: $p = 0.050$, all other tested samples: $p > 0.05$). *BMP2* gene expression tended to be increased for all the tested samples in comparison to HOB alone (all tested samples: $p > 0.05$) and for the combination of PRF and the respective material in comparison to the native BSM (all tested samples: $p > 0.05$). Allogeneic BSM significantly decreased the *COL1A1* expression in comparison to HOB alone ($p = 0.050$), but other samples did not (all other tested samples: $p > 0.05$). In comparison to the native BSM, the *COL1A1* expression was significantly increased for PRF in combination with the combination of xenogeneic material 2 with PRF ($p = 0.050$, all other tested samples:

differences (p = *0.467*). However, the percentage of HOB migrated into the gap after 24 h was slightly higher for all groups when PRF was added and was the highest for APKM (almost doubled in comparison to APKM alone) but failed to show statistical significance when compared to HOB alone (all tested samples: p > *0.05*). In comparison to their native BSM, PRF tended *to increase cell migration* for alloplastic material but no statistical significance differences where found (all tested samples: p > *0.05*, **Table 2C**).

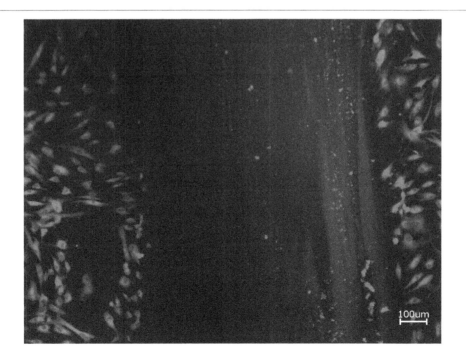

FIGURE 5 | Exemplary micrographs of migrated HOBs assessed via scratch test assay for allogeneic BSM without the addition of PRF (10× magnification).

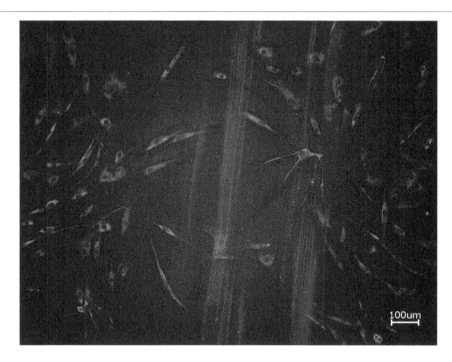

FIGURE 6 | Exemplary micrographs of migrated HOBs assessed via scratch test assay for allogeneic BSM with the addition of PRF (10× magnification).

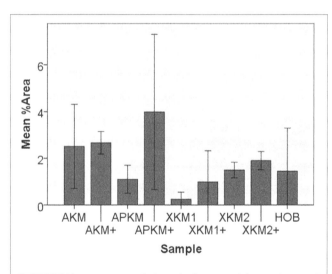

FIGURE 7 | Mean percentage of migrated cells assessed via scratch assay of HOB after co-incubation with the respective samples with (+)/without PRF (each $p > 0.05$, Mann–Whitney U testing in comparison to HOB and native BSM).

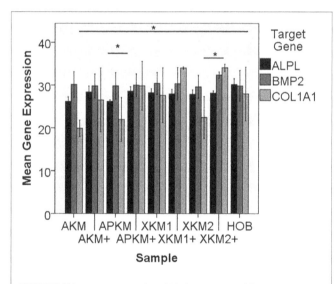

FIGURE 8 | Mean gene expression of *ALPL, BMP2, and COL1A1* after co-incubation of HOB with the respective samples with (+)/without PRF (*$p < 0.05$, Mann–Whitney U testing in comparison to HOB and native BSM, *ALPL:* APKM vs. APKM+: $p = 0.050$, *COL1A1:*AKM vs. HOB: $p = 0.050$, XKM2 vs. XKM2+: $p = 0.050$).

$p > 0.05$). For *OCN* expression, no significant difference for the tested material in comparison to HOB alone (all tested samples: $p > 0.05$) and between bio-activated and native BSM (all tested samples: $p > 0.05$) was found. Allogeneic and alloplastic BSM displayed a significant increase in the *RUNX2* expression, whereas the other analyzed BSM did not show noteworthy differences (AKM: $p = 0.050$, APKM: $p = 0.050$, all other tested samples: $p > 0.05$). Combination of the respective sample with PRF did

not significantly increase the RUNX-2 expression vs. the native BSM (all tested samples: $p > 0.05$).

Protein Expression

Next, ELISA quantification (five samples in triplets each per antibody, $n = 60$, **Figures 10, 11**) was done to analyze the

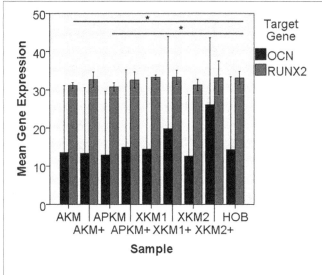

FIGURE 9 | Mean gene expression of *OCN* and *RUNX2* after co-incubation of HOB with the respective samples with (+)/without PRF (*$p < 0.05$, Mann–Whitney *U* testing in comparison to HOB and native BSM, *RUNX2*: AKM vs. HOB: $p = 0.050$, APKM vs. HOB: $p = 0.050$).

TABLE 3 | Gene expression of **(A)** *ALPL,* **(B)** *BMP2,* **(C)** *COL1A1,* **(D)** *OCN,* **(E)** *RUNX2* assessed via PCR for the respective samples and respective *p*-values vs. HOB alone and native BSM.

(A)

Sample	Mean *ALPL* expression	*p*-Value (respective sample vs. HOB, Mann–Whitney *U* test)	*p*-Value (respective sample with PRF vs. native control, Mann–Whitney *U* test)
HOB	30.14 ± 1.37	–	–
AKM	26.02 ± 1.02	0.083	0.127
AKM+	28.382 ± 1.37	0.248	
APKM	26.234 ± 0.350	0.083	0.050
APKM+	28.5595 ± 1.05	0.248	
XKM1	28.266 ± 0.902	0.121	0.564
XKM1+	27.963 ± 1.039	0. 439	
XKM2	27.859 ± 1,04	0.083	0.827
XKM2+	28.147 ± 0.54	0.083	

(B)

Sample	Mean *BMP2* expression	*p*-Value (respective sample vs. HOB, Mann–Whitney *U* test)	*p*-Value (respective sample with PRF vs. native control, Mann–Whitney *U* test)
HOB	29.837 ± 3.572	–	–
AKM	30.151 ± 2.992	0.827	0.827
AKM+	29.813 ± 2.77	0.827	
APKM	29.834 ± 3.065	0.827	0.827
APKM+	29.998 ± 2.642	0.827	
XKM1	30.420 ± 2.57	0.827	1.00
XKM1+	30.336 ± 3.780	1.00	
XKM2	29.623 ± 2.651	0.827	0.127
XKM2+	32.356 ± 0.747	0.513	

(C)

Sample	Mean *COL1A1* expression	*p*-Value (respective sample vs. HOB, Mann–Whitney *U* test)	*p*-Value (respective sample with PRF vs. native control, Mann–Whitney *U* test)
HOB	27.981 ± 6.247	–	–
AKM	19.897 ± 1.918	0.050	0.127
AKM+	26.546 ± 7.4264	0.827	
APKM	22.0 ± 5.1184	0.275	0.127
APKM+	29.85 ± 5.688	0. 513	
XKM1	27.641 ± 6.406	0.513	0.564
XKM1+	33.996 ± 0.280	0. 564	
XKM2	22.466 ± 4.931	0.275	0.050
XKM2+	34.064 ± 0.841	0.513	

(Continued)

differences on protein basis. There was no significant difference between all the tested samples (p = 0.069, **Tables 4A–D**).

ALP expression was found to be highest for HOB alone with a significant decrease for allogeneic and xenogeneic samples (AKM: *p* = 0.050, XKM1: *p* = 0.050, XKM2: *p* = 0.050, all other samples: *p* > 0.05). Furthermore, all BSM in combination with PRF tended to increase ALP expression (all tested samples: *p* > 0.05). For COL expression, there were no statistical significant differences of the respective samples in comparison to HOB alone (all tested samples: *p* > 0.05) and the native BSM (all tested samples: *p* > 0.05). Similarly, OCN expression did not have a significant statistical difference in comparison to HOB alone (all tested samples: *p* > 0.05) and combination of PRF and the respective BSM vs. native material (all tested samples: *p* > 0.05). BMP expression was increased for allogeneic (*p* = 0.050) and the combination of PRF and xenogeneic materials in comparison to HOB alone (XKM1+: *p* = 0.050, XKM2+: *p* = 0.050). Furthermore, PRF addition tended to increase BMP expression for the respective BSM vs. native material, however without reaching statistical significance (all tested samples: *p* > 0.05).

DISCUSSION

Within this study, a comparative analysis of the initial interaction of the combination of different BSM with PRF and its possible influence on early osteoblast viability, proliferation, and migration were performed *in vitro*.

As a major result, the combination of PRF with different BSM increases initial viability of HOBs. Furthermore, marker of proliferation and differentiation on gene and protein level, especially *RUNX2*, alkaline phosphatase, and collagen-1 demonstrated a noteworthy increase after co-incubation

TABLE 3 | Continued

(D)

Sample	Mean *OCN* expression	*p*-Value (respective sample vs. HOB, Mann–Whitney *U* test)	*p*-Value (respective sample with PRF vs. native control, Mann–Whitney *U* test)
HOB	14.340 ± 19.083	–	–
AKM	13.595 ± 17.499	0.827	0.827
AKM+	13.3773 ± 17.186	0.827	
APKM	12.965 ± 16.68	0.827	0.827
APKM+	14.988 ± 20.209	0.827	
XKM1	14.474 ± 18.596	0.827	0.564
XKM1+	19.809 ± 24.069	0.564	
XKM2	12.68 ± 16.060	0.827	0.127
XKM2+	26.05 ± 17.529	0.275	

(E)

Sample	Mean *RUNX2* expression	*p*-Value (respective sample vs. HOB, Mann–Whitney *U* test)	*p*-Value (respective sample with PRF vs. native control, Mann–Whitney *U* test)
HOB	33.095 ± 1.7340	–	–
AKM	31.143 ± 0.744	0.050	0.513
AKM+	32.668 ± 2.008	0.827	
APKM	30.758 ± 1.082	0.050	0.257
APKM+	32.556 ± 2.109	0.275	
XKM1	33.265 ± 0.599	0.513	1.00
XKM1+	33.273 ± 1.859	0.564	
XKM2	31.285 ± 1.488	0.275	0.513
XKM2+	33.113 ± 4.418	0.827	

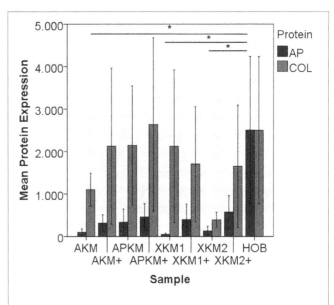

FIGURE 10 | Mean protein expression of AP and COL after co-incubation of HOB with the respective samples with (+)/without PRF (*$p < 0.05$, Mann–Whitney *U* testing in comparison to HOB and native BSM, AP: AKM vs. HOB: $p = 0.050$, XKM1 vs. HOB: $p = 0.050$, XKM2 vs. HOB: $p = 0.050$).

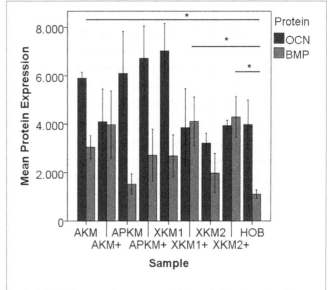

FIGURE 11 | Mean protein expression of OCN and BMP after co-incubation of HOB with the respective samples with (+)/without PRF (*$p < 0.05$, BMP: AKM vs. HOB: $p = 0.050$, XKM1+ vs. HOB: $p = 0.050$, XKM2+ vs. HOB: $p = 0.050$).

with BSM in addition to PRF and HOB in comparison to HOB alone for 24 h.

Other *in vitro* studies demonstrate ambivalent results where PRF did not significantly affect the expression of osteoblastic marker genes for differentiation, encoding ALP, RUNX2, or BMP2 (Sumida et al., 2019). Here, ALP mRNA levels were even decreased in comparison to premature osteoblasts alone. As a possible explanation, the authors state that ALP activity is high in mature osteoblasts and PRF did not inhibit, but rather delay the peak of osteoblast differentiation. This regulation may optimize bone remodeling to an osteogenic state during the early osteoblastic differentiation stages before ALP expression gradually increased over time (Sumida et al., 2019). This is in line with the presented results, where PRF led to an increase of the ALPL gene expression after 24 h. In addition, other studies found that TGF-β and PDGF, both growth factors released by PRF, may even reduce alkaline phosphatase and consequently delay differentiation (Strauss et al., 2020). Therefore, it can be discussed if PRF predominately assists in early stage osteogenesis by optimizing primarily osteoblast differentiation (Sumida

et al., 2019). The increased collagen expression found in this study is also in accordance with the literature where other *in vitro* studies proved that PRF increased osteoblast attachment and proliferation via upregulating collagen-related protein production (Wu et al., 2012). Furthermore, the elevated BMP and *RUNX2* expressions in the combination of PRF especially with allogeneic BSM may additionally induce osteoprotegerin and promote bone forming activity by increased collagen or osteocalcin production (Engler-Pinto et al., 2019; Sumida et al., 2019).

This is seen in the presented significant increased cell viability via MTT assay especially for xenogeneic BSM. In a recent analysis, the negative effect of zoledronic acid on the viability and proliferation of osteoblasts could partly be reversed by the application of PRF (Steller et al., 2019). In this study, differentiation and proliferation of osteoblasts tended to be increased when BSMs were combined with PRF but failed to show significant differences. Here, further immunological features should be addressed in subsequent studies to understand the cellular background. Using a first generation PC (Platelet Rich Plasma, PRP), the combination of PC and carbonated hydroxyapatite tended to decrease pro-inflammatory cell inflammation and subsequently showed a histologically increased bone formation (Oley et al., 2018).

This study suffers from some limitations. First and foremost, *in vitro* studies lack the general bias that results cannot reflect complex interactions in a biological system that may distort the effects. However, only *in vitro* analysis allows drawing conclusions about single cell-cell interaction. Next and in accordance with the literature, only one human osteoblast cell line was used for analysis. Surely, a multi cell line approach could strengthen the discussed hypothesis and should therefore be included in future studies. Additionally, this study solemnly focuses on the initial and early interaction of PRF and BSM and implications for HOB's viability proliferation and differentiation. This way, new insights in the underlying intercellular processes and protein release kinetics may be gained in comparison to the complemented data in the literature. However, subsequent time points are not validated in this analysis. Finally, most of the given results did not reach statistical significance. However, since only small sample sizes (as a further limitation) were analyzed, statistical significance should be treated with caution and may reflect overall limited validity. Taken together, future *in vivo* studies are much in need to validate the found tendencies.

Within the named limitation of the presented approach, no recommendation can be given which BSM may best optimize bony regeneration in combination with PRF. However, without reaching statistical significance, alloplastic and especially xenogeneic BSM interacted strongly with PRF and did influence osteoblast features the most.

The possible underlying intercellular mechanism and early angiogenic interactions of the PRF with the respective BSM were evaluated in another study by our working group (Blatt et al., 2021). Here, it was demonstrated that PRF initially interacts with its respective BSM via platelet activation *in vitro*. Furthermore, PRF had a significant positive pro-angiogenic effect, especially in combination with alloplastic and xenogeneic materials *in vivo*. Here, validated by scanning electron microscopy, a "storage" of the respective growth factors of the PRF via the close spatial relationship between the fibrin network and the BSM and a consecutive slow release that triggers vasoformative responses was hypothesized

TABLE 4 | textbf(A) AP, **(B)** COL, **(C)** OCN, **(D)** BMP protein expression assessed via ELISA for the respective samples and respective *p*-values vs. HOB alone and native BSM.

(A)

Sample	Mean AP protein expression	*p*-Value (respective sample vs. HOB, Mann–Whitney *U* test)	*p*-Value (respective sample with PRF vs. native control, Mann–Whitney *U* test)
HOB	3980.53 ± 1751.86	–	–
AKM	5893.47 ± 437.749	0.050	0.275
AKM+	4091.66 ± 2352.30	0.127	
APKM	6099.42 ± 3006.82	0.127	0.275
APKM+	6713.18 ± 2330.33	0.127	
XKM1	7031.43 ± 1955.22	0.050	0.275
XKM1+	3855.01 ± 2789.08	0.127	
XKM2	3219.49 ± 706.21	0.050	0.275
XKM2+	3935.84 ± 392.31	0.275	

(B)

Sample	Mean COL protein expression	*p*-Value (respective sample vs. HOB, Mann–Whitney *U* test)	*p*-Value (respective sample with PRF vs. native control, Mann–Whitney *U* test)
HOB	2502.06 ± 3004.99	–	–
AKM	1101.07 ± 666.66	0.827	0.513
AKM+	2126.60 ± 3181.29	0.275	
APKM	2146.64 ± 2427.82	0.827	0.127
APKM+	2634.02 ± 3533.55	0.827	
XKM1	2124.46 ± 3113.57	0.513	0.275
XKM1+	1705.80 ± 2339.48	0. 439	
XKM2	394.48 ± 305.84	0.127	0.439
XKM2+	1652.37 ± 2495.20	0.275	

(C)

Sample	Mean OCN protein expression	*p*-Value (respective sample vs. HOB, Mann–Whitney *U* test)	*p*-Value (respective sample with PRF vs. native control, Mann–Whitney *U* test)
HOB	1107.52 ± 310.94	–	–
AKM	3048.80 ± 824.21	0.127	0.513
AKM+	3971.44 ± 2436.41	0.827	
APKM	1524.62 ± 734.12	0.275	0.827
APKM+	2715.51 ± 1862.22	0.127	
XKM1	2689.14 ± 1504.79	0.127	0.275
XKM1+	4117.33 ± 1746.73	0.827	
XKM2	1977.93 ± 1412.79	0.513	0.127
XKM2+	4300.08 ± 1460.49	0.513	

(Continued)

TABLE 4 | Continued

(D)

Sample	Mean BMP2 protein expression	p-Value (respective sample vs. HOB, Mann–Whitney U test)	p-Value (respective sample with PRF vs. native control, Mann–Whitney U test)
HOB	2503.98 ± 3001.88	–	–
AKM	103.56 ± 132.29	0.050	0.513
AKM+	315.06 ± 336.14	0.127	
APKM	336.50 ± 536.87	0.513	0.275
APKM+	456.91 ± 540.82	0.275	
XKM1	50.21 ± 42.82	0.127	0.275
XKM1+	396.22 ± 634.17	0.050	
XKM2	132.69 ± 181.62	0.275	0.275
XKM2+	575.36 ± 661.23	0.050	

(Blatt et al., 2021). This assumption may be transferred to the implications of bony regeneration and could explain the release kinetics and expression of the above investigated markers found in this study: initially, PRF boosts primary viability of HOBs and subsequently releases differentiation and migration marker. This hypothesis also explains the fact that migration assay did demonstrate a noteworthy influence of the PRF but failed to reach statistical significance at this early time point.

This postulation is validated by another recent analysis by Kyyak et al. (2020) that investigated if the combination of an allogeneic or a xenogeneic BSM in combination with PRF may influence osteoblast activity after longer incubation time points (after 3, 7, and 14 days). It was shown that the addition of PRF to allogeneic and, to a minor content, to xenogeneic BSM revealed a significant increase of HOB viability, migration, proliferation, and differentiation (Kyyak et al., 2020 In a bone remodeling animal study, the incorporation of PRF into a carbonated hydroxyapatite loaded hydrogel demonstrated a higher number of osteoblasts and decreased osteoclast activity in comparison to BSM alone after 14 and 21 days (Alhasyimi et al., 2018). Therefore, it can be discussed if the combination of PRF and BSM predominately optimizes early stage osteogenesis whereas a significantly increased expression is seen at later time points after the passive release of the growth factors physically entrapped within the fibrin network. At this point in time, allogeneic BSMs that seem to bear osteoconductive properties may be in favor to increase

angiogenesis and new vessel sprouting (Kyyak et al., 2020). In context with the above-mentioned hypothesis, future studies should investigate if biomechanical aspects of the investigated BSM may influence interactions with PRF to a greater extent than what was previously assumed. This may broaden the indications of bioceramics and other BSM in regenerative medicine (Ana et al., 2018).

CONCLUSION

To conclude, PRF in combination with different BSM led to a noteworthy early influence on osteoblast proliferation, differentiation, and viability *in vitro*. In contrast to other bone-engineering methods that are hardly integrated in clinical workflow (mostly due to regulatory and practically restrictions), PC and especially PRF are autologous materials that are easy to produce and use chair-side. As shown, they seem capable to enhance the features that optimize bony regeneration. Therefore, translation in the clinical pathway seems feasible.

ETHICS STATEMENT

The studies involving human participants were reviewed and approved by Ärztekammer Rheinland-Pfalz, vote no. "2019-14705_1." The patients/participants provided their written informed consent to participate in this study.

AUTHOR CONTRIBUTIONS

SB and AP contributed to the conceptualization. PK and SK contributed to the methodology. SB, DT, and AP contributed to the validation. BA-N and PK contributed to the formal analysis and supervision. SB, DT, and AP contributed to the investigation. PK and SK contributed to the data curation. SB and PK contributed to the writing—original draft preparation. DT, AP, and BA-N contributed to the writing—review and editing. SK contributed to the visualization. AP contributed to the project administration. PK contributed to the funding acquisition. All authors have read and agreed to the published version of the manuscript.

ACKNOWLEDGMENTS

The authors would like to thank Dr. Jutta Goldschmidt and Christina Babel for their technical support as well as Mr. Wellbe Bartsma for the language editing. The data from this study are part of the dissertation work submitted to the Johannes-Gutenberg University, Mainz, as part of the medical doctoral thesis of SB.

REFERENCES

1. Alhasyimi, A. A., Pudyani, P. P., Asmara, W., and Ana, I. D. (2018). Enhancement of post-orthodontic tooth stability by carbonated hydroxyapatite-incorporated advanced platelet-rich fibrin in rabbits. *Orthod. Craniofac. Res.* 21, 112–118. doi: 10.1111/ocr.12224

2. Ana, I. D., Satria, G. A. P., Dewi, A. H., and Ardhani, R. (2018). Bioceramics for clinical application in regenerative dentistry. *Adv. Exp. Med. Biol.* 1077, 309–316. doi: 10.1007/978-981-13-0947-2_16

3. Blatt, S., Burkhardt, V., Kämmerer, P. W., Pabst, A. M., Sagheb, K., Heller, M., et al. (2020). Biofunctionalization of porcine-derived collagen matrices with

platelet rich fibrin: influence on angiogenesis in vitro and in vivo. *Clin. Oral Investig.* 24, 3425–3436. doi: 10.1007/s00784-020-03213-8

4. Blatt, S., Thiem, D. G. E., Pabst, A., Al-Nawas, B., and Kämmerer, P. W. (2021). Does platelet-rich fibrin enhance the early angiogenetic potential of different bone substitute materials? An in vitro and in vivo analysis. *Biomedicines* 9:61. doi: 10.3390/biomedicines9010061

5. Dohan, D. M., Choukroun, J., Diss, A., Dohan, S. L., Dohan, A. J., Mouhyi, J., et al. (2006). Platelet-rich fibrin (PRF): a second-generation platelet concentrate. Part I: technological concepts and evolution. *Oral Surg. Oral Med. Oral Pathol. Oral Radiol. Endod.* 101, e37–e44.

6. Dohle, E., El Bagdadi, K., Sader, R., Choukroun, J., James Kirkpatrick, C., and Ghanaati, S. (2018). Platelet-rich fibrin-based matrices to improve angiogenesis in an in vitro co-culture model for bone tissue engineering. *J. Tissue Eng. Regen. Med.* 12, 598–610. doi: 10.1002/term.2475

7. Engler-Pinto, A., Siéssere, S., Calefi, A., Oliveira, L., Ervolino, E., de Souza, S., et al. (2019). Effects of leukocyte- and platelet-rich fibrin associated or not with bovine bone graft on the healing of bone defects in rats with osteoporosis induced by ovariectomy. *Clin. Oral. Implants Res.* 30, 962–976. doi: 10.1111/ clr.13503

8. Ghanaati, S., Herrera-Vizcaino, C., Al-Maawi, S., Lorenz, J., Miron, R. J., Nelson, K., et al. (2018). Fifteen years of platelet rich fibrin in dentistry and oromaxillofacial surgery: how high is the level of scientific evidence? *J. Oral Implantol.* 44, 471–492. doi: 10.1563/aaid-joi-d-17-00179

9. Grosso, A., Burger, M. G., Lunger, A., Schaefer, D. J., Banfi, A., and Di Maggio, N. (2017). It takes two to tango: coupling of angiogenesis and osteogenesis for bone regeneration. *Front. Bioeng Biotechnol.* 5:68. doi: 10.3389/fbioe.2017.00068

10. Hinze, M. C., Wiedmann-Al-Ahmad, M., Glaum, R., Gutwald, R., Schmelzeisen, R., and Sauerbier, S. (2010). Bone engineering-vitalisation of alloplastic and allogenic bone grafts by human osteoblast-like cells. *Br. J. Oral Maxillofac. Surg.* 48, 369–373. doi: 10.1016/j.bjoms.2009.06.011

11. Khosropanah, H., Lashkarizadeh, N., Ayatollahi, M., Kaviani, M., and Mostafavipour, Z. (2018). The impact of calcium hydroxide on the osteoinductive capacity of demineralized freeze-dried bone allograft: an in-vitro study. *J. Dent. (Shiraz)* 19, 19–27.

12. Kyyak, S., Blatt, S., Pabst, A., Thiem, D., Al-Nawas, B., and Kämmerer, P. W. (2020). Combination of an allogenic and a xenogenic bone substitute material with injectable platelet-rich fibrin - A comparative in vitro study. *J. Biomater. Appl.* 35, 83–96. doi: 10.1177/0885328220914407

13. Miron, R. J., Zhang, Q., Sculean, A., Buser, D., Pippenger, B. E., Dard, M., et al. (2016). Osteoinductive potential of 4 commonly employed bone grafts. *Clin. Oral Investig.* 20, 2259–2265. doi: 10.1007/s00784-016-1724-4

14. Miron, R. J., Zucchelli, G., Pikos, M. A., Salama, M., Lee, S., Guillemette, V., et al. (2017). Use of platelet-rich fibrin in regenerative dentistry: a systematic review. *Clin. Oral Investig.* 21, 1913–1927.

15. Oley, M. C., Islam, A. A., Hatta, M., Hardjo, M., Nirmalasari, L., Rendy, L., et al. (2018). Effects of platelet-rich plasma and carbonated hydroxyapatite combination on cranial defect Bone Regeneration: an animal study. *Wound Med.* 21, 12–15. doi: 10.1016/j.wndm.2018.05.001

16. Pabst, A. M., Kruger, M., Ziebart, T., Jacobs, C., Sagheb, K., and Walter, C. (2015). The influence of geranylgeraniol on human oral keratinocytes after bisphosphonate treatment: an in vitro study. *J. Craniomaxillofac Surg.* 43, 688–695. doi: 10.1016/j.jcms.2015.03.014

17. Pripatnanont, P., Nuntanaranont, T., Vongvatcharanon, S., and Phurisat, K. (2013). The primacy of platelet-rich fibrin on bone regeneration of various grafts in rabbit's calvarial defects. *J. Craniomaxillofac Surg.* 41, e191–e200.

18. Rather, H. A., Jhala, D., and Vasita, R. (2019). Dual functional approaches for osteogenesis coupled angiogenesis in bone tissue engineering. *Mater Sci. Eng. C Mater Biol. Appl.* 103:109761. doi: 10.1016/j.msec.2019.109761

19. Steller, D., Herbst, N., Pries, R., Juhl, D., and Hakim, S. G. (2019). Positive impact of Platelet-rich plasma and Platelet-rich fibrin on viability, migration and proliferation of osteoblasts and fibroblasts treated with zoledronic acid. *Sci. Rep.* 9:8310.

20. Strauss, F. J., Nasirzade, J., Kargarpoor, Z., Stahli, A., and Gruber, R. (2020). Effect of platelet-rich fibrin on cell proliferation, migration, differentiation, inflammation, and osteoclastogenesis: a systematic review of in vitro studies. *Clin. Oral Investig.* 24, 569–584. doi: 10.1007/s00784-019-03156-9

21. Sumida, R., Maeda, T., Kawahara, I., Yusa, J., and Kato, Y. (2019). Platelet-rich fibrin increases the osteoprotegerin/receptor activator of nuclear factor-kappaB ligand ratio in osteoblasts. *Exp. Ther. Med.* 18, 358–365.

22. Tatullo, M., Marrelli, M., Cassetta, M., Pacifici, A., Stefanelli, L. V., Scacco, S., et al. (2012). Platelet Rich Fibrin (P.R.F.) in reconstructive surgery of atrophied maxillary bones: clinical and histological evaluations. *Int. J. Med. Sci.* 9, 872– 880. doi: 10.7150/ijms.5119

23. von Arx, T., Cochran, D. L., Hermann, J. S., Schenk, R. K., and Buser, D. (2001). Lateral ridge augmentation using different bone fillers and barrier membrane application. A histologic and histomorphometric pilot study in the canine mandible. *Clin. Oral Implants Res.* 12, 260–269. doi: 10.1034/j.1600-0501.2001. 012003260.x

24. Wu, C. L., Lee, S. S., Tsai, C. H., Lu, K. H., Zhao, J. H., and Chang, Y. C. (2012). Platelet-rich fibrin increases cell attachment, proliferation and collagen- related protein expression of human osteoblasts. *Aust. Dent. J.* 57, 207–212. doi: 10.1111/j.1834-7819.2012.01686.x

25. Yoon, J. S., Lee, S. H., and Yoon, H. J. (2014). The influence of platelet-rich fibrin on angiogenesis in guided bone regeneration using xenogenic bone substitutes: a study of rabbit cranial defects. *J. Craniomaxillofac Surg.* 42, 1071–1077. doi: 10.1016/j.jcms.2014.01.034

12

Efficacy and Safety of Ligation Combined with Sclerotherapy for Patients with Acute Esophageal Variceal Bleeding in Cirrhosis

Juan Su[1], Huilin Zhang[2]*, Maifang Ren[3], Yanan Xing[1], Yuefei Yin[3] and Lihua Liu[1]

[1] Department of Gastrology Ward III, Xi'an International Medical Center Hospital, Xi'an, China, [2] Department of Digestive Endoscopy and Treatment Center, Xi'an International Medical Center Hospital, Xi'an, China, [3] Department of Gastrology Ward I, Xi'an International Medical Center Hospital, Xi'an, China

*Correspondence:
Huilin Zhang
profhlzhang@163.com

Objective: To evaluate the efficacy and safety of endoscopic variceal ligation + endoscopic injection sclerotherapy (EVL+EIS) to control acute variceal bleeding (AVB).

Methods: Online databases, including Web of Science, PubMed, the Cochrane Library, Chinese National Knowledge Infrastructure (CNKI), China Biology Medicine (CBM) disc, VIP, and Wanfang, were searched to identify the studies comparing the differences between EVB+EIS and EVB, EIS from the inception of the databases up to December 30, 2020. STATA 13.0 was used for the meta-analysis.

Results: A total of eight studies involving 595 patients (317 patients in the EVL group and 278 patients in the EVL+EIS group) were included. The results of the meta-analysis did not reveal any statistically significant differences in the efficacy of acute bleeding control ($P = 0.981$), overall rebleeding ($P = 0.415$), variceal eradication ($P = 0.960$), and overall mortality ($P = 0.314$), but a significant difference was noted in the overall complications ($P = 0.01$).

Conclusion: EVL is superior to the combination of EVL and EIS in safety, while no statistically significant differences were detected in efficacy. Further studies should be designed with a large sample size, multiple centers, and randomized controlled trials to assess both clinical interventions.

Keywords: esophagogastric variceal bleeding, endoscopic variceal ligation, endoscopic injection sclerotherapy, cirrhosis, meta- analysis

BACKGROUND

Esophagogastric variceal bleeding (EVB) is the most dangerous complication of decompensated cirrhosis (1). Most of the patients with liver cirrhosis have symptoms of esophagogastric varices, with an increase in the incidence by 7% per year (2). EVB is the main influencing factor for the increased mortality in patients with liver cirrhosis (3). The mortality of the first bleeding was about 20–30% if an active intervention was not carried out (4). Within 2 years after the first bleeding, the rebleeding rate and mortality increased significantly, which threatened the safety of patients (5).

However, the secondary prevention of EVB in liver cirrhosis mainly includes endoscopic treatment, non-selective beta-blocker drugs (NSBBs), transjugular intrahepatic portosystemic shunt (TIPS), and surgical treatment (6); all these methods have limited curative effects. Although the evidence is not convincing, guidelines recommend the use of ligation and vasoactive drugs as first-line therapy for acute variceal bleeding (AVB) (7).

In the development of endoscopic therapy technology, sclerosing agent injection, tissue glue injection, vein ligation, and several other technical methods have emerged gradually to control acute bleeding and prevent rebleeding (8). Previous studies and meta-analyses have shown that vasoactive drugs and sclerotherapy are better than sclerotherapy alone (9). However, the clinical outcomes were not evaluated with respect

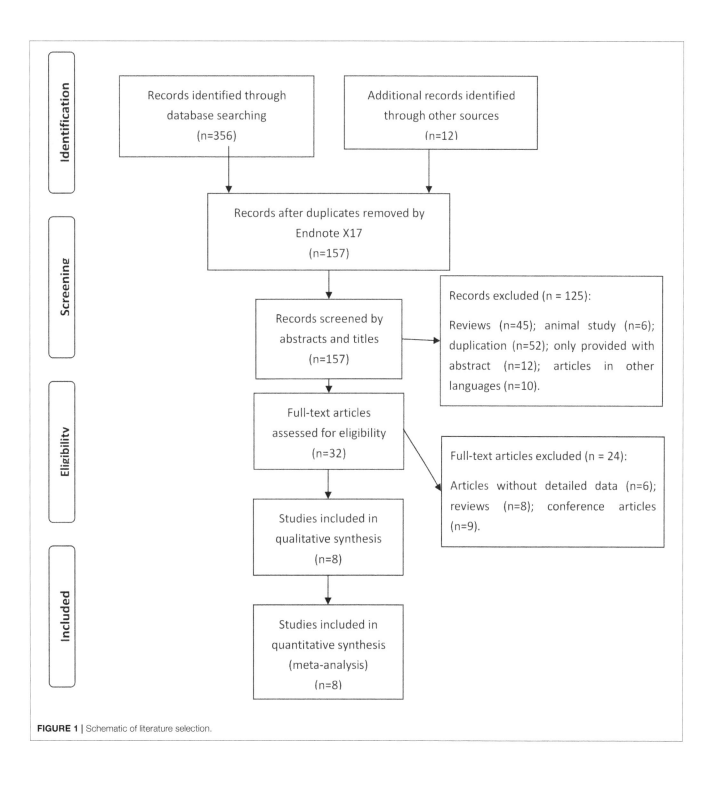

FIGURE 1 | Schematic of literature selection.

to endoscopic variceal ligation (EVL) combined with endoscopic injection sclerotherapy (EIS). Thus, we conducted a meta-analysis to investigate the efficacy and safety of EVL+EIS to control AVB.

METHODS
Inclusion and Exclusion Criteria
Inclusion Criteria
(1) Patients: Liver cirrhosis patients with AVB >18 years old. Among them, nationality and race. are not limited.
(2) Interventions: Clinical interventions are EVB combined with EIS, EVB, or EIS.
(3) Outcomes: Bleeding control rate, risk of overall rebleeding, rebleeding rate, overall mortality, and complications.
(4) Study design: Types of included studies are retrospective, prospective, and randomized controlled trials (RCTs).

Exclusion Criteria
(1) Patients with hepatocellular cell carcinoma or other malignancies.
(2) Publications based on animal experiments.
(3) Duplication, abstract, conference papers, and articles without detailed data were also excluded.

Database Search Strategy
The online databases, including Web of Science, PubMed, the Cochrane Library, Chinese National Knowledge Infrastructure (CNKI), China Biology Medicine disc (CBM), VIP, and Wanfang, were searched, and the studies that compared the differences between EVB combined with EIS and EVB, EIS were identified from the inception of the databases up to December 30, 2020. Free terms and subject terms were combined, and the language was restricted to English and Chinese. The key search words were "endoscopic variceal ligation," "endoscopic injection sclerotherapy," "EVL," "EIS," "cirrhosis," "esophageal variceal bleeding."

Data Extraction
Two researchers extracted the data from the studies independently. The information included the following: (1) General characteristics of the included studies: authors, country, study design, sample size, mean age, the main cause of cirrhosis, and Child–Pugh score; (2) Outcomes: efficacy of bleeding control, overall rebleeding rate, overall mortality, variceal eradication, and complications.

Risk of Bias Assessment
The methodological quality and bias assessment were completed by two reviewers. The risk of bias was assessed using the

TABLE 1 | The characteristics of included studies.

Study	Country	Study design	No. of patients (n)		Mean age	Male	Main cause of cirrhosis		Child–Pugh class C (n, %)	
			EVL	EVL+EIS	(Years)	(%)	EVL	EVL+EIS	EVL	EVL+EIS
Laine et al. (11)	USA	RCT	20	21	47	73.2	Alcohol	Alcohol	9 (45.00)	9 (42.86)
Saeed et al. (12)	USA	RCT	25	22	53.1	91.5	Alcohol	Alcohol	15 (16.00)	9 (40.91)
Traif et al. (13)	Saudi Arabia	RCT	31	29	48.8	61.7	HCV	HCV	10 (32.26)	5 (17.24)
Djurdjevic et al. (14)	USA	Prospective study	51	52	55.6	61.2	Alcohol	Alcohol	12 (23.23)	10 (19.23)
Umehara et al. (15)	Japan	RCT	26	25	58.2	62.3	HBV	HBV	6 (23.07)	4 (16.00)
Harras et al. (16)	Egypt	Prospective study	50	50	48.9	46.9	HCV	HCV	4 (0.08)	2 (0.04)
Mansour et al. (17)	Egypt	RCT	60	60	NA	65	HCV	HCV	32 (53.33)	24 (40.00)
Zheng et al. (18)	China	Prospective study	54	19	55.2	65.4	HBV	HBV	14 (9.21)	

RCT, randomized controlled trail; HCV, Hepatitis C virus; HBV, Hepatitis B virus.

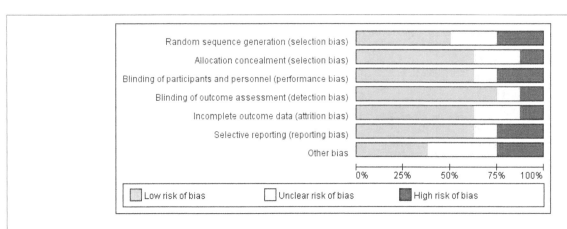

FIGURE 2 | Summary of the assessment of risk of bias.

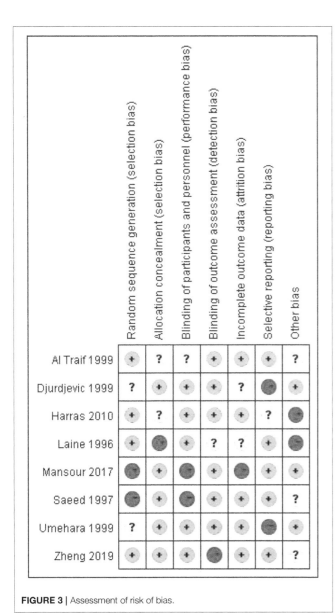

FIGURE 3 | Assessment of risk of bias.

Cochrane Collaboration tool, which rates seven items as high, low, or unclear for risk of bias (10). These items include random sequence generation, allocation concealment, blinding of participants and personnel, blinding of outcome assessment, incomplete outcome data, selective outcome reporting, and other potential sources of bias.

Data Analysis
STATA 13.0 was used for the meta-analysis. χ^2-test and I^2-test are used to determine the heterogeneity among the studies. If $I^2 < 50\%$, $P > 0.1$, there is no heterogeneity in the data analysis, and a fixed-effects model was used; if not, the random-effects model assessed the different causes of heterogeneity. Sensitivity analysis was carried out when the subgroup analysis was not satisfactory,

and it was employed to evaluate the robustness of the main results.

RESULTS
Characteristics of the Included Studies
A total of 368 records were searched in online databases. After assessing the titles and abstracts, 211 studies were identified as eligible citations. Full-text reading retrieved eight studies (11–18) involving 595 patients (317 patients in the EVL group and 278 patients in the EVL+EIS group) (**Figure 1**).

Among the eight included studies, three were from the USA, and five were designed as RCTs. The main courses of cirrhosis were hepatitis B virus (HBV), hepatitis C virus (HCV), and alcohol. The characteristics of the included studies are listed in **Table 1**.

None of the included studies were assessed to have a low risk of bias in all the seven items of the Cochrane Collaboration tool (**Figure 2**). The majority of the studies were high risk for random sequence generation and for other sources of bias (**Figure 3**). Studies scored high risk for other sources of bias with respect to concerns, such as baseline differences and industry funding. Most of the studies had an unclear risk of bias for selective outcome reporting, and a few had registered protocols.

Results of the Meta-Analysis
Efficacy of Acute Bleeding Control
In this meta-analysis, three studies reported the efficacy of acute bleeding control. No heterogeneity was detected between studies ($I^2 = 0.0\%$, $P = 0.933$), and the meta-analysis was conducted using a fixed-effects model. The results did not show any significant difference between EVL and EVL+EIS interventions (risk ratio (RR) = 0.99, 95% CI: 0.63–1.56, $P = 0.981$; **Figure 4**).

Overall Rebleeding
An overall rebleeding was reported in seven included studies, and no heterogeneity was observed between studies ($I^2 = 0.0\%$, $P = 0.873$). The meta-analysis was conducted using a fixed-effects model. No statistically significant difference was detected in EVL and EVL+EIS (RR = 0.83, 95% CI: 0.52–1.31, $P = 0.415$; **Figure 5**).

Variceal Eradication
Among the included studies, four reported variceal eradication. The meta-analysis using a fixed-effects model (study heterogeneity: $I^2 = 0.0\%$, $P = 0.985$) did not detect any statistically significant difference in EVL and EVL+EIS (RR = 1.01, 95% CI: 0.82–1.23, $P = 0.960$; **Figure 6**).

Overall Mortality
The overall mortality was reported in six included studies. No heterogeneity test was observed between studies ($I^2 = 0.0\%$, $P = 0.630$), and hence, a fixed-effects model was used to analyze the data. Strikingly, no statistically significant difference was detected in EVL and EVL+EIS (RR = 0.80, 95% CI: 0.52–1.24, $P = 0.314$; **Figure 7**).

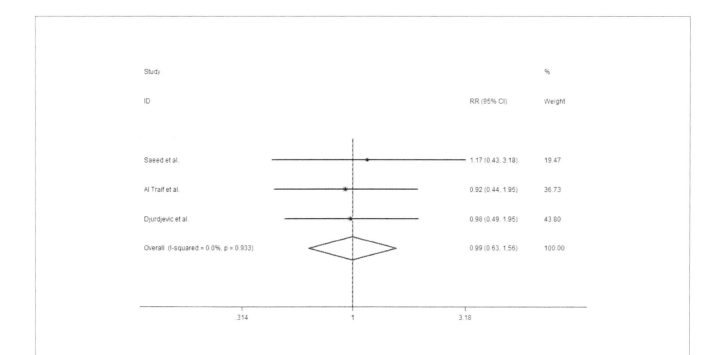

FIGURE 4 | Forest plot of the meta-analysis comparing EVL and EVL+EIS with respect to the efficacy of acute bleeding control. EIS, endoscopic injection sclerotherapy; EVL, endoscopic variceal ligation.

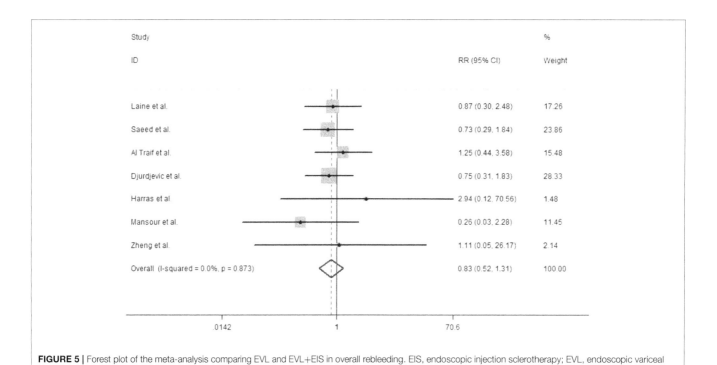

FIGURE 5 | Forest plot of the meta-analysis comparing EVL and EVL+EIS in overall rebleeding. EIS, endoscopic injection sclerotherapy; EVL, endoscopic variceal ligation.

Complications

Complications were reported in the included studies. The results of the meta-analysis show that deep ulcers (RR = 0.97, 95% CI: 0.53–1.79, P = 0.247), dysphagia (RR = 0.43, 95% CI: 0.18–1.01, P = 0.106), strictures dilated (RR = 0.15, 95% CI: 0.02–1.17, P = 0.353), and pain (RR = 0.56, 95% CI: 0.31–1.03, P = 0.124) did not show any significant difference between EVL and EVL+EIS, but the overall complication rate (RR = 0.60, 95% CI: 0.41–0.87, P = 0.01) had a statistically significant difference between EVL and EVL+EIS interventions (**Figure 8**).

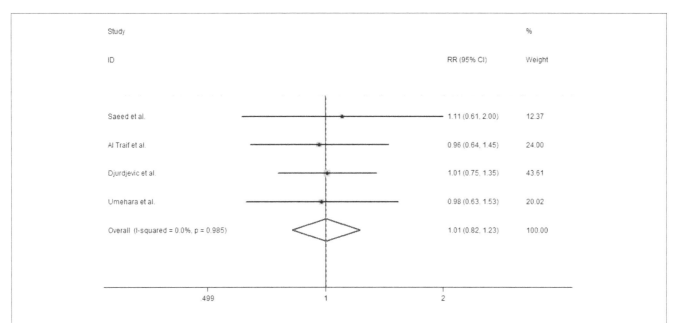

FIGURE 6 | Forest plot of the meta-analysis comparing EVL and EVL+EIS in variceal eradication. EIS, endoscopic injection sclerotherapy; EVL, endoscopic variceal ligation.

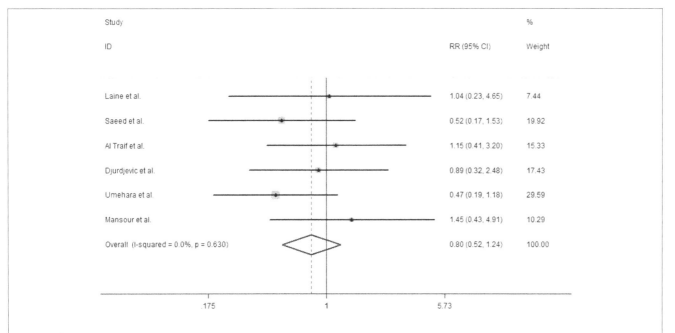

FIGURE 7 | Forest plot of the meta-analysis comparing EVL and EVL+EIS in overall mortality. EIS, endoscopic injection sclerotherapy; EVL, endoscopic variceal ligation.

DISCUSSION

EVB patients have a high risk of rebleeding and death after bleeding control (19). If the EVB patients do not receive secondary preventive treatment for 1–2 years, the rebleeding rate is elevated to about 60%, and the mortality rate is 33% (20). At present, EVL and EIS are indispensable in the endoscopic treatment of the secondary prevention of EVB. The basic goal of the treatment is to eradicate or reduce the degree of esophageal varices in order to reduce the recurrence rate and mortality (21). Patients with a history of EVB should be treated routinely by endoscopy, and patients with acute EVB should continue to receive corresponding endoscopic treatment after the termination of bleeding (22).

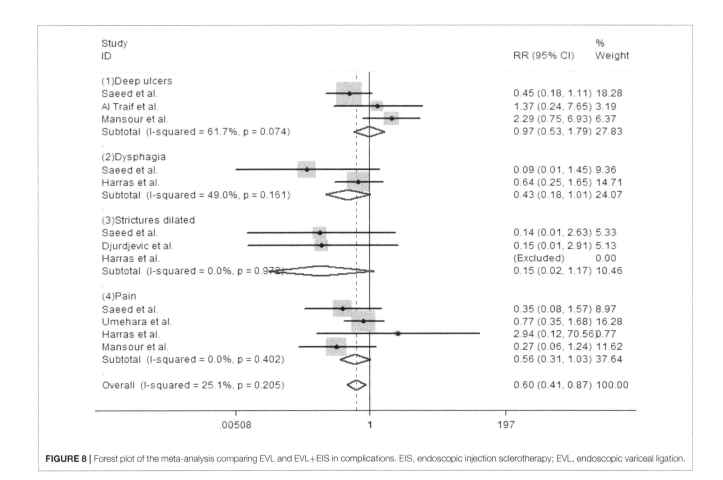

FIGURE 8 | Forest plot of the meta-analysis comparing EVL and EVL+EIS in complications. EIS, endoscopic injection sclerotherapy; EVL, endoscopic variceal ligation.

In EVL technology, the negative pressure at the front end of the endoscope is inhaled into the esophageal varices that are then ligated with a rubber ring in the transparent cap (7). The physical ligation blocks the blood supply of the varices, resulting in thrombosis, tissue necrosis, and ulcers, finally leaving healing scars for the treatment and elimination of varices (23). EIS refers to the injection of a sclerosing agent into the tissue of varicose vein or adjacent to varicose vein, which shows ischemia and necrosis in the tissue of varicose vein, and then produces fibrosis, to eliminate varicose veins (24). With the continuous development of endoscopic technology and the evolution of sclerosing agents, the clinical application of EVL and EVs is also evolving (25).

The present meta-analysis did not detect any statistically significant difference in the efficacy of acute bleeding control (RR = 0.99, 95% CI: 0.63–1.56, P = 0.981), overall rebleeding (RR = 0.83, 95% CI: 0.52–1.31, P = 0.415), variceal eradication (RR = 1.01, 95% CI: 0.82–1.23, P = 0.960), and overall mortality (RR = 0.80, 95% CI: 0.52–1.24, P = 0.314), but a significant difference was observed in the overall complications (RR = 0.60, 95% CI: 0.41–0.87, P = 0.01). The

main complications of EVL include chest pain or discomfort, dysphagia or pain, and erosion or ulcer at the ligation site, infection, or bacteremia (26). Rubber bands falling off and sliding can also form ulcers and after rebleeding (27). Compared to EVL alone, the effect of EIS combined with EVL varies in different studies. In patients with active bleeding, EVL uses ligation device, which limits the intraoperative field of vision, raising the technical requirements of endoscopic operators (28).

Due to various conditions, the present meta-analysis has some limitations. Firstly, the included studies were from different countries. Secondly, the frequency of follow-up and the total duration of follow-up were also incompatible. Thirdly, some disparities in medical technology and medical facilities were observed in the included literature. Therefore, EVL and EVs may show similar results in the treatment of esophageal variceal bleeding.

In conclusion, EVL is superior to the combination of EVL and EIS in safety, while no significant differences were noted in efficacy. Nonetheless, further studies should be designed based on a large sample size, multiple centers, RCTs to substantiate these two clinical interventions.

AUTHOR CONTRIBUTIONS

JS and HZ contributed to the conceptualization, project administration, and writing and review. JS and MR contributed to the data curation. YX and YY contributed to the data analysis. JS, HZ, and LL contributed to the methodology. HZ and MR contributed resources. YX and LL contributed the software. HZ contributed to the supervision. All authors contributed to the article and approved the submitted version.

REFERENCES

1. Wu LF, Xiang XX, Bai DS, Jin SJ, Zhang C, Zhou BH, et al. Novel noninvasive liver fibrotic markers to predict postoperative re-bleeding after laparoscopic splenectomy and azygoportal disconnection: a 1-year prospective study. *Surg Endosc.* (2020). doi: 10.1007/s00464-020-08111-4

2. Moon AM, Green PK, Rockey DC, Berry K, Ioannou GN. Hepatitis C eradication with direct-acting anti-virals reduces the risk of variceal bleeding. *Alimentary Pharmacol Therap.* (2020) 51:364–73. doi: 10.1111/apt.15586

3. Tantai XX, Liu N, Yang LB, Wei ZC, Xiao CL, Song YH, et al. Prognostic value of risk scoring systems for cirrhotic patients with variceal bleeding. *World J Gastroenterol.* (2019) 25:6668–80. doi: 10.3748/wjg.v25.i45.6668

4. Lin L, Cui B, Deng Y, Jiang X, Liu W, Sun C. The efficacy of proton pump inhibitor in cirrhotics with variceal bleeding: a systemic review and meta-analysis. *Digestion.* (2020) 102:117–27. doi: 10.1159/000505059

5. Rogalski P, Rogalska-Plonska M, Wroblewski E, Kostecka-Roslen I, Dabrowska M. Laboratory evidence for hypercoagulability in cirrhotic patients with history of variceal bleeding. *Thromb Res.* (2019) 178:41–6. doi: 10.1016/j.thromres.2019.03.021

6. Sohn H, Park S, Kang Y, Koh H, Han SJ, Kim S. Predicting variceal bleeding in patients with biliary atresia. *Scand J Gastroenterol.* (2019) 54:1385–90. doi: 10.1080/00365521.2019.1683225

7. Onofrio FQ, Pereira-Lima JC, Valença FM, Azeredo-da-Silva ALF, Tetelbom Stein A. Efficacy of endoscopic treatments for acute esophageal variceal bleeding in cirrhotic patients: systematic review and meta-analysis. *Endosc Int Open.* (2019) 7:E1503–14. doi: 10.1055/a-0901-7146

8. Yoo JJ, Kim SG, Kim YS, Lee B, Jeong SW, Jang JY, et al. Propranolol plus endoscopic ligation for variceal bleeding in patients with significant ascites: propensity score matching analysis. *Medicine.* (2020) 99:e18913. doi: 10.1097/MD.0000000000018913

9. Xu HB, An ZT, Xuan J, Wen W. Evidence-based endoscopic treatment of esophagogastric variceal bleeding. *World Chin J Digestol.* (2017) 25:1558. doi: 10.11569/wcjd.v25.i17.1558

10. Higgins JPT, Green S (editors.). *Cochrane Handbook for Systematic Reviews of Interventions, version 5.1.0 [updated March 2011].* The Cochrane Collaboration (2011). Available online at: http:// handbook.cochrane.org/ (accessed November 2, 2017).

11. Laine L, Stein C, Sharma V. Randomized comparison of ligation versus ligation plus sclerotherapy in patients with bleeding esophageal varices. *Gastroenterology.* (1996) 110:529–33. doi: 10.1053/gast.1996.v110.pm8566601

12. Saeed ZA, Stiegmann GV, Ramirez FC, Reveille RM, Goff JS, Hepps KS. Endoscopic variceal ligation is superior to combined ligation and sclerotherapy for esophageal varices: a multicenter prospective randomized trial. *Hepatology.* (1997) 25:71–4 doi: 10.1002/hep.510250113

13. Traif IA, Fachartz FS, Jumah AA, Johan MA, Omair AA, Bakr FA, et al. Randomized trial of ligation versus combined ligation and sclerotherapy for bleeding esophageal varices. *Gastrointestinal Endosc.* (1999) 50:1–6. doi: 10.1016/S0016-5107(99)70335-4

14. Djurdjevic D, Janosevic S, Dapcevic B, Vukcevic V, Djordjevic D, Svorcan P, et al. Combined ligation and sclerotherapy versus ligation alone for eradication of bleeding esophageal varices: a randomized and prospective trial. *Endoscopy.* (1999) 31:286–90. doi: 10.1055/s-1999-22

15. Umehara M, Onda M, Tajiri T, Toba M, Yoshida H, Yamashita K. Sclerotherapy plus ligation versus ligation for the treatment of esophageal varices: a prospective randomized study. *Gastrointest Endoscopy.* (1999) 50:7–12. doi: 10.1016/s0016-5107(99)70336-6

16. Harras F, Shetael S, Shehata M, El Saadany S, Selim M, Mansour L. Endoscopic band ligation plus argon plasma coagulation versus scleroligation for eradication of esophageal varices. *J Gastroenterol Hepatol.* (2010) 25:1058–65. doi: 10.1111/j.1440-1746.2010.06265.x

17. Mansour L, El-Kalla F, El-Bassat H, Abd-Elsalam S, El-Bedewy M, Kobtan A, et al. Randomized controlled trial of scleroligation versus band ligation alone for eradication of gastroesophageal varices. *Gastrointest Endosc.* (2017) 86:307–15. doi: 10.1016/j.gie.2016.12.026

18. Zheng J, Zhang Y, Li P, Zhang S, Li Y, Li L, et al. The endoscopic ultrasound probe findings in prediction of esophageal variceal recurrence after endoscopic variceal eradication therapies in cirrhotic patients: a cohort prospective study]. *BMC Gastroenterol.* (2019) 19:32. doi: 10.1186/s12876-019-0943-y

19. Miao Z, Lu J, Yan J, Lu L, Ye B, Gu M. Comparison of therapies for primary prevention of esophageal variceal bleeding: a systematic review and network meta-analysis. *Hepatology.* (2019) 69:1657–75. doi: 10.1002/hep.30220

20. Koya Y, Shibata M, Watanabe T, Kumei S, Miyagawa K, Oe S, et al. Influence of gastroesophageal flap valve on esophageal variceal bleeding in patients with liver cirrhosis. *Dig Endosc.* (2021) 33:100–9. doi: 10.1111/den.13685

21. Bledar K, Iris M, Akshija I, Koçollari A, Prifti S, Burazeri G. Predictors of esophageal varices and first variceal bleeding in liver cirrhosis patient. *World J Gastroenterol.* (2017) 23:4806–14. doi: 10.3748/wjg.v23.i26.4806

22. Carolina Mangas-Sanjuan, Belén Martínez-Moreno, Bozhychko M. Over-the-scope clip for acute esophageal variceal bleeding. *Dig Endosc.* (2019) 31:712–6. doi: 10.1111/den.13493

23. Suh JI. Are there seasonal variations in the incidence and mortality of esophageal variceal bleeding?. *Clin Endosc.* (2020) 53:107–9. doi: 10.5946/ce.2020.042

24. Lu Z, Sun X, Zhang W, Jin B, Han J, Wang Y. Second urgent endoscopy within 48-hour benefits cirrhosis patients with acute esophageal variceal bleeding. *Medicine.* (2020) 99:e19485. doi: 10.1097/MD.0000000000019485

25. Laine L. Primary prophylaxis of esophageal variceal bleeding: an endoscopic approach. *J Hepatol.* (2010) 52:944–5. doi: 10.1016/j.jhep.2009.12.035

26. Salman AA, Shaaban ED, Atallah M, Yousef M, Ahmed RA, Ashoush O, et al. Long-term outcome after endoscopic ligation of acute esophageal variceal bleeding in patients with liver cirrhosis. *Acta Gerontol.* (2020) 83:373–80.

27. Dy SM, Cromwell DM, Thuluvath PJ, Bass EB. Hospital experience and outcomes for esophageal variceal bleeding. *Int J Qual Health Care.* (2003) 15:139–46. doi: 10.1093/intqhc/mzg016

28. Rush B, Deol N, Teriyaki A, Sey M, Jairath V, Walley KR, et al. Lower 90-day hospital readmission rates for esophageal variceal bleeding after TIPS: a nationwide linked analysis. *J Clin Gastroenterol.* (2020) 54:90–5. doi: 10.1097/MCG.0000000000001199

13

Corrective Osteotomy of Upper Extremity Malunions Using Three-Dimensional Planning and Patient-Specific Surgical Guides

Babak Saravi[1]*, Gernot Lang[1], Rebecca Steger[1], Andreas Vollmer[2] and Jörn Zwingmann[3]

[1] Department of Orthopedics and Trauma Surgery, Faculty of Medicine, Medical Centre, Albert-Ludwigs-University of Freiburg, Freiburg, Germany, [2] Department of Oral and Maxillofacial Surgery, Faculty of Medicine, Medical Centre, Albert-Ludwigs-University of Freiburg, Freiburg, Germany, [3] Department of Orthopedics and Trauma Surgery, St. Elisabeth Hospital Ravensburg, Ravensburg, Germany

*Correspondence:
Babak Saravi
babak.saravi@jupiter.uni-freiburg.de

Malunions of the upper extremity can result in severe functional problems and increase the risk of osteoarthritis. The surgical reconstruction of complex malunions can be technically challenging. Recent advances in computer-assisted orthopedic surgery provide an innovative solution for complex three-dimensional (3-D) reconstructions. This study aims to evaluate the clinical applicability of 3-D computer-assisted planning and surgery for upper extremity malunions. Hence, we provide a summary of evidence on this topic and highlight recent advances in this field. Further, we provide a practical implementation of this therapeutic approach based on three cases of malunited forearm fractures treated with corrective osteotomy using preoperative three-dimensional simulation and patient-specific surgical guides. All three cases, one female (56 years old) and two males (18 and 26 years old), had painful restrictions in range of motion (ROM) due to forearm malunions and took part in clinical and radiologic assessments. Postoperative evaluation of patient outcomes showed a substantial increase in range of motion, reduction of preoperatively reported pain, and an overall improvement of patients' satisfaction. The therapeutic approach used in these cases resulted in an excellent anatomical and functional reconstruction and was assessed as precise, safe, and reliable. Based on current evidence and our results, the 3-D preoperative planning technique could be the new gold standard in the treatment of complex upper extremity malunions in the future.

Keywords: three-dimensional (3D), patient-specific 3D preoperative templating, surgical guides, corrective osteotomy, malunion, upper extremity (arm)

INTRODUCTION

The forearm is a complex anatomical and functional unit, including the radius, the ulna, the interosseous membrane (IOM), the triangular fibrocartilage complex (TFCC), the proximal (PRUJ) and the distal (DRUJ) radioulnar joint. Forearm malunions represent a disruption of this functional system, which could lead to limited forearm range of motion, loss of power, visible cosmetic changes, painful forearm rotations due to bony impingement of the IOM, and instability of the DRUJ (1, 2). Further, the malunion can increase the risk for osteoarthritis, especially if intra-articular structures are involved (3, 4). A range of motion in pronation and supination of $50°$ is reported to be required for most daily activities. Malunions with rotational deformities lead to losses in the motion range of pronation and supination and thus, significantly affect the quality of life (1, 5). The anatomical and functional reconstruction of diaphyseal forearm fractures with compression plate and screw-fixation is a well-established surgical intervention with a relatively low complication rate (6–9). A more difficult surgical challenge is the reconstructive surgery of malunited fractures that may occur after conservative or operative treatment of the fracture (1). The multidimensional reconstruction of the axial alignment, the restoration of the normal length, and correction of angular deformities is a demanding challenge for the surgeon. Precise preoperative planning is known to be essential in the correction of complex diaphyseal malunions (2). However, it is very difficult to fully assess these deformities via two-dimensional x-ray images. Computer-aided planning based on preoperatively acquired computer tomography (CT) data allows the surgeon to accurately visualize the operation via computer simulation and to produce patient-specific surgical guides based on the three-dimensional imagery of patients' anatomy (2, 10). The workflow for the application of the 3-D planning technique is shown in **Figure 1**. Preoperative three-dimensional planning and use of patient-specific guides were already known for many years in dental implant surgery and total knee arthroplasty and there is clear evidence that highlight the benefits compared to 2D techniques (15–17). However, there is no summary of evidence regarding the applicability of three-dimensional preoperative planning techniques and application in the surgery of upper extremity malunions.

Here, we provide evidence from recent advances and present three cases of forearm malunions treated with corrective osteotomy using preoperative three-dimensional planning and patient-specific surgical guides to evaluate the outcomes of this innovative technique and close the present evidence gap.

THREE-DIMENSIONAL VIRTUAL PLANNING OF CORRECTIVE OSTEOTOMIES OF UPPER EXTREMITY MALUNIONS: PREVIOUS STUDIES

First studies on the application and accuracy of preoperative simulation and production of computer-designed bone models of the upper extremity based on patients' CT data were provided by the workgroup of Oka et al. (18) and Oka et al. (19). In 22 patients, including patients with malunited forearm fractures, malunited distal radial fractures, and cubitus varus deformity, preoperative simulation, and design of a custom made osteotomy template to reproduce the simulation during the actual surgery resulted in satisfying outcomes with an osseous union in all patients within 6 months and a full anatomical reconstruction of the angular deformities (20). Further, intra-articular fracture

of the distal radius could be successfully treated through an extra-articular approach with this technique (19). The majority of studies in the literature since then focus on three-dimensional corrective osteotomy, particularly for distal radius fractures. In a systematic review and meta-analysis conducted by Keizer et al. (11), including 15 studies with a total of 68 patients, the authors concluded that preoperatively present palmar tilt, radial inclination, and ulnar variance in 96% of the observed cases with distal radius malunions could be significantly improved with the 3-D planning technique (11). The restoration reached $5°$ or $2\,mm$ of their normal values. Despite these promising results, complications occurred in 11 out of 68 patients (16%) of the patients, including postoperative hardware-related pain or discomfort with subsequent hardware removal ($n = 6$), postoperative screw loosening ($n = 2$), a persistent distal radioulnar subluxation ($n = 2$), and partial laceration of the extensor pollicis longus tendon ($n = 1$). The authors argued that especially corrective osteotomies of distal radius malunions tend to show higher percentages of complications compared to less complex elective wrist surgery (11, 21). In a case series of four patients with combined intra- and extraarticular malunion of the distal radius, the accuracy of the correction quantified by comparing the virtual three-dimensional planning models with the corresponding postoperative 3-D bone model was $-1° \pm 5°$ for the radial inclination, $0 \pm 1\,mm$ for the ulnar variance, respectively (22). However, the volar tilt was under-corrected in all cases, with an average of $-6 \pm 6°$. Corrective osteotomy of Monteggia lesions, in which the dislocation of the radial head is associated with a malunited fracture of the ulna, was examined in two case reports conducted by Oka et al. (23). The combined radius and ulnar fracture in both patients were initially treated non-operatively with closed reduction and casting, which resulted in malunion with chronic radial head dislocation. The preoperative planning and evaluation of the kinematics of joint motion and the use of CT bone models and surgical guides to transfer the simulation into the surgical situation resulted in a restoration of forearm rotation and absence of preoperatively reported elbow pain. 3-D corrective osteotomy in both forearm bones, ulna and radius, was performed by Miyake et al., reporting results from 14 patients with a median follow-up of 29 months (10). The authors reported excellent radiographic and clinical outcomes with an improvement of the mean arc of forearm motion from $76°$ preoperatively to $152°$ postoperatively, and improved grip strength from 82 to 94%, compared to that of the contralateral non-affected side.

One of the main advantages of three-dimensional corrective osteotomy is the preoperative assessment of the 3-D anatomy, which need to be taken into account for complex deformities such as cubitus varus or valgus deformities. This therapeutic approach allows the surgeon, therefore, to not only preferentially focus on the coronal plane but also precisely take into account internal rotation, flexion-extension deformities of the elbow, and lateral protrusion of the distal fragments in such complex deformities (24, 25). In a study conducted by Chung et al., 3-D corrective osteotomy of cubitus varus deformities in 23 adult patients resulted in an improvement of humeral-elbow-wrist angle from a mean of $26°$ preoperatively to a mean

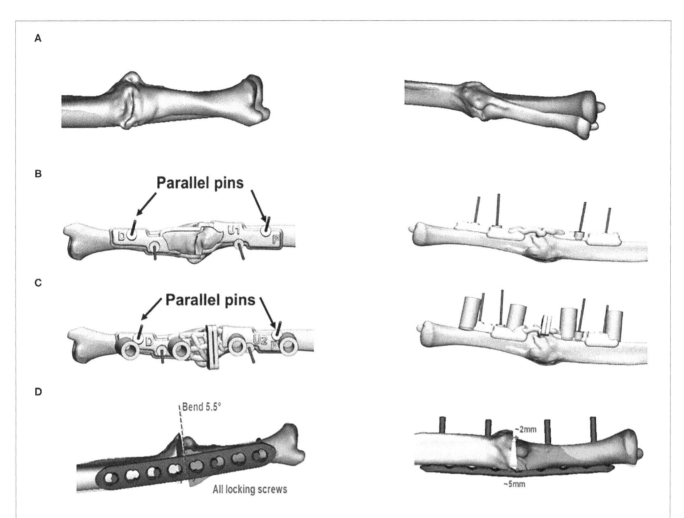

FIGURE 1 | Preoperative planning for the corrective osteotomy. 3-D- planned corrective osteotomy of forearm malunions typically involves the following steps: (1) obtaining CT data from malunited and contralateral non-affected forearm (2) creation of virtual models of both forearms (3) construction of patient-specific surgical guides to transform the digital process into the actual surgery. Rapid prototyping of the digital bone models can be used to compare the fitting of the guides during surgery (11–14). The workflow is shown for case 2 in our study: **(A)** Preoperative situation with the contralateral bone template shown in blue. Construction of bone models was based on preoperative CT data of both forearms; **(B)** Bone marking guide to mark the area in the window for verification of the drilling and cutting guides' position; **(C)** Drilling and cutting guide affixed to the bone using K-wires; verification of the desired position can be made by comparison with the guide outline on the bone model; **(D)** Simulated outcome model with the size of the bone wedges and the bending angle of the plate osteosynthesis.

of 3° postoperatively, whereas the mean internal rotation angle improved from 25° to 5° (25). No recurrence of the deformity was observed in the averaged 1 year and 10 months follow-up period after osteotomy, and the authors recommended this technique with regards to these satisfactory outcomes. Outcomes of 3-Dimensional corrective osteotomy for supracondylar cubitus valgus, and cubitus varus deformities, respectively, and diaphyseal malunions were analyzed in a case series of nine patients conducted by Kataoka et al. (26). The error in corrective osteotomy between the preoperative simulation and postoperative bone model manufactured by rapid prototyping was <3 mm and 2°. Patients who experienced wrist pain before surgery reported a substantial decrease in pain after surgery. The authors rated this technique as precise, relatively easily performable, and satisfactory for the treatment of complex supracondylar malunions with regards to the clinical

outcome. In another cohort study including 30 consecutive patients with a cubitus varus resulting from malunion of distal supracondylar fractures, the mean humerus-elbow-wrist angle and tilting angle improved significantly from 18.2° (varus), and 25°, respectively, preoperatively to 5.8° (valgus) and 38°, respectively, postoperatively (27). Preoperatively reported hyperextension of the elbow and internal rotation of the shoulder were normalized in all included patients, and the authors judged this technique to be a feasible treatment option for cubitus varus deformity. Finally, in a case series including 17 patients with cubitus varus deformities after supracondylar fractures, comparison of postoperative 3-D bone models with preoperative simulation revealed an improvement of 15° in varus before surgery to 6° in valgus after surgery, whereas the mean tilting angle of the affected side improved from 31° preoperatively to 40° postoperatively (28). The authors concluded that varus

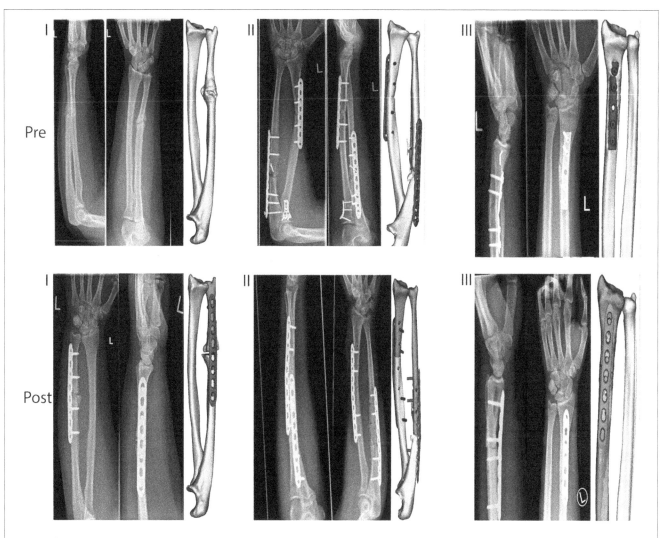

FIGURE 2 | Preoperative ("Pre") and postoperative ("Post") simulation model and radiography of three cases (I., II., and III.), treated with three-dimensional preoperative planning and corrective osteotomy of the forearm malunions.

deformities could be corrected accurately with the 3-D corrective osteotomy technique. Overall, these studies provide evidence that three-dimensional corrective osteotomy techniques for complex upper extremity malunion, such as cubitus varus and valgus deformities, respectively, can accurately and reliably restore the normal anatomical condition.

PRELIMINARY RESULTS FROM THREE CASES

All three cases, one female (56 years old) and two males (18 and 26 years old), had painful restrictions in range of motion (ROM) due to forearm malunions and took part in clinical and radiologic assessments (**Figure 2**). Based on this situation, corrective osteotomy with three-dimensional planning and patient-specific guides was proposed (*Materialise* NV, Leuven, Belgium). Based on patients' CT data, three-dimensional bone models were created to assess the deformity and plan the corrective osteotomy.

Malunions of the affected bones were further evaluated with the contralateral non-affected bone as a mirrored and precisely aligned ideal template for the correction. The planning of the corrective osteotomy was conducted with a clinical engineer to superimpose the contralateral template and simulate the corrective osteotomy. For both bones, ulna and radius, a closing osteotomy after removing a wedge of bone and consecutive plate fixation was simulated. According to the simulation, we determined the plate bending angle for the radius and the ulna, to fixate the fragments in the desired position, appropriately. One patient-specific drilling guide and one patient-specific combined drilling and cutting guide were designed for radius and ulna, respectively, to reproduce the simulation to the surgery. Guides' cutting slots were designed to orient the saw blade, and guiding holes served to orient K-wires as a reference during fragment reduction. Furthermore, drilling holes helped predrilling screw holes as an additional reference during fragment reduction and plate fixation. Fixation was performed with screws on each side of the osteotomy line. Follow-up of up to 9 months revealed a significant improvement of range of motion, which reached the level of the non-affected side in the first 2 months. The patients reported a significant improvement in pain and satisfaction compared to the preoperative situation. Fist closure and finger spreading were possible without restriction. No sensorimotor deficits were observed in clinical examination.

DISCUSSION

In the three presented cases, three-dimensional corrective osteotomy of forearm malunions resulted in excellent results. There is currently limited evidence from studies comparing three-dimensional surgical planning techniques with conventional planning methods with regards to forearm malunions to the best of our knowledge. One important reason is that three-dimensional planning techniques are often used for more complex cases, therefore making it difficult to compare cohorts (11). Vroemen et al. retrospectively investigated postoperative position after corrective osteotomy using two-dimensional vs. three-dimensional preoperative planning techniques of forearm malunions (29). They reported a significant correlation of malposition (assessed with malalignment parameters, such as palmar tilt, radial inclination, and ulnar variance) with the clinical outcome only for the three-dimensional rotational deficits but not between 2-D standard radiographs and the respective malalignment parameters. Therefore, this suggests that 3-D planning technique can more precisely assess misalignment and thus predict the clinical outcome to a higher degree compared to preoperative planning with conventional 2-D radiography. Buijze et al. recently published a randomized controlled trial comparing three-dimensional with two-dimensional preoperative planning techniques for corrective osteotomy of distal radius malunions (30). They reported a trend toward a minimal clinically important difference in patient-reported outcomes, such as pain and satisfaction scores in favor of the 3-D computer-assisted technique. However, the results were not significant, and the authors could not draw a definitive conclusion. According to these results, conventional surgical techniques and preoperative 2D fluoroscopy might be sufficient in many cases, but more complex cases involving combined intra- and extraarticular corrective osteotomies and multidimensional correction could be primarily managed by the 3-D technology in the future (22).

Patient-specific guides based on preoperative three-dimensional techniques have been reported to be accurate and easier to handle, and integration into the surgical workflow is simple to implement with structured training and the help of clinical engineers (12, 31). Another advantage is that additional conventional bending of the plates is avoided as the bending angle can be preoperatively simulated and therefore be reproduced during surgery. This leads to a reduced mean operative time and may reduce intraoperative bleeding, thus leading to a better functional recovery, as suggested previously (32). Errors of <1° and 1 mm for simulated osteotomies have been described for osteotomies with patient-specific guides (33). However, these measurements were taken in dry cadaver bones, and there could

be a discrepancy between these results and the realistic clinical accuracy as, in most cases, soft tissue envelope will block the vision when checking for the fit of patient-specific guides in the actual surgery setting (22). Promising results regarding the accuracy of three-dimensional corrective osteotomies of the forearm, especially for closed wedge osteotomies, have been reported by authors, such as less postoperative rotational deformity and less residual translation (33). Nevertheless, open wedge osteotomies (8.3 ± 5.35°) showed significant higher residual rotational deformity when compared to closing wedge (3.47 ± 1.09°) osteotomies. Campe et al. reported that restoration of the radius alignment to within 5° angular deformity and 2 mm ulnar variance in patients with malunion of the distal radius could be achieved in only 40% of the patients with the conventional technique (34). In contrast, 3-D virtual planning of corrective osteotomies of the distal radius has been reported to reach significant improvements in 96% of the cases with restorations to within 5° or 2 mm of their normal values in a systematic review and meta-analysis, including 15 studies with a total of 68 patients (11). Further, ulnar variances of 0 ± 1 mm and precise angular reconstruction in all included patients with distal radius malunions were reported by Stockmans et al. with the 3-D virtual planning (22). As stated by the same workgroup, volar tilt was more difficult to correct than the radial inclination and ulnar variance, as there was a tendency of under-correction of the fragment orientation, which hinged around the intraarticular osteotomy line (22). Despite these strengths of this innovative technique, there are some limitations that need to be addressed. The technique must be learned, and cooperation with clinical engineers to understand and apply the simulation procedure is required. In this case, the tendency to achieve higher accuracy is directly connected to experience on both, surgeons' and clinical design engineering side (22). Nevertheless, as a better visualization and guidance are associated with the 3-D preoperative planning technique, and the results in the literature suggest a high acceptance of the applicability by surgeons, the acquired experience could lead to an increased application of this technique, especially in highly complex cases in which the surgeon might not take the risk of the conventional surgery (35). Furthermore, the three-dimensional-planned technique is more expensive than the conventional method. Although the 3-D planning technique has been implemented in most radiology departments, the special software and the working hours of the clinical engineer for the planning process need to be taken into account (36). Additionally, cooperation with the specialized commercial companies is often required for the 3-D printing process, as the 3-D technology is time-consuming and yet not fully adapted in all hospital settings (11, 36). The costs for the three-dimensional corrective osteotomy technique for upper extremities have been noted to range from $2,000 to $4,000 depending on patients' preoperative situation (30). In contrast, the virtual surgery planning can be done multiple times with different virtual trials if once learned from the clinical engineer and thus is done at no additional cost, if no 3-D bone models are constructed. Moreover, the virtual project can be used with navigation systems already implemented at the respective surgery department. However, the use of patient-specific surgical guides is reported to be more time-saving than computer navigation techniques, and navigation systems for upper extremity corrective osteotomies are not easily applicable because of size-limiting factors of tracking markers and instruments (22, 37). One more point that has to be taken into account is the virtual planning and production time of the patient-specific guides, which takes between 6 and 8 weeks, depending on the complexity of the malunions (11, 22). The prolonged time between diagnosis of the malunion and surgery date could impair the functional disturbance and therefore be prognostically relevant for the outcome. Another disadvantage is that CT scans of both forearms are required for the three-dimensional planning technique, resulting in a higher radiation burden for the patients. However, the radiation exposure from CT scanning is considerably reduced below the normal dose used for diagnostic purposes because of the lower volume of the upper extremity compared to the thorax, abdomen, and pelvis (18). Computer simulation systems have been introduced in which 3-D bone models constructed from low dose radiation systems reached the same level of accuracy to those constructed from normal radiation doses CT data for three-dimensional corrective osteotomies techniques (18). In the future, the accuracy of such systems could be improved, resulting in a lower required radiation burden for the patients and a more precise bone surface model with lower errors. Finally, as described above, more randomized controlled trials evaluating the outcome in comparison with conventional techniques are required to account for this innovative but more expensive technique. To the author's best knowledge, there is only one randomized controlled trial comparing the computer-assisted vs. non-computer-assisted preoperative planning technique with regards to the corrective osteotomy of forearm malunions (30). Thus, the authors call for more well-designed randomized controlled trials comparing

the two-dimensional and three-dimensional preoperative planning techniques to provide sufficient evidence regarding the correction of complex forearm malunions in modern surgical therapy approaches.

Three-dimensional corrective osteotomy based on preoperative computerized planning and patient-specific surgical guides resulted in excellent results in this case series.

The promising evidence from the current literature and our case series suggest that preoperative computer-assisted three-dimensional planning techniques for corrective osteotomies of complex upper extremity malunion could be the new gold standard in the future.

ETHICS STATEMENT

The studies involving human participants were reviewed and approved by Local institutional review board at the University Medical Center Freiburg, Freiburg, Germany. The patients/participants provided their written informed consent to participate in this study. Written informed consent was obtained from the individual(s) for the publication of any potentially identifiable images or data included in this article.

AUTHOR CONTRIBUTIONS

BS and GL did the literature search and wrote the first draft of the manuscript. JZ performed the surgery of the three cases, designed the study, proofread the manuscript, and made corrections. RS and AV did the literature search, proofread the manuscript, designed figures, and edited the manuscript. All authors contributed to the article and approved the submitted version.

REFERENCES

1. Jayakumar P, Jupiter JB. Reconstruction of malunited diaphyseal fractures of the forearm. *Hand (New York, N,Y)*. (2014) 9:265–73. doi: 10.1007/s11552-014-9635-9
2. Mader K, Koolen M, Flipsen M, van der Zwan A, Pennig D, Ham J. Complex forearm deformities: operative strategy in posttraumatic pathology. *Obere Extremität*. (2015) 10:229–39. doi: 10.1007/s11678-015-0341-1
3. Delclaux S, Trang Pham TT, Bonnevialle N, Aprédoaei C, Rongières M, Bonnevialle P, et al. Distal radius fracture malunion: importance of managing injuries of the distal radio-ulnar joint. *Orthopaed Traumatol Surg Res*. (2016) 102:327–32. doi: 10.1016/j.otsr.2015.12.010
4. Duparc F. Malunion of the proximal humerus. *Orthopaed Traumatol Surg Res*. (2013) 99:S1–S1. doi: 10.1016/j.otsr.2012.11.006
5. Morrey BF, Askew LJ, Chao EY. A biomechanical study of normal functional elbow motion. *J Bone Joint Surg Am*. (1981) 63:872–7.
6. Anderson LD, Sisk D, Tooms RE, Park WI. Compression-plate fixation in acute diaphyseal fractures of the radius and ulna. *J Bone Joint Surg Am*. (1975) 57:287–97.
7. Chapman MW, Gordon JE, Zissimos AG. Compression-plate fixation of acute fractures of the diaphyses of the radius and ulna. *J Bone Joint Surg Am*. (1989) 71:159–69.
8. Dodge HS, Cady GW. Treatment of fractures of the radius and ulna with compression plates. *J Bone Joint Surg Am*. (1972) 54:1167–76.
9. Ross ER, Gourevitch D, Hastings GW, Wynn-Jones CE, Ali S. Retrospective analysis of plate fixation of diaphyseal fractures of the forearm bones. *Injury*. (1989) 20:211–4. doi: 10.1016/0020-1383(89)90114-9
10. Miyake J, Murase T, Oka K, Moritomo H, Sugamoto K, Yoshikawa H.

Computer-assisted corrective osteotomy for malunited diaphyseal forearm fractures. *J Bone Joint Surg Am*. (2012) 94:e150. doi: 10.2106/JBJS.K.00829
11. Eygendaal D, de Muinck Keizer RJO, Goslings JC, Schep NWL, Lechner KM, Mulders MAM. Three-dimensional virtual planning of corrective osteotomies of distal radius malunions: a systematic review and meta-analysis. *Stra Trauma Limb Reconstruct*. (2017) 12:77–89. doi: 10.1007/s11751-017-0284-8
12. Kunz M, Ma B, Rudan JF, Ellis RE, Pichora DR. Image-guided distal radius osteotomy using patient-specific instrument guides. *J Hand Surg Am*. (2013) 38:1618–24. doi: 10.1016/j.jhsa.2013.05.018
13. Schweizer A, Fürnstahl P, Nagy L. 3D kontrollierte planung und durchführung von osteotomien an vorderarm und hand. *Therapeutische Umschau*. (2014) 71:391–396. doi: 10.1024/0040-5930/a000528
14. Athwal GS, Ellis RE, Small CF, Pichora DR. Computer-assisted distal radius osteotomy. *J Hand Surg*. (2003) 28:951. doi: 10.1016/S0363-5023(03)00375-7
15. Lombardi AV, Berend KR, Adams JB. Patient-Specific Approach in Total Knee Arthroplasty. *Orthopedics*. (2008) 31:927–930. doi: 10.3928/01477447-20080901-21
16. Verstreken K, Van Cleynenbreugel J, Martens K, Marchal G, van Steenberghe D, Suetens P. An image-guided planning system for endosseous oral implants. *IEEE Trans Med Imaging*. (1998) 17:842–52. doi: 10.1109/42.736056
17. Vrielinck L, Politis C, Schepers S, Pauwels M, Naert I. Image-based planning and clinical validation of zygoma and pterygoid implant placement in patients with severe bone atrophy using customized drill guides. Preliminary results from a prospective clinical follow-up study. *Int J Oral Maxillofac Surg*. (2003) 32:7–14. doi: 10.1054/ijom.2002.0337
18. Oka K, Murase T, Moritomo H, Goto A, Sugamoto K, Yoshikawa H. Accuracy analysis of three-dimensional bone surface models of the forearm constructed

from multidetector computed tomography data. *Int J Med Robotics Comput Assist Surg.* (2009) 5:452–7. doi: 10.1002/rcs.277

19. Oka K, Moritomo H, Goto A, Sugamoto K, Yoshikawa H, Murase T. Corrective osteotomy for malunited intra-articular fracture of the distal radius using a custom-made surgical guide based on three-dimensional computer simulation: case report. *J Hand Surg.* (2008) 33:835–40. doi: 10.1016/j.jhsa.2008.02.008

20. Murase T, Oka K, Moritomo H, Goto A, Yoshikawa H, Sugamoto K. Three-dimensional corrective osteotomy of malunited fractures of the upper extremity with use of a computer simulation system. *J Bone Joint Surg Am.* (2008) 90:2375–89. doi: 10.2106/JBJS.G.01299

21. Mulders MAM, d'Ailly PN, Cleffken BI, Schep NWL. Corrective osteotomy is an effective method of treating distal radius malunions with good long-term functional results. *Injury.* (2017) 48:731–7. doi: 10.1016/j.injury.2017.01.045

22. Stockmans F, Dezillie M, Vanhaecke J. Accuracy of 3d virtual planning of corrective osteotomies of the distal radius. *Jnl Wrist Surg.* (2013) 02:306–14. doi: 10.1055/s-0033-1359307

23. Oka K, Murase T, Moritomo H, Yoshikawa H. Corrective osteotomy for malunited both bones fractures of the forearm with radial head dislocations using a custom-made surgical guide: two case reports. *J Shoulder Elbow Surg.* (2012) 21:e1–e8. doi: 10.1016/j.jse.2012.05.035

24. Gao S, Stephens JD, Piatt C, Hockman T, Hills A, Thompson J, et al. Chapter 8 - 3D printing in orthopedics: upper extremity trauma deformity. In: Dipaola M, Wodajo FM, editors. *3D Printing in Orthopaedic Surgery* (Amsterdam:Elsevier), 85–94. doi: 10.1016/B978-0-323-58118-9.00008-7

25. Chung MS, Baek GH. Three-dimensional corrective osteotomy for cubitus varus in adults. *J Shoul Elbow Surg.* (2003) 12:472–5. doi: 10.1016/S1058-2746(03)00090-9

26. Kataoka T, Oka K, Miyake J, Omori S, Tanaka H, Murase T. 3-dimensional prebent plate fixation in corrective osteotomy of malunited upper extremity fractures using a real-sized plastic bone model prepared by preoperative computer simulation. *J Hand Surg.* (2013) 38:909–19. doi: 10.1016/j.jhsa.2013.02.024

27. Takeyasu Y, Oka K, Miyake J, Kataoka T, Moritomo H, Murase T. Preoperative, Computer Simulation-Based, Three-Dimensional Corrective Osteotomy for Cubitus Varus Deformity with Use of a Custom-Designed Surgical Device: *The Journal of Bone & Joint Surgery.* (2013) 95:e173. doi: 10.2106/JBJS.L.01622

28. Omori S, Murase T, Oka K, Kawanishi Y, Oura K, Tanaka H, et al. Postoperative accuracy analysis of three-dimensional corrective osteotomy for cubitus varus deformity with a custom-made surgical guide based on computer simulation. *J Should Elbow Surg.* (2015) 24:242–9. doi: 10.1016/j.jse.2014.08.020

29. Vroemen JC, Dobbe JGG, Strackee SD, Streekstra GJ. Positioning evaluation of corrective osteotomy for the malunited radius: 3-D CT versus 2-D radiographs. *Orthopedics.* (2013) 36:e193–9. doi: 10.3928/01477447-20130122-22

30. Buijze GA, Leong NL, Stockmans F, Axelsson P, Moreno R, Ibsen Sörensen A, et al. Three-dimensional compared with two-dimensional preoperative planning of corrective osteotomy for extra-articular distal radial malunion: a multicenter randomized controlled trial. *J Bone Joint Surgery.* (2018) 100:1191–202. doi: 10.2106/JBJS.17.00544

31. Ma B, Kunz M, Gammon B, Ellis RE, Pichora DR. A laboratory comparison of computer navigation and individualized guides for distal radius osteotomy. *Int J Comput Assist Radiol Surg.* (2014) 9:713–24. doi: 10.1007/s11548-013-0966-8

32. Shuang F, Hu W, Shao Y, Li H, Zou H. Treatment of intercondylar humeral fractures with 3D-printed osteosynthesis plates. *Medicine.* (2016) 95:e2461. doi: 10.1097/MD.0000000000002461

33. Vlachopoulos L, Schweizer A, Graf M, Nagy L, Fürnstahl P. Three-dimensional postoperative accuracy of extra-articular forearm osteotomies using CT-scan based patient-specific surgical guides. *BMC Musculoskelet Disord.* (2015) 16:336. doi: 10.1186/s12891-015-0793-x

34. Campe A von, Nagy L, Arbab D, Dumont CE. Corrective Osteotomies in Malunions of the Distal Radius: Do We Get What We Planned? *Clin Orthop Related Res.* (2006) 450:179–185. doi: 10.1097/01.blo.0000223994.79894.17

35. Jupiter JB, Ruder J, Roth DA. Computer-generated bone models in the planning of osteotomy of multidirectional distal radius malunions. *J Hand Surg.* (1992) 17:406–15. doi: 10.1016/0363-5023(92)90340-U

36. Michielsen M, Van Haver A, Vanhees M, van Riet R, Verstreken F. Use of three-dimensional technology for complications of upper limb fracture treatment. *EFORT Open Reviews.* (2019) 4:302–12. doi: 10.1302/2058-5241.4.180074

37. Radermacher K, Portheine F, Anton M, Zimolong A, Kaspers G, Rau G, et al. Computer Assisted Orthopaedic Surgery With Image Based Individual Templates. *Clin Orthop Related Research.* (1998) 354:28–38. doi: 10.1097/00003086-199809000-00005

14

Volume of Surgical Freedom: The Most Applicable Anatomical Measurement for Surgical Assessment and 3-Dimensional Modeling

Lena Mary Houlihan, David Naughton and Mark C. Preul*

The Loyal and Edith Davis Neurosurgical Research Laboratory, Department of Neurosurgery, Barrow Neurological Institute,
St. Joseph's Hospital and Medical Center, Phoenix, AZ, United States

Correspondence:
Mark C. Preul
Neuropub@barrowneuro.org

Surgical freedom is the most important metric at the disposal of the surgeon. The volume of surgical freedom (VSF) is a new methodology that produces an optimal qualitative and quantitative representation of an access corridor and provides the surgeon with an anatomical, spatially accurate, and clinically applicable metric. In this study, illustrative dissection examples were completed using two of the most common surgical approaches, the pterional craniotomy and the supraorbital craniotomy. The VSF methodology models the surgical corridor as a cone with an irregular base. The measurement data are fitted to the cone model, and from these fitted data, the volume of the cone is calculated as a volumetric measurement of the surgical corridor. A normalized VSF compensates for inaccurate measurements that may occur as a result of dependence on probe length during data acquisition and provides a fixed reference metric that is applicable across studies. The VSF compensates for multiple inaccuracies in the practical and mathematical methods currently used for quantitative assessment, thereby enabling the production of 3-dimensional models of the surgical corridor. The VSF is therefore an improved standard for assessment of surgical freedom.

Keywords: neuroanatomical quantitation, surgical target structure, surgical access corridor, volume of surgical freedom, 3D modeling

INTRODUCTION

Importance of Quantitative Anatomy

Anatomy is the foundation of medical understanding. Medical practice has evolved through the continual scrutiny of biological structure and physiologic function (Acar et al., 2005; Elhadi et al., 2012; Arraez-Aybar et al., 2015). As the merits of anatomical scrutiny in disease therapy were elucidated, the drive to be able to discriminate between "normal" and "abnormal" biological arrangement increased. This development resulted in the advent of quantitative anatomical research, the objective of which was to measure the complexity of human architecture.

Abbreviations: ACoA, anterior communicating artery; ICA, internal carotid artery; SD, standard deviation; STS, surgical target structure; VSF, volume of surgical freedom; 2D, 2-dimensional; 3D, 3-dimensional.

Biological variability is an accepted reality (Kreutz and Timmer, 2009; Higdon, 2013) and a key aspect of managing pathologic processes. The aim of quantifying anatomy has been to identify the most reproducible homogenous model of specific organ systems, thereby establishing principles in biological structure and physiology. The establishment of these principles allowed for the appreciation of abnormal morphology and pathologic processes. The criteria for what now constitutes the so-called normal anatomy has been used in every aspect of medical education, investigation, translational research, and treatment development (Iaizzo et al., 2013).

Anatomical competency is of the utmost importance in surgical practice (Aziz and Mansor, 2006; Burgess and Ramsey-Stewart, 2015). It is the cardinal infrastructure upon which the knowledge base for all surgeons is founded and subsequently evolves (Selcuk et al., 2019). The surgeon must be aware of standardized structures and their spatial positioning, associated variations, and physiologic sequelae. The efforts and discoveries of anatomists have spurred pivotal breakthroughs in surgical and medical treatment (Melly et al., 2018; Iorio-Morin and Mathieu, 2020) as well as in the development of basic scientific progression and understanding of the disease process (Barth and Ray, 2019).

Quantitation of Surgical Feasibility

Quantitative anatomy is the method the surgeon uses to assess the surgical benefits and disadvantages of different surgical approaches. Studying quantitative anatomy improves the techniques of neurosurgery and other related surgery disciplines. This process allows the surgeon and related personnel to assess, plan, and select the optimal intervention or surgical approach specific to the pathology, thereby improving surgical outcomes for patients. Neuroanatomy is especially relevant and critical because the structural, functional, and physiologic components are often small in dimensional relation and are particularly intertwined. There is little room for error in neurosurgery; all system components represent a significant function, usually reflected in their structural integrity. The intricacy of preserving structural eloquence in the nervous system is further echoed in the surgical parameters the neurosurgeon must use. Dr. Albert Rhoton Jr. revolutionized the field of neuroanatomy, making neurosurgery "more accurate, gentle and safe" (Matsushima et al., 2018) not only by establishing key concepts in microsurgical anatomy but also by extrapolating the findings to a surgical approach-specific setting. This innovation enhanced the relevance of anatomy in surgical planning and led to the development of integral concepts that surgeons now use to determine the efficacy of the surgical approach.

The ability to manipulate surgical instruments is an important criterion in comparing surgical approaches and selecting the optimal one. Freedom of movement is especially relevant in neurosurgery, where surgical access through the cranium and into the deep areas of the brain is often restricted. When accessing the most extreme limitations of a surgical corridor, the neurosurgeon encounters parenchymal, bony, musculocutaneous, and neurovascular structures that define the boundaries. The degree of manipulation within these parameters is specific to the approach and delicacy of the structure, the appreciation of which is only possible with extensive

knowledge of the circumferential anatomy. An appreciation of these anatomical confines is second nature for the trained neurosurgeon; nonetheless, the mapping of surgical corridors specific to these structures has not yet been robustly completed.

When neurosurgery is performed using an operating microscope for magnification, the movement of surgical instruments to work on pathoanatomical structures may be in increments of millimeters. Small surgical corridors, microscopic anatomy, surgical depth, and impaired visualization all impose limitations on neurosurgical interventions. These are the principal surgical criteria that influence the neurosurgical decision-making process. Technological advances have broadened the available visualization options, with the microscope, endoscope, and exoscope all possessing specific benefits and disadvantages. This additional component must be assimilated into the surgical decision-making process (Jane, 2013; Belykh et al., 2018; Herlan et al., 2019). Only through quantitative anatomical assessment specific to these surgical parameters can neurosurgeons increase their insight and proficiency in neurosurgical techniques and operative interventions.

Analysis of the surgical corridor is critical to assessing the validity of any surgical approach. From a neurosurgical perspective, the ideal corridor to the structure of interest should be minimally invasive, with minimal morbidity and mortality, and it should be cosmetically satisfactory (Castelnuovo et al., 2013). Conceptually, the best surgical corridor combines the maximal room for instrument maneuverability and maximal visualization with the shortest distance to the target of interest. Instrument maneuverability and visualization are primary concerns; thus, a means is required for quantitatively assessing the spatial and morphometric advantages of the surgical corridor, in addition to considering the distance to the STS. This metric enables consideration of the influence of neuroanatomical structures on the feasibility of the corridor, as well as the ability of the neurosurgeon to function and complete the specific intervention. How well the neurosurgeon can operate and manipulate instruments with respect to the surgical approach directly influences the patient's outcome.

The measurement by which instrument maneuverability is quantified is termed "surgical freedom." The first description of surgical freedom was noted in 2000 (Horgan et al., 2000; Spektor et al., 2000). Stereotactic data gathered using a frameless stereotactic navigation device was used to produce a quantitative measurement of the area available for instrument maneuverability. The 3D coordinate data of the region were used to calculate the area by the summation of triangular areas. Twenty years later, this method remains the crux of neuroanatomical quantitation and a key determinant of the feasibility of any surgical approach (Pillai et al., 2009; Elhadi et al., 2014, 2015).

Surgical Freedom

Surgical freedom is defined in the medical literature as the maximum allowable working area at the proximal end of a probe with the distal end on the target structure (Horgan et al., 2000; Spektor et al., 2000; Noiphithak et al., 2018). The goal of this procedure is to assess the maneuverability of an instrument and provide the operator with insight into how realistic and

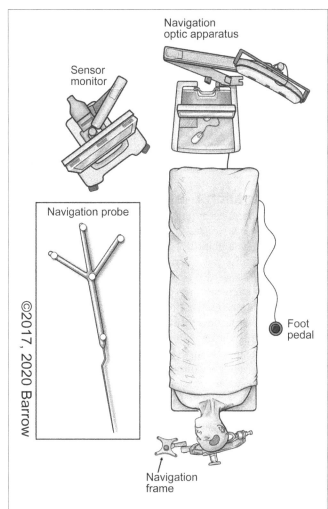

FIGURE 1 | Illustration of the neuronavigation system in the surgical setup commonly used to localize both pathologic and anatomically pertinent structures using stereotaxis. Used with permission from Barrow Neurological Institute, Phoenix, Arizona.

appropriate it is to use a specific access corridor while also allowing for the comparison of surgical approaches.

Neuroanatomists and neurosurgeons use specific methods to measure surgical freedom:

- The cadaveric head specimen is fixed in a rigid head holder.
- A stereotactic navigation system (**Figure 1**) is used to acquire the 3D coordinates of the target points for each surgical approach being analyzed, specific to the intracranial structure or region of interest.
- The distal end of the surgical instrument is placed on the target structure.
- For a quadrangular area measurement, the surgical instrument is moved as far mediocranially, mediocaudally, laterocranially, and laterocaudally as possible for four or more points to represent the most extreme limits of the surgical corridor specific to the approach. At all times, the distal end of the probe is not moved from the target structure.

- The coordinates of the surgical instrument's proximal tip are obtained with the navigation probe when the tip of the instrument is at the most extreme position.
- The area bounded by the coordinate data points from the probe's proximal tip at the extreme limits is calculated by dividing the bounded area into triangles in which the data points form the triangle vertices, then calculating the sum of the areas of all the triangles using Heron's formula (Weisstein).
- The result is represented in either square millimeters or square centimeters.

This method produces an area that is used as a metric for surgical freedom. The standard process is to collect four, but occasionally six, data points. The distribution of these points, as dictated by the measuring researcher, is usually along the extrema of the surgical corridor, which does not necessarily take into account any structural components, or the lack thereof, between the points. Previous methods have tended to impose regular, symmetrical shapes on the measurement data to simplify the shape of the access corridor. In reality, however, the borders of any surgical corridor are never symmetrical, and they are never a perfect shape that can be represented by conventional shapes.

This method aims to quantitatively portray the range of motion of an instrument during a surgical intervention to illustrate the feasibility and functionality of the surgical approach and the surgical corridor specific to the target structure. However, multiple inaccuracies are associated with this calculation method from a practical, mathematical, and application perspective: (1) The measured data points are not coplanar, which distorts the perceived area of surgical freedom. (2) The surgical freedom metric is dependent on the length of the probe that is used to capture data. This variation across the literature precludes interstudy comparisons, which weakens the scientific robustness of such studies and impairs reproducibility. (3) Measurement inaccuracy can result in substantial variation in the measured area. (4) Surgical corridors are irregular and cannot be fully expressed using simple shapes. (5) A 2-dimensional (2D) shape does not allow for visualization of a 3D surgical corridor.

In terms of visualization, the area of surgical freedom is not an optimal representational concept of the surgical approach corridor because the area is a 2D measurement, and neurosurgical approaches and corridors are volumetric, or 3D, shapes. Surgical freedom is arguably the most important technical parameter dictating the surgical approach and selection process specific to an anatomical target. Quantitatively analyzing surgical freedom allows the neurosurgeon to proceed in a more informed fashion by comparing the numerical values with those of different approaches to the same anatomical target. What is not taken into consideration by this method is the fact that surgical instruments are not deployed in a 2D area but rather in an irregularly shaped 3D corridor.

Due to the nature of the surgical site, the surgical corridor transitions from a region of large maneuverability at the surgical entry point to an apex of minimal freedom at the target structure. At present, an instrument's maneuverability within the surgical corridor is estimated by the angle formed at the apex of the corridor (the angle of attack) in one or two planes, usually vertical or horizontal. The angle of attack is another anatomical metric neurosurgeons use to evaluate an instrument's maximal working ability in one or more planes where the instrument will be most frequently deployed. This information gives specific insight regarding the instrument's operational freedom, which may not be evident when assessing the numerical value produced by the present method of calculating surgical freedom. However, this method produces a limited representation of the 3D shape of the surgical corridor.

The deficits in estimating this surgical principle are exemplified by the illustrations published in the neurosurgery literature. These illustrations broadly represent the surgical corridors, denoting general shapes and trajectories garnered from the neurosurgeon's experience, but they lack anatomical, spatial, and surgical accuracy. Surgical freedom should be defined by the whole expanse of the surgical corridor and should not be limited to its 2D infrastructure. For all these reasons, we have endeavored to improve upon the imprecision in currently accepted methodology for this crucial method of quantitative surgical anatomy.

Volume of Surgical Freedom

The volume of surgical freedom (VSF) is defined as the maximal available working volume with respect to a specific surgical corridor and target structure. VSF is a new methodology that produces the optimal qualitative and quantitative representation of an access corridor and provides the neurosurgeon with an anatomical, spatially accurate, and clinically applicable metric. From this representation, 3D visualization of the surgical corridor is possible.

The VSF metric uses a normalized calculation to reduce error and allow for direct comparison among measurements. This calculation is achieved by measuring the volume of the irregular-based cone model of the surgical corridor, with the irregular base of the cone at a fixed distance from the apex. This report details a novel approach for surgical anatomy quantitation, the anatomical experiment used to investigate its validity, and the key steps in producing a mathematically and spatially superior model of the approach corridor.

MATERIALS AND EQUIPMENT

Anatomical Specimen Preparation

Cranial dissections of 14 cadaveric specimens were completed to investigate the data-collection process and for logistical and surgical representation. The cadaveric heads were fixed with a customized alcohol-based solution as a preservative. Colored silicone was incrementally injected into the cerebral vasculature, with the arteries represented by red and the veins represented by blue. This differentiation allowed for clearer interrogation of the intracranial structures and surgical target structure (STS). Each head was rigidly fixed in a head holder while measurements were obtained.

Dissections were completed by the first author, a neurosurgery resident competent in the two selected approaches. Dissection

was completed using a clinical-grade neurosurgical operating microscope (Zeiss OPMI Pentero, Carl Zeiss Meditec AG, Oberkochen, Germany). The two open transcranial neurosurgical approaches selected to model this quantitative methodology were the standard pterional craniotomy and the supraorbital craniotomy (**Figure 2**). These approaches are two of the most common neurosurgical corridors used to access deep paramedian structures and regions of surgical complexity. These anatomical areas are of particular interest in the context of anatomical quantitation because of the need to avoid injury to critical neurovascular structures.

Neuronavigation System

A neuronavigation system (StealthStation S7 Surgical Navigation System; Medtronic, Dublin, Ireland) was used to acquire predetermined data points. Neuronavigation uses the principle of stereotaxis. The neuronavigation system uses Cartesian coordinates to divide the geometric volume of the brain into three imaginary intersecting spatial planes (axial, sagittal, and coronal) that are orthogonal to each other. Any point within the brain can be specified by measuring its distance along these three intersecting planes. Neuronavigation uses the reference of this coordinate system in parallel with 3D images of the brain displayed on the console of the computer workstation to provide guidance to the corresponding anatomical locations using medical images (Başarslan and Cüneyt, 2014).

Institutional review board approval was not required for this cadaveric laboratory investigation.

Methodology Calculator and 3D Modeling Software

The methodology described herein was implemented as a calculation tool in Excel for Office 365 (Microsoft, Redmond, WA, United States). An Excel spreadsheet was used to perform all of the calculation steps described in this paper, apart from the calculation of the best-fit plane. The generalized reduced gradient nonlinear engine of Microsoft Excel Solver was used to calculate the least-squares best-fit plane for the data points. The Excel spreadsheet calculation tool was used to calculate the normalized volume of the surgical corridor (normalized VSF) using the measurement data as an input. In addition to calculating the VSF metric using Excel, the VSF data were modeled using a student license for the 3D modeling software Solidworks 2020 (Dassault Systèmes, Vélizy-Villacoublay, France). The modeling software was used to create 3D renderings of the surgical corridors from the measurement data to visualize the surgical corridor for each dataset. The 3D models were also superimposed onto microscope images of anatomical approaches to illustrate the surgical corridor to the structure of interest.

METHODS

Data Collection

A pterional craniotomy was conducted on seven cadaveric specimens, and a supraorbital craniotomy was conducted on

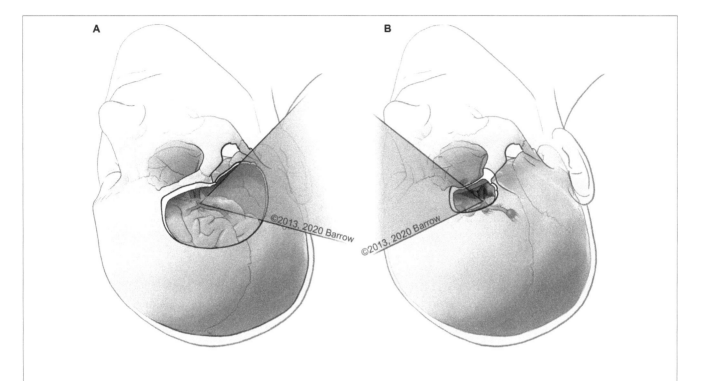

FIGURE 2 | (A) Example of a pterional transcranial approach, in which the surgeon uses a lateral trajectory that usually traverses the natural fissures of the brain to access complex paramedian regions. **(B)** Example of a supraorbital approach, with an incision made along the eyebrow approaching the skull base from a more anterolateral perspective, tracking medially along the bone of the anterior cranial fossa that represents the roof of the orbit. Used with permission from Barrow Neurological Institute, Phoenix, Arizona.

seven cadaveric specimens. Predetermined STSs were selected by the first author. To illustrate the methodology, three surgical targets (**Figure 3**) were identified that are common to both approaches: (1) paraclinoid internal carotid artery (ICA), (2) terminal ICA, and (3) anterior communicating artery (ACoA) complex.

The data points required to calculate the VSF and produce a spatially and anatomically accurate model were collected for each STS and both the pterional and supraorbital surgical approaches. **Figure 4** depicts the collection process for all data points.

Interrater and intrarater variability were accounted for by recording the STS VSF for each specimen and approach a minimum of three times by multiple qualified neurosurgery residents. This replication ensured reproducibility of the method, as well as a larger pool of measurements to assess our methodology's advantages and limitations. VSF results are reported as cubic millimeters, and each result was normalized to a height of 10 mm from the STS.

Mathematical Methodology

The VSF was calculated by modeling the surgical corridor as a cone with an irregular base. The STS is the apex of the cone, and the points measured at the extrema of the maneuverability of the instrument compose the base of the cone. For this study, we measured eight extrema points around the base of the cone, but the calculation methodology is equally applicable to more or less than 8 points. The 3D coordinate

data from the measurements were used to calculate the volume of the irregular-based cone. This method can be summarized as follows:

(1) Calculate a best-fit plane to the extrema data points, which best represents the plane of the base of the cone.
(2) Translate the best-fit plane in 3D space to a fixed perpendicular distance from the apex point (normalized height), maintaining the slope of the plane.
(3) Translate the extrema data points onto the best-fit plane, along the line between the measured point and the apex point.
(4) Convert the 3D coordinates of the data points to a 2D coordinate system on the best-fit plane.
(5) Use the 2D coordinates to calculate the area of the irregular polygon enclosed by the data points.
(6) Calculate the perpendicular height from the best-fit plane to the apex point.
(7) Calculate the volume of the irregular-based cone from the area and the perpendicular height.

This methodology calculates a normalized volume by calculating the volume of the cone with an irregular base, modeling the surgical corridor at a fixed height from the apex point (**Figure 5**). This methodology was conceived to reduce the effects of measurement inaccuracy and measurement probe length on the calculated VSF value.

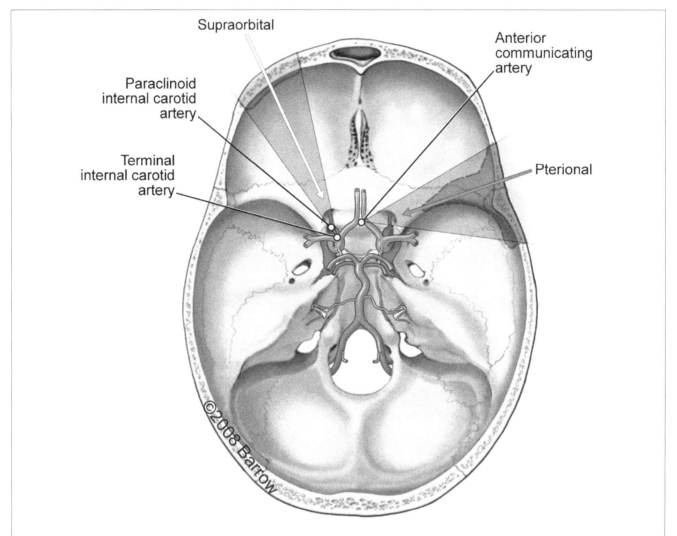

FIGURE 3 | Axial view illustration of the skull base showing the primary vasculature supplying the brain. The three surgical structures of interest accessible using either a pterional craniotomy (*orange arrow and shading; dashed line*) or supraorbital craniotomy (*yellow arrow and shading; solid line*) are the paraclinoid internal carotid artery (ICA), the terminal ICA, and the anterior communicating artery. Used with permission from Barrow Neurological Institute, Phoenix, Arizona.

Calculation of Best-Fit Plane

The best-fit plane was fitted to the data points using the least-squares method. The best-fit plane was considered to be the plane that results in the minimum sum of the squares of the perpendicular distances between each data point and the plane.

The problem is nonlinear, so a nonlinear solver was used to optimize the best-fit plane. An average plane was first calculated to use as an initial condition in the solver. The plane intersecting each subset of three points was calculated using various combinations of three data points from the set of extrema data points. The average plane equation coefficients of all the calculated planes were used as the coefficients of the average for the initial condition in the solver.

Calculating a Plane From Three Points

The general equation of a plane can be expressed as follows:

$$Ax + By + Cz + D = 0,$$

where A, B, and C are the coefficients of the slope in the directions of the x, y, and z axes, respectively, and D is the coefficient representing the distance from the plane to the origin.

Calculating a plane from three points $P_1 = (x_1, y_1, z_1)$, $P_2 = (x_2, y_2, z_2)$, and $P_3 = (x_3, y_3, z_3)$ first requires calculating the two vectors between the three points:

$$\overrightarrow{P_1P_2} = P_2 - P_1,$$

$$\overrightarrow{P_1P_3} = P_3 - P_1.$$

The A, B, and C coefficients of the plane can then be calculated from the cross-product of the two vectors:

$$[A\,B\,C] = \overrightarrow{P_1P_2} \times \overrightarrow{P_1P_3}.$$

The coefficient D can then be calculated from the plane equation by using one of the points (P_1):

$$D = -(Ax_1 + By_1 + Cz_1)$$

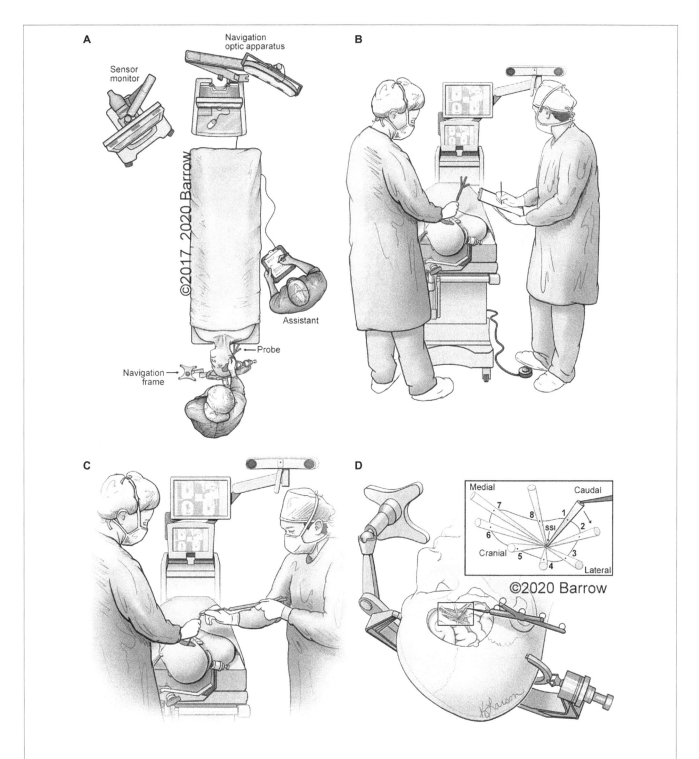

FIGURE 4 | Illustrative depiction of the data collection process. **(A)** Position of the neuronavigation system, the cadaver, the neurosurgeon with probe, and the assistant recording data. **(B)** The neurosurgeon obtains coordinates of the STS with the tip of the neuronavigation probe on the STS. The coordinates, as depicted on the monitor, are recorded by the assistant. **(C)** While the surgeon holds an instrument with its distal end on the STS, the assistant holds the neuronavigation probe and places its distal tip on the proximal end of the surgeon's instrument to obtain the 3D coordinates of the instrument's proximal end in space. **(D)** Eight data points are sequentially collected that represent the maximal allowable parameters of the surgical corridor. The data points are obtained by placing the tip of the navigation probe on the proximal end of the surgical instrument in the position marking a specific boundary point. Points 1 and 5 represent the craniocaudal maximal angle of attack, whereas points 3 and 7 can be used to represent the mediolateral angle of attack. STS, surgical target structure. Used with permission from Barrow Neurological Institute, Phoenix, Arizona.

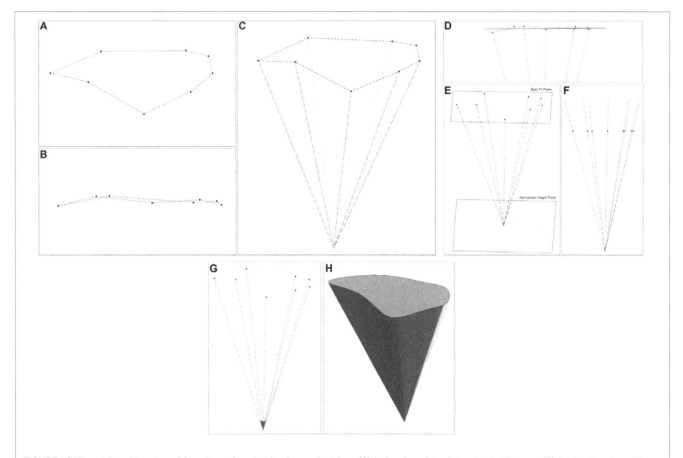

FIGURE 5 | 3D modeling of the steps of the volume of surgical freedom methodology. **(A)** A plan view of the data points in 3D space. **(B)** An elevation view of the points, illustrating that they are not on a single plane. **(C)** A view of the data points and apex point in space. **(D)** The best plane fitted to the data points. **(E)** A view of the normalized-height plane, at a fixed distance from the apex. **(F)** An elevation view of the data points after translation to the normalized-height plane. **(G,H)** The 3D representation of the shape of the surgical corridor **(G)** relative to the measured data points **(H)** standalone view of the corridor model. Used with permission from Barrow Neurological Institute, Phoenix, Arizona.

Calculating the Average Plane

After the plane equation of n planes has been calculated, the average plane can be calculated from the average coefficients:

$$A_{\text{average}}x + B_{\text{average}}y + C_{\text{average}}z + D_{\text{average}} = 0,$$

where

$$A_{\text{average}} = \frac{A_1 + A_2 + \ldots + A_n}{n},$$

$$B_{\text{average}} = \frac{B_1 + B_2 + \ldots + B_n}{56},$$

$$C_{\text{average}} = \frac{C_1 + C_2 + \ldots + C_n}{n}, \text{ and}$$

$$D_{\text{average}} = \frac{D_1 + D_2 + \ldots + D_n}{n}.$$

Running the Excel Solver to Calculate the Least-Squares Best-Fit Plane

Because the least-squares calculation of the best-fit plane is a nonlinear problem, a nonlinear solver was used to calculate the

coefficients of the least-squares fitting plane. The coefficients A_{average}, B_{average}, C_{average}, and D_{average} were used as the initial conditions for the solver. The distance d between each point $P = (x, y, z)$ and the plane $Ax + By + Cz + D = 0$ is obtained by

$$d = \frac{|Ax + By + Cz + D|}{\sqrt{A^2 + B^2 + C^2}}.$$

The nonlinear solver then solved for the coefficients A, B, C, and D, which minimized the expression

$$\sum_{p=1}^{n} \left(\frac{Ax_p + By_p + Cz_p + D}{\sqrt{A^2 + B^2 + C^2}} \right)^2,$$

where n is the number of data points to which the plane is being fitted.

Normalizing the Best-Fit Plane

Calculating the cone's cross-sectional area at a fixed distance from the apex required a new normalized-height plane, which is parallel to the cone's base, at the required distance from the apex point. After the best-fit plane $Ax + By + Cz + D = 0$ is calculated using the nonlinear solver, this plane is translated into 3D space so that the perpendicular distance between the apex point and the plane is the required normalized height of the cone.

Because the plane is parallel to the base of the cone (i.e., the calculated best-fit plane for the data points), the A, B, and C plane coefficients will be the same for both planes. Given this constraint, the formula for the perpendicular distance between the normalized-height plane $Ax + By + Cz + D_{\text{norm}} = 0$ and the apex point $P_a = (x_a, y_a, z_a)$ can be rearranged to give the following:

$$D_{\text{norm}} = h_{\text{norm}} \left(\sqrt{A^2 + B^2 + C^2} \right) - \left(Ax_a + By_a + Cz_a \right).$$

The least-squares best-fit plane was used as the plane for the base of the cone model.

Translating the Points to the Best-Fit Plane

After the normalized-height plane is calculated, the points must be translated onto this plane to calculate the area of the base of the cone model. Maintaining the shape of the cone requires the points to be translated onto the normalized-height plane along the line between each point and the apex. This method ensures that the cross-section profile of the shape of the cone is unaltered when the points are translated.

The vector between each data point $P = (x, y, z)$ and the apex point $P_a = (x_a, y_a, z_a)$ is given by the following:

$$\overrightarrow{PP_a} = P_a - P.$$

A multiplication factor, t, representing the distance between the point and the best-fit plane $Ax + By + Cz + D_{\text{norm}} = 0$ is calculated as follows:

$$t = \frac{-\left(Ax_a + By_a + Cz_a + D_{\text{norm}} \right)}{Ax_0 + By_0 + Cz_0}.$$

The coordinates of the point after translation onto the best-fit plane are then calculated by

$$P' = [x' \; y' \; z'] = [tx \; ty \; tz].$$

The translation was performed for all n data points to obtain the translated points $P'_1, P'_2 \ldots P'_n$.

Calculating the Area Enclosed by the Translated Points

The shoelace formula (Weisstein) was used to calculate the area of the base of the cone model. This formula calculates the enclosed area of an irregular polygon from the 2D coordinates of the vertices of the polygon. Calculating the area using this method required mapping the translated 3D points to a 2D coordinate system on the normalized-height plane.

The choice of the origin was arbitrary, so the 2D plots of the data points were simplified by taking the centroid of the data points as the new origin. The centroid is calculated by taking average x, y, and z coordinates of all data points as follows:

$$\text{Centroid } O = \begin{bmatrix} x_O & y_O & z_O \end{bmatrix}$$
$$= \left[\frac{x_1 + x_2 + \ldots + x_n}{n} \; \frac{y_1 + y_2 + \ldots + y_n}{n} \; \frac{z_1 + z_2 + \ldots + z_n}{n} \right].$$

Two perpendicular axes on the plane were created by defining two vectors on the normalized-height plane using the centroid O, and two of the translated points P'_1 and P'_2:

$$\overrightarrow{v} = P'_1 - O,$$
$$\overrightarrow{u} = P'_2 - O.$$

A vector $\overrightarrow{w}$ is calculated that is perpendicular to both $\overrightarrow{u}$ and $\overrightarrow{v}$:

$$\overrightarrow{w} = \overrightarrow{u} = \overrightarrow{v}.$$

A new vector, $\overrightarrow{u'}$, is then calculated perpendicular to both $\overrightarrow{v}$ and $\overrightarrow{w}$:

$$\overrightarrow{u'} = \overrightarrow{v} = \overrightarrow{w}.$$

The unit vectors $\hat{v}$ and $\widehat{u'}$ are then calculated:

$$\hat{v} = \frac{v}{|v|}, \; \widehat{u'} = \frac{u'}{|u'|}.$$

This series of calculations results in two perpendicular vectors on the normalized-height plane that are then used as the axes for the 2D coordinate system. Each 3D data point P' is converted to a 2D point P_{2D} by calculating the dot product of each axis vector with the vector between the origin and the point $\overrightarrow{OP'}$:

$$P_{2D} = \left(x_{2D} \; y_{2D} \right) = \left(\widehat{u'}.\overrightarrow{OP'} \; \hat{v}.\overrightarrow{OP'} \right).$$

With the data points mapped to a 2D coordinate system, the area of the shape enclosed by the points is calculated using the shoestring formula:

$$A = \frac{1}{2} \left(\left| x_1 \; x_2 \; y_1 \; y_2 \right| + \left| x_2 \; x_3 \; y_2 \; y_3 \right| + + \left| x_n \; x_1 \; y_n \; y_1 \right| \right),$$

where $\left| x_n \; x_{n+1} \; y_n \; y_{n+1} \right|$ is the determinant of the matrix, given by

$$\left| x_n \; x_{n+1} \; y_n \; y_{n+1} \right| = x_n y_{n+1} - y_n x_{n+1}.$$

Calculating the Perpendicular Height of the Cone Shape

The perpendicular height of the cone shape, h, is simply the perpendicular distance between the best-fit plane $Ax + By + Cz + D = 0$ and the apex point $P_a = (x_a, y_a, z_a)$:

$$h = \frac{|Ax_a + By_a + Cz_a + D|}{\sqrt{A^2 + B^2 + C^2}}.$$

Calculating the Volume of the Cone Shape

The volume of the cone shape can be calculated from the area enclosed by the points on the best-fit plane (A) and the perpendicular height of the cone shape (h):

$$\text{Volume} = \frac{1}{3} = A = h.$$

This volume is reported as cubic millimeters.

Normalized Volume of Surgical Freedom

The volume calculation depends on the length of the probe used to obtain the point data because the length of the probe determines the height of the cone shape. If this factor is removed from the calculation, then the resulting VSF values will be directly comparable to all other calculations using this spreadsheet or methodology, regardless of the length of the probe used to take the measurements.

Modeling Methodology

The 3D models of the surgical corridors were generated from the coordinates of the extrema points after translation onto the normalized-height plane and from the coordinates of the apex point. Although the mathematical calculation of the area assumes straight lines between each of the extrema data points when calculating the enclosed area of the base of the cone, the 3D model of the surgical corridor used curved splines between each of the extrema points to better visualize the shape of the surgical corridor observed in the specimen.

Measurement Inaccuracy Analysis

Because the original measurement data points were not coplanar, we investigated their effect on the calculation of the area bounded by the points. For an illustrative data set, the area bounded by the measured data points was calculated using Heron's formula. The data points were then translated onto the best-fit plane, and the area bounded by these translated points was calculated using the same method.

As of this writing, 174 individual VSF measurements have been completed in the neurosurgical research laboratory to explore multiple neurosurgical approaches. A 190-mm probe was used for all measurements. For each set of measurement data, the average probe length was calculated by averaging the calculated distance from each of the eight coordinates to the apex coordinate. The average minimum and maximum probe lengths with standard deviations (SDs) were identified for the 174 measurement samples.

Analysis of the effect of the probe length on the calculated volume of the surgical corridor required the calculation of the volume of a cone from the best-fit plane of the measurement data points to the apex point. The cone shape was maintained while the cone height was increased by 5 mm, and the data points were translated onto the plane 5 mm farther away from the apex. This translation created a new data set representing the same surgical corridor as that measured by a longer probe. The volume of the cone was then calculated again from the best-fit plane to the new data set representing a longer probe. Data analysis was completed in Microsoft Excel.

RESULTS

Quantitation and Modeling

This methodology generated two useful products: a mathematically robust quantitation of the surgical freedom of a neurosurgery instrument and a 3D spatially accurate model of the surgical corridor that takes into account irregular neuroanatomical parameters. This process gives direct quantitative information to allow for the comparison of surgical approaches. VSF is expressed in cubic millimeters. By default, the VSF also produces the craniocaudal and mediolateral angles of attack. The spatially accurate model obtained with the VSF provides a visual representation of this information, elucidating the breadth of maneuverability specific to all planes.

Table 1 depicts the comparative quantitative results of a set of measurements for specific anatomical STSs and pterional and supraorbital approaches. These illustrative examples show that the pterional craniotomy provides a larger VSF for all three STSs than the VSF provided by the supraorbital craniotomy. Thus, if any of these structures must be accessed, the pterional craniotomy would be the superior corridor because it provides an increased VSF and an increased angle of attack in both the craniocaudal and mediolateral dimensions.

Figures 6–8 demonstrate the 3D models of the surgical corridors available for deployment of neurosurgery instruments, specific to the pterional and supraorbital approaches and the STSs. This methodology provides an increased body of quantitative and visual information on surgical approach metrics to aid the neurosurgeon in the decision-making process.

TABLE 1 | Comparative volumetric results of the VSF for measuring instrument maneuverability specific to the surgical target structure and approach*.

Surgical target structure	VSF, mm³ NU		Craniocaudal Angle of Attack, degrees		Mediolateral Angle of Attack, degrees	
	Pterional	Supraorbital	Pterional	Supraorbital	Pterional	Supraorbital
Paraclinoid ICA	165.88	43.83	36.72	20.86	50.55	37.40
Terminal ICA	50.69	31.01	22.63	16.29	27.59	31.62
ACoA complex	38.34	15.66	12.64	14.50	31.69	17.44

ACoA, anterior communicating artery; ICA, internal carotid artery; NU, normalized unit; VSF, volume of surgical freedom.
Craniocaudal and mediolateral angles of attack were also produced using this measurement system.

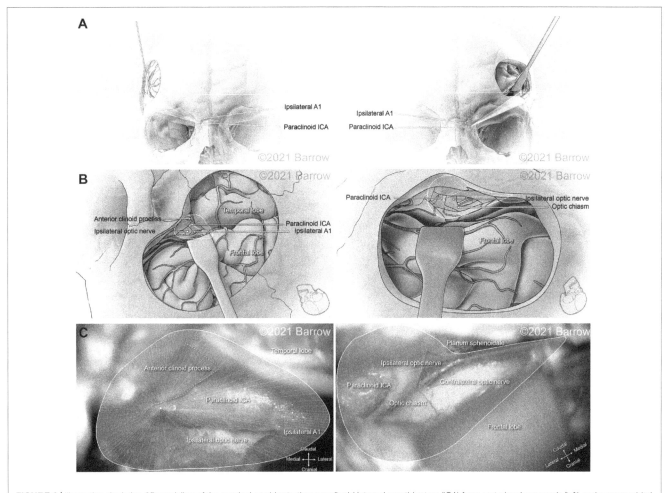

FIGURE 6 | Illustration depicting 3D modeling of the surgical corridor to the paraclinoid internal carotid artery (ICA) from a pterional approach (left) and a supraorbital approach (right). **(A)** The anterior of the surgical corridor. **(B)** The surgical anatomy as visualized specific to the surgical corridor model. **(C)** The surgical view of the cadaveric anatomy, which is in continuity with the surgical corridor model parameters (pterional: VSF = 165.88 mm³, craniocaudal angle of attack = 36.72°, mediolateral angle of attack = 50.55°; supraorbital: VSF = 43.83 mm³, craniocaudal angle of attack = 20.86°, mediolateral angle of attack = 30.40°). VSF, volume of surgical freedom; 3D, 3-dimensional. Used with permission from Barrow Neurological Institute, Phoenix, Arizona.

Measurement Inaccuracy

The illustrative data set for **Figure 5** was used to compare the calculated area bounded by the original measurement data points to the calculated area bounded by the points after translation onto the best-fit plane. The sample data set comprised measurements for a supraorbital craniotomy surgical corridor to the anterior communicating artery. It represented the area calculated by the previous surgical freedom method (Heron's Formula) and the area after translation onto the best-fit plane. The calculation of the area bounded by this sample set of data point measurements was 1,489 mm², and the calculation of the area bounded by the data points after translation onto the best-fit plane for the data set was 1,418 mm². To illustrate the effect of probe length on the calculated volume, we used this same data set to calculate the volume from the best-fit plane of the measured data points to the apex. A cone height of 183.6 mm gave a volume of 119,386 mm³. The points representing data of the same corridor as measured were then translated to a plane 5 mm farther away from the apex. This 5-mm increase in the height

of the same cone shape, to 188.6 mm, gave a cone volume of 129,448 mm³.

Figure 9 shows the frequency distribution of the probe lengths of the 8 data points for the 174 sets of measurements. The mean (SD) probe length was 190.4 (5.0) mm, with a minimum of 168.3 mm and a maximum of 212.0 mm.

DISCUSSION

Surgical Application Advantages of the VSF

The VSF compensates for multiple defects in the established method of producing a quantitative result to assess surgical instrument freedom. The process incorporates various spatial, anatomical, and technical components pertinent for the accurate and insightful analysis of a surgical corridor. This quantitative approach resolves issues in assessing this surgically imperative parameter that are cause by multiple planes,

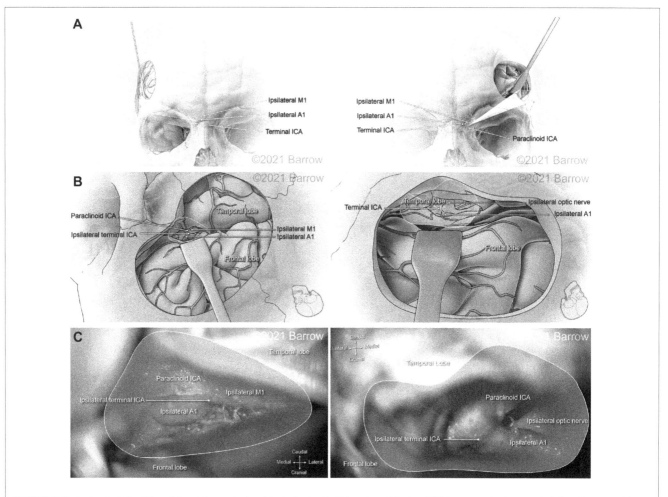

FIGURE 7 | Illustration depicting 3D modeling of the surgical corridor to the terminal internal carotid artery (ICA) from a pterional approach (left) and a supraorbital approach (right). **(A)** The anterior of the surgical corridor. **(B)** An illustration of the surgical anatomy as visualized specific to the surgical corridor model. **(C)** The surgical view of the cadaveric anatomy, which is in continuity with the surgical corridor model parameters (pterional: VSF = 50.69 mm^3, craniocaudal angle of attack = 22.63°, mediolateral angle of attack = 27.59°; supraorbital: VSF = 31.01 mm^3, craniocaudal angle of attack = 16.29°, mediolateral angle of attack = 31.62°). ACoA, anterior communicating artery; VSF, volume of surgical freedom; 3D, 3-dimensional. Used with permission from Barrow Neurological Institute, Phoenix, Arizona.

irregularly shaped access corridors, procedural variability, and mathematical inaccuracies.

This methodology comprises the various embodiments of a system and an associated mathematical method to determine a 3D VSF before operating on neurosurgical structures. The system characterizes, assesses, and models a 3D volumetric measurement of the maneuverability of a surgical instrument within a surgical corridor with respect to STS access, thereby providing new insight into the accessibility of an intracranial structure via a specific approach. It is explicitly advantageous to medical specialties, such as neurosurgery, that deal with microanatomical structure and require competency in microsurgical techniques. Dealing with small structures that have definitive targets is inherent in the microsurgery of STSs that lie at a depth from the surgical entry point.

Neurosurgeons try to maximize the potential physiologic space at their disposal to minimize circumferential damage. The VSF is a metric that enables a more accurate assessment of the freedom of this physiologic space in conjunction with specific surgical maneuvers. Anatomically, this concept and the basis behind neurosurgical corridor modeling can be characterized by examining the pathologic processes encountered by the neurosurgeon. For example, vascular aneurysms are abnormal protrusions or weaknesses in the wall of a blood vessel. Obliteration of these weaknesses is imperative to prevent intracranial hemorrhage and potential morbidity and mortality. Minimizing the degree of brain retraction is an important factor in decision-making when selecting a surgical approach. With the VSF, the degree of retraction can be quantitatively measured with respect to each approach and each STS. Another example is the midline tumor, such as the pituitary lesion, which often produces complex surgical conditions because of the need to cross neurovascular structures and overcome difficult angles of attack produced by the anatomy. As with vascular lesions, the VSF can provide a more accurate quantitative assessment of midline tumors and better anatomical visualization of the

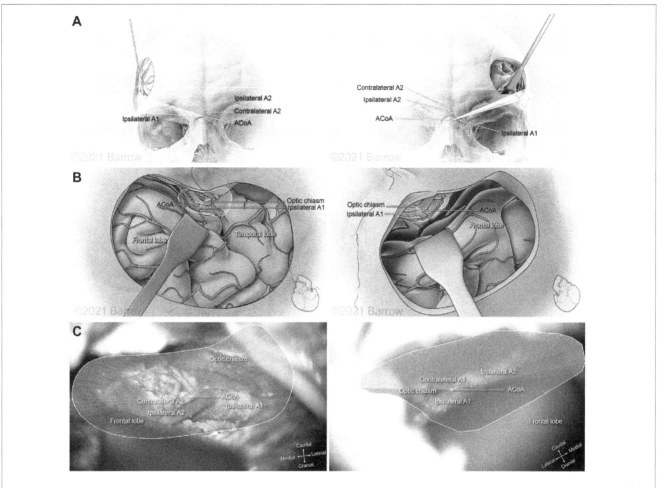

FIGURE 8 | Illustration depicting 3D modeling of the surgical corridor to the anterior communicating artery (ACoA) from a pterional approach (left) and a supraorbital approach (right). **(A)** The anterior of the surgical corridor. **(B)** The surgical anatomy as visualized specific to the surgical corridor model. **(C)** The surgical view of the cadaveric anatomy, which is in continuity with the surgical corridor model parameters (pterional: VSF = 38.34 mm³, craniocaudal angle of attack = 12.64°, mediolateral angle of attack = 31.69°; supraorbital: VSF = 15.66 mm³, craniocaudal angle of attack = 14.50°, mediolateral angle of attack = 17.44°). ICA, internal carotid artery; VSF, volume of surgical freedom; 3D, 3-dimensional. Used with permission from Barrow Neurological Institute, Phoenix, Arizona.

different surgical corridors to reach this region of interest. Finally, a third example is the abnormal lesion of the nerves, such as an acoustic neuroma growing at the deep apex of the cerebellopontine angle of the skull base, the trajectory of which naturally follows the conical structure of our model when the potential physiologic space is created by brain retraction and the release of cisternal cerebrospinal fluid.

Given that neurovascular structures tend to traverse the fossae floors along their pathway, the use of this surgical corridor modeling method is particularly relevant in surgical interventions of the skull base, where the STSs are usually bounded inferiorly by the skull base. Skull base surgery usually entails both anatomical and technical obstacles: deep STSs, multiple eloquent structure boundaries, dural tethering, and skull base canal insertion. These influential factors substantially limit maneuverability, which is extremely precious. The VSF is a valuable tool for evaluating surgical corridors that allow only restricted movement and therefore is a particularly useful metric for the assessment of skull base surgical approaches.

This methodology generates the first spatially accurate model of an irregular surgical corridor that also considers actual anatomical boundaries. Furthermore, it allows the influence of the different visualization techniques used in surgical intervention to be examined. For example, the operating microscope, although limited in image expanse and illuminating capabilities, does not function within the approach corridor. In contrast, the endoscope is used within the surgical corridor, where, as an extra instrument or a space-occupying entity, it will impede the freedom of other instrumentation. Experimental scrutiny of this variable has not been completed, although it is common knowledge among endoscopic surgical specialists who have proposed multiportal endoscopic approaches to combat instrument crowding or "swording" (Dallan et al., 2015; Lim et al., 2020). The VSF not only provides a numerical representation of the effect of the endoscope on instrument freedom but also creates a 3D representation of this influence. Notably, the endoscope is dynamic and can be moved out of the trajectory of attack as dictated by the operating surgeon, but the numeric

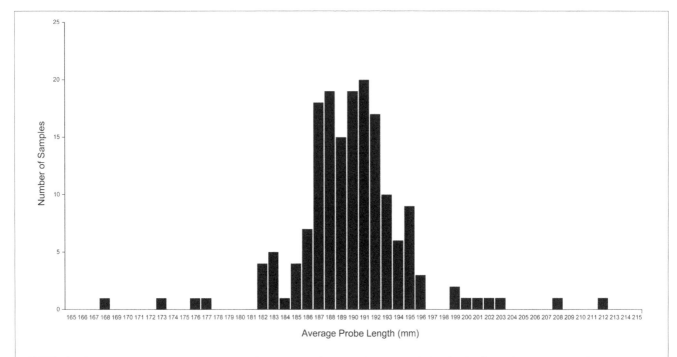

FIGURE 9 | A plot of the average probe length of each set of measurement data. Probe length was calculated as the distance between the coordinates of each extrema point and the apex point. The plot shows considerable variation in the calculated probe length, although the same fixed-length probe was used in all measurements. This variation is caused by measurement error that can be mitigated by using the normalized volume of surgical freedom metric. Used with permission from Barrow Neurological Institute, Phoenix, Arizona.

change in the VSF caused by its presence remains valid. Given the dynamic nature of the endoscope, mapping its optimal position in the context of different STSs and angles of attack could pose a useful predictive model for improving the efficiency of surgical movement and minimizing exposure.

The system and the associated method provide the surgeon with a volumetric metric to determine the appropriateness and utility of a surgical approach to access a specific pathology. It would, therefore, potentially allow the neurosurgeon to select approaches and define a safe access corridor for guidance during both the planning and the conduct of surgery. This metric can also elucidate the appropriateness of surgically attainable targets specific to an approach. Like all attempts at neuroanatomical quantitation, the VSF functions as a quantifiable metric for assessing the likelihood of surgical risk and injury to anatomical STSs, but it achieves this with substantially superior accuracy and volumetric spatial computation.

Procedural Superiority of the VSF

The VSF methodology includes the calculation of the area bounded by the surgical corridor extrema coordinate points. Perpendicular to the central axis of the surgical corridor, this area is bounded by the surgical corridor extrema points that are measured.

Previous methods also measured the bounded area and used this area calculation as the metric of surgical freedom. These methods used Heron's formula to calculate the area, which involved subdividing the bounded area into triangles, with the measured points as the vertices of the triangles. With the

coordinates of each vertex known, the lengths of the three sides of each triangle were calculated using Heron's formula, and the areas were summed to give the total bounded area.

In our proposed VSF methodology, the bounded area is used in calculating the VSF because the base of the cone shape is formed by the bounded area and the area value is used to calculate the volume of the cone shape. The VSF methodology uses a different method—the shoelace formula—to calculate the area. The shoelace formula was used instead of Heron's formula because it can calculate the area of irregular shapes more accurately. Heron's formula inherently requires choosing how to divide the area into triangles, which is important, as illustrated in **Figure 10**. This figure illustrates two methods of dividing an ideal shape and a shape determined from measurement data into triangles. The first choice of division of the shape results in an accurate calculation of the bounded area of each shape. However, the second choice of division, while calculating the area of the ideal shape correctly, overestimates the area of the shape from the measurement data and results in an area outside the bounds of the shape being included in the calculation.

A method that requires a choice, or the validation of a choice, for each set of data is not conducive to creating a calculator that will give repeatable and accurate results because each calculation requires user input to review and determine how the shape will be divided into triangles. To avoid this dilemma, we selected the shoelace formula to use in calculating the area for the VSF methodology. This formula uses coordinate data of the vertices of a closed, irregular shape to calculate the enclosed area. This method accounts for irregular shapes and does not overestimate

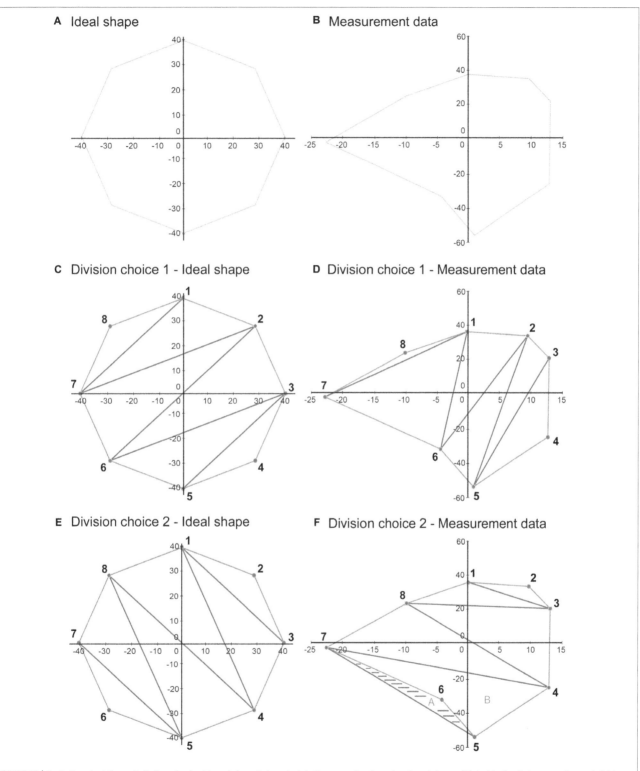

FIGURE 10 | Illustration depicting a limitation of using Heron's formula to calculate the area of an irregular closed shape. **(A)** An idealized shape made up of eight data points. **(B)** A shape plotted from a sample measurement, also with eight data points. **(C)** An example of a choice of division of the area into component triangles for application of Heron's formula. **(D)** This division choice applied to the sample data. In this case, using Heron's formula on each of the triangles results in a correct calculation of the total area. **(E)** Another example of a choice of division of the area into component triangles. **(F)** This division choice applied to the sample data. In this case, using Heron's formula on each of the triangles results in an overestimation of the bounded area, as the shaded area is included twice in the calculated area, as part of triangles A (5-6-7) and B (4-5-7), although it is outside the area bounded by the data points. Used with permission from Barrow Neurological Institute, Phoenix, Arizona.

the area, as the Heron's formula method does. Because the VSF method includes the identification of a normalized-height plane for the base of the cone, and the measured points are translated onto this plane, the points can be converted into a 2D coordinate system on the normalized-height plane, and the 2D shoelace formula can be used. Converting the 3D coordinates to 2D coordinates has the advantage of allowing the creation of 2D plots of the cone base that can be used to verify the measurement data.

Translating the original measurement points onto a plane and calculating the area using the translated points also increases the accuracy of the calculated area over a calculation using the original 3D measurement points. The area of interest is the area of the surgical corridor perpendicular to the central axis of the surgical corridor, which is the truest representation of the accessibility of the surgical approach. Because the best-fit plane is perpendicular to the central axis of the surgical corridor, the area bounded by the translated points is perpendicular to the axis of the surgical corridor and thus represents a true cross-section of the surgical corridor. As noted previously, the 3D coordinate data that are measured are not in a single plane because of inaccuracies in measurement, meaning that the triangles formed for measuring the bounded area using Heron's formula are not perpendicular to the central axis of the surgical corridor. As a result, calculating the total area by summing the areas of the triangles would be an overestimation. The sample data set of **Figure 5** illustrates this as the area calculated using Heron's formula on the original measurement data points (1,489 mm^2) was 5% higher than the perpendicular area measured from the data points after translation onto the best-fit plane (1,418 mm^2).

Benefits of Using Normalized Height

Although the concept of volumetric quantification of surgical freedom is novel, we further refined the concept to a normalized volumetric quantification of surgical freedom to compensate for several inaccuracies inherent in the measurement process. The measurement process involves measuring the coordinate data points for the extrema of the surgical corridor at the end of a surgical instrument of fixed length (**Figure 4**). Doing so resulted in the coordinate data being measured outside the cadaveric specimen, such that the area being measured was not a measurement of the surgical entrance but rather an abstract measurement of surgical freedom that could only be compared to other measurements that used a surgical instrument of equal length. Measuring with a shorter probe would result in a smaller measurement of surgical freedom for the same surgical corridor because of the conical shape of the surgical corridor, whereas measuring with a longer probe would result in a larger measurement of surgical freedom because the length of the probe defines the vertical height of the cone shape from base to apex.

The depth of the structure from the surgical entry point is of secondary importance to the degree of freedom of the instruments within the surgical corridor, which is why this method of measurement can be used at the end of a fixed probe. With the use of this method, surgical corridors and their

quantitative measurements with respect to STSs can be directly compared only if the probe length is exactly equal across studies. This limitation raises questions about the scientific validity of these studies and restricts replication of results and large-scale analysis of anatomical surgical corridor data. The limitation is equally applicable to a volumetric measurement of surgical freedom; for the same surgical corridor, a shorter probe results in a smaller volume measurement, and a longer probe results in a larger volume measurement. Measuring the volume of the surgical corridor up to a fixed distance from the apex (a normalized height) can mitigate this issue. The measurement data from any length of probe can be used to calculate the VSF at a fixed distance from the apex, so the normalized VSF calculation allows the direct comparison of VSF data from any measurement that uses this method.

This decoupling of cone height from probe length also improves the accuracy of the VSF measurement. In our experimental data, human error in collecting coordinate data led to variation in the distance between the apex point and each of the extrema data points of the surgical corridor. This inaccuracy in the data existed in all three dimensions, and there is little that can be done in processing the data to improve the accuracy in the two dimensions on the plane of the base of the cone. However, the normalized VSF measurement, by defining a fixed distance from the apex to the base of the cone, can reduce the inaccuracy in the third dimension along the axis of the cone. The inaccuracy in this dimension has a large effect on resultant calculations. The SD of the average probe length data for all measurement data sets was identified as 5 mm from the plot (**Figure 9**). The effect of this variation on the calculated volume can be seen in our sample data set analysis. In this case, the height of the cone shape increased from 183.6 to 188.6 mm, for an increase of 5 mm (2.7%). The resultant calculation of the cone volume increased by 8.4%. This outcome demonstrates how errors in probe length measurements can be exaggerated in the calculated surgical freedom metric, and thus may translate to important surgical implications. The use of a normalized cone height eliminates this variation in the calculated volume and leads to a more consistent result that can be compared to other normalized VSF data with a much higher degree of confidence.

3D Modeling of the Operative Corridor

Visualization is a critical skill. From the surgeon's perspective, being able to orient and envision the structures and any restrictions and obstacles in the surgical corridor is imperative to selecting the most appropriate approach and planning specifically for the selected surgical strategy. As previously noted, neuroanatomy has been extensively analyzed and neurosurgeons have a well-established knowledge base about anatomical sites and the sizes and arrangements of specialized regions. Less explicitly defined are the physiologic and surgical corridors created by operators, the architecture of these potential or created spaces, and how the circumferential anatomy affects these crucial aspects in surgical decision-making.

The novel design of the VSF results in an improved concept constructing a configuration that embodies the actual geometry of the surgical approach corridor, which is illustrated by our models. When incorporated with the clinical, anatomical, and surgical application, this volumetric model yields better assessment and prediction of the ability to manipulate surgical instruments, while providing spatially and anatomically accurate representation that can aid the surgeon in decision-making. These images accentuate the importance of not only anatomical considerations but also the critical principles of microsurgery: technique, instrument maneuverability, and the predicted primary instrument axis. The VSF methodology provides an anatomically and spatially accurate 3D depiction illustrating all these key surgical ideals, which proves its substantial clinical applicability.

Limitations

Ideally, this quantitative analysis and modeling should be conducted *in vivo* in human patients rather than in cadaveric specimens because the brain parenchyma can harden in cadavers with fixed tissue, resulting in decreased surgical maneuverability. However, cadaveric brain tissue is the best model available; although it may not be exactly representative, the quantitative results are proportionate. Although the surgical corridor may be larger *in vivo*, the anatomical parameters are the same, and the 3D models of the surgical corridor are therefore still reflective of real-time surgical views.

Ideally, the VSF measurements should be made in relation to pathologic processes, such as a vascular weakness like an aneurysm or an intracranial mass lesion, which was not possible in the current study. We therefore could not take into account the potential mass effect influence of intracranial pathology on surrounding brain parenchyma and structures, nor could we predict the pathologic decrease in intracranial potential space. Again, this limitation is inherent in all cadaveric modeling because the accessible anatomy is generally physiologically normal. The reproducible STSs are reasonable representations of delicate neurovascular components of high priority to the neurosurgeon who must select the optimal approach on the basis of quantitative metrics that are critical to the decision-making process. What can be extrapolated from our analysis is the predictable numeric value and anatomical shape of surgical access corridors used to reach the pathologic target. In addition, the VSF quantitatively and visually allows for the comparison of approaches, and it ultimately provides increased multifaceted information for surgical decision-making that is comparable to other available metrics.

The VSF methodology is based on the assumption that the surgical corridor traverses from a region of large freedom and maneuverability to an apex or an STS. This assumption produces the cone shape that supports the mathematical and modeling structure of this system. This is the accepted surgical trajectory of transcranial surgical interventions and potentially that of other surgical interventions, where instruments proceed from areas of large surgical freedom to small, confined regions necessitating microsurgical technique. However, this model is not applicable for comparison with all approaches. The caveat of this quantitative and visual estimator is the assumption of the surgical apex; the corridor ends at the point represented by the STS. For quantitatively and spatially comparable results, the comparison of different surgical approaches is possible only when both approaches abide by this assumption. For example, the comparison of a transcranial pterional approach and an endonasal transplanum-cavernous approach to the paraclinoid internal carotid artery is not an equivalent assessment, because an endonasal approach creates a large amount of deep surgical exposure, and its parameters do not converge to an apex as in a transcranial approach (**Figure 11**). Conversely, it is acceptable to quantify and model specific to an STS if both approaches have the same surgical boundaries (i.e., both use a deep transsphenoidal approach) and if an assumption has been established that the STS represents the conical apex. For example, a comparison of a transnasal approach and a transmaxillary approach is possible because both produce the same deep surgical exposure, although they are restricted more superficially by different anatomical structures at the surgical entrance. In this scenario, the VSF is a useful metric and a helpful surgical corridor modeling tool for visualizing these restrictions.

Future Directions

This report describes in detail an improved and more representational mathematical and modeling methodology for quantitatively assessing surgical freedom. Our rationale was to produce a robust, multifaceted tool that neurosurgeons can use to estimate the benefits and disadvantages of different surgical approaches specific to various STSs.

Although we have illustrated quantitatively and visually how the various constituents of this novel design are superior to the previous method, comparative analysis has yet to be completed. Our next step in proving the scientific, mathematical, logistical, and applicable advantages of the VSF will be to complete cadaveric quantitation of the same surgical approaches specific to various STSs and to analyze the results. Specifically, three areas should be examined in detail when comparing this VSF methodology with previous methodologies: (1) the increase in accuracy of the measured area when measuring the area on a single plane versus on points in 3D space because of the measurement of only the perpendicular area; (2) the reduction in the variation in results because of the calculated probe length using the normalized unit of the VSF and how variations in probe length affect the calculated area or the VSF metric; and (3) further analysis of the limitations of Heron's formula, specifically regarding the choice of division of the bounded area of irregular shapes.

Our interdisciplinary research group also intends to replicate this experimental methodology with multiple neurosurgical approaches. We will then quantitatively analyze the benefits and disadvantages of different operative corridors to specific STSs, which will ultimately increase the body of reproducible, standardized, and comparable surgical freedom data and promote optimal surgical techniques and practices.

In regard to comparing the VSF with the previously used method, we predict that the quantitative results will correlate and will be approximately proportionate. It is important to highlight that the merits of the VSF are a result of two key features: the increased accuracy of this multifaceted biomedically orientated mathematical methodology and the ability to produce

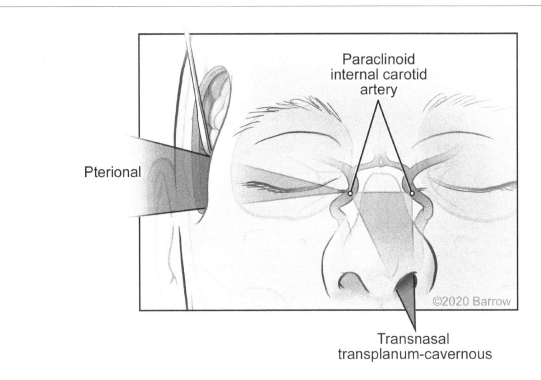

FIGURE 11 | Surgical maneuverability of an instrument using a transcranial pterional approach compared with a transnasal transplanum-cavernous approach to the paraclinoid internal carotid artery. In the transcranial approach, the surgical corridor progresses from a superficial region of large maneuverability to a small deep apex, whereas in the transnasal approach, a significant amount of deep volume is created by traversing the ethmoid and sphenoid sinuses. Used with permission from Barrow Neurological Institute, Phoenix, Arizona.

anatomically and spatially accurate 3D models. These two components have coalesced to produce an effective translational tool that combines anatomical, clinical, and surgically pertinent principles for improved operative decision-making.

Although our report details the use of this methodology for neurosurgical operative corridors, this system can likely be used in its current form to quantitatively analyze and spatially visualize the surgical approaches of different surgical specialties. Doing so would require that they abide by the structural parameters of this measurement process: that the instrument freedom of the surgeon traverses from a region of larger maneuverability at the surgical entrance to a target apex of minimal maneuverability. As denoted when referencing skull base surgical concepts, it is in fixed domains of minimal freedom that knowledge and insight about the movement capabilities of an instrument are most important. Quantitation of spinal surgical corridors and specific STSs is certainly feasible using this methodology, and it is worthy of further investigation.

Our method for determining the VSF provides the surgeon with a diverse metric and a useful tool for improved surgical preoperative planning and decision-making. Current neurosurgical navigational systems plan surgical routes along a direct trajectory based on a linear display. These navigational approaches portray the trajectory line to the STSs in different views (e.g., axial, coronal, sagittal, and probe view), which is not always the optimal approach and does not incorporate any criteria relevant to surgical corridor analysis. These planning

navigation systems also do not incorporate any modeling, which would elucidate or illustrate the degree of surgical freedom. By compiling a substantial body of data, we hope to develop standardized reproducible surgical approach principles specific to operative corridors and STSs and thereby establish predictive surgical theory. Consequently, the integration of the VSF into intraoperative planning, as well as into surgical navigation software and systems, could prove to be a powerful tool for improving surgical decision-making and techniques, while ultimately minimizing surgical morbidity and mortality.

CONCLUSION

The VSF is a superior method of quantitative anatomical measurement. This innovative concept can be used to develop an actual geometric model of a surgical corridor that yields better assessment and prediction of the ability to manipulate surgical instruments. The VSF accounts for multiple inaccuracies in the practical and mathematical method of assessment, and it also enables the production of 3D models. For this reason, the VSF is a preferable and clinically applicable standard for the assessment of surgical freedom. This quantitative measurement can establish surgically attainable targets for specific approaches and also assess the suitability of a specific surgical approach compared to alternative operative options, thereby acting as a pivotal tool in the decision-making armamentarium of the neurosurgeon.

AUTHOR CONTRIBUTIONS

LMH: conception, design, data collection, data analysis, manuscript write-up, review, and revisions. DN: conception, design, data Analysis, manuscript write-up, review, and revisions. MCP: supervision, review, and revisions. All authors contributed to the article and approved the submitted version.

ACKNOWLEDGMENTS

We acknowledge the support of Richard O' Shea, Ph.D., and Behrooz Kousari. We thank the staff of Neuroscience Publications at Barrow Neurological Institute for assistance with manuscript preparation.

REFERENCES

1. Acar, F., Naderi, S., Guvencer, M., Ture, U., and Arda, M. N. (2005). Herophilus of chalcedon: a pioneer in neuroscience. *Neurosurgery* 56, 861–867; discussion – 7.

2. Arraez-Aybar, L. A., Navia-Alvarez, P., Fuentes-Redondo, T., and Bueno-Lopez, J. L. (2015). Thomas Willis, a pioneer in translational research in anatomy (on the 350th anniversary of Cerebri anatome). *J. Anat.* 226, 289–300. doi: 10.1111/joa.12273

3. Aziz, N., and Mansor, O. (2006). The role of anatomists and surgeons in clinical anatomy instruction inside and outside the operating room. *Malays. J. Med. Sci.* 13, 76–77.

4. Barth, A. L., and Ray, A. (2019). Progressive circuit changes during learning and disease. *Neuron* 104, 37–46. doi: 10.1016/j.neuron.2019.09.032

5. Başarslan, S. K., and Cüneyt, G. (2014). Neuronavigation: a revolutionary step of neurosurgery and its education. *Derleme Rev.* 5, 24–31. doi: 10.17944/mkutfd. 15885

6. Belykh, E. G., Zhao, X., Cavallo, C., Bohl, M. A., Yagmurlu, K., Aklinski, J. L., et al. (2018). Laboratory evaluation of a robotic operative microscope : visualization platform for neurosurgery. *Cureus* 10:e3072.

7. Burgess, A. W., and Ramsey-Stewart, G. (2015). The importance of surgeons teaching anatomy, especially by whole-body dissection. *Med. J. Aust.* 202, 18–19. doi: 10.5694/mja14.00410

8. Castelnuovo, P., Lepera, D., Turri-Zanoni, M., Battaglia, P., Bolzoni Villaret, A., Bignami, M., et al. (2013). Quality of life following endoscopic endonasal resection of anterior skull base cancers. *J. Neurosurg.* 119, 1401–1409. doi: 10.3171/2013.8.jns13296

9. Dallan, I., Castelnuovo, P., Locatelli, D., Turri-Zanoni, M., AlQahtani, A., Battaglia, P., et al. (2015). Multiportal combined transorbital transnasal endoscopic approach for the management of selected skull base lesions: preliminary experience. *World Neurosurg.* 84, 97–107. doi: 10.1016/j.wneu.2015.02.034

10. Elhadi, A. M., Almefty, K. K., Mendes, G. A., Kalani, M. Y., Nakaji, P., Dru, A., et al. (2014). Comparison of surgical freedom and area of exposure in three endoscopic transmaxillary approaches to the anterolateral cranial base. *J. Neurol. Surg. B Skull Base* 75, 346–353. doi: 10.1055/s-0034-1372467

11. Elhadi, A. M., Hardesty, D. A., Zaidi, H. A., Kalani, M. Y., Nakaji, P., White, W. L., et al. (2015). Evaluation of surgical freedom for microscopic and endoscopic transsphenoidal approaches to the sella. *Neurosurgery* 11(Suppl 2), 69–78; discussion – 9.

12. Elhadi, A. M., Kalb, S., Perez-Orribo, L., Little, A. S., Spetzler, R. F., and Preul, M. C. (2012). The journey of discovering skull base anatomy in ancient Egypt and the special influence of Alexandria. *Neurosurg. Focus* 33:E2.

13. Herlan, S., Marquardt, J. S., Hirt, B., Tatagiba, M., and Ebner, F. H. (2019). 3D exoscope system in neurosurgery: comparison of a standard operating microscope with a new 3D exoscope in the cadaver lab. *Oper. Neurosurg. (Hagerstown)* 17, 518–524. doi: 10.1093/ons/opz081

14. Higdon, R. (2013). "Experimental design, variability," in *Encyclopedia of Systems Biology*, eds W. Dubitzky, O. Wolkenhauer, K.-H. Cho, and H. Yokota (New York, NY: Springer), 704–705. doi: 10.1007/978-1-4419-9863-7_1191

15. Horgan, M. A., Anderson, G. J., Kellogg, J. X., Schwartz, M. S., Spektor, S., McMenomey, S. O., et al. (2000). Classification and quantification of the petrosal approach to the petroclival region. *J. Neurosurg.* 93, 108–112. doi: 10.3171/jns.2000.93.1.0108

16. Iaizzo, P. A., Anderson, R. H., and Hill, A. J. (2013). The importance of human cardiac anatomy for translational research. *J. Cardiovasc. Transl. Res.* 6, 105– 106. doi: 10.1007/s12265-012-9419-y

17. Iorio-Morin, C., and Mathieu, D. (2020). Perspective on the homunculus, the history of cerebral localization, and evolving modes of data representation. *World Neurosurg.* 135, 42–47. doi: 10.1016/j.wneu.2019.11.104

18. Jane, J. A. Jr. (2013). Endoscopy versus microscopy. *J. Neurosurg.* 118:611; discussion – 2.

19. Kreutz, C., and Timmer, J. (2009). Systems biology: experimental design. *FEBS J.*

20. 276, 923–942. doi: 10.1111/j.1742-4658.2008.06843.x

21. Lim, J., Roh, T. H., Kim, W., Kim, J. S., Hong, J. B., Sung, K. S., et al. (2020). Biportal endoscopic transorbital approach: a quantitative anatomical study and clinical application. *Acta Neurochir. (Wien)* 162, 2119–2128. doi: 10.1007/s00701-020- 04339-0

22. Matsushima, T., Kobayashi, S., Inoue, T., Rhoton, A. S., Vlasak, A. L., and Oliveira, E. (2018). Albert L. Rhoton Jr., MD: his philosophy and education of neurosurgeons. *Neurol. Med. Chir. (Tokyo)* 58, 279–289. doi: 10.2176/nmc. ra. 2018-0082

23. Melly, L., Torregrossa, G., Lee, T., Jansens, J. L., and Puskas, J. D. (2018). Fifty years of coronary artery bypass grafting. *J. Thorac. Dis.* 10, 1960–1967.

24. Noiphithak, R., Yanez-Siller, J. C., Revuelta Barbero, J. M., Otto, B. A., Carrau, R. L., and Prevedello, D. M. (2018). Quantitative analysis of the surgical exposure and surgical freedom between transcranial and transorbital endoscopic anterior petrosectomies to the posterior fossa. *J. Neurosurg.* 131, 569–577. doi: 10.3171/ 2018.2.jns172334

25. Pillai, P., Baig, M. N., Karas, C. S., and Ammirati, M. (2009). Endoscopic image- guided transoral approach to the craniovertebral junction: an anatomic study comparing surgical exposure and surgical freedom obtained with the endoscope and the operating microscope. *Neurosurgery* 64(5 Suppl 2), 437–442; discussion 442–4.

26. Selcuk, I., Tatar, I., and Huri, E. (2019). Cadaveric anatomy and dissection in surgical training. *Turk. J. Obstet. Gynecol.* 16, 72–75.

27. Spektor, S., Anderson, G. J., McMenomey, S. O., Horgan, M. A., Kellogg, J. X., and Delashaw, J. B. Jr. (2000). Quantitative description of the far- lateral transcondylar transtubercular approach to the foramen magnum and clivus. *J. Neurosurg.* 92, 824–831. doi: 10.3171/jns.2000.92.5. 0824

28. Weisstein, E. W. (0000). *Heron's Formula*. Available online at: https://mathworld. wolfram.com/HeronsFormula.html (accessed January 10, 2020).

29. Weisstein, E. W. (0000). *Polygon Area*. Available Online at: https://mathworld. wolfram.com/PolygonArea.html (accessed January 10, 2020).

15

A Case Report of the Reconstruction of a Bone Defect Following Resection of a Comminuted Fracture of the Lateral Clavicle Using a Titanium Prosthesis

Sahar Ahmed Abdalbary[1]*, Sherif M. Amr[2], Khaled Abdelghany[3], Amr A. Nssef[4] and Ehab A. A. El-Shaarawy[5]

[1] Department of Orthopaedic Physical Therapy, Faculty of Physical Therapy, Nahda University, Beni Suef, Egypt, [2] Department of Orthopaedic Surgery, Faculty of Medicine, Cairo University, Giza, Egypt, [3] Advanced Manufacturing Division, The Central Metallurgical Research and Development Institute, Helwan, Egypt, [4] Department of Intervention Radiology, Radiology and Vascular Imaging, Faculty of Medicine, Cairo University, Giza, Egypt, [5] Department of Anatomy and Embryology, Faculty of Medicine, Cairo University, Giza, Egypt

*Correspondence:
Sahar Ahmed Abdalbary
saharabdalbary@yahoo.com
orcid.org/0000-0003-1346-6750

Introduction: This case report describes the reconstruction of a severe comminuted fracture and bone defect in the lateral half of the clavicle using a novel titanium prosthesis. This unique prosthesis has been specifically designed and three dimensionally printed for the clavicle, as opposed to the Oklahoma cemented composite prosthesis used in common practice. The aims of this study were to: (1) describe the prosthesis, its stress analysis, and its surgical fixation and (2) to demonstrate the results of the 2-year follow-up of the patient with the lateral clavicle prosthesis.

Patient's Main Concerns: A 20-year-old, right-handed woman complaining of severe pain in the right shoulder was admitted to our hospital following a traffic accident. Physical examination revealed pain, swelling, tenderness, limb weakness, asymmetric posturing, and loss of function in the right shoulder.

Diagnosis, Intervention, and Outcomes: Radiographic evaluation in the emergency room showed complete destruction with a comminuted fracture of the lateral half of the right clavicle and a comminuted fracture of the coracoid. We designed a new prosthesis for the lateral half of the clavicle, which was then tested by finite element analysis and implanted. Use of the new prosthesis was effective in the reconstruction of the comminuted fracture in the lateral half of the clavicle. After 2 years of follow-up, the patient had an aesthetically acceptable curve and was able to perform her activities of daily living. Her pain was relieved, and the disabilities of the arm, shoulder, and hand score improved. Active range of motion of the shoulder joint and muscle strength were also improved.

Conclusion: This novel prosthesis is recommended for reconstruction of the lateral half of the clavicle following development of bony defects due to fracture. Our patient achieved functional and aesthetic satisfaction with this prosthesis.

Keywords: finite element analysis, comminuted fracture, clavicle, fracture, clavicle prosthesis

INTRODUCTION

The clavicle, acting as a strut between the scapula and the sternum, articulates with the sternal manubrium medially and with the acromion of the scapula laterally (1). The clavicle contributes to the strength, coordinated scapulohumeral rhythm, and overall range of motion (ROM) of the shoulder girdle (2).

Fractures of the clavicle are common in adults and represent about 4% of all fractures. Further, 21% of clavicle fractures affect the lateral half (3). Clavicular fractures are caused mostly from direct injury, accompanied by a fall on the point of the shoulder, which is the most clinical and biomechanical mechanism of fracture (4).

Recently, to decrease the high rate of surgical complications after claviculectomy, some surgeons suggest a new method for reconstruction of bony defects with autogenous bone or allografts bone to protect the subclavian vessels and brachial plexus, restore the shape of the shoulder, and decrease pain (5). Outcomes of midshaft clavicular malunion, including restoration of length and alignment, soft-tissue preservation, use of local bone graft, and plate fixation, is a reliable treatment option, regardless of the time since fracture (6). Vartanian et al. (7), report the use of an Oklahoma prosthesis, which is a cemented composite prosthesis used to reconstruct bony defects after metastatic tumor resection of the medial third of the clavicle.

Computer-aided engineering technology has many applications in the medical field to generate a surface model of the prosthesis mirrored from the contralateral healthy side (8). Finite element analysis is used to examine the biomechanics of the clavicle reconstruction plate, which are calculated by the quantity of the forces applied by the muscles as a result of the surgical technique (9).

We present the case of a severe comminuted bony defect following fracture in the lateral half of the clavicle treated using a titanium prosthesis. To resolve the bony defect, we designed a novel titanium prosthesis for the lateral half of the clavicle.

In this study, we designed the titanium prosthesis and tested it by finite element stress analysis and inserted it to fill the defect at the site of bone loss in the clavicle. The aims of this study were to: (1) describe the prosthesis, its stress analysis, and its surgical fixation and (2) to demonstrate the results of the 2-year follow-up of the patient with the lateral clavicle prosthesis. To our knowledge, the presentation, findings, and management of this case have not been previously described in the literature.

CASE REPORT

A 20-year-old, right-handed woman complaining of severe pain in the right shoulder was admitted to our hospital following a traffic accident. Physical examination revealed pain, swelling, tenderness, limb weakness, asymmetric posturing, and loss of function in the right shoulder.

Abbreviations: 3D, three-dimensional; CT, computed tomography; DASH, disabilities of the arm, shoulder, and hand; DICOM, digital imaging and communication in medicine; FEA, finite element analysis; ROM, range of motion; VAS, visual analog scale.

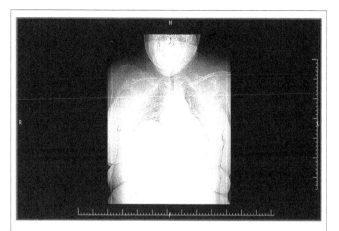

FIGURE 1 | Preoperative computed tomography scan revealing the scope of the lesion. This was essential in identifying the small bone fragments separated from the fracture.

Radiographic evaluation in the emergency room showed complete destruction with a comminuted fracture of the lateral half of the right clavicle and a comminuted fracture of the coracoid. A computed tomography (CT) scan revealed the scope of the lesion and was essential in identifying the small bone fragments separated from the fracture (**Figure 1**).

A preoperative assessment was performed for pain using the visual analog scale (VAS) score with a result of 9. The preoperative disabilities of the arm, shoulder, and hand (DASH) score (10) was 98.3. A higher score means greater disability, with 100 points indicating a complete disability of the extremity and 0 points indicating a perfect extremity.

The patient was informed that data concerning her status would be submitted for publication and the patient agreed and signed the form providing written informed consent to participate in the study. The study was registered on ClinicalTrials.gov (NCT03577678).

Manufacturing of Prosthesis and Finite Element Analysis

A normal clavicle three-dimensional (3D) geometry model was designed using data extracted from the CT scan. The 3D model of the clavicle was developed using the digital imaging and communication in medicine format, and image segmentation was performed using the Mimics software (Materialize NV) (**Figure 2**). The size of the prosthesis corresponded to that of the lost portion of the clavicle,

The Prosthesis was manufactured by using 3D printer selective laser melting. The material used was Ti-6Al-4V alloy powder. The prosthesis Size of pores were 900 microns air and 100 microns solid, and the Volume of pores to the e whole implant was 60% while Weight of pores to whole implant body is 38%. The prosthesis was structured from mesh and 2 holes on the medial part of both sides to reduce the modulus. The surface of the prosthesis was polished without any coating (**Figure 3**). We created three designs to reach the best one which simulate bony part of clavicle.

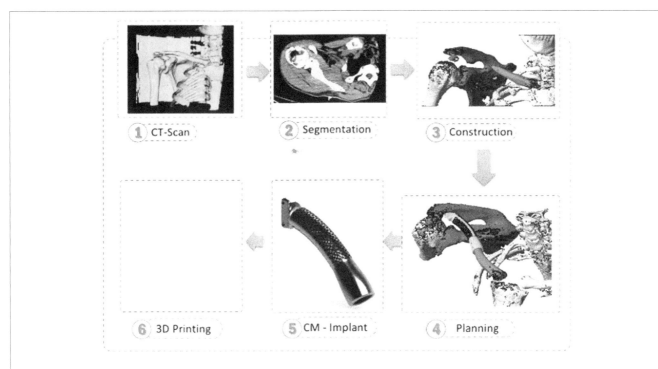

FIGURE 2 | The process of manufacturing of the prosthesis. The three-dimensional model of the clavicle was developed using the digital imaging and communication in medicine format, and image segmentation was performed using the Mimics software (Materialize NV).

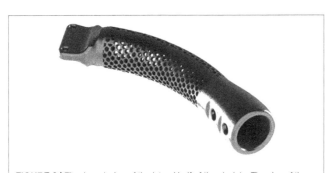

FIGURE 3 | Titanium design of the lateral half of the clavicle. The size of the prosthesis corresponded to that of the lost portion of the clavicle, and the prosthesis had a porous structure to reduce the modulus.

After completion, the 3D computer models and the designed model were imported into the ANSYS Workbench 15.0 (ANSYS Inc., Canonsburg, PA, USA) for finite element analysis. The stress distribution and deformation were calculated using the ANSYS Workbench. The boundary conditions applied are two fixed points at the ends of the implant on the lateral side and medial side. Thereafter, the effect of dynamic load location on the clavicle is applied with tension loads in two directions of the later side and medial side with an amount assumed to be 150 N to simulate the real case. The maximum stress was tested. The maximum stress was present at the middle third of the clavicle length, which is a characteristic of clavicle fractures in real life. While the maximum elongation was 50 microns and 75 microns in the lateral and medial sides, respectively. Thus, a comparison of the stresses predicted and the load location by finite element

analysis suggested that the results could be in the same range (**Figure 4**).

We validated the results of FEA to check the results given by FEA software. This was done by comparison with experimental data, and comparison with other similar computation techniques.

Surgical Technique

The patient underwent the operation in the supine position. The operative site was sterilized from the lateral border of the acromion to the sternum, and then a horizontal skin incision was made on the superior surface of the clavicle. The skin, platysma, and subcutaneous tissue were raised, with care taken to avoid injury to the supraclavicular nerves. The fracture site was exposed and inspected; thereafter, the small fragments and sharp fracture ends were removed.

The prosthesis was fixed with the remaining normal portion of the clavicle using a press fit, and the entire prosthesis was filled with a synthetic bone substitute (**Figure 5**). The prosthesis was implanted and fixed to the acromion with non-absorbable sutures through small holes on the surface of the prosthesis. Thereafter, the wound was closed. The operating time was 1.5 h, the blood loss was 1 L, and there were no intra-operative complications.

Postoperative Care

The arm was maintained in a sling throughout the day for 2 weeks. Thereafter, active assisted ROM exercises of the shoulder at the scapular plane were initiated. Full active motion was started at 4 weeks, and strengthening and resistive exercises of the shoulder girdle were started at 6 weeks up to 12 weeks. The

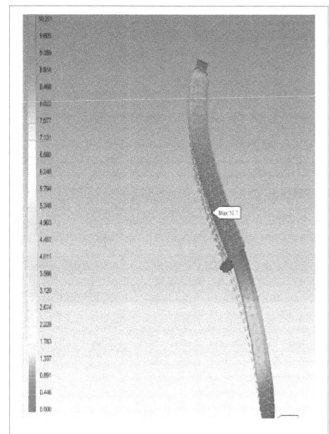

FIGURE 4 | Finite element analysis. A comparison of the stresses predicted and the load location suggest that the results could be in the same range.

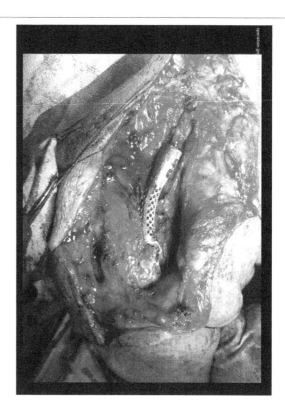

FIGURE 5 | Implantation of the prosthesis. The prosthesis was fixed with the remaining normal portion of the clavicle using a press fit, and the entire prosthesis was filled with a synthetic bone substitute.

progress of the exercises was dependent on the tolerance of the patient. By 6 months, the patient resumed her normal activities of daily living.

Outcomes

The VAS score for pain was 2, while the DASH score was 28, after 2 years post operation. The CT scan 6 months after the operation (**Figure 6**) revealed a good position for the prosthesis and no evidence of a stress fracture. Active ROM results of the shoulder at 1-year follow-up were flexion 125°, abduction 110°, external rotation 50°, and internal rotation 70°.

A radiographic examination at 2-year follow-up (**Figure 7**) revealed a good position of the prosthesis and no bony changes found. Muscle strengths compared with the uninjured shoulder at 2-year follow-up were maximum flexion strength 73%, maximum abduction strength 71%, maximum external rotation strength 65%, and maximum internal rotation strength 77%. Our patient was able to perform her activities of daily living but was not able to participate in sports activities that required a wider shoulder ROM, such as throwing.

DISCUSSION

This study described a case with comminuted lateral half clavicle fracture that was reconstructed using a 3D printed prosthesis

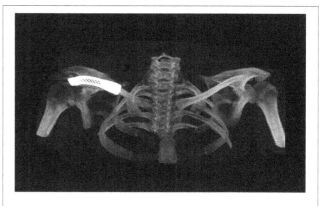

FIGURE 6 | Postoperative computed tomography scan 6 months after the operation revealed a good position for the prosthesis and no evidence of a stress fracture.

for treatment of the bone defect. The postoperative contours of the shoulder were acceptable to the patient, and there was no evidence of related complications, like infection or a rejection reaction. The procedure maintained the supportive function of the shoulder and protection for the major vessels and nerves at the base of neck.

The clavicle provides protection for the major vessels and nerves at the base of the neck and maintains an aesthetic

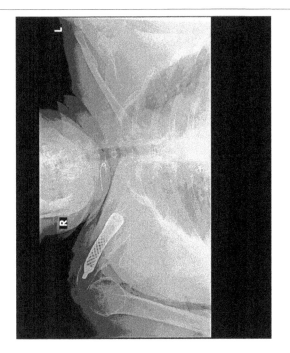

FIGURE 7 | Postoperative radiograph at 2-year follow-up revealed a good position of the prosthesis.

function by defining graceful curves. It also works as a support to hold the glenohumeral joint and increase the ROM (11). To our knowledge, there are two studies regarding bone defect reconstruction with cement prosthesis after clavicle tumor resections (5, 7), and 1 about a titanium prosthesis after total claviculectomy (11). The use of customized 3D printing prostheses has proved beneficial in many surgeries (12). In this study, 3D printing was used to construct a lateral half model of the clavicle, and the geometrical borders of the contralateral healthy clavicle were used to design the prosthesis. The largest differences between the reconstructed portion and the normal one were seen at the insertion sites of the tendons and ligaments, because the action of the muscles was limited in the reconstruction of the lateral half of the clavicle (13).

The Ti-6Al-4V alloy is considered biocompatible to the human body. One of the main desirable properties of biomaterials for orthopedic implants is the low modulus of elasticity due to bone reabsorption, besides biocompatibility, corrosion resistance, mechanical strength, fatigue resistance and wear resistance, which is especially the case of metallic materials.

The surface of prosthesis has a direct influence on its anchorage in bone. It is responsible for direct contact with patient tissues and is a key factor for Osseo integration (14); we designed the prosthesis from Ti-6Al-4V alloy.

Selective laser melting is one of the most widely used additive manufacturing processes for metallic materials, based on powder-bed fusion. It can be defined as a process whereby 3D functional parts can be produced by selectively scanning and consolidating a powder bed in a layer-wise manner. SLM provides many advantages over conventional processes such as ability to create complex geometries with internal cavities

or features without specific dies or tools, reduced lead time from design to testing, reduced need for assemblies, and joining processes resulting in less production costs (15). We use the selective laser melting at manufacturing of our prosthesis.

A good and lasting connection of the implant with the bone tissue is possible when there are sufficient conditions for the bone to grow into the pores of the material, therefore the use of a porous implant may be helpful in solving this problem Surface morphology is an important factor determining long-term implant stability, especially if bone quality is poor. A porous surface improves mechanical interlocking between the implant biomaterial and the surrounding natural tissue, providing greater mechanical stability at this critical interface (16), our prosthesis had Size of pores shape 900 microns air and 100 microns solid, Volume of pores shape to the whole implant shape is 60% and Weight of pores shape to whole implant body is 38%.

Finite element simulation techniques are being developed to provide mechanical responses and are used without any risks. These techniques provide definition about the load and material, as well as the value of the forces, using computation to investigate the biomechanics of the clavicle as a result of the surgical technique (17). Maximum stress occurs at the middle third of the clavicle length, which is a characteristic of clavicle fractures in normal life. During the dynamic strength analysis, the prosthesis in our study showed similar characteristics and resulted in the same range. The bone substitutes also had similar structural properties and compression strength, indicating that they are suitable for different clinical conditions (18, 19).

Finite element method (FEM) is a highly convenient and effective method to analyze near-real situations with the help of real-time, anticipated boundary and loading conditions, especially for biomedical applications. Computational structural analysis provides many approaches to successfully achieve the target. It is very difficult to analyze and predict exact mechanical behavior of adjacent tissues and implant inside the body (*in-vivo*), during the process of healing in orthopedic applications. Therefore, FEA is very helpful in designing and analyzing any medical device for optimality (20).

Using the FE method in our study was to provide a model allowing detecting the changes in bone characteristics leading to the manifestation of pathological conditions. Therefore, the focus in FE analysis is on creating an optimal FE model.

Validating the results of FEA it is extremely important to check the results given by FEA software (21). This was done by comparison with experimental data, and comparison with other similar computation techniques.

Limitations of this technique are the cost because it is custom made and is therefore more expensive, and, if the patient has any contraindications for CT scans or even surgery, this technique will be limited.

In conclusion, we advocate the use of this novel prosthesis for reconstruction of the lateral half of the clavicle after bone defects due to fracture. The advantages of the new prosthesis are that it replicates the dimensions of the normal bone; the patient could use her shoulder and return to activities of daily living and was satisfied with the aesthetics of the shoulder.

ETHICS STATEMENT

Written informed consent was obtained from the relevant individual for the publication of any potentially identifiable images or data included in this article.

AUTHOR CONTRIBUTIONS

SA did the finite element analysis and the design of the prosthesis. SMA did the surgery. KA manufacturing the prosthesis. AN

and EE-S substantial contributions to the conception and design of the work, drafting the work or revising it for important intellectual content, and final approval of the version to be published. All authors contributed to the article and approved the submitted version.

ACKNOWLEDGMENTS

The authors would like to acknowledge Mr. Abdallah A. Selim who opened the world of science to us and who helped us to get started.

REFERENCES

1. Sheehan SE, Gaviola G, Sacks A, Gordon R, Shi LL, Smith SE. Traumatic shoulder injuries: a force mechanism analysis of complex injuries to the shoulder girdle and proximal humerus. *Am J Roentgenol.* (2013) 201:409–24. doi: 10.2214/AJR.12.9986
2. Rubright J, Kelleher P, Beardsley C, Paller D, Shackford S, Beynnon B, et al. Long-term clinical outcomes, motion, strength, and function after total claviculectomy. *J Shoulder Elbow Surg.* (2014) 23:236–44. doi: 10.1016/j.jse.2013.05.011
3. Ieong E, Ferran NA. Lateral clavicle fracture fixation using a superiorly placed locking plate. *J Bone Joint Surg.* (2016) 6:e40. doi: 10.2106/JBJS.ST.16.00013
4. Stanley D, Trowbridge EA, Norris SH. The mechanism of clavicular fracture: a clinical and biomechanical analysis. *J Bone Joint Surg Br.* (1988) 70:461–4. doi: 10.1302/0301-620X.70B3.3372571
5. Lin B, He Y, Xu Y, Sha M. Outcome of bone defect reconstruction with clavicle bone cement prosthesis after tumor resection: a case series study. *BMC Musculoskel Dis.* (2014) 15:183. doi: 10.1186/1471-2474-15-183
6. Strong DH, Strong MW, Hermans D, Duckworth D. Operative management of clavicular malunion in midshaft clavicular fractures: a report of 59 cases. *JSES.* (2019) 28:2343–9. doi: 10.1016/j.jse.2019.04.058
7. Vartanian SM, Colaco S, Orloff LE, Theodore PR. Oklahoma prosthesis: resection of tumor of clavicle and chest wall reconstructed with a custom composite graft. *Ann Thorac Surg.* (2006) 82:332–4. doi: 10.1016/j.athoracsur.2005.09.029
8. Zou Y, Yang Y, Han Q, Yang K, Zhang K, Wang J, et al. Novel exploration of customized 3D printed shoulder prosthesis in revision of total shoulder arthroplasty: a case report. *Medicine.* (2018) 97:e13282. doi: 10.1097/MD.0000000000013282
9. Cronskär M, Rasmussen J, Tinnsten M. Combined finite element and multibody musculoskeletal investigation of a fractured clavicle with reconstruction plate. *Comput Method Biomech.* (2015) 18:740–8. doi: 10.1080/10255842.2013.845175
10. Smith MV, Calfee RP, Baumgarten KM, Brophy RH, Wright RW. Upper extremity-specific measures of disability and outcomes in orthopaedic surgery. *J Bone Joint Surg Am.* (2012) 94:277–85. doi: 10.2106/JBJS.J.01744

11. Fan H, Fu J, Li X, Pei Y, Li X, Pei G, et al. Implantation of customized 3-D printed titanium Prosthesis in limb salvage surgery: a case series and review of the literature. *World J Surg Oncol.* (2015) 13:308. doi: 10.1186/s12957-015-0723-2
12. Cheah JW, Goodman JZ, Dang AC. Clavicle fracture malunion treated with an osteotomy guided by a three-dimensional-printed model: a case report. *J Bone Joint Surg.* (2018) 8:1–4. doi: 10.2106/JBJS.CC.17.00304
13. Benazzi S, Orlandi M, Gruppioni G. Technical note: virtual reconstruction of a fragmentary clavicle. *Am J Phys Anthropol.* (2009) 138:507–14. doi: 10.1002/ajpa.20997
14. Jardini AL, Larosa MA, Maciel R Fo, Zavaglia CAC, Bernardes LF, Lambert CS, et al. Cranial reconstruction: 3D biomodel and custom-built implant created using additive manufacturing. *J Cranio Maxillo Fac Surg.* (2014) 42:1877–84. doi: 10.1016/j.jcms.2014.07.006
15. Yang J, Yu H, Yin J, Gao M, Wang Z, Zeng X. Formation and control of martensite in Ti-6Al-4V alloy produced by selective laser melting. *Mater Des.* (2016) 108:308–18. doi: 10.1016/j.matdes.2016.06.117
16. Mierzejewska ZA, Hudák R, Sidun J. Mechanical properties and microstructure of DMLS Ti6Al4V alloy dedicated to biomedical applications. *Materials.* (2019) 12:1–17. doi: 10.3390/ma12010176
17. Marie C. Strength analysis of clavicle fracture fixation devices and fixation technique using finite element analysis with musculoskeletal force input. *Med Biol Eng Comput.* (2015) 53:759–69. doi: 10.1007/s11517-015-1288-5
18. Webb JC, Spencer RF. The role of polymethylmethacrylate bone cement in modern orthopaedic surgery. *J Bone Joint Surg Br.* (2007) 89:851–7. doi: 10.1302/0301-620X.89B7.19148
19. Saito T, Kumagai K, Akamatsu Y, Kobayashi H, Kusayama Y. Five-to ten-year outcome following medial opening-wedge high tibial osteotomy with rigid plate fixation in combination with an artificial bone substitute. *Bone Joint J.* (2014) 96:339–44. doi: 10.1302/0301-620X.96B3.32525
20. Ruffoni D, Van Lenthe GH. 3.10 Finite element analysis in bone research: a computational method relating structure to mechanical function. *Compr Biomater II.* (2017) 3:169–96. doi: 10.1016/B978-0-12-803581-8.09798-8
21. Taddei F, Schileo E, Helgason B, Cristofolini L, Viceconti M. The material mapping strategy influences the accuracy of CT-based finite element models of bones: an evaluation against experimental measurements. *Med Eng Phys.* (2007) 29:973–9. doi: 10.1016/j.medengphy.2006.10.014

16

Complicated Postoperative Flat Back Deformity Correction with the Aid of Virtual and 3D Printed Anatomical Models

Jennifer Fayad [1,2,3], Mate Turbucz [2,4], Benjamin Hajnal [2], Ferenc Bereczki [2,4], Marton Bartos [5], Andras Bank [6], Aron Lazary [3,6†] and Peter Endre Eltes [2,3†]*

[1] *In Silico Biomechanics Laboratory, National Center for Spinal Disorders, Buda Health Center, Budapest, Hungary,*
[2] *Department of Industrial Engineering, Alma Mater Studiorum, Universita di Bologna, Bologna, Italy,* [3] *Department of Spine Surgery, Semmelweis University, Budapest, Hungary,* [4] *School of PhD Studies, Semmelweis University, Budapest, Hungary,* [5] *Do3D Innovations Ltd., Budapest, Hungary,* [6] *National Center for Spinal Disorders, Buda Health Center, Budapest, Hungary*

Correspondence:
Aron Lazary
aron.lazary@bhc.hu

[†] *These authors have contributed equally to this work*

Introduction: The number of patients with iatrogenic spinal deformities is increasing due to the increase in instrumented spinal surgeries globally. Correcting a deformity could be challenging due to the complex anatomical and geometrical irregularities caused by previous surgeries and spine degeneration. Virtual and 3D printed models have the potential to illuminate the unique and complex anatomical-geometrical problems found in these patients.

Case Presentation: We present a case report with 6-months follow-up (FU) of a 71 year old female patient with severe sagittal and coronal malalignment due to repetitive discectomy, decompression, laminectomy, and stabilization surgeries over the last 39 years. The patient suffered from severe low back pain (VAS = 9, ODI = 80). Deformity correction by performing asymmetric 3-column pedicle subtraction osteotomy (PSO) and stabilization were decided as the required surgical treatment. To better understand the complex anatomical condition, a patient-specific virtual geometry was defined by segmentation based on the preoperative CT. The geometrical accuracy was tested using the Dice Similarity Index (DSI). A complex 3D virtual plan was created for the surgery from the segmented geometry in addition to a 3D printed model.

Discussion: The segmentation process provided a highly accurate geometry (L1 to S2) with a DSI value of 0.92. The virtual model was shared in the internal clinical database in 3DPDF format. The printed physical model was used in the preoperative planning phase, patient education/communication and during the surgery. The surgery was performed successfully, and no complications were registered. The measured change in the sagittal vertical axis was 7 cm, in the coronal plane the distance between the C7 plumb line and the central sacral vertical line was reduced by 4 cm. A 30° correction was achieved for the lumbar lordosis due to the PSO at the L4 vertebra. The patient ODI was reduced to 20 points at the 6-months FU.

Conclusions: The printed physical model was considered advantageous by the surgical team in the pre-surgical phase and during the surgery as well. The model was able to simplify the geometrical problems and potentially improve the outcome of the surgery by preventing complications and reducing surgical time.

Keywords: 3D printed anatomical models, flat back deformity, 3D virtual model, 3DPDF, fused deposition modeling

INTRODUCTION

As the number of instrumented spinal operations increases globally, the group of patients with iatrogenic spinal deformities is growing (1). Loss of lordosis, development of segmental or global kyphosis after a shorter or longer thoracolumbar stabilization are the most common form of iatrogenic (so called "flat back") deformities (2). Beyond the consequent spinal canal stenosis, the disturbance of global balance can result in severe disability and pain where only surgical correction of the spinal alignment can provide significant functional improvement (2). The common sagittal balance problem in some cases is complicated with coronal imbalance, making the surgical correction procedure more complex. Further anatomical and geometrical irregularities caused by the previous surgeries (e.g., lack of anatomical landmarks, segmental bony deformations) makes the situation more challenging. In such cases, meticulous preoperative planning and proper implementation of the surgical plan are the keys to success and advanced scientific tools are needed to support the process and improve the outcome.

Here, we present the case of an elderly female patient with severe sagittal and coronal malalignment due to repetitive spine surgical interventions for over 39 years. Virtual and 3D printed patient-specific models were used to understand the unique and complex anatomical-geometrical problem and to plan the proper surgical correction.

CASE PRESENTATION

Medical History

A 71-year-old female patient was admitted to our institution. She suffered from severe low back pain, irradiating to the left leg, and an inability to walk more than 50 m due to fatigue in both lower extremities. There were some significant, treated comorbidities in her medical history: chronic hypertension, non-insulin-dependent (type II) diabetes, and ischemic heart disease. Previously, the patient's back problems were treated in other hospitals. The first discectomy surgery at the level of L4/S1 was performed 39 years ago, since then a mild L5 sensory-motor deficit persisted on the right side. Sixteen years later, L4/5

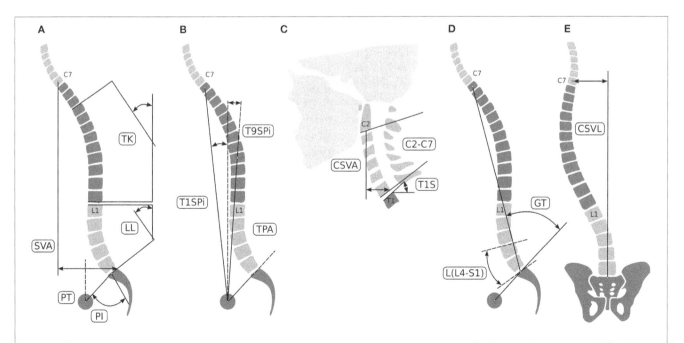

FIGURE 1 | Spinal alignment evaluation. Sagittal spino-pelvic parameters **(A–C)** for the assessment of the alignment [A–C adopted from Lafage et al. (4)]: pelvic parameters measured were PI, PT, and SS. Regional spinal parameters included PI-LL mismatch, LL, and TK. Global alignment was assessed linearly by SVA and the angular measurements of T1SPI, T9SPI, and TPA. Cervical parameters were composed of T1 slope, C2–C7 cervical lordosis, and C2–C7 SVA. **(D)** For the GAP score L4-S1 lordosis L(L4-S1) and the global tilt (GT) were defined. **(E)** Coronal alignment is assessed by measuring the distance between the center of the C7 vertebral body and the CSVL.

discectomy was performed followed by an L3/4 discectomy a year later. A repeated discectomy was done at L4/5 level 4 years ago, followed by a discectomy/decompression at the L2/3 level due to signs of cauda syndrome. The last surgical intervention in another hospital was done a year later (3 years ago), when an L2-L4 posterior stabilization and L3 laminectomy without intervertebral fusion was performed.

Evaluation and Analysis

Physical examination showed severe sagittal and coronal imbalance, compromised gait, tenderness at the lower back area and spastic muscles. She suffered from mild distal motor weakness in both lower extremities and numbness of the left leg. Based on her examination and imaging studies [full spine X-ray, lumbar CT (**Supplementary Figure 1**) and MRI (**Supplementary Figure 2**)], the severe lumbar sagittal and coronal malalignment was identified as the primary source of pain. Beside the deformity, non-union and partial implant loosening at the L2-L4 segments, and degenerative instability at the L1/2 and L3/4 segments were diagnosed. Patient's pain was assessed by Visual Analog Scale (VAS = 9 preoperatively), and disability was measured using the Oswestry Disability Index (ODI = 80% preoperatively) (3). Surgical treatment was indicated considering the spinal pathology, severe pain, disability, and life quality deterioration.

Analysis of Spinopelvic Alignment in Terms of Surgical Correction

Global balance and spinopelvic alignment were analyzed to determine the objective of the correction. Parameters describing the spinopelvic alignment were calculated from standing X-ray using the Surgimap software (Nemaris Inc., New York, NY, USA). Pelvic incidence (PI), pelvic tilt (PT), sacral slope (SS), lumbar lordosis (LL), and thoracic kyphosis (TK) were measured (4) (**Figure 1**). Global sagittal alignment parameters such as the sagittal vertical axis (SVA), T1 spinopelvic inclination (T1SPi), T9 spinopelvic inclination (T9SPi), and T1 pelvic angle (TPA) were also calculated (5). The Global Alignment and Proportion (GAP) Score was calculated according to the method published by Yilgor et al. (6). The coronal alignment was assessed by measuring the distance between the center of C7 vertebral body and the central sacral vertical line (CSVL) (7). The measurements are summarized in **Table 1**.

The central origin of the patient's complaint was the loss of lordosis at the lumbar spine due to the degenerative and iatrogenic processes. The patient's global balance was characterized as an imbalance both in the sagittal and coronal planes. The GAP score was 8 preoperatively, corresponding to severely disproportioned alignment. Therefore, the aim of the surgical correction was the 3D correction of the lumbar alignment. To calculate the degree of the desired lordosis correction, different approaches were sequentially applied. First, we used the formula published by Le Huec et al. (8) to calculate the ideal lumbar lordosis (ILL) corresponding to the pelvic anatomy of the patient. According to their formula (LL = $0.54*PI + 27.6°$) the ILL was $57°$. Second, the ILL was adjusted by the patient's age to avoid overcorrection and to decrease

TABLE 1 | Parameters for the evaluation of the spinal alignment pre- and postoperatively.

Parameter	Preop	Postop
PI (°)	55	55
PT (°)	27	21
SS (°)	28	34
LL (°)	17	47
PI-LL (°)	38	8
TL (°)	2	5
TK (°)	16	30
T9SPI (°)	0	6
T1SPI (°)	7	1
TPA (°)	34	22
T1S (°)	41	31
CL (°)	39	32
GT (°)	12	28
L(L4-S1) (°)	14	31
C2-C7 SVA (mm)	12	20
SVA C7-S1 (mm)	156	82
C7 to CSVL distance (mm)	48	5
GAP score	8	3

surgical invasiveness (4, 9, 10). In the age-group of 65–74-year-old, the threshold of spino- pelvic alignment parameters to avoid significant disability (ODI > 40%) are SVA = 9 cm, PI-LL = 18°, PT = 26°. The threshold values for minimal disability (ODI < 20%) are SVA = 5 cm, PI-LL = 6°, PT = 23°. According to these data (10), target values of SVA between 5 and 9 cm, PI-LL between 6 and 18° and PT between 23 and 25° were determined for the alignment correction. A LL between 37° and 49° corresponded to these parameters, therefore the desired total lordosis correction was 20–32°. Considering all of the surgical issues, and the optimal lordosis distribution, an L1/L2 and L3/L4 transforaminal lumbar interbody fusions (TLIF) and alignment correction by performing an asymmetric pedicle substraction osteotomy (PSO) of about 20° at the L4 level as well as stabilization from Th9 to the iliac bone with posterior fusion was decided as the required surgical intervention to treat the patient.

Virtual and 3D Printed Models of the Surgery

To better understand the complex anatomical condition at the lower lumbar level, especially in the neuro foraminal and central spinal canal area, patient-specific virtual and physical models were created based on the pre-op CT (**Figure 2**). The CT data were exported from the hospital PACS in DICOM file format. To comply with the ethical approval and the patient data protection policies, anonymization of the DICOM data was performed using Clinical Trial Processor software (CTP, RSNA, USA) (11). The segmentation process was performed on the 2D CT images (12). The thresholding algorithm and manual segmentation tools (erase, paint, fill etc.) were used in 3D Slicer 4.1.1 free

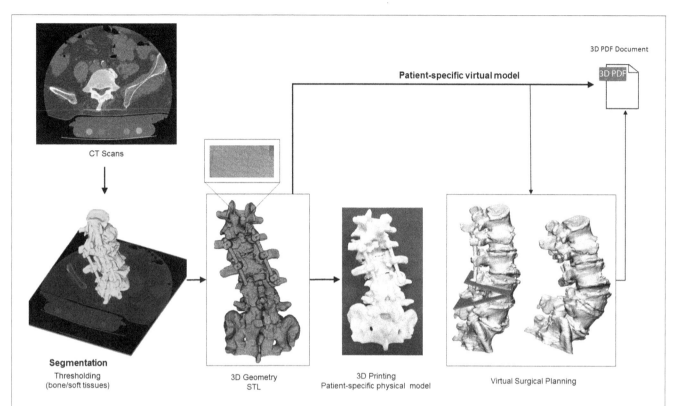

FIGURE 2 | Definition of virtual 3D geometry from CT scan. During the segmentation process the bone volume is first separated from the surrounding soft tissue by thresholding of the greyscale levels of the CT images. The resulting mask (green) voxels represent the 3D volume of the L1-S1 spine segment. Then, from the mask, a triangulated surface mesh is generated in STL format. The STL file serves as an input for 3D printing, with FDM technology. The virtual patient-specific geometry can be edited in CAD software in order to perform virtual surgical intervention (L4 PSO). The virtual geometries are then integrated in the clinical communication as a 3DPDF document.

software (Brigham and Women's Hospital, Boston, MA, USA) (13), **Figure 2**. To evaluate the accuracy of the segmentation process, the Dice Similarity Index (DSI) was calculated (14), obtaining a value of 0.92 and thus providing a highly accurate geometry. Inspection and correction of the 3D geometry was performed with MeshLab 1.3.2 free software (CNR, Pisa, Italy) (15) and universal remeshing with contour preservation was applied. The virtual geometry of the patient's spine [triangulated surface mesh, STereoLithography (STL) format] was printed with a *Fused Deposition Modeling* (FDM) device (Dimension 1200es 3D Printer; Stratasys, Israel; filament type: ABS*plus* in ivory,/scaffold: Soluble Support Technology, SST). In parallel to the printing process, a complex 3D virtual plan was created for the surgery in Autodesk Fusion 360 (Autodesk Inc., California, U.S.A.) Computer Aided Design (CAD) software. First the STL model was converted into a solid body, and then virtually we cut out a wedge shape from the L4 vertebra for an asymmetric 3-column pedicle subtraction osteotomy (PSO) with 20° correction in the sagittal plane. The virtual model and virtual surgical plan was imported in STL format to MeshLab 1.3.2 and subsequently saved as a Universal 3D File (U3D). A 3D Portable Document Format (3DPDF) file, containing the U3D mesh, was created using Adobe Acrobat (version 10 Pro Extended) 3D tools with default activation settings. The 3D visualization parameters were set as follows: CAD optimized lights, white background, solid rendering style, and default 3D conversion settings. The 3DPDF file was then incorporated in the institutional web browser-based SQL database (Oracle Database 12c) as previously described in the literature (16). The document was accessible by clinicians from any institutional desktop PC or mobile device.

Surgical Treatment and Outcome

The surgery was successfully performed without any complications (OR time: 270 min, blood loss: 750 ml). The patient was discharged from the hospital in good condition, 4 days after surgery. 30 degrees of lumbar lordosis correction was achieved, the majority at the L4-S1 levels (17°) (**Figure 3**, **Table 1**). The measured change in the sagittal vertical axis (SVA) was 7 cm. In the coronal plane, the C7 to CSVL distance was reduced by 4 cm. The GAP score decreased significantly from 8 to 3. ODI decreased at the 6-months FU to 20 points from 80, the VAS for the LBP decreased to 3 from 9 (17).

DISCUSSION

Clinical studies about the benefits of new visualization and 3D printing techniques are still very rare worldwide (18). Patient-specific tangible, 3D printed physical models can improve

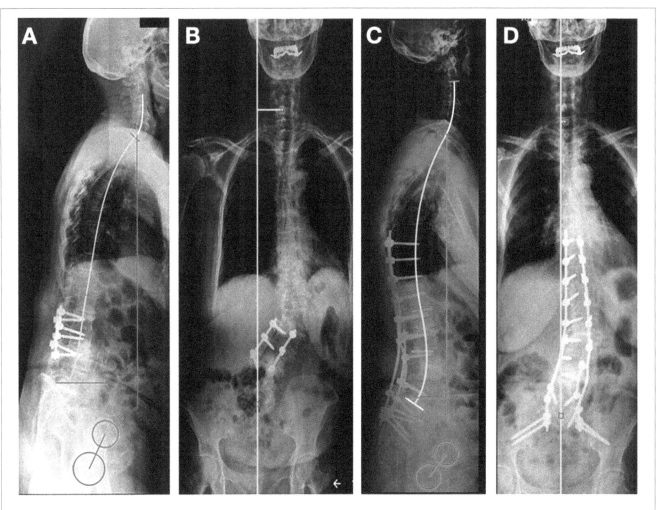

FIGURE 3 | Preoperative **(A,B)** and postoperative **(C,D)** standing X-rays for sagittal **(A,C)** and coronal **(B,D)** spinal alignment evaluation, using the Surgimap software sagittal alignment tools. In the sagittal plane, the SVA was reduced by 7.4 cm compared to the preoperative X-rays due to the Th9-Ileum fixation, correction with the L3-L4 intervertebral fusion (TLIF) and the 3-column osteotomy at the L4 level. The coronal alignment was corrected by reducing the distance between C7 to CSVL from 4.8 cm pre-op **(B)** to 0.5 cm post-op **(D)**.

surgical performance and outcome compared to the sole on-screen inspection of the virtual models (19). 3D printed physical models through haptic perception improve understanding of 3D shapes compared to visual perception only (20–22). In a survey based study among the members of AOSpine (23), a high interest among spine surgeons toward the incorporation of 3D technologies (virtual or 3D printed models) into the clinical practice was recorded. The Radiological Society of North America (RSNA) 3D printing Special Interest Group (SIG) published (24) guidelines for medical 3D printing and appropriateness for clinical scenarios. The recommended scenarios do not include the iatrogenic adolescent spinal deformity; although this case demonstrates the benefits.

In a recent systematic review by Lopez et al. (25), in adult spinal deformity, the usage of 3D printing in preoperative planning and in the manufacturing of surgical guides is associated with increased screw accuracy and favorable deformity correction outcomes. In our study, the physical model not only

provided guidance in the preoperative planning phase, but also aided the surgeon in understanding the complex anatomy during the surgery.

It is challenging in the surgical management of adult spinal deformity to determine the degree of planned correction, particularly in patients with severe preoperative malalignment. Less aggressive correction may constitute a reasonable compromise between radiographic alignment goals and perioperative and postoperative risk (9). The Surgimap software allowed the measurement of pre- and postoperative X-rays with ease and speed, providing a vast array of opportunities for assessment of spinal deformity and surgical planning. The aid of 3D virtual and 3D printed models, and X-ray based planning software allowed us to achieve a LL of 47° after the surgery providing the restoration of global balance showed by the improvement of the GAP score. The well-planned surgical correction of the lumbar alignment provided the restoration of the global spinopelvic balance, resulting in the reduction in pain and disability as well as improvement in health-related quality of life. The improved global parameter (GAP score of 3) corresponds to a moderately disproportioned alignment with low chance of postoperative mechanical complication (6).

The limitation of the described approach is that currently it is uncommon for medical centers to have access to a 3D printing facility or lack the know-how for image processing needed for model preparation. The time needed for the presented visualization, printing, and planning is also a limitation as it is not always available before surgery.

CONCLUSION

A patient-specific 3D virtual and printed physical geometry as well as computer-aided surgical planning were used to develop the optimal surgical plan for the deformity correction in a complicated iatrogenic adult spinel deformity case. The surgery was successfully implemented providing the planned correction of the lumbar alignment. The printed physical model was considered advantageous by the surgical team in the pre-surgical phase and during the surgery as well. The chosen FDM technology provided an accurate, robust, and affordable physical model. The model not only clarifies the geometrical problems, but it can also improve the outcome of the surgery by preventing complications and reducing surgical time.

ETHICS STATEMENT

The study was approved by the National Ethics Committee of Hungary, the National Institute of Pharmacy and Nutrition (Reference Number: ETT TUKEB IV/6329-1/2020/EKU). Informed consent was obtained from the participant. The patients/participants provided their written informed consent to participate in this study. Written informed consent was obtained from the individual(s) for the publication of any potentially identifiable images or data included in this article.

AUTHOR CONTRIBUTIONS

PE and AL contributed to the conception and design of the study. PE, JF, FB, MT, and BH did the CT based image analyses which provided the 3D visualizations, the virtual model, and the CAD design. PE, JF, and AL performed the pre and postoperative X-ray measurements. MB and MT provided the 3D print. AL, AB, and PE performed the surgery described in this case report. PE and JF wrote the first draft of the manuscript and prepared the pictures together with AL. All authors contributed to manuscript revision, read, and approved the submitted version.

REFERENCES

1. Diebo BG, Shah NV, Boachie-Adjei O, Zhu F, Rothenfluh DA, Paulino CB, et al. Adult spinal deformity. *Lancet.* (2019) 394:160–72. doi: 10.1016/S0140-6736(19)31125-0
2. Potter BK, Lenke LG, Kuklo TR. Prevention and management of iatrogenic flatback deformity. *JBJS.* (2004) 86:1793–808. doi: 10.2106/00004623-200408000-00027
3. Valasek T, Varga PP, Szövérfi Z, Kümin M, Fairbank J, Lazary A. Reliability and validity study on the Hungarian versions of the Oswestry Disability Index and the Quebec Back Pain Disability Scale. *Eur Spine J.* (2013) 22:1010–8. doi: 10.1007/s00586-012-2645-9
4. Lafage R, Ferrero E, Henry JK, Challier V, Diebo B, Liabaud B, et al. Validation of a new computer-assisted tool to measure spino-pelvic parameters. *Spine J.* (2015) 15:2493–502. doi: 10.1016/j.spinee.2015.08.067
5. Protopsaltis TS, Schwab FJ, Smith JS, Klineberg EO, Mundis GM, Hostin RA, et al. The T1 pelvic angle (TPA), a novel radiographic parameter of sagittal deformity, correlates strongly with clinical measures of disability. *Spine J.* (2013) 13:S61. doi: 10.1016/j.spinee.2013.07.173
6. Yilgor C, Sogunmez N, Yavuz Y, Boissiere L, Obeid I, Acaroglu E, et al. Global alignment and proportion (GAP) score: development and validation of a new method of analyzing spinopelvic alignment to predict mechanical complications after adult spinal deformity surgery. *Spine J.* (2017) 17:S155–6. doi: 10.1016/j.spinee.2017.07.234
7. Bess S, Protopsaltis TS, Lafage V, Lafage R, Ames CP, Errico T, et al. Clinical and radiographic evaluation of adult spinal deformity. *J Spinal Disord Tech.* (2016) 29:6–16. doi: 10.1097/BSD.0000000000000352
8. Le Huec JC, Thompson W, Mohsinaly Y, Barrey C, Faundez A. Sagittal balance of the spine. *Eur Spine J.* (2019) 28:1889–905. doi: 10.1007/s00586-019-06083-1
9. Ailon T, Smith JS, Shaffrey CI, Lenke LG, Brodke D, Harrop JS, et al. Degenerative spinal deformity. *Neurosurgery.* (2015) 77:S75–91. doi: 10.1227/NEU.0000000000000938
10. Lafage R, Schwab F, Challier V, Henry JK, Gum J, Smith J, et al. Defining Spino-pelvic alignment thresholds: should operative goals in adult spinal deformity surgery account for age? *Spine.* (2016) 41: 62–8. doi: 10.1097/BRS.0000000000001171
11. Aryanto KYE, Oudkerk M, van Ooijen PMA. Free DICOM de-identification tools in clinical research: functioning and safety of patient privacy. *Eur Radiol.* (2015) 25:3685–95. doi: 10.1007/s00330-015-3794-0
12. Bozic KJ, Keyak JH, Skinner HB, Bueff HU, Bradford DS. Three-dimensional finite element modeling of a cervical vertebra: an investigation of burst fracture mechanism. *J Spinal Disord.* (1994) 7:102–10. doi: 10.1097/00002517-199407020-00002
13. Kikinis R, Pieper SD, Vosburgh KG. 3D Slicer: a platform for subject-specific image analysis, visualization, clinical support. In: *Intraoperative Imaging and Image-Guided Therapy.* New York, NY: Springer New York (2014). p. 277–89.
14. Zou KH, Warfield SK, Bharatha A, Tempany CMC, Kaus MR, Haker SJ, et al. Statistical validation of image segmentation quality based on a spatial overlap index. *Acad Radiol.* (2004) 11:178–89. doi: 10.1016/S1076-6332(03)00671-8
15. Cignoni P, Callieri M, Corsini M, Dellepiane M, Ganovelli F, Ranzuglia G. Meshlab: an open-source mesh processing tool. In: *Eurographics Italian Chapter Conference.* Salerno (2008). p. 129–36.
16. Eltes PE, Bartos M, Hajnal B, Pokorni AJ, Kiss L, Lacroix D, et al. Development of a computer-aided design and finite element analysis combined method for affordable spine surgical navigation with 3D-printed customized template. *Front Surg.* (2021) 7:1–10. doi: 10.3389/fsurg.2020.583386
17. Rocchi MB, Sisti D, Benedetti P, Valentini M, Bellagamba S, Federici A. Critical comparison of nine different self-administered questionnaires for the evaluation of disability caused by low back pain. *Eura Medicophys.* (2005) 41:275–81.
18. Wilcox B, Mobbs RJ, Wu A-M, Phan K. Systematic review of 3D printing in spinal surgery: the current state of play. *J spine Surg.* (2017) 3:433–43. doi: 10.21037/jss.2017.09.01
19. Zheng Y, Yu D, Zhao J, Wu Y, Zheng B. 3D printout models vs. 3D-rendered images: which is better for preoperative planning? *J Surg Educ.* (2016) 73:518–23. doi: 10.1016/j.jsurg.2016.01.003
20. Wijntjes MWA, Volcic R, Pont SC, Koenderink JJ, Kappers AML. Haptic perception disambiguates visual perception of 3D shape. *Exp Brain Res.* (2009) 193:639–44. doi: 10.1007/s00221-009-1713-9
21. Norman JF, Norman HF, Clayton AM, Lianekhammy J, Zielke G. The visual and haptic perception of natural object shape. *Percept Psychophys.* (2004) 66:342–51. doi: 10.3758/BF03194883

22. Norman JF, Clayton AM, Norman HF, Crabtree CE. Learning to perceive differences in solid shape through vision and touch. *Perception.* (2008) 37:185–96. doi: 10.1068/p5679

23. Eltes PE, Kiss L, Bartos M, Eösze Z, Szövérfi Z, Varga PP, et al. Attitude of spine surgeons towards the application of 3D technologies-a survey of AOSpine members. *Ideggyogy Sz.* (2019) 72:227–35. doi: 10.18071/isz.72.0227

24. Chepelev L, Wake N, Ryan J, Althobaity W, Gupta A, Arribas E, et al. Radiological Society of North America (RSNA) 3D printing Special Interest Group (SIG): guidelines for medical 3D printing and appropriateness for clinical scenarios. *3D Print Med.* (2018) 4:1–38. doi: 10.1186/s41205-018-0030-y

25. Lopez CD, Boddapati V, Lee NJ, Dyrszka MD, Sardar ZM, Lehman RA, et al. Three-dimensional printing for preoperative planning and pedicle screw placement in adult spinal deformity: a systematic review. *Glob Spine J.* (2020) 7:2192568220944170. doi: 10.1177/2192568220944170

17

Feasibility of Microwave-Based Scissors and Tweezers in Partial Hepatectomy: An Initial Assessment on Canine Model

Khiem Tran Dang[1,2], Shigeyuki Naka[3,4], Atsushi Yamada[1] and Tohru Tani[1*]

[1] Department of Research and Development for Innovative Medical Devices and Systems, Shiga University of Medical Science, Otsu, Japan, [2] Department of Surgery, University of Medicine and Pharmacy at Ho Chi Minh City, Ho Chi Minh City, Vietnam, [3] Department of Surgery, Shiga University of Medical Science, Otsu, Japan, [4] Department of Surgery, Hino Memorial Hospital, Hino, Japan

Correspondence:
Tohru Tani
tan@belle.shiga-med.ac.jp

Purpose: This study aimed to assess the feasibility of partial hepatectomy (PH) simplified by using microwave-based devices in animal experiments.

Methods: PH was performed on 16 beagles using either Acrosurg Scissors (AS) or Acrosurg Tweezers (AT) without hepatic pedicle (HP) control. Parenchymal transection time, Glissonean pedicle (GP) seal time, bleeding volume, bile leak, and burst pressure were recorded. Probable complications were investigated after 4 weeks.

Results: Transection time (6.5 [6.0–7.6] vs. 11.8 [10.5–20.2] min, $p < 0.001$) with AT were significantly shorter than with AS. GP sealing times (60 [55–60] vs. 57 [46–91] s, $p = 0.859$) by both devices were nearly similar. Bleeding volume in the AT group was approximately one-fourth of that in the AS group (6.7 [1.4–22] vs. 28.8 [5.8–48] mL, $p = 0.247$). AT created higher burst pressure on the bile duct stumps ($p = 0.0161$). The two devices did not differ significantly in morbidity and mortality after four-week follow-up.

Conclusion: Acrosurg devices achieved a safe PH without HP control owing to microwave-based sealing. AS could be used alone in PH, whereas the clamp-crushing function of AT seemed more advantageous in reducing the transection time and blood loss.

Keywords: microwave surgical device, scissors-type, tweezers-type, clamp crushing, partial hepatectomy

INTRODUCTION

Hepatectomy is the main surgical intervention for several liver diseases, especially liver tumors. When performing partial hepatectomy (PH), the most common problems that surgeons encounter are hemorrhage and bile leak (1, 2). Various strategies, including vascular control (Pringle maneuver, total hepatic vascular exclusion, low central venous pressure), and transection techniques (finger fracture, clamp crushing), are used to prevent intraoperative bleeding (3–5). In recent decades, many advanced surgical tools, such as ultrasonically activated devices (UAD), electrothermal bipolar vessel sealers (EBVS), Habib's coagulator, CUSA®, and staplers have also been introduced during liver surgery to reduce the risk associated with PH (6–10). However, none of the latest advanced energy devices could achieve a complete transection of both the hepatic parenchyma and the Glissonean pedicle (GP) safely without the assistance of other surgical tools or hemostatic agents (5, 11–15). The role of such energy devices in the occurrence of post-operative bile leak also remains controversial (16, 17). In practice, the clamp-crush technique under GP clamping is still favored for liver resection at many surgical centers (3, 5, 13, 15, 18), and PH still requires several surgical energy devices so far.

Amid the booming development of modern energy devices, our group invented microwave coagulation surgical instruments (MWCX) for use in many surgical procedures (19–21). The unique microwave dielectric heating by these original MWCX has demonstrated advantages of sealing sizable vessels (20, 22) as well as coagulating fragile parenchyma (spleen, liver) (21, 23). In 2017, two types of microwave surgical devices with improved coagulation power and energy efficiency of MWCX were released commercially: a scissors-type for seamless "seal-and-cut" dissection and a tweezers-type for forceful grasping and sealing of tissues. However, both the old MWCX and the updated scissors and tweezers have never been formally approved for PH as the main surgical instrument. In fact, due to the limitations of currently-used energy devices, hepatectomy needs several surgical tools for dissection, coagulation and cutting of the liver parenchyma as well as the Glissonean pedicle. Our devices could be the solution to this thorny problem.

Based on MWCXs' excellent tissue coagulation reported in previous studies (19–23), we hypothesized that using the new microwave scissors alone would enable PH and GP sealing, whereas the single microwave tweezers would be sufficient to reduce blood loss in this procedure. Therefore, this experimental study was set up to assess the feasibility of using the scissors-type or tweezers-type microwave devices as a single surgical instrument to achieve a safe and simple PH with respect to less bleeding, less risk of bile leaks, and the use of fewer instruments.

MATERIALS AND METHODS

Instruments

Two microwave surgical devices (Acrosurg, Nikkiso Co., Ltd., Tokyo, Japan), which have been commercialized based on our MWCX, were used in this study (20, 22, 23). One was the Acrosurg Scissors S09 (AS), and the other was the Acrosurg Tweezers S22 (AT). AS is comprised of a pistol-type handgrip with a microwave emitting button, a 90-mm-long shaft covering a microwave antenna, a 15-mm fixed lower blade, and a 15-mm rotating upper blade (**Figure 1A**). The thickness of the lower and upper blades is 2.5 and 1.4 mm, respectively. The central and outer electrodes of the microwave antenna are integrated into the fixed and rotating blades, respectively. Thus, microwaves can be emitted from the lower blade to the upper one while performing resection (**Figure 1C**). In contrast, AT has a pair of fine-serrated jaws whose width and length are 3.2 and 10 mm, respectively, similar to surgical thumb forceps (**Figure 1B**). Each jaw contains two outer electrodes placed in parallel alongside a central electrode of the microwave antenna so that microwaves circulate around each jaw independently when grasping or clamping tissues (**Figure 1D**). Both microwave devices are connected to a generator (ASG-01, Nikkiso Co.,

Ltd., Tokyo, Japan) that produces microwaves at 2,450 MHz (12-cm wavelength).

Animals

All procedures for the animal experiments were approved by Shiga University of Medical Science (SUMS) Ethical Committee for Animal Research. Sixteen female beagles weighing from 8.5 to 10.5 kg were raised in pathogen-free conditions according to the institutional regulations of SUMS Research Center for Animal Life Science (RCALS). We chose female beagles to facilitate the PH procedure because the male animal has a penis attached alongside the mid-line of the lower half of the abdomen, hindering an extended incision of the abdominal wall. Otherwise, animal sex does not affect the PH short-term outcomes. The beagles underwent general anesthesia with mixed medications: subcutaneous injection of ketamine hydrochloride (Ketalar 500 mg/10 mL, Daiichi Sankyo, Tokyo, Japan) at a dose of 25 mg/kg body weight and medetomidine chloride (Domitor 10 mg/10 mL, Orion Pharma, Espoo, Finland) at a dose of 20 µg/kg body weight. Anesthesia was maintained by inhaled insoflurane 1–2% via an endotracheal tube. The animal were mechanically ventilated with an oxygen-mixed inflow of positive-pressure air to keep the tidal volume in the range of 12–15 mL/kg (24). Physiologic saline 0.9% was intravenously infused at a rate of 180–200 mL/h for intraoperative resuscitation.

Procedures

All surgical procedures were performed by a single senior surgeon specialized in hepatic surgery (SN) with the assistance of a surgical fellow (KD). Sixteen beagles were allocated to two groups using either AS or AT. After receiving general anesthesia, the beagle was placed in the supine position. A 20-cm-midline incision from the xiphisternum to the umbilicus was made to expose the left lateral lobe (LLL) of the liver. The inner portion of the LLL, which had a separate GP, was selected for PH. The operation included three steps: (1) cut-line marking on the LLL surface; (2) parenchymal transection without hepatic pedicle (HP) occlusion; (3) GP sealing and cutting of the treated portion (**Figure 2**). The second and third steps depended on which device was employed.

When AS was used, the surgeon performed PH by using only this device. The power output was set at 60 W. The hepatic parenchyma was coagulated and cut seamlessly from the free edge toward the radical end of LLL adjacent to its proper GP. The corresponding GP was, in turn, sealed and cut afterward. When AT was used, the power output was set at 80 W. The hepatic parenchyma was grasped and gently crushed by the AT to isolate crossing vessels and bile ducts inside, while microwaves were concomitantly released from the AT jaws to coagulate the fragmented tissue. The coagulated part was then cut by using Metzenbaum scissors. This cycle was repeated toward the LLL radical end. Similarly, the GP was also sealed by AT and cut with Metzenbaum scissors.

In both protocols, parenchymal transection time and GP seal time were recorded separately. Bleeding volume was estimated in milliliters by subtracting the weight of new gauzes from the blood-soaked gauzes after the surgery using a conversion rate of

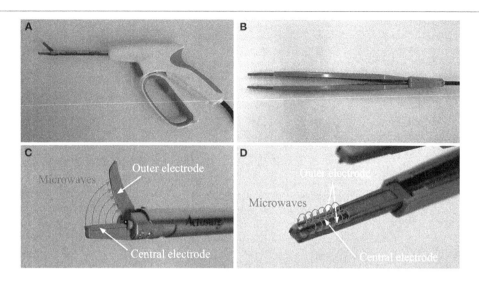

FIGURE 1 | Acrosurg Scissors: the central electrode of the microwave antenna is integrated within the lower blade and the upper blade contains the outer electrode **(A,C)**. Acrosurg Tweezers consists of two branches connected to each other at the hinged end and a bipolar forceps-styled tip. Each serrated jaw includes a central electrode and two parallel outer electrodes of the microwave antenna **(B,D)**.

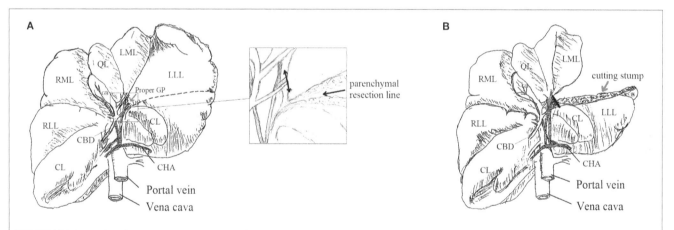

FIGURE 2 | Schema of partial hepatectomy (PH): beagle's liver with demarcated line for parenchymal transection [black dashed line, **(A)**]; parenchymal transection of the inner portion of LLL and its proper GP [double-headed arrow, squared image **(A)**]; liver remnant after PH and the sealed GP stump [black line, **(B)**]. LLL, Left Lateral Lobe; LML, Left Medial Lobe; QL, Quadrate Lobe; RML, Right Medial Lobe; RLL, Right Lateral Lobe; CL, Caudate Lobe; CBD, Common Bile Duct; GB, Gallbladder; CHA, Common Hepatic Artery; GP, Glissonean Pedicle.

$1\,g = 1\,mL$ (25). If excessive bleeding occurred, the lost blood was to be harvested by a suction system and its volume added to the total volume. The length and thickness of the resected portions and GP diameter were measured.

Before abdominal closure, new gauze was applied on the cutting stump of the remnant liver to check the bile-leak coloration; leaking was confirmed if yellowish fluid tinged the gauze. The dog was then transferred back to RCALS for post-operative follow-up. After 4 weeks, re-laparotomy was conducted to confirm any chronic adverse events (bleeding, abscess, ascites, adhesion). The extrahepatic bile ducts (EBDs) were harvested to test *ex vivo* the EBD sealing. In this test, a small catheter was inserted into the open lumen of the EBD. Physiologic saline 0.9% was administered gradually by an electric pump (KDJ20, KD Scientific, Inc., Holliston, Massachusetts) connected to a pressure amplifier (PA-001, Star Medical, Inc., Tokyo, Japan). Burst pressure was defined as the highest intraluminal pressure prior to EBD stump leakage (16).

All resected portions containing the GP stump and sealed EBDs were fixed in 10% neutral-buffered formalin, paraffinized, and sectioned into 2-μm-thick slides for hematoxylin and eosin (H&E) staining. Histological features were evaluated under a light microscope (Nikon Eclipse 90i, Nikon Corp., Tokyo, Japan) with image processing software (Image-Pro Plus version 7.0J, Media Cybernetics, Inc., Bethesda, Maryland).

Statistical Analyses

The data are presented as medians with interquartile ranges for continuous variables and as actual numbers for categorical variables. The cutting surface of the liver was approximated

TABLE 1 | Outcomes of partial hepatectomy using Acrosurg Scissors (AS) and Tweezers (AT).

Outcome	AS	AT	p*
Total operated cases	8	8	
Parenchymal transection			
Transection area (cm²)	12 [11.2–12.4]	12.7 [12.2–15.9]	0.082
Transection time (min)	11.8 [10.5–20.2]	6.5 [6.0–7.6]	0.0008
Transection speed (cm²/min)	0.9 [0.7–1.2]	2.1 [1.9–2.2]	0.0007
GP sealing			
GP diameter (mm)	7.9 [7.7–8.9]	11.1 [10–12.8]	0.003
GP seal time (s)	57 [46–91]	60 [55–60]	0.859
Intraoperative bleeding			
Bleeding volume (mL)	28.8 [5.8–48]	6.7 [1.4–22]	0.247
Bleeding rate (mL/cm²)§	2.4 [0.5–3.5]	0.5 [0.1–1.7]	0.292
Bile leak after hepatectomy	0	0	1.0
After 4-week follow-up			
Total cases observed	8	8	
Adhesion	6	3	0.351
Complication	1 (Ascites)	1 (Bile leak)	1.0
Death	1 (Gallbladder bed bleeding)	0	1.0

*p-value calculated by the Wilcoxon rank-sum test for quantitative data represented as median [interquartile range]; and by Fisher's exact test for qualitative data.
§ Bleeding rate calculated from the bleeding volume and transection area.
GP, Glissonean pedicle.

by an ellipsoidal shape. Thus, the transection area S (cm²) and transection speed v (cm²/min) were calculated by the following equations:

$$S = \pi ab \quad (a \text{ and } b \text{ represent half of the section length and thickness})$$

$$v = S/t \quad (t \text{ represents the transection time})$$

The bleeding rate (mL/cm²) was also calculated by dividing the bleeding volume by the transection area. All data were analyzed by a statistical software package (Stata 12.0, StataCorp., Lakeway Drive, Texas). Fisher's exact test was applied to compare two categorical variables, whereas the Wilcoxon rank-sum test was applied to test the difference between two quantitative groups; $p < 0.05$ was considered significant.

RESULTS

The PH outcomes using the Acrosurg devices (AS and AT) are presented in **Table 1**. The transection areas by both devices were not significantly different ($p = 0.082$). AT required only half of the transection time of AS to finish the parenchymal dissection (median: 6.5 vs. 11.8 min, $p < 0.001$). As a result, the transection speed of AT was two-fold higher than that of AS (median: 2.1 vs. 0.9 cm²/min, $p < 0.001$). AT sealed GP that had a larger diameter (median: 11.1 vs. 7.9 mm, $p = 0.003$) within a similar seal time (median: 60 vs. 57 s, $p = 0.859$) compared to AS.

TABLE 2 | Extrahepatic bile duct (EBD) sealing by two acrosurg devices.

Outcome	AS	AT	p*
Number of trials	6	6	
Diameter (mm)	1.8 [1.8–1.8]	3.4 [2.8–3.4]	0.0045
Burst pressure (mmHg)	607.5 [472–705]	806.5 [776–889]	0.0161

*p-value from Wilcoxon's ranksum test, data represented as median [interquartile range]. AS, Acrosurg Scissors; AT, Acrosurg Tweezers.

The bleeding volume in the AT group was estimated at less than one-fourth of that in the AS group (median: 6.7 vs. 28.8 mL, $p = 0.247$). PH using AS often encountered more oozing of blood than with AT (median bleeding rate: 2.4 vs. 0.5 mL/cm²). Most blood loss collected during the operation were determined to be parenchymal transection-related bleeding because all GP sealing was accomplished by both devices without any considerable bleeding. No blood loss was harvested by using a suction system. There was no bile leak at the cutting surface immediately after PH in both groups.

All dogs in the AT group were healthy after 4 weeks, whereas one dog from the AS group died on the 2nd post-operative day. Autopsy revealed many clots had accumulated at the infrahepatic recess, surrounding the gallbladder bed. The gallbladder of this dog had been removed because of a gallbladder laceration when performing PH. The old cutting stump remained dry without clotting or ongoing bleeding. There were no differences regarding complications between the two groups ($p = 1.0$). A pale bile-tinged coloration of the cutting stump was discovered in one case in the AT group that implied a probable bile leak. Adhesions were observed more frequently when using AS than with AT ($p = 0.351$).

Ex vivo experimental data are shown in **Table 2**. Although the EBD stumps sealed by both devices exhibited excellent burst pressure, AT-induced seals withstood a significantly higher burst pressure than that of AS-induced seals (median: 806.5 vs. 607.5 mmHg, $p = 0.0161$), and AT could seal larger EBDs ($p = 0.0045$).

Microscopic examination revealed that the GP stumps sealed by both devices showed complete fusion of the pedicle as well as its inside components, which were histologically indistinguishable. The surrounding area was covered by a layer of destroyed hepatocytes (**Figure 3A**). It was possible to observe the vacuolization in the interstitial zone alongside the GP, which indicated the unique characteristic of microwave coagulation in the tubal structures. The EBD samples revealed similar pathological features: all layers were denatured and fixed with interlayer vacuole-like spaces that created total occlusion of the sealed edges (**Figure 3C**). In particular, there was a flattened, well-coagulated segment in specimens sealed by AT due to the forceful compression from the serrated jaws of the tweezers (dashed lines, **Figures 3B,D**).

DISCUSSION

In this study, we assessed the contribution of two Acrosurg devices separately to achieve safe and simple PH. To date, one of the most widely-accepted strategies to control blood loss in

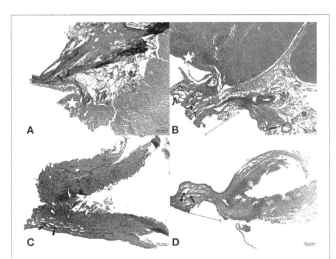

FIGURE 3 | Upper images: a microscopic view of a sealed Glissonean pedicle (GP) by AS **(A)** and AT **(B)**; Lower images: sealed EBD using AS **(C)** and AT **(D)**. The GP stumps in both groups were fused; their structures were histologically indistinct (H&E stain, x40). The vicinity of the GP was covered by a layer of deformed hepatocytes, which lost their normal texture [star mark, **(A,B)**]. Vacuolization caused by microwave energy existed along the GP's interstitial zones [black arrow, **(A,B)**]. Vacuole-like spaces also appeared in the EBD stumps [black arrow, **(C,D)**, x40] whose sealed edges revealed a deformed segment that fitted the serrated-jaws of the tweezers-type device [dashed lines, **(B,D)**]. AS, Acrosurg Scissors; AT, Acrosurg Tweezers; EBD, Extrahepatic bile duct; H&E, Hematoxylin and Eosin.

PH is the combination of inflow occlusion (Pringle maneuver) with some energy devices (EBVS, UAD) or a dissector (CUSA®, water jet) (7, 8, 18, 26, 27). As a result, a PH procedure requires several surgical instruments (dissectors, energy-based sealers, stapler etc.). Acrosurg devices have already proven their sealing capability in previous studies (19–21, 23). Hence, it was reasonable to test AS and AT as new instruments to reduce the number of instruments used for a PH.

In the present study, both AS and AT could achieve a complete parenchymal transection with minor bleeding (<30 mL). Even when adding up to 25% of the estimated blood loss, which was considered the "concealed" bleeding during the operation (25), to the total volume, the subsequent amount of bleeding remained <50 mL. The bleeding rates when using AS or AT were lower than those reported by recent studies that employed conventional energy devices in open hepatectomy. Although it is difficult to compare experimental data with clinical outcomes, the use of AT resulted in a bleeding rate that was less than one-sixth of the published clinical data (0.5 vs. 6.6, 5.04, 3.19, or 3.4 mL/cm^2) (7, 8, 15, 28). Both AS and AT gave positive outcomes in terms of transection speed. Although the speed with AS seemed equivalent to other energy devices, AT outperformed energy devices applied in previous studies (2.1 vs. 1.07, 1.11, and 1.16 cm^2/min) (7, 8, 28). The overwhelming cutting speed and minor bleeding associated with the use of AT compared to other energy devices (even with AS) might be explained by its sealing process. AT has serrated jaws to grasp and crush the tissue, which is then flattened under forceful compression. Owing to the crushing of the 3.2-mm-wide jaws, intrahepatic structures (artery, portal

vein, bile duct) were skeletonized within a narrow strip (equal to 3.2 mm) that allowed the surgeon to observe them clearly before conducting the coagulation. The use of AS precluded the identification of the underlying structures that were sandwiched by the hepatic parenchyma during the seamless transection. Therefore, the sealing zone could sometimes undergo premature resection that caused the oozing of blood on the cutting surface, requiring more time for recoagulation during the transection phase. Clinically, AS is suitable to perform a simple hepatectomy such as wedge resection whereas AT could be used for large liver resections which need firm hemostases. It is also possible to combine AT and AS to shorten the transection time.

The good results of Acrosurg devices are also attributed to the heating mechanism of microwaves. Microwaves are able to penetrate to the core of the induced liver portion and enable homogenous coagulation of the targeted tissue from inside to outside (29). Their dielectric heating also engenders less thermal injury, avoiding undesirable destruction of collateral structures (21, 23). The microwave sealing process, combined with the scissors-like design, helped AS achieve PH without instrument exchanges. If such excellent sealing is accompanied by the use of the clamp-crushing AT, a surgeon only needs a pair of Metzenbaum scissors to perform nearly bloodless PH within a short transection period. In practice, there are some energy devices, such as EBVS or UAD, that are available for parenchymal dissection, but neither has been applied as the sole instrument for the whole procedure of PH (7, 8, 18). Hence, using Acrosurg devices might be likely to simplify the PH procedure.

Besides parenchymal dissection, the GP, which consists of portal triads, is often ligated separately by tying knots, placing sutures, or using staplers in a conventional PH (5, 9, 10, 13, 18). In contrast, Acrosurg alone could seal the GP as well as EBDs flawlessly. In the experimental condition, our study reported the creation of an EBD stump capable of withstanding significantly higher burst pressure compared to other EBVS/UAD instruments reported in a previous study (16). This finding was consolidated by histological examination where the GP and EBD stumps, deemed to be single large vessels, were shown to be definitely fused and fixed, demonstrating seal integrity. During this experiment, regardless of whether AS or AT was used, the large GP was slowly sealed and cut sequentially in two or three overlapping cycles with only a less-than-5-mm, intervening GP segment to ensure an adequate seal. These results showed that Acrosurg devices were able to seal these structures perfectly. Furthermore, the results with EBDs demonstrated that Acrosurg devices could secure the coagulation of smaller intrahepatic bile ducts, which showed no cholorrhea immediately after the operation.

The 4-week follow-up also revealed positive endpoints. The dead beagle in the AS group was attributed to intra-abdominal hemorrhage due to excessive bleeding from the gallbladder bed. This case was considered a PH complication, but it was not directly related to the bleeding from the parenchyma or GP stump. This indicated that all stumps had been completely sealed. Nevertheless, a bile leak was still detected with the naked-eye in one case in the AT group. To eliminate the drawback of macroscopic assessment, we recommend that bilirubin tests of ascites or abdominal fluid should be carried out in both the acute and chronic post-operative stages.

In this study, we did not perform a comparative experiment between our devices and other conventional energy devices (Harmonic, LigaSure or CUSA®) because there was no one currently available device that could be used to perform the entire PH procedure by itself. Also, the function of Acrosurg for hepatectomy has not been presented earlier. Our work is the first study to prove that PH and Glissonean pedicle dissection could be achieved safely and simply with a single microwave device in an experimental model. We used a number of 16 beagles to comply with the principles of 3Rs in animal experiments (implemented by SUMS) but still ensure the statistical significance of the research. These preclinical data are the essential evidence to introduce Acrosurg to PHs on humans.

The primary limitation of this study was the lack of intraoperative monitoring of blood pressure and central venous pressure whose fluctuations might affect bleeding during liver resection (14). This study was performed on a normal liver, whereas performing PH on a cirrhotic liver is not an exceptional circumstance (30). Therefore, functional assessment of Acrosurg on abnormal liver texture should be conducted, especially focusing on the potential of a non-bleeding parenchymal dissection without prior HP control. A safe PH without inflow occlusions helps patients avoid the risk of liver function impairment as well as hemodynamic disturbance, both life-threatening events in cirrhotic or chemotherapy-induced livers.

In conclusion, two microwave-based Acrosurg devices were able to achieve a complete parenchymal transection as well as a GP seal without prior HP occlusion in an experimental model. AS could be employed as a sole instrument to perform PH whereas AT, which combined a clamp-crushing maneuver with microwave sealing, demonstrated a quasi-bloodless PH in a shorter operation time than the seamless transection achieved using AS. Both devices allow surgeons to perform a safer PH with very few instruments. The results of this study indicate that these Acrosurg devices could be tested for PH in clinical trials.

ETHICS STATEMENT

The animal study was reviewed and approved by Shiga University of Medical Science (SUMS) Ethical Committee for Animal Research.

AUTHOR CONTRIBUTIONS

KD: participated in study design, performed the experiment, collected and analyzed the data, and wrote the manuscript. SN: designed the study, performed the experiment, provided critical comments, and revised the manuscript. AY: participated in the experiment and data collection, provided critical comments, and edited the manuscript. TT: designed the study, performed the experiment, critically revised the manuscript, and approved the submission. All authors contributed to the article and approved the submitted version.

ACKNOWLEDGMENTS

The authors would like to express special thanks to Ms. Ikuko Arikawa and Ms. Miho Yamamoto, laboratory technicians at the Department of Surgery of SUMS for their assistance in sample preparation.

REFERENCES

1. Rahbari NN, Garden OJ, Padbury R, Maddern G, Koch M, Hugh TJ, et al. Post-hepatectomy haemorrhage: a definition and grading by the International study group of liver surgery (ISGLS). *HPB.* (2011) 13:528–35. doi: 10.1111/j.1477-2574.2011.00319.x

2. Martin AN, Narayanan S, Turrentine FE, Bauer TW, Adams RB, Stukenborg GJ, et al. Clinical factors and postoperative impact of bile leak after liver resection. *J Gastrointest Surg.* (2018) 22:661–7. doi: 10.1007/s11605-017-3650-4

3. Scalzone R, Lopez-Ben S, Figueras J. How to transect the liver? A history lasting more than a century. *Dig Surg.* (2012) 29:30–4. doi: 10.1159/000335719

4. Yamamoto M, Ariizumi S. Glissonean pedicle approach in liver surgery. *Ann Gastroenterol Surg.* (2018) 2:124–28. doi: 10.1002/ags 3.12062

5. Romano F, Garancini M, Uggeri F, Degarte L, Nespoli L, Gianotti L, et al. Bleeding in hepatic surgery: sorting through methods to prevent it. *HBP Surg.* (2012) 2012:169351. doi: 10.1155/2012/169351

6. Pai M, Spalding D, Jiao L, Habib N. Use of bipolar radiofrequency in parenchymal transection of the liver, pancreas and kidney. *Dig Surg.* (2012) 29:43–7. doi: 10.1159/000335732

7. Ichida A, Hasegawa K, Takayama T, Kudo H, Sakamoto Y, Yamazaki S, et al. Randomized clinical trial comparing two vessel-sealing devices with crush clamping during liver transection. *Br J Surg.* (2016) 103:1795–803. doi: 10.1002/bjs.10297

8. Ikeda M, Hasegawa K, Sano K, Imamura H, Beck Y, Sugawara Y, et al. The vessel sealing system (LigaSure) in hepatic resection a Randomized controlled trial. *Ann Surg.* (2009) 250:199–203. doi: 10.1097/SLA.0b013e3181 334f9

9. Reddy SK, Barbas AS, Gan TJ, Hill SE, Roche AM, Clary BM. Hepatic parenchymal transection with vascular staplers:a comparative analysis with the crush-clamp technique. *Am J Surg.* (2008) 196:760–67. doi: 10.1016/j.amjsurg.2007.12.054

10. Schemmer P, Bruns H, Weitz J, Schmidt J, Buchler MW. Liver transection using vascular stapler: a review. *HPB.* (2008) 10:249–52. doi: 10.1080/13651820802166930

11. Koffron AJ, Stein JA. Laparoscopic liver surgery: parenchymal transection using saline-enhanced electrosurgery. *HPB.* (2008) 10:225–8. doi: 10.1080/13651820802166864

12. Scatton O, Brustia R, Belli G, Pekolj J, Wakabayashi G, Gayet B. What kind of energy devices should be used for laparoscopic liver resection? Recommendations from a systematic review. *J Hepatobiliary Pancreat Sci.* (2015) 22:327–34. doi: 10.1002/jhbp.213

13. Poon RTP. Current techniques of liver transection. *HPB.* (2007) 9:166–73. doi: 10.1080/13651820701216182

14. Huntington JT, Royall NA, Schmidt CR. Minimizing blood loss during hepatectomy: a literature review. *J Surg Oncol.* (2014) 109:81–8. doi: 10.1002/jso.23455

15. Lesurtel M, Selzner M, Petrowsky H, McCormack L, Clavien PA. How should

transection of the liver be performed a prospective randomized study in 100 consecutive patients comparing four different transection strategies. *Ann Surg.* (2005) 242:814–22. doi: 10.1097/01.sla.0000189121.35617.d7

16. Hope WW, Padma S, Newcomb WL, Schmelzer TM, Heath JJ, Lincourt AE, et al. An evaluation of electrosurgical vessel-sealing devices in biliary tract surgery in a porcine model. *HPB.* (2010) 12:703–8. doi: 10.1111/j.1477-2574.2010.00240.x

17. Gotohda N, Yamanaka T, Saiura A, Uesaka K, Hashimoto M, Konishi M, et al. Impact of energy devices during liver parenchymal transection: a multicenter randomized controlled trial. *World J Surg.* (2015) 39:1543–49. doi: 10.1007/s00268-015-2967-y

18. Aragon RJ, Solomon NL. Techniques of hepatic resection. *J Gastrointest Oncol.* (2012) 3:28–40. doi: 10.3978/j.issn.2078-6891.2012.006

19. Tani T, Naka S, Murakami K, Higashiguchi T, Tani S, Akabori H, et al. Comparative study between newly developed microwave surgical devices and commercialized energy devices in animal model. *Tan Sui.* (2016) 37:581–88. Available online at: http://www.igakutosho.co.jp/magazine/t_s/2016/zt3706.html

20. Tani T, Naka S, Tani S, Shiomi H, Murakami K, Yamada A, et al. The invention of microwave surgical scissors for seamless coagulation and cutting. *Surg Today.* (2018) 48:856–64. doi: 10.1007/s00595-018-1662-7

21. Nguyen VQ, Tani T, Naka S, Yamada A, Murakami K. Thermal tissue change induced by a microwave surgical instrument in a rat hepatectomy model. *Am J Surg.* (2016) 211:189–96. doi: 10.1016/j.amjsurg.2015.07.008

22. Dang KT, Tani T, Naka S, Yamada A, Tani S. Comparative study of novel microwave coagulation surgical instrument and currently commercialized energy devices in an animal model. In: *7th International Conference on the Development of Biomedical Engineering in Vietnam (BME7).* Vietnam (2018).

23. Dang KT, Naka S, Nguyen VQ, Yamada A, Tani T. Functional evaluation of a novel microwave surgical device in a canine splenectomy model. *J Invest Surg.* (2019) 34:164–71. doi: 10.1080/08941939.2019.1619884

24. Hopper K, Powell LL. Basics of mechanical ventilation for dogs and cats. *Vet Clin North Am Small Anim Pract.* (2013) 43:955–69. doi: 10.1016/j.cvsm.2013.03.009

25. Thornton JA. Estimation of blood loss during surgery. *Ann R Coll Surg Engl.* (1963) 33:164–74.

26. Rau HG, Duessel AP, Wurzbacher S. The use of water-jet dissection in open and laparoscopic liver resection. *HPB.* (2008) 10:275–80. doi: 10.1080/13651820802167706

27. Bodzin AS, Leiby BE, Ramirez CG, Frank AM, Doria C. Liver resection using cavitron ultrasonic surgical aspirator (CUSA) versus harmonic scalpel: a retrospective cohort study. *Int J Surg.* (2014) 12:500–3. doi: 10.1016/j.ijsu.2014.02.007

28. Oba A, Ishizawa T, Mise Y, Inoue Y, Ito H, Ono Y, et al. Possible underestimation of blood loss during laparoscopic hepatectomy. *BJS Open.* (2019) 3:336–43. doi: 10.1002/bjs5.50145

29. Brace CL. Microwave tissue ablation: biophysics, technology and applications. *Crit Rev Biomed Eng.* (2010) 38:65–78. doi: 10.1615/CritRevBiomedEng.v38.i1.60

30. Li M, Zhang W, Li Y, Li P, Li J, Gong J, et al. Radiofrequency-assisted versus clamp-crushing parenchyma transection in cirrhotic patients with hepatocellular carcinoma: a randomized clinical trial. *Dig Dis Sci.* (2013) 58:835–40. doi: 10.1007/s10620-012-2394-y

18

Radiopaque Chitosan Ducts Fabricated by Extrusion-Based 3D Printing to Promote Healing After Pancreaticoenterostomy

Maoen Pan[1†], Chaoqian Zhao[2†], Zeya Xu[2], Yuanyuan Yang[1], Tianhong Teng[1], Jinxin Lin[2*] and Heguang Huang[1*]

[1] Department of General Surgery, Fujian Medical University Union Hospital, Fuzhou, China, [2] Key Laboratory of Optoelectronic Materials Chemical and Physics, Fujian Institute of Research on the Structure of Matter, Chinese Academy of Sciences, Fuzhou, China

*Correspondence:
Jinxin Lin
franklin@fjirsm.ac.cn
Heguang Huang
heguanghuang123@163.com

[†] Thes authors have contributed equally to this work

Long-term placement of non-degradable silicone rubber pancreatic duct stents in the body is likely to cause inflammation and injury. Therefore, it is necessary to develop degradable and biocompatible stents to replace silicone rubber tubes as pancreatic duct stents. The purpose of our research was to verify the feasibility and biological safety of extrusion-based 3D printed radiopaque chitosan (CS) ducts for pancreaticojejunostomy. Chitosan-barium sulfate (CS-Ba) ducts with different molecular weights (low-, medium-, and high-molecular weight CS-Ba: LCS-Ba, MCS-Ba, and HCS-Ba, respectively) were soaked *in vitro* in simulated pancreatic juice (SPJ) (pH 8.0) with or without pancreatin for 16 weeks. Changes in their weight, water absorption rate and mechanical properties were tested regularly. The biocompatibility, degradation and radiopaque performance were verified by *in vivo* and *in vitro* experiments. The results showed that CS-Ba ducts prepared by this method had regular compact structures and good molding effects. In addition, the lower the molecular weight of the CS-Ba ducts was, the faster the degradation rate was. Extrusion-based 3D-printed CS-Ba ducts have mechanical properties that match those of soft tissue, good biocompatibility and radioopacity. *In vitro* studies have also shown that CS-Ba ducts can promote the growth of fibroblasts. These stents have great potential for use in pancreatic duct stent applications in the future.

Keywords: 3D printing, chitosan, pancreatic duct stent, biocompatible, degradation

INTRODUCTION

Pancreaticoduodenectomy (PD) is still the classic method of treatment of benign and malignant tumors of the pancreas, ampullary and duodenum. However, the incidence of postoperative complications is still higher than 30–40% due to complicated procedures (Gouma et al., 2000; Bassi et al., 2001). Pancreaticojejunostomy is the most important and complicated procedure in PD surgery. Pancreatic fistula is the most serious complication after pancreaticojejunostomy (Karim et al., 2018). Severe pancreatic fistula can cause abdominal infection and hemorrhage, and even progress to severe sepsis. Therefore, it is recommended to use pancreatic duct stents to reduce complications and mortality during PD and middle segment pancreatectomy. To drain pancreatic fluid, placement of a silicone rubber stent into the main pancreatic duct has been proven to be an ideal method to promote anastomotic healing by preventing trypsin from corroding the anastomosis in the early postoperative stage and by reducing the incidence of postoperative pancreatic fistula (Isayama et al., 2016). However, as these materials are non-degradable and easily cause inflammation after long-term use, their applications are limited. Some studies have used polylactic acid (PLA) to prepare pancreatic duct stents (Yang et al., 2019). However, the high modulus of this material, which is not consistent with that of soft tissue, is prone to induce damage and inflammation during its use, and it takes a long time to degrade. Therefore, it is necessary to develop a material with a suitable degradation time and Young's modulus for the preparation of pancreatic duct stents.

Various methods have been used to prevent anastomotic fistula, but the study results show that they produced little difference in the rate of pancreatic fistula, and the incidence of B-grade and C-grade pancreatic fistula is still as high as 19.8% (Peng et al., 2002; Bassi et al., 2017). Therefore, it is of great significance to reduce the incidence of early pancreatic fistula by developing a new pancreatic duct stent material. Traditional silicone rubber tubes are inert materials and have no biological activity. However, with the increasing application of natural biodegradable materials in clinical practice, this shortcoming can be effectively solved.

Chitosan (CS), which is the deacetylated form of chitin (degree of deacetylation >50%), is a naturally occurring polymer and the second most abundant natural biopolymer after cellulose (Ahmed and Ikram, 2016). CS is an excellent biocompatible polymer with a range of properties, such as non-toxicity, biodegradability, antimicrobial and immune-modulatory activities (Anitha et al., 2014). Most importantly, CS has the potential to promote soft tissue healing (Ahmed and Ikram, 2016). Our previous research (Zhao et al., 2020) studied the preparation of extrusion-based 3D printing of CS ducts for soft tissue engineering. It was found that the mechanical properties of these CS ducts matched well with those of soft tissue and had great potential in soft tissue engineering.

When a biodegradable stent is developed, it is essential to know how long it will take to degrade. This means that we must be able to track its degradation in vivo. In future clinical applications, postoperative follow-up observation of patients is very important. X-ray imaging technology is an effective and convenient method for detecting and evaluating the position and shape of implant materials (Sang et al., 2014; Houston et al., 2017). Traditional polymer molecules should be endowed with radiopaque properties to meet medical requirements. Barium sulfate is the common imaging agent used to enhance the imaging effects of polymers in the body and facilitate the dynamic observation of implant material changes after surgery.

It is very difficult to prepare the complicated structures of ducts by traditional manufacturing technologies, whereas the emergence of 3D printing provides vast opportunities for personalized medicine (Shi and Huang, 2020). In this study, based on clinical requirements, radiopaque pancreatic duct stents using degradable CS and barium sulfate were prepared by extrusion-based 3D printing technology for the first time. To evaluate the mechanical matching of CS-BaSO$_4$ (CS-Ba) to pancreatic tissue, the mechanical properties of CS-Ba were tested during its degradation in simulated pancreatic juice (SPJ). The biosafety and applicability of the CS-Ba composites were evaluated by biocompatibility testing in vitro and in vivo. In addition, the radiopaque effects of CS-Ba ducts were studied in vivo. Overall, this study will verify the advantages of extrusion-based 3D-printed CS-Ba ducts as pancreatic duct stents in many aspects.

EXPERIMENTAL

Materials

Three CS samples (deacetylation: 95%) with different molecular weights, including low molecular weight (50,000 g/mol, LCS), medium molecular weight (200,000 g/mol, MCS), and high molecular weight (500,000 g/mol, HCS) CS, were purchased from Cool Chemical Science and Technology Co., Ltd., China. Barium sulfate (BaSO$_4$, 99%), glycolic acid (GA) (C$_2$H$_4$O$_3$, 98%) (GA), potassium hydroxide (KOH, 85%), sodium chloride (NaCl, 99.5%), and the analytical reagent ethanol (C$_2$H$_6$O, 99.7%) were purchased from Sinopharm Chemical Reagents Co., Ltd., China. Additionally, pancreatin from porcine pancreas was purchased from Sigma-Aldrich, St. Louis, MO, United States; the Live-Dead Cell Staining Kit was from Dalian Meilun Biotechnology Co., Ltd., China; the mouse TNF-α/IL-10 Quantikine ELISA Kit was purchased from R&D Systems, United States; and the DNA Content Quantitation Assay Kit (Cell Cycle) and lipopolysaccharide (LPS) were purchased from Beijing Solarbio Science & Technology Co., Ltd., China. Mouse fibroblasts (L929 cells) and mouse RAW264.7 macrophages were purchased from Shanghai Cell Bank, Chinese Academy of Sciences, and Sprague-Dawley (SD) rats were purchased from Experimental Animal Center, Fujian Medical University.

Preparation of the solution of artificial SPJ was performed according to Charteris et al. (1998) and Del Piano et al. (2008). A solution containing 0.1% pancreatin and 0.5% sodium chloride was prepared using deionized water, and the pH was adjusted to 8.0 by the addition of NaOH.

Duct Preparation

CS-Ba ducts were prepared with a weight mixing ratio of 23% barium sulfate to CS with different molecular weights. GA was added for dissolution at a ratio of solute to solvent of 1:4, and the mixture was stirred evenly. Combination with rotation-axis and slurry-extrusion 3D printing (cRS3DP) was used to fabricate CS-Ba ducts. A stepping motor was used to drive the quartz rod to match the speed. In this study, the 3D printing parameters were as follows: the printing layer (d_c) was 0.4 mm in each layer, the printing speed (υ_e) was 4 mm/s, and the air pressure was 0.8 MPa, the diameter of the rotary axis (d) was 2 mm, the moving speed of the syringe needle (υ) was 0.12 mm/s and the rotary speed of the rotary axis (x) was 0.29 r/s (Zhao et al., 2020). The number of printing layers was adjusted according to the required diameter of the ducts. The duct cavity diameter was determined by the diameter of the quartz rod. The function of the quartz rod was to act as a rotary axis driven by a stepper motor for slurry deposition. The printed quartz rod and CS-Ba ducts were soaked in KOH for 12 h and then transferred to deionized water for 12 h. Finally, the quartz rod in the middle of the ducts were removed, and the shaped ducts were stored in deionized water for later use (diagram shown in **Figure 1**). Because the quartz rod is smooth, it is easy to remove from the ducts.

X-ray Diffraction (XRD) Patterns and Fourier Transform Infrared Spectroscopy of CS-Ba Ducts

The sample was placed on a sample stage for analysis. A Cu target, a tube voltage of 40 kV, a tube current of 5 mA, continuous scanning at $2\theta = 5–85°$, a scanning speed of $5°/min$, and a step size of $0.02°$ were used. Fourier transform infrared (FTIR) was used to characterize functional groups with the following parameters: infrared scanning range, wavelength range of $4,000–650\ cm^{-1}$, resolution of $4\ cm^{-1}$, and 16 scans.

In vitro Swelling and Degradation Tests of the CS-Ba Ducts

Different molecular weights of CS mixtures (LCS-Ba, MCS-Ba, and HCS-Ba) ($n \geq 15$ per group) were accurately weighed after drying at 65°C for 24 h and soaked in SPJ solution. The ratio of mass to solvent was 1:30 g/mL, and the solution was changed every other day to maintain the activity of pancreatin. At 2, 4, 8, 12, and 16 weeks, three samples from each group were removed and weighed after washing and drying at 65°C for 24 h. The degradation rate was calculated as the degradation rate = $[(W_0 - W')/W_0] \times 100\%$ (where W_0 is the original weight and W' is the dried weight). To observe the degradation of CS-Ba by pancreatin in this study, an SPJ solution without pancreatin was created (with the other conditions remaining the same), and the degradation rates of the samples in the SPJ solutions were compared.

To evaluate the changes in the water swelling rates of the samples during the degradation process, samples from different groups were removed at 4, 8, and 16 weeks, and after the water on the surface of the samples was wiped dry with filter paper, W_0 was recorded. The samples were placed in an oven and weighed upon reaching a constant weight to determine W_d. The swelling percentage was calculated as follows: $S\% = [(W_0 - W_d)/W_0] \times 100\%$.

Mechanical Strength Measurements of the CS-Ba Rods

The samples were made into cylindrical tensile samples with cross sections approximately 1.5 mm in diameter. A universal testing machine (CMT4304 and SANS) with a tensile speed of 10 mm/s was used to test each sample's original tensile strength, Young's modulus and fracture stress according to ISO 527-1 2012. Samples were soaked in the alkaline SPJ solution. The mechanical properties of the samples were tested at 4, 8, and 16 weeks and compared with the original mechanical properties to observe the mechanical strength changes during the degradation process.

CS-Ba Duct Cell Viability Assays

The MTT method was used to test the *in vitro* cytotoxicity of different molecular weight of samples. Extraction of the sample: According to ISO 10993-12:2012 (E), the extraction ratio was 0.2 g/mL, the extraction medium was modified Eagle medium (MEM) medium containing 10% fetal bovine serum (FBS), the extraction temperature was $(37 \pm 1)°C$, and the extraction time was (24 ± 2) h. The blank control group used MEM containing 10% FBS, the negative control group was a high-density polyethylene (HDPE) extract group, and the positive control was a complete medium containing 0.64% phenol. The absorbance was measured at 570 nm with a microplate reader, and the survival rate (%) was calculated according to the following formula:

$$\text{Cell viability (\%)} = (\text{OD}_{570e}/\text{OD}_{570b}) \times 100\%,$$

where OD_{570e} is the absorbance of the 100% extract and OD_{570b} is the absorbance of the blank group. If the cell survival rate is less than 70% that of the blank cells, the compound is potentially cytotoxic.

Live/Dead Fluorescence Staining

One hundred microliters of L929 cells were inoculated into a 96-well plate at a density of 1×105 cells/mL per well. The cells were incubated with complete medium for 24 h, and then the complete medium was replaced with the corresponding sample extract. After incubation for 24 or 48 h, the extract was discarded and the cells were washed with PBS twice. The dyes calcein-AM and propidium iodide (PI) were added followed by incubation at 37°C in the dark for 30 min. The staining solution was discarded, and 100 μL of PBS was added. The morphology and viability of the cells were observed under an inverted fluorescence microscope. Green fluorescence indicated living cells, and red fluorescence indicated dead cells.

Cell Cycle Detection

L929 cells were cultured with extracts of the three kinds of ducts (The extraction method of sample extract was shown in section "CS-Ba Duct Cell Viability Assays"), and the control group was cultured with complete medium. After 24 h, the cells were digested with 0.25% trypsin to prepare a single cell suspension, which was fixed with 70% ice ethanol for 24 h. After centrifugation at 1000 rpm, the cells were washed with PBS twice and incubated at 37°C for 30 min after the addition of 0.25 mg/mL RNase. Next, PI solution was added followed by incubation at 4°C for 30 min. The supernatant was discarded after centrifugation, and 500 μL of PBS was added. Cell cycle changes were measured with a BD Accuri C6 Plus cytometer (United States).

Hemolysis Assay

Rat blood (1 mL) was centrifuged for 10 min at 3000 rpm, the upper serum was discarded, and the samples were washed three times with PBS. Then, 20 μL of red blood cells were treated by the addition of 500 μL of PBS extract with different molecular weights of CS-Ba samples, which were exposed to ionizing water and PBS as positive and negative controls, respectively, for 4 h at 37°C. The absorption sensitivity of the hemoglobin in the liquid was monitored with an ultraviolet spectrometer after centrifugation for 10 min at a speed of 3000 rpm, and the hemolysis rate (HR) of the solution was calculated using the following formula. In the formula, A_t, A_{pc}, and A_{nc} are the absorbance of the supernatant at 540 nm for the test sample and the positive and negative controls, respectively. $HR\,(\%) = (A_t - A_{nc})/(A_{pc} - A_{nc}) \times 100\%$.

Measurement of the Production of Inflammatory Factors *in vitro*

Mouse RAW 264.7 macrophages were cultured in Dulbecco's modified Eagle medium (DMEM) containing 10% FBS. The concentration of the cells was adjusted to 1×10^5/mL in complete culture medium. The cells were inoculated into 96-well plates at 100 μL per well. After 24 h of culture, the original culture medium in the wells was discarded. The negative control group was supplemented with 100 μL of complete culture medium, and the positive control group was supplemented with complete culture medium containing 1 μg/mL LPS. Then, the LCS-Ba, MCS-Ba, and HCS-Ba samples were added to the extract solution. The supernatant of the cell culture was extracted 24 h later, and the TNF-α and IL-10 contents were determined with ELISA kits.

Animal Experiment

The animal research protocol was approved by the Experimental Animal Ethical Committee of Fujian Medical University (No: 2020-0022). Thirty-two SD rats weighing 200–250 g were randomly divided into four groups. The control group was implanted with inert silicone rubber tubes, and the other groups were implanted with LCS-Ba, MCS-Ba, and HCS-Ba ducts. Each duct was placed in the abdominal cavity and fixed to the surface of the pancreas with 5–0 non-absorbable sutures (as shown in **Figure 4A**). Serum amylase was then measured in blood from the tail vein of three rats in each group 1 day before surgery and 1, 3, and 7 days after surgery. Eight and sixteen weeks after the operation, the radiopaque performance and degradation of the CS-Ba ducts in each group of rats were observed by X-ray, and venous blood was taken for the detection of liver and kidney function. Then, four rats from each group were euthanized, and the pancreatic tissues around the ducts were taken as pathological sections to observe the inflammation of the tissues around the ducts. During the 16th week, the hearts, liver, spleen, lungs and kidneys of the rats were taken for hemoxylin-eosin (HE) staining to observe the toxicity of the test materials *in vivo* after long-term implantation. Finally, the removed ducts were cleaned and dried to a constant weight, and the duct degradation rate was determined after comparison with the weight before implantation. The surface morphologies of the materials were observed by scanning electron microscopy (SEM).

Statistical Analysis

All experiments were repeated three or more times ($n \geq 3$) and the data are presented as mean ± SD. Statistical analysis was performed using one-way ANOVA, and $P < 0.05$ was considered statistically significant.

RESULTS AND DISCUSSION

Due to the limitations of biodegradable materials, many stents that have been researched have a long degradation time and high Young's modulus, which restricts their scope of clinical use (Parviainen et al., 2000; Laukkarinen et al., 2008; Nordback et al., 2012). Therefore, it is necessary to constantly explore new materials and develop pancreatic duct stents that are more suitable for clinical needs. As a natural biopolymer material, CS has been widely studied and used in various disciplines due to its excellent biological properties (Griffon et al., 2005; Biazar and Heidari Keshel, 2014; Dan et al., 2016). However, there are few studies on its use as a pancreatic duct stent. Based on the above experimental results, this study will verify the feasibility and safety of CS as a pancreatic duct stent from multiple aspects, such as its degradation performance, mechanical properties and biocompatibility.

Preparation and Identification of CS-Ba Ducts

The preparation of 3D CS ducts is currently difficult. Due to the characteristics of CS, it cannot be 3D printed by thermal processing, and CS ducts prepared by the freeze-drying method are not suitable for pancreatic duct stents due to their irregularities and large porosity (Ao et al., 2006; Nawrotek et al., 2016). Irregular and large pores may cause pancreatic fluid to leak from the lateral wall of the catheter and thus corrode the surrounding anastomotic tissue, causing anastomotic damage. Therefore, CS ducts were prepared by 3D printing by extrusion molding and it was verified that the use of GA to dissolve CS can achieve the best biocompatibility (Zhao et al., 2020). To implant CS in the body and obtain good visualization, we added barium sulfate to the CS to prepare a slurry. The infrared spectra of CS and different molecular weights of CS-Ba samples are shown in **Figure 2A**. The main functional groups of CS included NH_2 (1596 cm^{-1}), C = O-NHR (1658 cm^{-1}), axial C-H (2868, 2922 cm^{-1}), and −OH and N-H (3400 cm^{-1}) (Barbosa et al., 2019). The characteristic peaks of SO_4^{2-} were located at 1195, 1120, and 983 cm^{-1}, corresponding to symmetrical vibrations, and the out-of-plane vibrations of SO_4^{2-} at to 610 and 636 cm^{-1} (Sivakumar et al., 2015). The CS-Ba ducts prepared in this study had obvious vibration peaks in both places, indicating that the synthesized product contained barium sulfate particles. In addition, comparison of the spectra of different molecular weights of CS showed that the basic skeleton structure of the CS molecules did not change, indicating that the molecular weight had little effect on the chemical structure. **Figure 2B** shows the XRD patterns of CS and CS-Ba with different molecular weights. The spectrum of pure CS showed two characteristic diffraction peaks at 11.40 and 20.20°. These are the characteristic peaks of

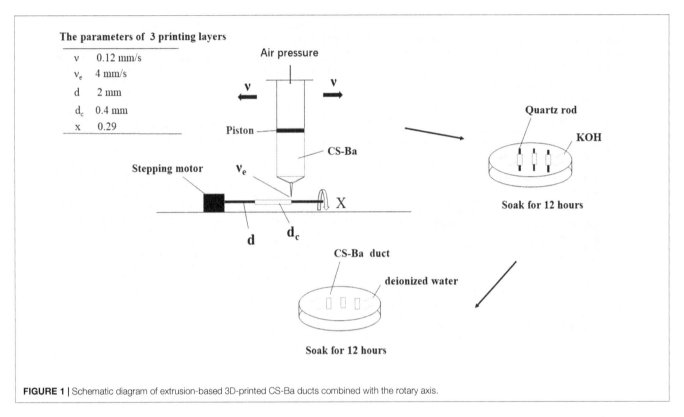

FIGURE 1 | Schematic diagram of extrusion-based 3D-printed CS-Ba ducts combined with the rotary axis.

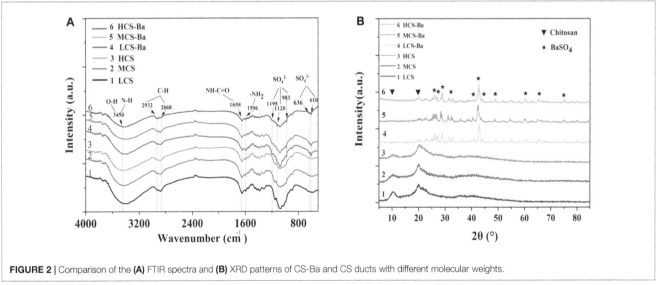

FIGURE 2 | Comparison of the **(A)** FTIR spectra and **(B)** XRD patterns of CS-Ba and CS ducts with different molecular weights.

the semicrystalline structure of CS (Samanta and Ray, 2014). The diffraction peaks from CS-Ba at 2θ = 25.8, 26.8, 28.7, 32.8, 41.6, 42.6, 45.9, 48.2, 60.8, 65.8, and 75.8° correspond to the barium sulfate standard diagram (210), (102), (211), (020), (022), (113), (411), (402), (232), (224), and (125) crystal planes (PDF#83-2053). The presence of these peaks indicated an increase in local crystallinity.

As shown in **Figure 3**, the color of the extrusion-based 3D printed CS-Ba ducts was light yellow, and there was no significant difference in the color between the different molecular weights

of CS-Ba ducts. The CS-Ba duct surfaces were relatively smooth, their shapes were regular, and they had good flexibility after the absorption of water and subsequent expansion. In the dry state, the duct walls became hard, and hollow ducts had good patency from the side view (**Figures 3A–E**). Electron microscopy observations showed that the surfaces of the ducts prepared by the extrusion method were uniform and flat with dense structures and little particle deposition (**Figures 3F–K**). It was found that the CS-Ba ducts prepared by this method had a dense structure with regular microfibers on the surface and few holes. This dense

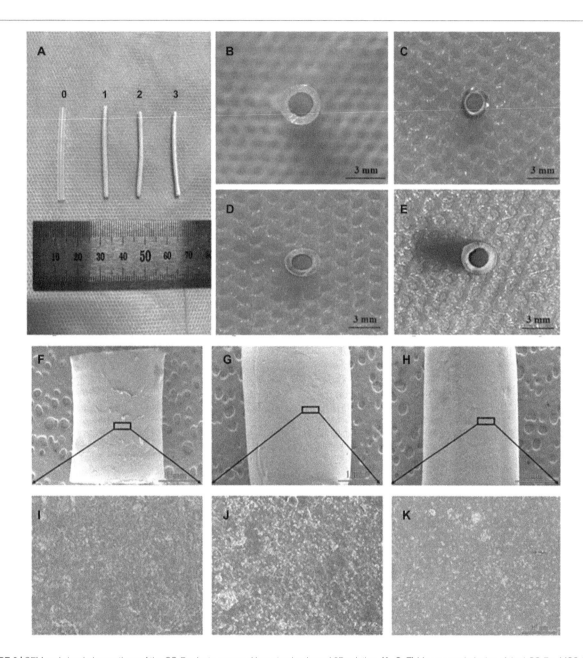

FIGURE 3 | SEM and visual observations of the CS-Ba ducts prepared by extrusion-based 3D printing. **(A, C–E)** Macro morphologies of the LCS-Ba, MCS-Ba, and HCS-Ba samples in different positions (0-silicone rubber, 1-LCS-Ba, 2-MCS-Ba, and 3-HCS-Ba). **(B)** A silicone rubber tube was used as a control. **(F–K)** Radial micromorphology of the LCS-Ba **(F)**, MCS-Ba **(G)**, and HCS-Ba **(H)** ducts.

structure can prevent pancreatic juice from leaking from the wall to the outer side and corroding anastomotic tissue. The microstructure confirmed that the CS-Ba ducts prepared by this method were suitable for use as pancreatic duct stents during pancreaticojejunostomy.

Degradation of CS-Ba in SPJ and *in vivo*

The ideal biomaterial needs a degradation rate that matches the rate of tissue regeneration to ensure normal healing of the anastomosis after pancreaticojejunostomy while avoiding complications such as anastomotic stenosis caused by rapid degradation of the stents. The most optimal degradation time of the pancreatic duct stent is approximately 3–6 months. Enzymatic hydrolysis is one of the important ways of chitosan degradation *in vivo*. In addition to specific enzymes such as chitinase, chitosanase, and lysozyme, chitosan can also be degraded by non-specific enzymes such as cellulase, lipase, pepsin and papain (Lee et al., 2008; Suwan et al., 2009; Pan et al., 2016). Lysozyme is the main chitosan degrading enzyme in the human body. However, pancreatin is the enzyme that is directly contact with the CS-Ba ducts. In this study, we compared the degradation of CS-Ba ducts in solutions both with and

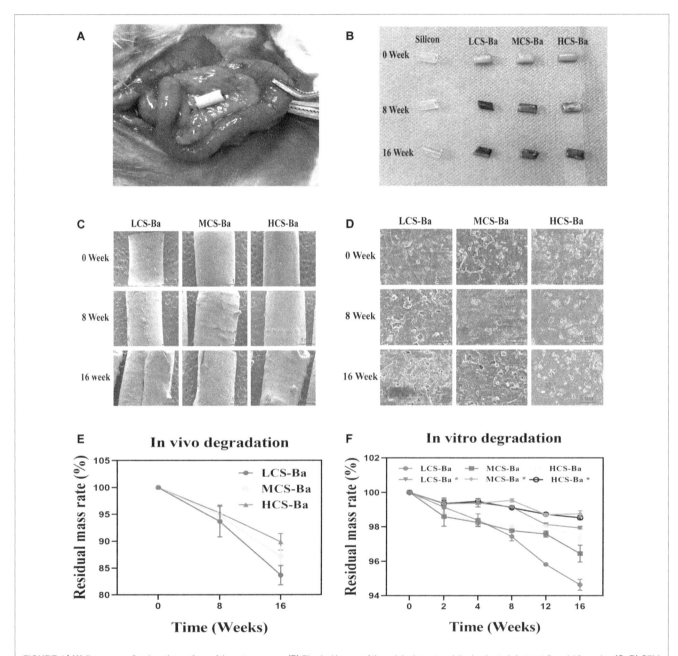

FIGURE 4 | (A) Ducts were fixed on the surface of the rat pancreas. (B) Physical image of the original stent and the implanted ducts at 8 and 16 weeks. (C, D) SEM images of the changes in the microstructures of the original ducts and the implanted ducts at 8 and 16 weeks (scales are 1 mm and 5 μm, respectively). (E) In vivo degradation rate. (F) The degradation rates of different molecular weights of CS-Ba ducts in vitro (* SPJ solution without pancreatin).

without pancreatin (**Figure 4F**). The results showed that the degradation of the three types of CS-Ba ducts in the SPJ solution containing pancreatin was significantly faster than that of the ducts in the SPJ solution without pancreatin ($P < 0.05$). In the SPJ solution containing pancreatin, the degradation rate of the LCS-Ba ducts was significantly faster than that of the MCS-Ba and HCS-Ba ducts ($P < 0.05$). The environment of human pancreatic juice is weakly alkaline (pH 7.8–8.4). Under weakly alkaline conditions, the digestive effects of pancreatin are the strongest. In a pH > 6 environment, the dissolution

rate of CS is reduced due to the deprotonation of the amino groups present (Matica et al., 2019). Therefore, under the combined effects of many factors, the SPJ solution containing pancreatin can degrade CS-Ba ducts faster than the SPJ solution without pancreatin. In addition, the molecular weight is an important factor that affects the degradation of CS—the lower the molecular weight is, the faster the degradation rate will be (Varoni et al., 2018). Therefore, the molecular weight of CS can be adjusted to meet the degradation time requirement of pancreatic duct stents.

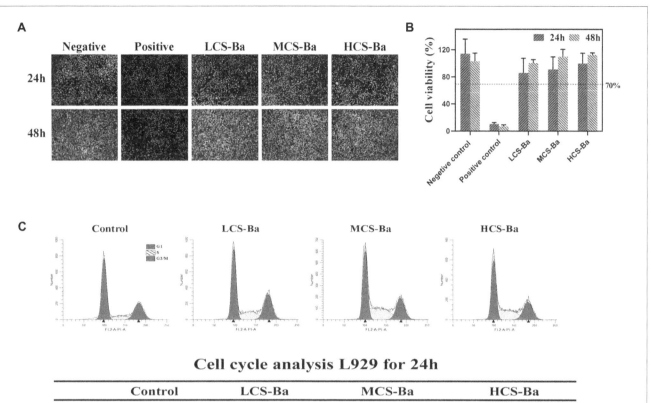

Cell cycle analysis L929 for 24h

	Control	LCS-Ba	MCS-Ba	HCS-Ba
G1	58.14±1.85%	45.99±1.68% *	42.02±2.18% *	43.58±2.48% *
S	14.49±0.86%	22.70±1.45% *	33.04±1.76% * #	30.87±1.64% *#
G2/M	27.37±2.4%	31.31±3.11%	24.94±1.54% #	25.55±1.91% #

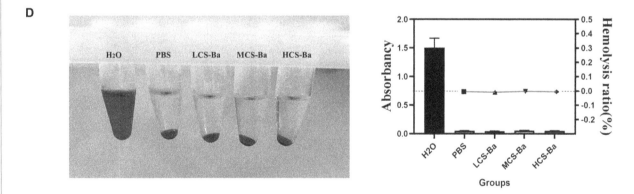

FIGURE 5 | Cytotoxicity and blood compatibility of CS-Ba ducts. **(A)** Live-dead fluorescence staining and **(B)** cell viability of CS-Ba ducts with original extract solutions. **(C)** Effects of CS-Ba duct extraction solution on the L929 cell proliferation cycle. **(D)** The hemolysis rate of CS-Ba ducts (* represents a significant result compared with the control group, $P < 0.05$; # represents significant results compared with the LCS-Ba group, $P < 0.05$).

Figure 4E displays the mass losses of the CS-Ba ducts after implantation. Compared with the original masses, the average mass losses of LCS-Ba, MCS-Ba, and HCS-Ba after 8 weeks of implantation were 6.37, 5.25, and 4.77%, respectively, and the average mass losses after 16 weeks were 16.34, 12.85, and 10.16%, respectively. We found that the degradation rate of LCS-Ba was significantly faster than the rates of MCS-Ba and HCS-Ba ($P < 0.05$). Moreover, the degradation rates of different molecular weights of CS-Ba ducts were found to be significantly faster *in vivo* than *in vitro*, which was related to the wet environment inside the body and the acidic nature of cellular metabolites. The body temperature and lysozymes also promoted the degradation of the materials. As shown in **Figure 4B**, images of the ducts after degradation showed that

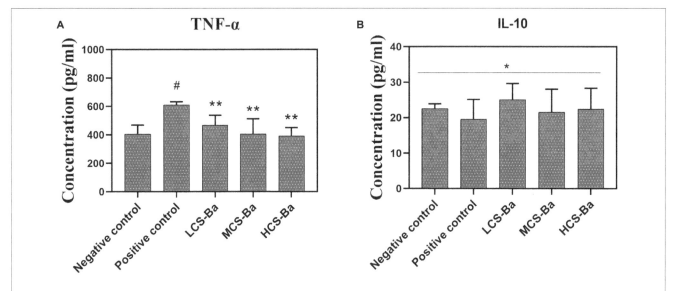

FIGURE 6 | Different molecular weights of CS-Ba ducts induced RAW 264.7 macrophages to secrete **(A)** TNF-α and **(B)** IL-10 (* represents $P > 0.05$, ** represents $P < 0.05$ compared with the positive control; # represents $P < 0.05$ compared with the negative control).

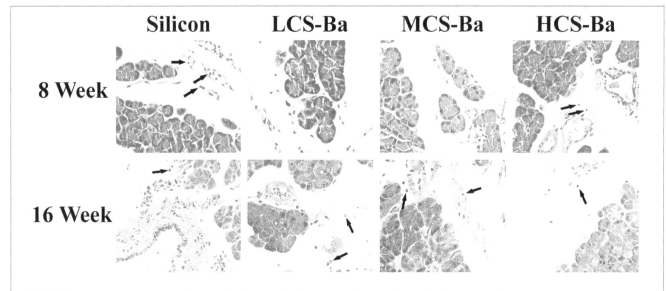

FIGURE 7 | HE staining of the pancreas and surrounding tissues at the duct contact site at 8 and 16 weeks. There was no obvious abnormality in the pancreatic tissue, and few inflammatory cells were found (↑) (magnification 400×).

the color became black, the texture became brittle, and part of the ducts appeared to be deformed and broken. The ducts at different time points were observed by SEM, and very small scaffold fragments and etched cavities appeared on the surface of each group at 8 weeks. With further degradation at 16 weeks, the surface cracks of the ducts deepened, parts of the ducts collapsed and the etched cavity increased. The changes in the LCS-Ba ducts were the most obvious among all of the ducts (**Figures 4C,D**). In addition, during degradation in the body, the surface of the material gradually turned from pale yellow to black. This phenomenon is very similar to the darkening of CS after heat treatment, radiation treatment or the Maillard reaction (Yue, 2014; Shamekhi et al., 2017). The essence of the

Maillard reaction is the condensation reaction between carbonyl ammonia. Since most of the enzymes in the body are proteins, their carboxyl group and the amino group of chitosan may react under certain conditions to produce the complex black polymer protein melanin, leading to blackening of the surface of the ducts.

In vitro and *in vivo* Biocompatibility of CS-Ba Ducts

Any medical device applied to the human body must undergo toxicity testing before clinical application. Chitosan has been proven to be a natural polymer material with good biocompatibility. Although barium sulfate has been widely used

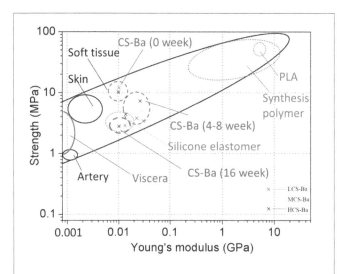

FIGURE 8 | Strength and Young's modulus of CS-Ba ducts during degradation in SPJ solution compared with viscera and other biopolymers.

as a gastrointestinal contrast agent, its toxicity as a CS-Ba mixed material duct is unclear. **Figure 5B** shows that the cell survival rate of L929 cells treated with CS-Ba with different molecular weights was greater than 70%. Moreover, the cell survival rate of each group was significantly better than that of the positive control group ($P < 0.05$). **Figure 5A** shows that the number of cells increased rapidly over time, and the cells were in the full state. From the above results, it was proven that the CS-Ba ducts had no obvious cell cytotoxicity. Additionally, hemolysis is regarded as a primary and credible method of judging the blood compatibility of implants, and values up to 5% are permissible for biomaterials (Liu et al., 2017). If the material of a pancreatic duct stent cause hemolysis, since it is in direct contact with the blood around the anastomotic site, it will affect the blood supply of the anastomotic site tissue, thus affecting healing. In this study, the red blood cells incubated with different CS-Ba compound extracts showed no obvious hemolysis (a HR of almost 0), indicating that the CS-Ba compounds had good blood compatibility (**Figure 5D**).

To further explain the effects of the CS-Ba degradation products on the proliferation cycle of L929 cells, we quantitatively analyzed the cell proportions in each phase of proliferation by flow cytometry. From **Figure 5C**, we found that the number of cells in the G0/G1 phase was significantly lower in the three CS-Ba groups than in the control group, while the proportion of cells entering the S and G2/M phases in the three CS-Ba groups was higher, indicating that the CS-Ba extract contains ingredients that promote cell proliferation. Muzzarelli et al. (1988) believed that CS functions similarly to glycosaminoglycans because of its structural properties. As important glycoproteins in the extracellular matrix, glycosaminoglycans play an important role in cell proliferation, differentiation and morphogenesis. Thus, CS could promote the growth of fibroblasts in the anastomotic tissue and accelerate anastomotic healing after pancreatoenterostomy.

Macrophages regulate tissue healing by secreting different inflammatory factors during the early and late stages of healing

(Mirza et al., 2009; Rodero and Khosrotehrani, 2010; Koh and DiPietro, 2011; Mahdavian Delavary et al., 2011). In the early stage of healing, macrophages secrete proinflammatory factors (TNF-α, IL-1, and IL-6, etc.), proteases and reactive oxygen radicals to enhance the inflammatory response against pathogens at the damaged site. In the stage of tissue formation, macrophages secrete anti-inflammatory factors (IL-10, etc.) and phagocytic apoptotic cells to promote the regression of wound inflammation and initiate tissue repair. However, overexpression of inflammatory factors will disrupt the balance of the local immune environment and cause the overexpression of fibroblasts in the late stage of healing, leading to the occurrence of anastomotic stenosis. Therefore, the *in vitro* inflammatory factor induction experimental results were studied. As shown in **Figure 6**, we found that LCS-Ba, MCS-Ba and HCS-Ba did not induce an excessive inflammatory response in macrophages ($P > 0.05$).

Rats have been widely used in animal studies of changes in acute pancreatitis (Gill et al., 1989). In animal experiments, CS-Ba ducts were fixed onto the surface of the pancreas in rats for evaluation so that they fully touched the pancreatic parenchyma. At the same time, we used the silicone tube for comparison, because it is an inert non-degradable material and is the most commonly used material for pancreatic duct stents. Serum amylase is the most sensitive hematological index in acute pancreatitis, and its changes mainly occur in the early stage. Therefore, rat serum amylase was tested in the first week after surgery. The results showed that except for a transient increase in amylase on the first day after the operation, the levels returned to near normal after 3 days (**Supplementary Figure 1b**). This result showed that the CS-Ba materials did not cause acute inflammation of the pancreas. Additionally, in the histological specimens at 8 and 16 weeks (**Figure 7**), pancreatic acinar cell vacuolation, fibrosis and granuloma were not found. However, a small amount of inflammatory cell infiltration was observed. This result does not reflect chronic toxicity of the material to the tissue. In addition, HE staining of the heart, liver, spleen, lung and kidney of the rats and blood biochemical indexes confirmed that CS-Ba did not have obvious toxicity to the important organs in the body after exposure for a long period of time (**Supplementary Figures 1c–f, 2**).

Mechanical Properties of CS-Ba Ducts and Their Matching With Soft Tissue

Mechanical properties are key factors that affect tissue regeneration in addition to biocompatibility. Matching of the Young's modulus of the implant material with that of the tissue can reduce complications such as tissue damage, inflammation, and necrosis and contribute to cell adhesion and tissue regeneration (Lee et al., 2019). **Figure 8** shows the comparison between the mechanical properties of CS-Ba in the degradation process with other polymers and soft tissues (Ashby, 2011; Jang et al., 2018; Liravi and Toyserkani, 2018). The elastic modulus and strength of soft tissues are generally low, as the Young's modulus of human internal organs is lower than 0.001 GPa. Currently, a silicone rubber stent is commonly

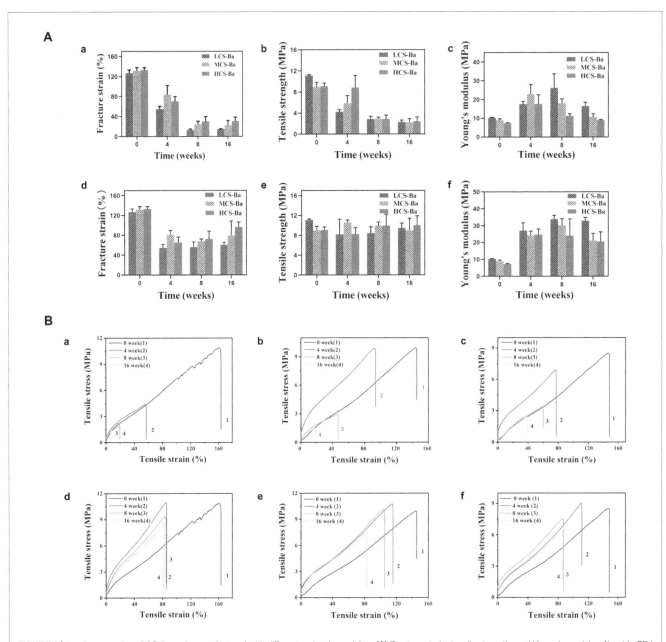

FIGURE 9 | Tensile properties of CS-Ba rods manufactured with different molecular weights. **(A)** Fracture strain, tensile strength, and Young's modulus. [(a–c) In SPJ solution with pancreatin. (d–f) In SPJ solution without pancreatin]. **(B)** Tensile stress and strain curves. [(a, d) LCS-Ba rods. (b, e) MCS-Ba rods. (c, f) HCS-Ba rods.].

used for pancreaticojejunostomy, and it has a Young's modulus of 0.006–0.02 GPa. Compared with other degradable polymers, such as PLA (Young's modulus of 2–4 GPa and strength of 40–70 MPa), the Young's modulus of silicone rubber is more suitable for the repair of soft tissues such as the pancreas, but its inability to degrade limits its further applications. In this study, the Young's modulus of CS-Ba increased in the early stage and then decreased but was still 0.01 GPa after 16 weeks, which is close to the modulus of the human viscera. During degradation, the strength continued to decline; however, it could be maintained at 3–4 MPa after 16 weeks, which represents a good supportive effect compared with internal organs. It could prevent the

anastomotic site from collapsing and causing stenosis. In this study, the original Young's modulus of three molecular weights of CS-Ba ducts was approximately 8–10 MPa, which is slightly lower than the mechanical properties of the pure CS previously studied (Zhao et al., 2020). This is because the blended system of the polymer and heavy metal salt cannot guarantee fusion of the two phases and is prone to incompatibility or two-phase separation, which will become a source of fracture and affect the mechanical properties of the final material (Rawls et al., 1990). At the 16th week of degradation, the tensile strengths and Young's modulus of the CS-Ba ducts were basically the same as those of silicone elastomers, which indicated that after 16 weeks

Radiopaque Chitosan Ducts Fabricated by Extrusion-Based 3D Printing to Promote Healing...

191

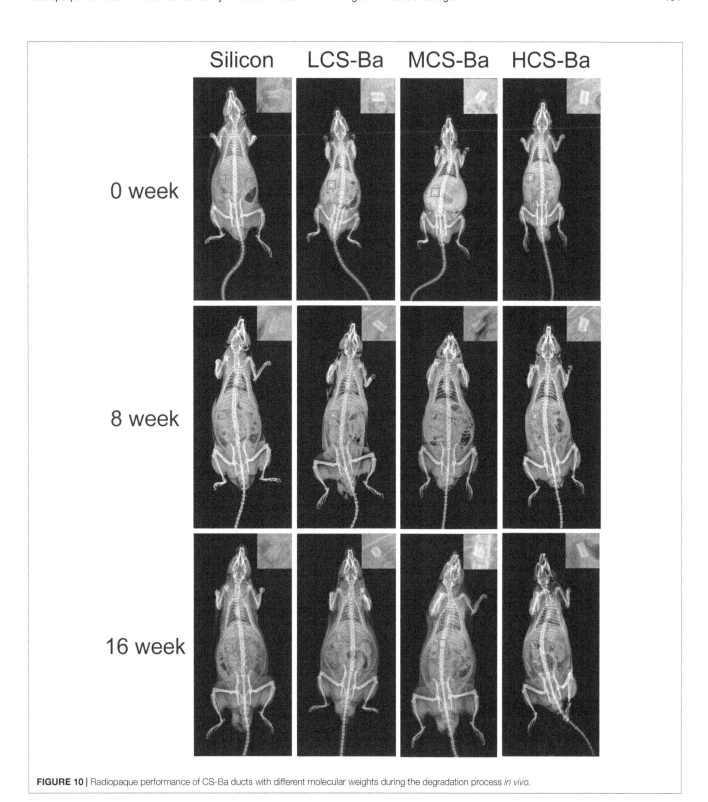

FIGURE 10 | Radiopaque performance of CS-Ba ducts with different molecular weights during the degradation process *in vivo.*

of degradation of CS-Ba ducts, their mechanical properties maintained sufficient support for the drainage of pancreatic fluid, and no corresponding collapse occurred.

An interesting phenomenon appeared in this study. As shown in **Figure 9A**, in SPJ solution, the breaking strain and tensile strength of CS-Ba with different molecular weights decreased with increasing degradation time, and the lower the molecular weight was, the faster was the rate of decline ($P < 0.05$). In the SPJ solution without pancreatin, the fracture strain decreased in the early stage but did not decrease further after 4 weeks. There were no obvious changes in the tensile strength, indicating that the degradation of the material was not obvious in the alkaline solution. Interestingly, the Young's modulus of the materials increased in the early stage but decreased in the late stage in the SPJ group containing pancreatin for the different molecular weights of CS-Ba samples. In the SPJ solution without pancreatin, the modulus remained unchanged after the initial increase and did not continue to decrease. This change rule can be clearly seen in the stress-strain curve (**Figure 9B**). This result was similar to the change trend of the water absorption rate of the material (**Supplementary Figure 3**). In the early stage, the water absorption rate decreased, and the material became hard. As degradation progressed, the water absorption rate slowly increased. This phenomenon also appeared during the degradation process of electrodeposited CS catheters in Nawrotek et al.'s (2020) study. This may be due to the deprotonation of the CS amine groups in the early stage under alkaline conditions, the reduction in ion repulsion, and the strengthening of molecular connections through hydrogen bonds and hydrophobic interactions, making the texture of the material harder, increasing the Young's modulus, and decreasing the water absorption rate. In the solution with pancreatin, as the degradation progressed, cracks or holes appeared on the surface of the material, allowing water to enter the inside of the material, causing the water absorption rate to increase and the modulus to decrease. In the alkaline solution without pancreatin, the tensile strength of CS-Ba did not change significantly, while the Young's modulus increased and did not decrease in the later stage. The results confirmed that pancreatin can accelerate the degradation of CS-Ba.

Cs-Ba Ducts With Good Radiopaque Properties

In most polymer materials, the macromolecular chain only contains elements with a low electron density and low specific gravity such as C, H, O, and N. There are no elements with a high electron cloud density (such as halogens or metal elements), so the materials cannot be radiographically tested. To overcome this inherent defect, traditional polymer molecules must be endowed with radiation-impermeable properties to meet medical needs. In this study, degradable radiopaque CS-Ba ducts were prepared so that the ducts could be detected by X-ray after implantation. Nordback et al. (2012) verified that PLA stents mixed with 23% barium sulfate have good radio-opacity effects. From **Figure 10**, X-ray observations indicated that the imaging effects of the ducts containing 23% barium sulfate were significantly better than those of the silicone rubber tube. With increasing implantation time, the duct radiopaque status was slightly decreased compared with the initial status, and the peripheral duct edge in the LCS-Ba group became blunt, but the outline was still not deformed, indicating that the CS-Ba ducts can maintain a certain radial support force after 16 weeks. In addition, the imaging performance was good, which is very beneficial for future observations and follow-up after the material is implanted in the human body.

As mentioned above, this study investigated the process, microstructure and performance of CS-Ba ducts for pancreaticojejunostomy tissue repair. The microstructure of the CS-Ba ducts was analyzed by SEM, FTIR, and XRD. The tensile strength, Young's modulus and fracture strain of CS-Ba ducts were measured to evaluate the degree of mechanical matching to pancreatic tissue. The degradation performance and biocompatibility of CS-Ba ducts of different molecular weights in SPJ *in vitro* and *in vivo* were also studied. The radioopacity of the CS-Ba ducts in the body was evaluated. There are still some shortcomings in this study. The best degradation time of the pancreatic duct stent is approximately 3–6 months, but the degradation rate of 50,000 g/mol molecular weight chitosan in this study was still unable to meet its needs. Therefore, in future work, we will try to further reduce its molecular weight to regulate the degradation time of the stent and use large animals, such as pigs, for further verification.

CONCLUSION

This study verified the advantages of extrusion-based 3D printed CS-Ba ducts as pancreatic duct stents. The following conclusions can be drawn:

1. CS-Ba ducts prepared by this method have the following advantages: compact and ordered structure, good molding effects, and a simple preparation method. The length and diameter of the CS-Ba ducts can be adjusted to customize personalized pancreatic duct stents for the patient.
2. CS-Ba ducts possess mechanical properties that match those of soft tissues, and they can meet the degradation time required for the healing of the pancreaticojejunostomy by controlling the molecular weight of CS. In an *in vitro* study, it was shown to have the potential to promote the growth of fibroblasts, which could accelerate anastomotic healing after pancreatoenterostomy.
3. The CS-Ba ducts had a good radiopaque performance and could be detected by X-ray after surgery. In conclusion, extrusion-based 3D-printed CS-Ba ducts can feasibly replace silicone rubber tubes as pancreatic duct stents and have considerable application potential in the future.

ETHICS STATEMENT

The animal study was reviewed and approved by the Experimental Animal Ethical Committee of Fujian Medical University.

AUTHOR CONTRIBUTIONS

MP: conceptualization, investigation, methodology, formal analysis, software, writing – original draft, and writing – review and editing. CZ: data curation, validation, methodology, and formal analysis. ZX and YY: investigation. TT: project administration. JL: funding acquisition and conceptualization. HH: funding acquisition, supervision, and writing – review and editing. All authors contributed to the article and approved the submitted version.

Science Foundation of China [No. 82001895]; Joint Funds of Scientific and Technological Innovation Program of Fujian Province [No. 2018Y9039]; and Startup Fund for scientific research, Fujian Medical University [No. 2019QH2017].

REFERENCES

1. Ahmed, S., and Ikram, S. (2016). Chitosan based scaffolds and their applications in wound healing. *Achiev. Life Sci.* 10, 27–37. doi: 10.1016/j.als.2016.04.001

2. Anitha, A., Sowmya, S., Kumar, P. T. S., Deepthi, S., and Jayakumar, R. (2014). Chitin and chitosan in selected biomedical applications. *Prog. Polym. Sci.* 39, 1644–1667.

3. Ao, Q., Wang, A., Cao, W., Zhang, L., Kong, L., He, Q., et al. (2006). Manufacture of multimicrotubule chitosan nerve conduits with novel molds and characterization in vitro. *J. Biomed. Mater. Res. A* 77, 11–18. doi: 10.1002/jbm.a.30593

4. Ashby, M. F. (2011). *Materials Selection in Mechanical Design*, 4th Edn. Oxford: Butterworth-Heinemann, 341–366.

5. Barbosa, H. F. G., Francisco, D. S., Ferreira, A. P. G., and Cavalheiro, E. T. G. (2019). A new look towards the thermal decomposition of chitins and chitosans with different degrees of deacetylation by coupled TG-FTIR. *Carbohydr. Polym.* 225:115232. doi: 10.1016/j.carbpol.2019.115232

6. Bassi, C., Falconi, M., Salvia, R., Mascetta, G., and Molinari, E. (2001). Management of complications after pancreaticoduodenectomy in a high volume centre: results on 150 consecutive patients/with invited commentary. *Dig. Surg.* 18, 453–458. doi: 10.1159/000050193

7. Bassi, C., Marchegiani, G., Dervenis, C., Sarr, M., Abu, H. M., Adham, M., et al. (2017). The 2016 update of the International Study Group (ISGPS) definition and grading of postoperative pancreatic fistula: 11 years after. *Surgery* 161, 584–591. doi: 10.1016/j.surg.2016.11.014

8. Biazar, E., and Heidari Keshel, S. (2014). Development of chitosan-crosslinked nanofibrous PHBV guide for repair of nerve defects. *Artif. Cells Nanomed. Biotechnol.* 42, 385–391. doi: 10.3109/21691401.2013.832686

9. Charteris, W. P., Kelly, P. M., Morelli, L., and Collins, J. K. (1998). Development and application of an in vitro methodology to determine the transit tolerance of potentially probiotic Lactobacillus and Bifidobacterium species in the upper human gastrointestinal tract. *J. Appl. Microbiol.* 84, 759–768. doi: 10.1046/j.1365-2672.1998.00407.x

10. Dan, Y., Liu, O., Liu, Y., Zhang, Y. Y., Li, S., Feng, X. B., et al. (2016). Development of novel biocomposite scaffold of chitosan-gelatin/nanohydroxyapatite for potential bone tissue engineering applications. *Nanoscale Res. Lett.* 11:487. doi: 10.1186/s11671-016-1669-1

11. Del Piano, M., Strozzi, P., Barba, M., Allesina, S., Deidda, F., Lorenzini, P., et al. (2008). In vitro sensitivity of probiotics to human pancreatic juice. *J. Clin. Gastroenterol.* 42(Suppl. 3), S170–S173. doi: 10.1097/MCG.0b013e3181815976

12. Gill, T. J., Smith, G. J., Wissler, R. W., and Kunz, H. W. (1989). The rat as an experimental animal. *Science* 245, 269–276. doi: 10.1126/science.2665079

13. Gouma, D. J., van Geenen, R. C., van Gulik, T. M., de Haan, R. J., de Wit, L. T., Busch, O. R., et al. (2000). Rates of complications and death after pancreaticoduodenectomy: risk factors and the impact of hospital volume. *Ann. Surg.* 232, 786–795. doi: 10.1097/00000658-200012000-00007

14. Griffon, D. J., Sedighi, M. R., Sendemir-Urkmez, A., Stewart, A. A., and Jamison, R. (2005). Evaluation of vacuum and dynamic cell seeding of polyglycolic acid and chitosan scaffolds for cartilage engineering. *Am. J. Vet. Res.* 66, 599–605. doi: 10.2460/ajvr.2005.66.599

15. Houston, K. R., Brosnan, S. M., Burk, L. M., Lee, Y. Z., Luft, J. C., Ashby, V. S., et al. (2017). Iodinated polyesters as a versatile platform for radiopaque biomaterials. *J. Polym. Sci. A Polym. Chem.* 55, 2171–2177. doi: 10.1002/pola.28596

16. Isayama, H., Nakai, Y., Hamada, T., Matsubara, S., Kogure, H., and Koike, K. (2016). Understanding the mechanical forces of self-expandable metal stents in the biliary ducts. *Curr. Gastroenterol. Rep.* 18:64. doi: 10.1007/s11894-016-0538-5

17. Jang, H. J., Park, S. B., Bedair, T. M., Oh, M. K., Ahn, D. J., Park, W., et al. (2018). Effect of various shaped magnesium hydroxide particles on mechanical and biological properties of poly(lactic-co-glycolic acid) composites. *J. Ind. Eng. Chem.* 59, 266–276. doi: 10.1016/j.jiec.2017.10.032

18. Karim, S. A. M., Abdulla, K. S., Abdulkarim, Q. H., and Rahim, F. H. (2018). The outcomes and complications of pancreaticoduodenectomy (Whipple procedure): cross sectional study. *Int. J. Surg.* 52, 383–387. doi: 10.1016/j.ijsu. 2018.01.041

19. Koh, T. J., and DiPietro, L. A. (2011). Inflammation and wound healing: the role of the macrophage. *Expert Rev. Mol. Med.* 13:e23. doi: 10.1017/S1462399411001943

20. Laukkarinen, J., Lamsa, T., Nordback, I., Mikkonen, J., and Sand, J. (2008). A novel biodegradable pancreatic stent for human pancreatic applications: a preclinical safety study in a large animal model. *Gastrointest. Endosc.* 67, 1106–1112. doi: 10.1016/j.gie.2007.10.013

21. Lee, D. X., Xia, W. S., and Zhang, J. L. (2008). Enzymatic preparation of chitooligosaccharides by commercial lipase. *Food Chem.* 111, 291–295. doi: 10.1016/j.foodchem.2008.03.054

22. Lee, J. E., Park, S. J., Yoon, Y., Son, Y., and Park, S. H. (2019). Fabrication of 3D freeform porous tubular constructs with mechanical flexibility mimicking that of soft vascular tissue. *J. Mech. Behav. Biomed. Mater.* 91, 193–201. doi: 10.1016/j.jmbbm.2018.12.020

23. Liravi, F., and Toyserkani, E. (2018). Additive manufacturing of silicone structures: a review and prospective. *Addit. Manuf.* 24, 232–242. doi: 10.1016/j.addma. 2018.10.002

24. Liu, J., Wang, P., Chu, C. C., and Xi, T. (2017). Arginine-leucine based poly (ester urea urethane) coating for Mg-Zn-Y-Nd alloy in cardiovascular stent applications. *Colloids Surf. B Biointerfaces* 159, 78–88. doi: 10.1016/j.colsurfb. 2017.07.031

25. Mahdavian Delavary, B., van der Veer, W. M., van Egmond, M., Niessen, F. B., and Beelen, R. H. (2011). Macrophages in skin injury and repair. *Immunobiology* 216, 753–762. doi: 10.1016/j.imbio.2011.01.001

26. Matica, M. A., Aachmann, F. L., Tondervik, A., Sletta, H., and Ostafe, V. (2019). Chitosan as a wound dressing starting material: antimicrobial properties and mode of action. *Int. J. Mol. Sci.* 20:5889. doi: 10.3390/ijms20235889

27. Mirza, R., DiPietro, L. A., and Koh, T. J. (2009). Selective and specific macrophage ablation is detrimental to wound healing in mice. *Am. J. Pathol.* 175, 2454–2462. doi: 10.2353/ajpath.2009.090248

28. Muzzarelli, R., Baldassarre, V., Conti, F., Ferrara, P., Biagini, G., Gazzanelli, G., et al. (1988). Biological activity of chitosan: ultrastructural study. *Biomaterials* 9, 247–252. doi: 10.1016/0142-9612(88)90092-0

29. Nawrotek, K., Tylman, M., Adamus-Wlodarczyk, A., Rudnicka, K., Gatkowska, J., Wieczorek, M., et al. (2020). Influence of chitosan average molecular weight on degradation and stability of electrodeposited conduits. *Carbohydr. Polym.* 244:116484. doi: 10.1016/j.carbpol.2020.116484

30. Nawrotek, K., Tylman, M., Decherchi, P., Marqueste, T., Rudnicka, K., Gatkowska, J., et al. (2016). Assessment of degradation and biocompatibility of electrodeposited chitosan and chitosan-carbon nanotube tubular implants. *J. Biomed. Mater. Res. A* 104, 2701–2711. doi: 10.1002/jbm.a.35812

31. Nordback, I., Raty, S., Laukkarinen, J., Jarvinen, S., Piironen, A., Leppiniemi, J., et al. (2012). A novel radiopaque biodegradable stent for pancreatobiliary applications–the first human phase I trial in the pancreas. *Pancreatology* 12, 264–271. doi: 10.1016/j.pan.2012.02.016

32. Pan, A. D., Zeng, H. Y., Foua, G. B., Alain, C., and Li, Y. Q. (2016). Enzymolysis of chitosan by papain and its kinetics. *Carbohydr. Polym.* 135, 199–206. doi: 10.1016/j.carbpol.2015.08.052

33. Parviainen, M., Sand, J., Harmoinen, A., Kainulainen, H., Valimaa, T., Tormala, P., et al. (2000). A new biodegradable stent for the pancreaticojejunal anastomosis after pancreaticoduodenal resection: in vitro examination and pilot experiences in humans. *Pancreas* 21, 14–21. doi: 10.1097/00006676-200007000-00047

34. Peng, S., Mou, Y., Cai, X., and Peng, C. (2002). Binding pancreaticojejunostomy is a new technique to minimize leakage. *Am. J. Surg.* 183, 283–285. doi: 10.1016/ s0002-9610(02)00792-4

35. Rawls, H. R., Starr, J., Kasten, F. H., Murray, M., Smid, J., and Cabasso, I. (1990). Radiopaque acrylic resins containing miscible heavy-metal compounds. *Dent. Mater.* 6, 250–255. doi: 10.1016/S0109-5641(05)80006-5

36. Rodero, M. P., and Khosrotehrani, K. (2010). Skin wound healing modulation by macrophages. *Int. J. Clin. Exp. Pathol.* 3, 643–653.

37. Samanta, H. S., and Ray, S. K. (2014). Controlled release of tinidazole and theophylline from chitosan based composite hydrogels. *Carbohydr. Polym.* 106, 109–120. doi: 10.1016/j.carbpol.2014.01.097

38. Sang, L., Wei, Z., Liu, K., Wang, X., Song, K., Wang, H., et al. (2014). Biodegradable radiopaque iodinated poly(ester urethane)s containing poly(epsilon-caprolactone) blocks: synthesis, characterization, and biocompatibility. *J. Biomed. Mater. Res. A* 102, 1121–1130. doi: 10.1002/jbm.a.34777

39. Shamekhi, M. A., Rabiee, A., Mirzadeh, H., Mahdavi, H., Mohebbi-Kalhori, D., and Baghaban Eslaminejad, M. (2017). Fabrication and characterization of hydrothermal cross-linked chitosan porous scaffolds for cartilage tissue engineering applications. *Mater. Sci. Eng. C Mater. Biol. Appl.* 80, 532–542. doi: 10.1016/j.msec.2017.03.194

40. Shi, B., and Huang, H. (2020). Computational technology for nasal cartilage-related clinical research and application. *Int. J. Oral Sci.* 12:21. doi: 10.1038/ s41368- 020-00089-y

41. Sivakumar, S., Soundhirarajan, P., Venkatesan, A., and Khatiwada, C. P. (2015). Spectroscopic studies and antibacterial activities of pure and various levels of Cu-doped BaSO(4) nanoparticles. *Spectrochim. Acta A Mol. Biomol. Spectrosc.* 151, 895–907. doi: 10.1016/j.saa.2015.07.048

42. Suwan, J., Zhang, Z., Li, B., Vongchan, P., Meepowpan, P., Zhang, F., et al. (2009). Sulfonation of papain-treated chitosan and its mechanism for anticoagulant activity. *Carbohydr. Res.* 344, 1190–1196. doi: 10.1016/j.carres.2009. 04.016

43. Varoni, E. M., Vijayakumar, S., Canciani, E., Cochis, A., De Nardo, L., Lodi, G., et al. (2018). Chitosan-based trilayer scaffold for multitissue periodontal regeneration. *J. Dent. Res.* 97, 303–311. doi: 10.1177/0022034517736255

44. Yang, Y. Y., Zhao, C. Q., Wang, L. S., Lin, J. X., Zhu, S. Z., and Huang, H. G. (2019). A novel biopolymer device fabricated by 3D printing for simplifying procedures of pancreaticojejunostomy. *Mater. Sci. Eng. C Mater. Biol. Appl.* 103:109786. doi: 10.1016/j.msec.2019.109786

45. Yue, W. (2014). Prevention of browning of depolymerized chitosan obtained by gamma irradiation. *Carbohydr. Polym.* 101, 857–863. doi: 10.1016/j. carbpol. 2013.10.011

46. Zhao, C. Q., Liu, W. G., Xu, Z. Y., Li, J. G., Huang, T. T., Lu, Y. J., et al. (2020). Chitosan ducts fabricated by extrusion-based 3D printing for soft-tissue engineering. *Carbohydr. Polym.* 236:16058. doi: 10.1016/j.carbpol.2020.116058

19

Tissue-Engineered Solutions in Plastic and Reconstructive Surgery

Sarah Al-Himdani[1,2†], Zita M. Jessop[1,2†], Ayesha Al-Sabah[1], Emman Combellack[1,2],
Amel Ibrahim[1,2,3], Shareen H. Doak[1,4], Andrew M. Hart[5], Charles W. Archer[1,6],
Catherine A. Thornton[1,7] and Iain S. Whitaker[1,2]*

[1] Reconstructive Surgery and Regenerative Medicine Research Group (ReconRegen), Institute of Life Science, Swansea University Medical School, Swansea, UK, [2] The Welsh Centre for Burns and Plastic Surgery, Morriston Hospital, Swansea, UK, [3] Institute of Child Health, University College London, London, UK, [4] In Vitro Toxicology Group, Institute of Life Science, Swansea University Medical School, Swansea, UK, [5] Canniesburn Plastic Surgery Unit, Centre for Cell Engineering, University of Glasgow, Glasgow, UK, [6] Cartilage Biology Research Group, Institute of Life Science, Swansea University Medical School, Swansea, UK, [7] Human Immunology Group, Institute of Life Science, Swansea University Medical School, Swansea, UK

*Correspondence:
Iain S. Whitaker
i.s.whitaker@swansea.ac.uk

†Joint first authors.

Recent advances in microsurgery, imaging, and transplantation have led to significant refinements in autologous reconstructive options; however, the morbidity of donor sites remains. This would be eliminated by successful clinical translation of tissue-engineered solutions into surgical practice. Plastic surgeons are uniquely placed to be intrinsically involved in the research and development of laboratory engineered tissues and their subsequent use. In this article, we present an overview of the field of tissue engineering, with the practicing plastic surgeon in mind. The Medical Research Council states that regenerative medicine and tissue engineering "holds the promise of revolutionizing patient care in the twenty-first century." The UK government highlighted regenerative medicine as one of the key eight great technologies in their industrial strategy worthy of significant investment. The long-term aim of successful biomanufacture to repair composite defects depends on interdisciplinary collaboration between cell biologists, material scientists, engineers, and associated medical specialties; however currently, there is a current lack of coordination in the field as a whole. Barriers to translation are deep rooted at the basic science level, manifested by a lack of consensus on the ideal cell source, scaffold, molecular cues, and environment and manufacturing strategy. There is also insufficient understanding of the long-term safety and durability of tissue-engineered constructs. This review aims to highlight that individualized approaches to the field are not adequate, and research collaboratives will be essential to bring together differing areas of expertise to expedite future clinical translation. The use of tissue engineering in reconstructive surgery would result in a paradigm shift but it is important to maintain realistic expectations. It is generally accepted that it takes 20–30 years from the start of basic science research to clinical utility, demonstrated by contemporary treatments such as bone marrow transplantation. Although great advances have been made in the tissue engineering field, we highlight the barriers that need to be overcome before we see the routine use of tissue-engineered solutions.

Keywords: tissue engineering, regenerative medicine, stem cells, translation, bioengineering, barriers to translation, translational research, plastic and reconstructive surgery

INTRODUCTION

Reconstructive plastic surgery aims to provide living tissue in order to restore both form and function following a wide range of congenital or acquired defects. Operations are complex, often transcending anatomic boundaries. Versatility resulting from surgery on a full range of tissues including skin, fat, nerve, muscle, bone, and cartilage promotes innovation, and with the recent advances in medical imaging (1), microsurgery (2), vascularized composite allotransplantation (3, 4), nanotechnology (5), cell biology, biomaterials (6), and 3D printing (7–10), treatment options for patients are wider than ever before. Even armed with new reconstructive options based on microsurgical principles and transplantation, surgeons have become increasingly cognizant that there is the real potential for a paradigm shift in reconstructive surgery in the medium term via tissue-engineered solutions. The implementation into practice could potentially eliminate the need for donor sites and their morbidity, reduce hospital stay and associated costs (11).

Relevance of This Article

Contrary to public perception, the diverse workload of reconstructive plastic surgeons comprises a relatively small proportion of purely esthetic procedures (12). The majority of operations undertaken pertain to neoplasia and wound management, with a significant health economic impact (12). Over one million patients are treated per year in NHS England by Plastic Surgeons (13, 14), with evidence suggesting that this workload will continue to increase (15). If you extrapolate these figures worldwide, it is easy to see the clinical need is vast. As a group, reconstructive surgeons are facing more challenging composite defects than ever before coupled with Internet and media savvy patients with increasing expectations (16). Technological innovation in reconstructive surgery in the twentieth century offered the possibility for surgeons to operate on microvascular structures enabling free tissue transfers (2) and extremity replantations. Despite these developments in practice, we are still confronted with shortcomings relating to the availability of donor tissues. In order to overcome this, novel approaches have been investigated. Among these approaches, the most attractive concept is tissue engineering.

Tissue engineering is a modern, interdisciplinary field combining principles of engineering, physics, and the life sciences. It shares a common objective with plastic and reconstructive surgery; "to restore form and function" (17, 18). The long-term aim of tissue engineering is to biomanufacture autologous, vascularized, physiologically relevant solutions to repair and restore complex defects. Successful biomanufacture will depend on the correct blend of cell source, suitable scaffold and ideal microenvironment (19). Answers to these fundamental questions rely on interdisciplinary collaboration between cell biologists, material scientists, biotechnologists, and associated medical specialties (20). Upscaling and widespread use in health services will need close interaction with the cell therapy industry and associated manufacturers.

The surgical community worldwide is becoming increasingly aware of the research landscape. The American Society of Plastic surgeons have highlighted the role of tissue engineering in the future of plastic surgery (21), particularly the need for a focus on translation from bench research to clinical practice. In the United Kingdom, the House of Lords recognized the potential of regenerative medicine to impact on the health service and highlighted the current "lack of coordination" in the field as a whole (22, 23). Recommendations included the development of multidisciplinary working groups (basic scientists, clinicians, investors, manufacturing experts, and regulators), as well as governmental support to drive forward the agenda on regenerative medicine.

There is a need to develop NHS capacity with regional facilities licensed for Good Laboratory Practice (GLP) and current Good Manufacturing Practices (cGMP), which are engaged with a clinical specialty skilled in the manipulation of cells and the viable insertion of tissue-engineered constructs. Skilled in vascularization and in tissue viability/transfer, plastic surgeons already fulfill this role as an interface specialty delivering complex reconstructive techniques to a broad range of other specialties. The regional service structure of plastic surgery within the NHS would further support their capacity to align with regional cGMP facilities and deliver tissue-engineering solutions to a range of medical and surgical specialties.

Objectives
Assess the Shortcomings Of
Traditional Reconstructive Options

Up till now, restoration of form and function has relied on the use of autologous (rarely allogeneic) tissue, alloplastic implants, or a combination of the two. Although effective, these options have disadvantages that merit highlighting (**Table 1**).

Tissue-Engineered Solutions

Although tissue-engineered solutions hold great promise, we must be realistic in that contemporary tissue-engineered constructs implanted into immune-competent animal models have been observed to undergo inflammation, fibrosis, foreign body reaction, and degradation (**Table 1**; **Figure 1**). One of the major problems remains vascularization of larger volume constructs (24), and an issue coming to the fore in modern literature is the potential for tumorigenesis (25).

Provide an Overview Of
Fundamental Principles of Tissue Engineering: Cell Source, Scaffold, Assembly Method, and Molecular and Mechanical Signaling

We discuss the multiple considerations for tissue engineering research in order to highlight the complexity of the field as a whole. This supports the argument for multidisciplinary coordination, which is required to take the field forward. The fundamental principles are summarized in **Figure 2**: cell source, scaffolds, assembly method, subsequent growth (molecular and mechanical signaling), and patient safety. These factors all contribute to the "environment" (19). In simple terms, the cell is required for synthesis of the new tissue matrix, while the scaffold, biomolecules, and the microenvironment provide trophic cues to guide proliferation and differentiation. Growth, induction, and

TABLE 1 | Advantages and shortcomings of reconstructive solutions for managing tissue defects.

Reconstructive solution	Advantages	Disadvantages
Autologous	• No immunological complications • No ethical constraints • Biologically compatible • Minimal degradation • Fewer legal restrictions • No disease transmission • Challenging harvesting cells in aged or diseased	• Donor site morbidity • Limited quantity of tissue available • Two separate operative sites—greater risk and cost
Allogeneic	• No donor site morbidity • Donor cells may have higher viability • Tissue always healthy • Greater quantity of available tissue	• Temporary (i.e., cadaveric skin used in extensive burns) • Tissue typing is required • Immunosuppression may be needed • Risk of disease transmission • Greater legal hurdles • Ethical and psychological challenges
Synthetic	• Maintain structural integrity • Predictable and reproducible physical and mechanical properties • Cost effective • Avoids concerns over disease transmission	• Extrusion • Infection • Cannot restore all of specialized tissue/organ functions • Do not respond to biological cues/grow with patient • May provoke an immune/inflammatory/fibrotic reaction • Materials safety testing and manufacturing governance
Tissue engineered	• Biocompatible • Good biofunctionality • Good retention of size and shape • No donor site morbidity • Unlimited expansion of cells/tissues • No immunological concerns • Mechanical stability	• Long-term effect unknown • Size often limited by vascularity • Costly • Tumorigenic potential • Difficult to engineer "physiologically relevant/mature tissue"

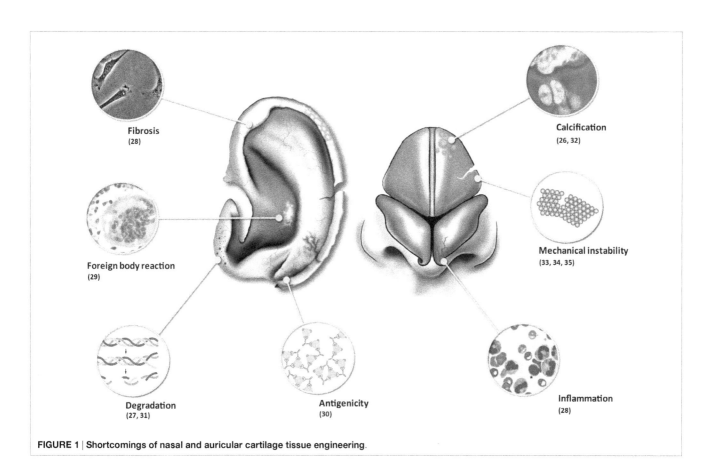

FIGURE 1 | Shortcomings of nasal and auricular cartilage tissue engineering.

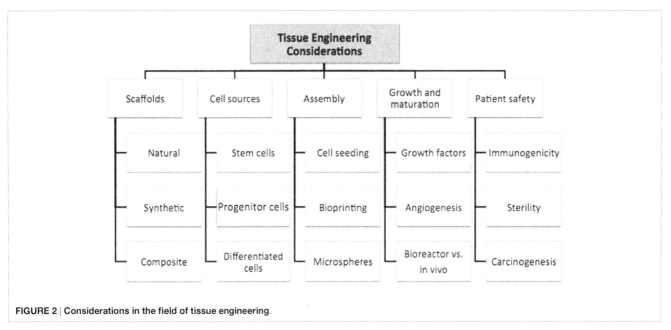

FIGURE 2 | Considerations in the field of tissue engineering.

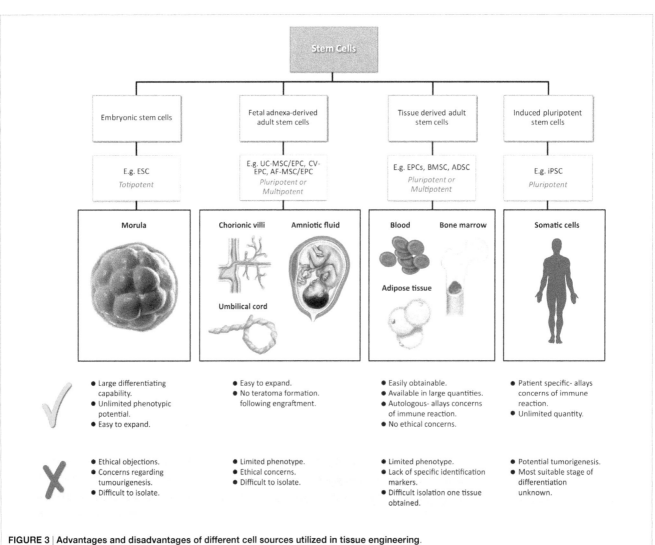

FIGURE 3 | Advantages and disadvantages of different cell sources utilized in tissue engineering.

maintenance of maturation are important for providing durability of the tissue-engineered construct.

Cell Sources

Classical tissue-engineering approaches use *tissue-derived cells* (*not necessarily stem cells*) seeded onto scaffolds (36). These cells may be autologous, allogenic, or xenogenic cells; however, autologous cells are the preferred choice due to the lack of immunogenicity. Cells may be further classified based on differences in their differentiating capabilities (**Figure 3**). Adult somatic cells are fully differentiated, and therefore have restricted future differentiation potential and relatively poor growth, limiting their usefulness for tissue-engineering purposes (37). Progenitor cells are more differentiated than stem cells and are therefore referred to as multipotent rather than pluripotent (38). Stem cells are non-differentiated cells, able to proliferate through multiple generations and differentiate into a variety of cell types (39, 40), and may overcome the limitations of differentiated cells (36) when used for tissue engineering. Pluripotent by definition, stem cells can be derived from embryonic, fetal, or adult (or postnatal somatic) tissue (39). Stem cells are the current preferred cell source for tissue-engineering endeavors and regenerative medicine therapies due to their high potency and capacity for expansion (41). Contemporary research efforts

have focused on adult stem cells or progenitor cells for tissue-engineering purposes. The use of embryonic and fetal tissue, although providing pluripotent stem cells with high proliferative potential, raises potential ethical issues as well as safety concerns over tumorigenic potential (42, 43). Adult derived stem cells, which are found among differentiated cells, have been isolated from an increasingly varied number of tissues over the past decade such as bone marrow (i.e., mesenchymal stem cells and hematopoietic stem cells), adipose [adipose-derived stem cells (44)], epithelial (epithelial-derived stem cells), and umbilical cord (cord blood stem cells) tissue (43). Developments made in isolation and culture of adult derived stem cells have improved cell yield during harvest. Subsequent research has focused on manipulating proliferation and differentiation into the desired cell type (45). Adult derived stem cells can only divide a finite number of times and accumulate genetic changes that can limit their supply for tissue-engineering purposes. The discovery of induced pluripotent stem cells (iPSCs) by Takahashi and Yamanaka (46) introduced the idea that a mature differentiated cell could be reverted to a state of pluripotency and multilineage potential (**Figure 4**). While this process, which has been shown to be possible with human cells, creates a potentially limitless source of easily accessible stem cells, it is not without drawbacks (47). Reprograming the cells has raised questions about

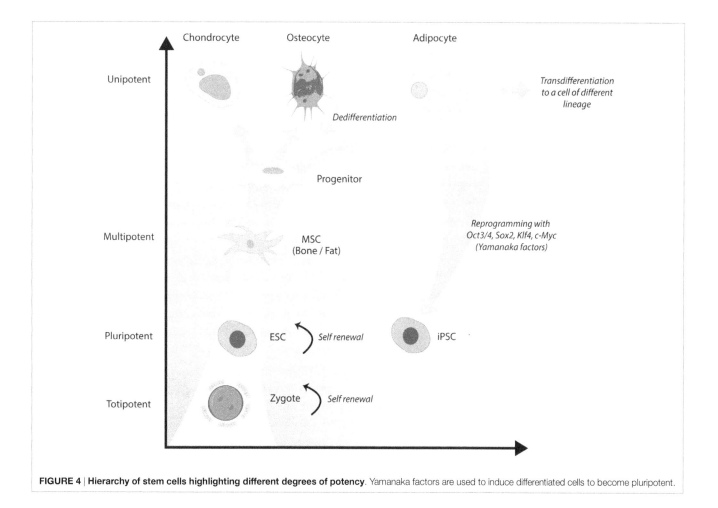

FIGURE 4 | Hierarchy of stem cells highlighting different degrees of potency. Yamanaka factors are used to induce differentiated cells to become pluripotent.

epigenetic effects in particular, with a number of papers purporting to show DNA errors that have arisen during the process of inducing pluripotency (47, 48). Questions have also been raised regarding immunogenicity of engineered tissues with iPSCs implanted into a genetically identical mouse able to provoke an unexpected T cell-mediated immune response (49).

To better understand the behavior of specific cell types and their utility for tissue-engineering purposes, there is an increased reliance on advanced technologies (41) to monitor cell phenotype, migration, proliferation, migration, and differentiation both *in vitro* and *in vivo*. Impedance-based systems such as iCELLigence system (ACEA Biosciences) as well as Seahorse XF^{e}24 Extracellular Flux Analyzer are allowing real-time monitoring of cellular processes and offer distinct and important advantages over traditional endpoint assays (**Figure 5**). Contemporary imaging modalities such as two photon excited fluorescence microscopy (50) and Raman spectroscopy (51), both with high resolution and depth of penetration (>100 nm, 300 nm and 1 mm, 0.4 mm, respectively) are giving researchers clearer insights into the behavior of different cell types (**Figure 5**).

Further complications arise from the wide donor-to-donor variation in the behavior of cells, particularly stem cell populations, that has become apparent. Human adipose-derived stem cells, an increasingly prevalent source of adult stem cells for studies in tissue engineering, exhibit high donor-to-donor variability with regard to proliferation and differentiation characteristics, and this is not explained simply by donor age (52).

Currently, there is no consensus on the *ideal* cell source for tissue-engineering purposes. A thorough understanding of the advantages and disadvantages of each cell type is crucial to decide on cell selection and the optimal culture conditions in order to engineer specific tissue types.

Scaffold Choices

An appropriate scaffold is crucial to any tissue-engineering strategy. The ideal scaffold provides a framework for cell growth and development, allowing cells to attach, migrate, proliferate, and differentiate while facilitating cellular reorganization into a functional 3D network (**Table 2**).

Desirable characteristics of scaffolds include the following:

- Biomimetic (53)
- Biodegradable (with site specific absorption kinetics) (54–56)
- Appropriate mechanical strength
- Optimal micropores: enabling vascularization and allowing metabolic needs to be met (oxygen and waste product transfer)
- Biocompatible (57)
- Non-immunogenic (58)
- Versatile with regard to manufacturing methods
- Functionalization potential (59)

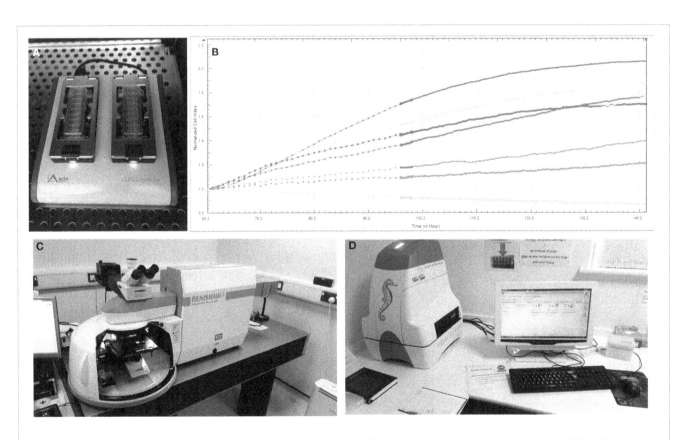

FIGURE 5 | Advanced technologies for monitoring cell behavior and survival. (A) ICELLigence impedance based cell assay machine. (B) Proliferation curves at different cell seeding densities generated by iCELLigence. (C) The Renishaw inVia confocal Raman microscope allows identification of stem cells based on the scattering of photons due to vibrations of molecular bonds. (D) Seahorse XF^{e}24 Extracellular Flux Analyzer is used for measurement of cellular bioenergetics.

TABLE 2 | Advantages and disadvantages of biomaterials utilized currently as scaffolds in tissue engineering.

Scaffold class	Scaffold subtype	Macrostructure	Microstructure	Chemical composition	Advantages	Disadvantages
Synthetic	Polylactic acid (PLA)				• More predictable and reproducible mechanical and physical properties • High tensile strength, degradation rate, and elastic modulus (7) • More readily available • Relatively inexpensive	• Immune reaction • Lack biological cues (8) • Toxicity • Infections
	Polyglycolic acid (PGA)					
	Polyethylene glycol derivatives (PEG)					
Biological	Fibrin				• Biocompatibility • Cell-controlled degradability • Intrinsic cellular interaction • Hydrated environment • Non-toxic • Mucoadhesive • Cytocompatible (9)	• Batch variations • Limited range of mechanical properties • Less reproducible • Costly • Specific processing conditions (10)
	Elastin					
	Collagen					

(Continued)

TABLE 2 | Continued

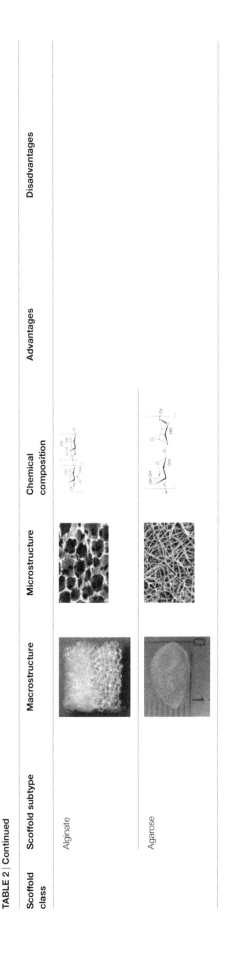

Scaffold class	Scaffold subtype	Macrostructure	Microstructure	Chemical composition	Advantages	Disadvantages
	Alginate					
	Agarose					

- 3D control of macroarchitecture
- Various nano- and micro-topographies, stiffnesses, and micro-environments appropriate to the proliferation, migration, and maturation of native or engrafted cells
- Suitable for clinical grade sterilization
- Suitable for industrial production.

Scaffolds are generally classified as biological (organic) or synthetic (inorganic). Engineering of the cell-scaffold construct can be undertaken *in vitro* in a bioreactor or *in vivo* by implanting the construct into the body. Advances in engineering, material science, and biomanufacturing technologies have enabled the design and development of more complex scaffolds using self assembly (60), computer modeling, bioprinting, and nanotechnology (60–62). "Functionalized," "decorated," or "smart" biomaterials that incorporate of biomolecular moieties on the surface, aim to orchestrate, and optimize the attachment and growth of cells and the synthesis of new tissue (61, 63). Scaffold size is largely limited by the lack of effective vascularization. Most successful work in the field focuses on understanding native tissue constituents and microarchitecture to allow accurate reproduction of functional tissue (64).

Environment

Consideration of the biophysiochemical 3D environment is crucial for tissue engineering. Cells not only require a scaffold for structural and biological support but also require an environment that provides the correct combination of growth supplements, differentiation signals, perfusion of nutrients, gaseous/waste exchange, pH regulation, and mechanical forces. The metabolic requirements of different tissues are varied and dictate the perfusion, gaseous/waste exchange, pH, and mechanical environment required. There is an increasing awareness that molecular and mechanical signaling is pivotal in the growth and differentiation of tissue-engineered constructs, and in addition to well-known growth factors such as bone morphogenetic proteins, vascular epithelial growth factor, basic fibroblast growth factor FGF-2, and transforming growth factor-β (65), "induction factors," including oxygen tension (66–68), mechanical (69), and electrical stimulation (70), guide subsequent proliferation and differentiation of cells. Cells participate in a web of multidirectional interactions within their niches and tissues of residence [interacting with various nanotopographically sized cues (71)]. This has implications during biomimetic tissue engineering, where the cellular environment (biomolecules), scaffold topography, and other external factors (mechanical and electrical stimulation) require regulation. This is complicated by the fact that cells not only respond to multiple stimuli but also have a direct impact on the environment themselves.

Research in this field is at the interface of cell biologists, engineers, materials scientists, and clinicians and is expanding rapidly. Multidisciplinary teams are working on bioreactor technology, which is vital for *in vitro* tissue engineering. Optimal conditions can to a great extent be applied and controlled through the use of bioreactors to mimic required conditions (72), and specialized bioreactors to help engineer a range of tissues have been developed in recent years (73, 74). Bioreactors are

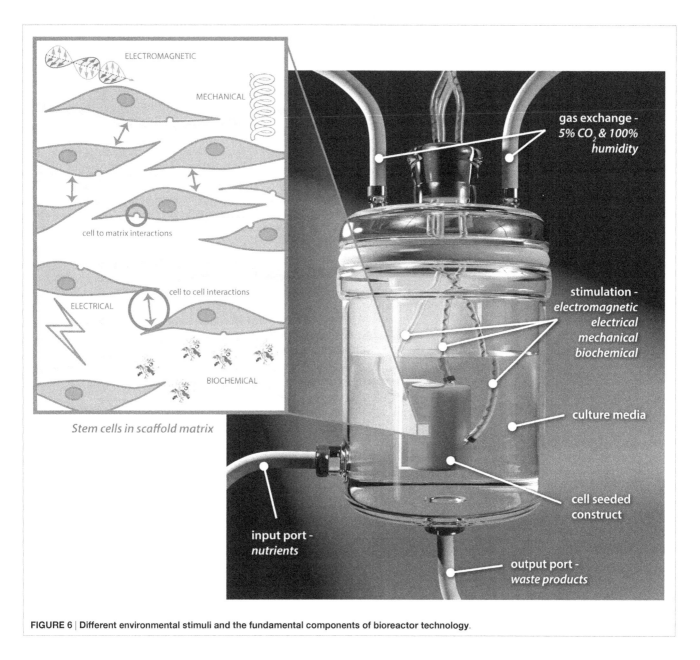

FIGURE 6 | Different environmental stimuli and the fundamental components of bioreactor technology.

increasingly being used to provide more complex environments, exposing cells to a range of controllable electrical, electromagnetic, biomolecular, and mechanical cues while varying cell–cell or cell–matrix interactions (**Figure 6**) (73).

CURRENT BARRIERS TO TRANSLATION

Tissue engineering has the potential for major clinical impact in plastic and reconstructive surgery. Some products using tissue-engineering concepts are already on the market; however, the panacea of functional vascularized composite tissue-engineered constructs is still theoretical. Translation of good basic science research from the laboratory to clinical reality remains a considerable challenge (**Figure 7**). In addition to meeting the scientific challenges of engineering durable and functional tissue

for implantation into patients (75), one must also navigate the complex regulatory processes. The regulations controlling the delivery of stem cell therapeutics to the clinic parallel many of those developed for the pharmaceutical industry (76, 77). Guidelines governing the development of cell-based products can be found on websites for the U.S. Food and Drug Administration (FDA),[1] the European Medicines Agency,[2] and related governmental regulatory authorities. The United States Pharmacopeia is an internationally recognized resource defining the currently accepted industry standards for product purity, potency, and quality assurance.[3] These targets are hard to meet outside a large,

---

[1] http://www.fda.gov/.
[2] http://www.ema.europa.eu/ema.
[3] http://www.usp.org/.

well-equipped commercial enterprise. Many research laboratories attached to clinical facilities do not produce mesenchymal stem cells in accordance with the criteria for either GLP or the more stringent cGMP, both requiring strict operational and certification records relating to all laboratory equipment and reagents used in the cell manufacture process (1, 4, 5).

A clear understanding of the manufacturing workflow is required to allow autologous and allogeneic tissue-engineered product integration into clinical practice (78). Once cells are obtained from a donor, they must be stored in specialized banks and both "scaled-up" (increasing batch size) and "scaled out" (increasing number of batches). There are several challenges in mass production alone including the monitoring of product yield and ensuring purity, potency, and viability throughout the process. Mass production of autologous tissue requires a facility allowing multiple, parallel, patient-specific production lines. Where scaffolds are required, testing and maintenance of quality attributes needs to be undertaken prior to seeding (78). Additional challenges include storage/transportation, contamination, and obtaining regulatory approval.

The long-term safety, efficacy, and functionality of the products also need to be closely assessed (79). Practical considerations

that need to be contemplated include the storage environment and shelf life of the manufactured products.

It is also of interest that tissue-engineered products do not easily conform to either of the traditional Food and Drug Administration classification: biologics or devices (80, 81). Combined scaffold and cell-containing devices may be in more than one classification category. For devices, a single confirmatory study is often sufficient for FDA approval. If the product is regulated as a biologic, it must be reviewed and approved by the FDA Center for Biologics Evaluation and Research. If regulated as a drug, several further phases are required prior to FDA approval. Although these regulatory processes above present significant challenges, many countries do have streamlined regulatory processes that might reduce the obstacles faced (82).

TISSUE ENGINEERING—WHERE ARE WE NOW?

Stable and physiologically relevant (74) tissue replacement with composite engineered tissue remains elusive. Allograft transplantation has been an exciting development for the reconstructive surgeon, but the requirement for long-term immunosuppressive therapy (83), health-care infrastructure, and funding streams means it is not mainstream practice (**Table 3**). Tissue engineering is a promising alternative and has yielded small successes so far. Atala et al. were the first to report tissue-engineered constructs being used in patients (84). This was followed by several reports between 2008 and 2014 in a range of tissues including the trachea (85, 86), urethra (87), and nasal cartilage (88). Results have been varied; tracheal work is currently under investigation due to the deaths of three out of six patients and for nasal cartilage in particular, there was a question mark whether the tissue was replaced by scar or native tissue (89). The current significant barriers to translation for large-volume tissue replacement are the inability to produce "physiologicallty relevant tissue" (74) and difficulties with vascularization (24). Small constructs may succeed based on local angiogenesis (84, 87); however, the metabolic needs of the implanted cells in larger constructs means prevascularisation or the use of vascular pedicles is likely to be necessary (87).

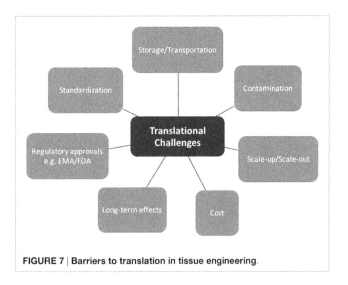

FIGURE 7 | Barriers to translation in tissue engineering.

TABLE 3 | Successful applications of tissue-engineered constructs in humans.

Organ/ tissue	No. of patients	Cell source	Outcomes	Reference
Bladder	7	Bladder urothelial and muscle cells	Improved volume and compliance with no metabolic consequences at mean 46 months follow-up	Atala et al. (84)
Trachea	1	Recipient MSCs	Functional airway with a normal appearance and mechanical properties at 4 months	Macchiarini et al. (85)
Urethra	5	Muscle and epithelial cells	Maintenance of wide urethral calibers without strictures, normal architecture on biopsy at 3 months following implantation	Raya-Rivera et al. (87)
Nasal cartilage	5	Autologous nasal chondrocytes	Good structural stability and respiratory function after 1 year	Fulco et al. (88)
Vaginal organs	4	Vulval biopsy—epithelial and muscle cells	Tri-layered structure on biopsy with phenotypically normal smooth muscle and epithelia with follow-up up to 8 years	Raya-Rivera et al. (90)

CONCLUSION AND FUTURE PERSPECTIVES

Surgical reconstruction using bioengineered tissues has the potential to revolutionize clinical practice. To be successful, one must be able to generate tissue constructs *in vitro* that are morphologically and functionally similar to native tissues. There has been a steady increase in basic science activity in cell therapy and a growing portfolio of cell therapy trials; however, this has not translated to commercial products available for clinical use. To achieve clinical translation, a multidisciplinary approach that successfully integrates engineering and biological methodologies is necessary. Ethical, regulatory, financial, and clinical considerations all present challenges in the translation of tissue-engineered constructs from the laboratory to mainstream clinical practice. Even though The Medical Research Council states that regenerative medicine and tissue engineering "holds the promise of revolutionizing patient care in the 21st century" (91) and that stem cell therapy is viewed as a future "game changer" by the plastic surgery community (92), many are yet to be convinced of this potential within the NHS, with major concerns involving cost-effectiveness, efficacy, reimbursement, and regulation (93). There is little doubt that tissue engineering offers great potential to reduce patient morbidity and mortality, and only co-ordinated and prolonged liaison between clinicians, scientists, and industry will move this from potential to reality.

GLOSSARY

Cell Biology

Differentiation—The process by which a cell becomes specialized in order to perform a specific function.

Commitment—When a cell becomes dedicated to a specific lineage.

Potency—The array of commitment opportunities available to a cell.

Totipotent—Cells capable of differentiating into any body cell type in addition to extraembryonic or placental cells.

Multipotent—Cells capable of differentiating into multiple cell types along one lineage (e.g., hematopoietic stem cells).

Pluripotent—Cells that may differentiate into tissues derived from all three germ cell layers.

Unipotent—Cells only capable of differentiating into one cell type (e.g., spermatogonial stem cells).

Clonal—A population of identical cells derived from the same cell.

Polyclonal—A population of cells derived from multiple clones.

Progenitor—A cell that has limited potency, but is able to differentiate to another cell type, or differentiate to its target cell lineage.

Embryonic stem cells—Embryonically derived pluripotent cells that are obtained from the inner cell mass.

Induced pluripotent stem cells—Differentiated cells that are reverted to their pluripotent state via a set of transcription factors.

Autologous—Cells or tissues obtained from the same individual.

Allogeneic—Cells or tissues obtained from a different individual of the same species.

Xenogeneic—Cells or tissues obtained from a different species.

Extracellular matrix—Biomolecules synthesized by the cell to provide a suitable environment to support surrounding cells and maintain tissue integrity in response to biochemical and mechanical cues.

Biomaterials/Scaffolds

Scaffold—A 3D biomaterial construct that defines the geometry of the replacement tissue and provides environmental cues that promote tissue regeneration.

Biomimetic—Human-made substances, e.g., scaffolds that imitate nature.

Functionalization—The modification of scaffolds with bioactive material to enhance the biocompatibility of the scaffold.

Nanotechnology—Technology that deals with dimensions and tolerances of less than 100 nm, especially the manipulation of individual atoms and molecules.

Biomolecular factors—Biomolecular factors include growth factors, transcription factors, and components of the extracellular matrix.

Mechanical factors—External environmental stimuli such as forces generated during everyday movement.

Manufacturing

Bioprinting—the process of generating spatially controlled cell patterns using 3D printing technologies.

Bioreactor—System in which conditions are closely controlled to permit or induce certain behavior in living cells or tissues.

Good Laboratory Practice (GLP)—System of management controls for laboratories conducting research to ensure consistency, reliability, reproducibility, and high quality of chemical (including pharmaceutical) tests.

Good Manufacturing Practice (GMP) guidelines—Regulatory guidelines that outline specific requirements for the handling and processing of human tissue, ensuring safe products of reliable quality.

Scale-out—Increasing the number of batches of an engineered product.

Scale-up—Increasing batch size on an engineered product.

AUTHOR CONTRIBUTIONS

SA-H and ZJ completed a literature search and contributed to preparing the manuscript. AA-S, EC, and AI contributed ideas and content to the manuscript. SD, AH, CT, and CA critically revised the manuscript. IW conceived, contributed to the preparation of, and critically revised the manuscript. All the authors read and approved the final manuscript and agreed to be accountable for all aspects of the work.

ACKNOWLEDGMENTS

The Reconstructive Surgery and Regenerative Medicine Research Group (ReconRegen) is currently supported by funding from the Royal College of Surgeons of England, British Association of Plastic, Reconstructive and Aesthetic Surgeons (BAPRAS), Medical Research Council (MR/N002431/1), ABMU Health Board, and Welsh Assembly Government. The authors thank Mr. Steve Atherton and Ms. Amy Shorter, medical illustrators, ABMU Health Board, for figures.

REFERENCES

1. Pratt GF, Rozen WM, Chubb D, Ashton MW, Alonso-Burgos A, Whitaker IS. Preoperative imaging for perforator flaps in reconstructive surgery: a systematic review of the evidence for current techniques. *Ann Plast Surg* (2012) 69(1):3–9. doi:10.1097/SPA.0b013e318222b7b7

2. Taylor GI, Daniel RK. The free flap: composite tissue transfer by vascular anastomosis. *Aust N Z J Surg* (1973) 43(1):1–3. doi:10.1111/j.1445-2197.1973. tb05659.x

3. Shores JT, Brandacher G, Lee WPA. Hand and upper extremity transplantation: an update of outcomes in the worldwide experience. *Plast Reconstr Surg* (2015) 135(2):351e–60e. doi:10.1097/PRS.0000000000000892

4. Khalifian S, Brazio PS, Mohan R, Shaffer C, Brandacher G, Barth RN, et al. Facial transplantation: the first 9 years. *Lancet* (2014) 384(9960):2153–63. doi:10.1016/S0140-6736(13)62632-X

5. Nodzo SR, Hohman DW, Chakravarthy K. Nanotechnology: why should we care? *Am J Orthop* (2015) 44(3):E87–8.

6. Naderi H, Matin MM, Bahrami AR. Review paper: critical issues in tissue engineering: biomaterials, cell sources, angiogenesis, and drug delivery systems. *J Biomater Appl* (2011) 26(4):383–417. doi:10.1177/0885328211408946

7. Murphy SV, Atala A. 3D bioprinting of tissues and organs. *Nat Biotechnol* (2014) 32(8):773–85. doi:10.1038/nbt.2958

8. Gerstle TL, Ibrahim AM, Kim PS, Lee BT, Lin SJ. A plastic surgery application in evolution: three-dimensional printing. *Plast Reconstr Surg* (2014) 133(2):446–51. doi:10.1097/01.prs.0000436844.92623.d3

9. Chae MP, Rozen WM, McMenamin PG, Findlay MW, Spychal RT, Hunter-Smith DJ. Emerging applications of bedside 3D printing in plastic surgery. *Front Surg* (2015) 2:25. doi:10.3389/fsurg.2015.00025

10. Kamali P, Dean D, Skoracki R, Koolen PG, Paul MA, Ibrahim AM, et al. The current role of three-dimensional (3D) printing in plastic surgery. *Plast Reconstr Surg* (2016). doi:10.1097/PRS.0000000000003106

11. Golas AR, Hernandez KA, Spector JA. Tissue engineering for plastic surgeons: a primer. *Aesthetic Plast Surg* (2014) 38(1):207–21. doi:10.1007/s00266-013-0255-5

12. Whitaker I, Boyce E. Dismissing the myths: an analysis of 12,483 procedures. All in a years work for a plastic surgical unit. *Internet J World Health Soc Politics* (2009) 6(2).

13. *Hospital Episode Statistics, Admitted Patient Care, England 2012–13.* Health and Social Care Information Centre (2015). Available from: http://www.hscic.gov.uk/catalogue/PUB12566

14. *Hospital Episode Statistics, Outpatient Care.* Health and Social Care Information Centre (2015). Available from: http://www.hscic.gov.uk/searchcatalogue?productid=18356&q=title%3a%22hospital+episode+statistics%22&sort=Relevance&size=10&page=1#top

15. *Recommendation for Plastic Surgery Training 2011.* UK: Centre for Workforce Intelligence a Report from the Royal College of Surgeons of England (2015). Available from: http://www.rcseng.ac.uk/surgeons/surgical-standards/docs/2011-surgical-workforce-census-report

16. Søreide K. Epidemiology of major trauma. *Br J Surg* (2009) 96(7):697–8. doi:10.1002/bjs.6643

17. Sterodimas A, De Faria J, Correa WE, Pitanguy I. Tissue engineering in plastic surgery: an up-to-date review of the current literature. *Ann Plast Surg* (2009) 62(1):97–103. doi:10.1097/SAP.0b013e3181788ec9

18. Skalak R, Fox CF. *Tissue Engineering: Proceeding of a Workshop Held at Granlibakken, Lake Tahoe, California.* New York: Liss (1998).

19. Ikada Y. Challenges in tissue engineering. *J R Soc Interface* (2006) 3(10):589–601. doi:10.1098/rsif.2006.0124

20. Pallua N, Gröger A. Tissue engineering and plastic surgery. In: Klein ME, Neuhann-Lorenz C, editors. *Innovations in Plastic and Aesthetic Surgery.* Berlin, Heidelberg: Springer (2008). p. 17–23.

21. D'Amico RA, Rubin JP. Regenerative medicine and the future of plastic surgery. *Plast Reconstr Surg* (2014) 133(6):1511–2. doi:10.1097/PRS.0000000000000212

22. Committee GBP HOLSAT. *House of Lords – Select Committee on Science and Technology – HL 76.* London: The Stationery Office Limited (2013).

23. O'Dowd A. Peers call for UK to harness "enormous" potential of regenerative medicine. *Br Med J* (2013) 347:f4248. doi:10.1136/bmj.f4248

24. Findlay MW, Dolderer JH, Trost N, Craft RO, Cao Y, Cooper-White J, et al. Tissue-engineered breast reconstruction: bridging the gap toward large-volume tissue engineering in humans. *Plast Reconstr Surg* (2011) 128(6):1206–15. doi:10.1097/PRS.0b013e318230c5b2

25. Freese KE, Kokai L, Edwards RP, Philips BJ, Sheikh MA, Kelley J, et al. Adipose-derived stems cells and their role in human cancer development, growth, progression, and metastasis: a systematic review. *Cancer Res* (2015) 75(7):1161–8. doi:10.1158/0008-5472.CAN-14-2744

26. Bichara DA, O'Sullivan NA, Pomerantseva I, Zhao X, Sundback CA, Vacanti JP, et al. The tissue-engineered auricle: past, present, and future. *Tissue Eng Part B Rev* (2012) 18:51–61. doi:10.1089/ten.TEB.2011.0326

27. Cao Y, Vacanti JP, Paige KT, Upton J, Vacanti CA. Transplantation of chondrocytes utilizing a polymer-cell construct to produce tissue-engineered cartilage in the shape of a human ear. *Plast Reconstr Surg* (1997) 100:297–302. doi:10.1097/00006534-199708000-00001

28. Kamil SH, Vacanti MP, Aminuddin BS, Jackson MJ, Vacanti CA, Eavey RD. Tissue engineering of a human sized and shaped auricle using a mold. *Laryngoscope* (2004) 114:867. doi:10.1097/00005537-200405000-00015

29. Christophel JJ, Chang JS, Park SS. Transplanted tissue-engineered cartilage. *Arch Facial Plast Surg* (2006) 8(2):117–22. doi:10.1001/archfaci.8.2.117

30. Nayyer L, Patel KH, Esmaeili A, Rippel RA, Birchall M, O'Toole G, et al. Tissue engineering: revolution and challenge in auricular cartilage reconstruction. *Plast Reconstr Surg* (2012) 129(5):1123–37. doi:10.1097/PRS.0b013e31824a2c1c

31. Brommer H, Brama PAJ, Laasanen MS, Helminen HJ, van Weeren PR, Jurvelin JS. Functional adaptation of articular cartilage from birth to maturity under the influence of loading: a biomechanical analysis. *Equine Vet J* (2005) 37(2):148–54. doi:10.2746/0425164054223769

32. Kusuhara H, Isogai N, Enjo M, Otani H, Ikada Y, Jacquet R, et al. Tissue engineering a model for the human ear: assessment of size, shape, morphology, and gene expression following seeding of different chondrocytes. *Wound Repair Regen* (2009) 17(1):136–46. doi:10.1111/j.1524-475X.2008.00451.x

33. Nabzdyk C, Pradhan L, Molina J, Perin E, Paniagua D, Rosenstrauch D. Auricular chondrocytes—from benchwork to clinical applications. *In Vivo* (2009) 23(3):369–80.

34. Homicz MR, Schumacher BL, Sah RH, Watson D. Effects of serial expansion of septal chondrocytes on tissue-engineered neocartilage composition. *Otolaryngol Head Neck Surg* (2002) 127:398–408. doi:10.1067/mhn.2002.129730

35. Jian-Wei X, Randolph MA, Peretti GM, Nazzal JA, Roses RE, Morse KR, et al. Producing a flexible tissue-engineered cartilage framework using expanded polytetrafluoroethylene membrane as a pseudoperichondrium. *Plastic Reconstr Surg* (2005) 116(2):577–89. doi:10.1097/01.prs.0000172985.81897.dc

36. Bianco P, Robey PG. Stem cells in tissue engineering. *Nature* (2001) 414(6859):118–21. doi:10.1038/35102181

37. Guillot PV, Cui W, Fisk NM, Polak DJ. Stem cell differentiation and expansion for clinical applications of tissue engineering. *J Cell Mol Med* (2007) 11(5):935–44. doi:10.1111/j.1582-4934.2007.00106.x

38. Shi Q, Rafii S, Wu MH, Wijelath ES, Yu C, Ishida A, et al. Evidence for circulating bone marrow-derived endothelial cells. *Blood* (1998) 92(2):362–7.

39. Thomson JA, Itskovitz-Eldor J, Shapiro SS, Waknitz MA, Swiergiel JJ, Marshall VS, et al. Embryonic stem cell lines derived from human blastocysts. *Science* (1998) 282(5391):1145–7. doi:10.1126/science.282.5391.1145

40. Dominici M, Le Blanc K, Mueller I, Slaper-Cortenbach I, Marini F, Krause D, et al. Minimal criteria for defining multipotent mesenchymal stromal cells. The International Society for Cellular Therapy position statement. *Cytotherapy* (2006) 8(4):315–7. doi:10.1080/14653240600855905

41. Kupfer ME, Ogle BM. Advanced imaging approaches for regenerative medicine: emerging technologies for monitoring stem cell fate in vitro

and in vivo. *Biotechnol J* (2015) 10(10):1515–28. doi:10.1002/biot. 201400760

42. Asano T, Sasaki K, Kitano Y, Terao K, Hanazono Y. In vivo tumor formation from primate embryonic stem cells. *Methods Mol Biol* (2006) 329: 459–67.

43. da Silva Meirelles L, Caplan AI, Nardi NB. In search of the in vivo identity of mesenchymal stem cells. *Stem Cells* (2008) 26(9):2287–99. doi:10.1634/stemcells.2007-1122

44. Zuk PA, Zhu M, Mizuno H, Huang J, Futrell JW, Katz AJ, et al. Multilineage cells from human adipose tissue: implications for cell-based therapies. *Tissue Eng* (2001) 7(2):211–28. doi:10.1089/107632701300062859

45. Stock UA, Vacanti JP. Tissue engineering: current state and prospects. *Annu Rev Med* (2001) 52(1):443–51. doi:10.1146/annurev.med.52.1.443

46. Takahashi K, Yamanaka S. Induction of pluripotent stem cells from mouse embryonic and adult fibroblast cultures by defined factors. *Cell* (2006) 126(4):663–76. doi:10.1016/j.cell.2006.07.024

47. Hayden EC. Stem cells: the growing pains of pluripotency. *Nature* (2011) 9:272–4. doi:10.1038/473272a

48. Laurent LC, Ulitsky I, Slavin I, Tran H, Schork A, Morey R, et al. Dynamic changes in the copy number of pluripotency and cell proliferation genes in human ESCs and iPSCs during reprogramming and time in culture. *Cell Stem Cell* (2011) 8(1):106–18. doi:10.1016/j.stem.2010.12.003

49. Zhao T, Zhang Z-N, Rong Z, Xu Y. Immunogenicity of induced pluripotent stem cells. *Nature* (2011) 474(7350):212–5. doi:10.1038/nature10135

50. Chang T, Zimmerley MS, Quinn KP, Lamarre-Jouenne I, Kaplan DL, Beaurepaire E, et al. Non-invasive monitoring of cell metabolism and lipid production in 3D engineered human adipose tissues using label-free multiphoton microscopy. *Biomater* (2013) 34(34):8607–16. doi:10.1016/j.biomaterials.2013.07.066

51. Erlach von TC, Hedegaard MAB, Stevens MM. High resolution Raman spectroscopy mapping of stem cell micropatterns. *Analyst* (2015) 140(6):1798–803. doi:10.1039/c4an02346c

52. Bodle JC, Teeter SD, Hluck BH, Hardin JW, Bernacki SH, Loboa EG. Age-related effects on the potency of human adipose-derived stem cells: creation and evaluation of superlots and implications for musculoskeletal tissue engineering applications. *Tissue Eng Part C Methods* (2014) 20(12):972–83. doi:10.1089/ten.TEC.2013.0683

53. Bhatnagar R, Li S. Biomimetic scaffolds for tissue engineering. *Conf Proc IEEE Eng Med Biol Soc* (2004) 7:5021–3. doi:10.1109/IEMBS.2004.1404387

54. Hollister SJ. Porous scaffold design for tissue engineering. *Nat Mater* (2005) 4(7):518–24. doi:10.1038/nmat1421

55. Hutmacher DW. Scaffolds in tissue engineering bone and cartilage. *Biomaterials* (2000) 21(24):2529–43. doi:10.1016/S0142-9612(00)00121-6

56. Rezwan K, Chen QZ, Blaker JJ, Boccaccini AR. Biodegradable and bioactive porous polymer/inorganic composite scaffolds for bone tissue engineering. *Biomaterials* (2006) 27(18):3413–31. doi:10.1016/j.biomaterials. 2006.01.039

57. Kim BS, Mooney DJ. Development of biocompatible synthetic extracellular matrices for tissue engineering. *Trends Biotechnol* (1998) 16(5):224–30. doi:10.1016/S0167-7799(98)01191-3

58. Lutolf MP, Hubbell JA. Synthetic biomaterials as instructive extracellular microenvironments for morphogenesis in tissue engineering. *Nat Biotechnol* (2005) 23(1):47–55. doi:10.1038/nbt1055

59. Sanghvi AB, Miller KP-H, Belcher AM, Schmidt CE. Biomaterials functionalization using a novel peptide that selectively binds to a conducting polymer. *Nat Mater* (2005) 4(6):496–502. doi:10.1038/nmat1397

60. Barnes CP, Sell SA, Boland ED, Simpson DG, Bowlin GL. Nanofiber technology: designing the next generation of tissue engineering scaffolds. *Adv Drug Deliv Rev* (2007) 59(14):1413–33. doi:10.1016/j.addr.2007.04.022

61. Furth ME, Atala A, Van Dyke ME. Smart biomaterials design for tissue engineering and regenerative medicine. *Biomaterials* (2007) 28(34):5068–73. doi:10.1016/j.biomaterials.2007.07.042

62. Wong YS, Tay CY, Wen F. Engineered polymeric biomaterials for tissue engineering. *Curr Tissue Eng* (2012) 1:41–53.

63. Anderson DG, Burdick JA, Langer R. Materials science. Smart biomaterials. *Science* (2004) 305(5692):1923–4. doi:10.1126/science.1099987

64. Lanza R, Langer R, Vacanti JP. *Principles of Tissue Engineering*. 4th ed. Academic Press (2013). 1 p.

65. Chen F-M, Zhang M, Wu Z-F. Toward delivery of multiple growth factors in tissue engineering. *Biomaterials* (2010) 31(24):6279–308. doi:10.1016/j. biomaterials.2010.04.053

66. Leijten J, Georgi N, Moreira Teixeira L, van Blitterswijk CA, Post JN, Karperien M. Metabolic programming of mesenchymal stromal cells by oxygen tension directs chondrogenic cell fate. *Proc Natl Acad Sci U S A* (2014) 111(38):13954–9. doi:10.1073/pnas.1410977111

67. Fotia C, Massa A, Boriani F, Baldini N, Granchi D. Prolonged exposure to hypoxic milieu improves the osteogenic potential of adipose derived stem cells. *J Cell Biochem* (2015) 116(7):1442–53. doi:10.1002/jcb. 25106

68. De Miguel MP, Alcaina Y, la Maza de DS, Lopez-Iglesias P. Cell metabolism under microenvironmental low oxygen tension levels in stemness, proliferation and pluripotency. *Curr Mol Med* (2015) 15(4):343–59. doi:10.2174/1 566524015666150505160406

69. Correia V, Panadero JA, Ribeiro C, Sencadas V, Rocha JG, Gomez Ribelles JL, et al. Design and validation of a biomechanical bioreactor for cartilage tissue culture. *Biomech Model Mechanobiol* (2016) 15(2):471–8. doi:10.1007/ s10237-015-0698-5

70. Hernández-Bule ML, Paíno CL, Trillo MÁ, Úbeda A. Electric stimulation at 448 kHz promotes proliferation of human mesenchymal stem cells. *Cell Physiol Biochem* (2014) 34(5):1741–55. doi:10.1159/000366375

71. Griffin MF, Butler PE, Seifalian AM, Kalaskar DM. Control of stem cell fate by engineering their micro and nanoenvironment. *World J Stem Cells* (2015) 7(1):37–50. doi:10.4252/wjsc.v7.i1.37

72. Pörtner R, Nagel-Heyer S, Goepfert C, Adamietz P, Meenen NM. Bioreactor design for tissue engineering. *J Biosci Bioeng* (2005) 100(3):235–45. doi:10.1263/jbb.100.235

73. Hansmann J, Groeber F, Kahlig A, Kleinhans C, Walles H. Bioreactors in tissue engineering – principles, applications and commercial constraints. *Biotechnol J* (2013) 8(3):298–307. doi:10.1002/biot.201200162

74. Abbott RD, Kaplan DL. Strategies for improving the physiological relevance of human engineered tissues. *Trends Biotechnol* (2015) 33(7):401–7. doi:10.1016/j.tibtech.2015.04.003

75. Hunziker E, Spector M, Libera J, Gertzman A, Woo SL-Y, Ratcliffe A, et al. Translation from research to applications. *Tissue Eng* (2006) 12(12):3341–64. doi:10.1089/ten.2006.12.3341

76. Halme DG, Kessler DA. FDA regulation of stem-cell-based therapies. *N Engl J Med* (2006) 355(16):1730–5. doi:10.1056/NEJMhpr063086

77. Fink DW. FDA regulation of stem cell-based products. *Science* (2009) 324(5935):1662–3. doi:10.1126/science.1173712

78. Hunsberger J, Harrysson O, Shirwaiker R, Starly B, Wysk R, Cohen P, et al. Manufacturing road map for tissue engineering and regenerative medicine technologies. *Stem Cells Transl Med* (2015) 4(2):130–5. doi:10.5966/ sctm.2014-0254

79. Berry MG, Stanek JJ. The PIP mammary prosthesis: a product recall study. *J Plast Reconstr Aesthet Surg* (2012) 65(6):697–704. doi:10.1016/j. bjps.2012.02.019

80. Lu L, Arbit HM, Herrick JL, Segovis SG, Maran A, Yaszemski MJ. Tissue engineered constructs: perspectives on clinical translation. *Ann Biomed Eng* (2015) 43(3):796–804. doi:10.1007/s10439-015-1280-0

81. Uppal RS, Sabbagh W, Chana J, Gault DT. Donor-site morbidity after autologous costal cartilage harvest in ear reconstruction and approaches to reducing donor-site contour deformity. *Plast Reconstr Surg* (2008) 121(6):1949–55. doi:10.1097/PRS.0b013e318170709e

82. Birchall MA, Seifalian AM. Tissue engineering's green shoots of disruptive innovation. *Lancet* (2014) 384(9940):288–90. doi:10.1016/ S0140-6736(14)60533-X

83. Whitaker IS, Duggan EM, Alloway RR, Brown C, McGuire S, Woodle ES, et al. Composite tissue allotransplantation: a review of relevant immunological issues for plastic surgeons. *J Plast Reconstr Aesthet Surg* (2008) 61(5):481–92. doi:10.1016/j.bjps.2007.11.019

84. Atala A, Bauer SB, Soker S, Yoo JJ, Retik AB. Tissue-engineered autologous bladders for patients needing cystoplasty. *Lancet* (2006) 367(9518):1241–6. doi:10.1016/S0140-6736(06)68438-9

85. Macchiarini P, Jungebluth P, Go T, Asnaghi MA, Rees LE, Cogan TA, et al. Clinical transplantation of a tissue-engineered airway. *Lancet* (2008) 372(9655):2023–30. doi:10.1016/S0140-6736(08)61598-6

86. Baiguera S, Birchall MA, Macchiarini P. Tissue-engineered tracheal transplantation. *Transplantation* (2010) 89(5):485–91. doi:10.1097/TP.0b013e3181cd4ad3

87. Raya-Rivera A, Esquiliano DR, Yoo JJ, Lopez-Bayghen E, Soker S, Atala A. Tissue-engineered autologous urethras for patients who need reconstruction: an observational study. *Lancet* (2011) 377(9772):1175–82. doi:10.1016/S0140-6736(10)62354-9

88. Fulco I, Miot S, Haug MD, Barbero A, Wixmerten A, Feliciano S, et al. Engineered autologous cartilage tissue for nasal reconstruction after tumour resection: an observational first-in-human trial. *Lancet* (2014) 384(9940):337–46. doi:10.1016/S0140-6736(14)60544-4

89. Russell AJ. The end of the beginning for tissue engineering. *Lancet* (2014) 383(9913):193–5. doi:10.1016/S0140-6736(13)62110-8

90. Raya-Rivera AM, Esquiliano D, Fierro-Pastrana R, López-Bayghen E, Valencia P, Ordorica-Flores R, et al. Tissue-engineered autologous vaginal organs in patients: a pilot cohort study. *Lancet* (2014) 384(9940):329–36. doi:10.1016/S0140-6736(14)60542-0

91. Medical Research Council. *Regenerative Medicine and Stem Cells*. Available from: http://www.mrc.ac.uk/research/initiatives/regenerative-medicine-stem-cells/ (accessed January 26, 2017).

92. Ozturk S, Karagoz H, Zor F. The future of plastic surgery: surgeon's perspective. *J Craniofac Surg* (2015) 26(8):e708–13. doi:10.1097/SCS.0000000000002204

93. Davies BM, Rikabi S, French A, Pinedo-Villanueva R, Morrey ME, Wartolowska K, et al. Quantitative assessment of barriers to the clinical development and adoption of cellular therapies: a pilot study. *J Tissue Eng* (2014) 5(0):2041731414551764. doi:10.1177/2041731414551764

Emerging Applications of Bedside 3D Printing in Plastic Surgery

Michael P. Chae[1,2], Warren M. Rozen[1,2], Paul G. McMenamin[3], Michael W. Findlay[1,4]*,
Robert T. Spychal[1] and David J. Hunter-Smith[1,2]

[1] 3D PRINT Laboratory, Department of Surgery, Peninsula Health, Frankston, VIC, Australia, [2] Monash University Plastic and
Reconstructive Surgery Group (Peninsula Clinical School), Peninsula Health, Frankston, VIC, Australia, [3] Department of
Anatomy and Developmental Biology, Centre for Human Anatomy Education, School of Biomedical Sciences, Faculty of
Medicine, Nursing and Health Sciences, Monash University, Clayton, VIC, Australia, [4] Department of Surgery, Stanford
University, Stanford, CA, USA

*Correspondence:
Michael W. Findlay,
3D PRINT Laboratory, Department of
Surgery, Peninsula Health, 2 Hastings
Road, Frankston, VIC 3199, Australia
mfindlay@stanford.edu

Modern imaging techniques are an essential component of preoperative planning in plastic and reconstructive surgery. However, conventional modalities, including three-dimensional (3D) reconstructions, are limited by their representation on 2D workstations. 3D printing, also known as rapid prototyping or additive manufacturing, was once the province of industry to fabricate models from a computer-aided design (CAD) in a layer-by-layer manner. The early adopters in clinical practice have embraced the medical imaging-guided 3D-printed biomodels for their ability to provide tactile feedback and a superior appreciation of visuospatial relationship between anatomical structures. With increasing accessibility, investigators are able to convert standard imaging data into a CAD file using various 3D reconstruction softwares and ultimately fabricate 3D models using 3D printing techniques, such as stereolithography, multijet modeling, selective laser sintering, binder jet technique, and fused deposition modeling. However, many clinicians have questioned whether the cost-to-benefit ratio justifies its ongoing use. The cost and size of 3D printers have rapidly decreased over the past decade in parallel with the expiration of key 3D printing patents. Significant improvements in clinical imaging and user-friendly 3D software have permitted computer-aided 3D modeling of anatomical structures and implants without outsourcing in many cases. These developments offer immense potential for the application of 3D printing at the bedside for a variety of clinical applications. In this review, existing uses of 3D printing in plastic surgery practice spanning the spectrum from templates for facial transplantation surgery through to the formation of bespoke craniofacial implants to optimize post-operative esthetics are described. Furthermore, we discuss the potential of 3D printing to become an essential office-based tool in plastic surgery to assist in preoperative planning, developing intraoperative guidance tools, teaching patients and surgical trainees, and producing patient-specific prosthetics in everyday surgical practice.

Keywords: 3D printing, bedside, desktop application, plastic and reconstructive surgery, cost, preoperative planning, intraoperative guidance, education

Introduction

Advanced medical imaging has become an essential component of preoperative planning in plastic surgery. In breast reconstructive surgery, the introduction of computed tomographic angiography (CTA) has enabled surgeons to improve clinical outcomes (1) through accurate and reliable prospective selection of the donor site, flap, perforators, and the optimal mode of dissection (2, 3). Recent development of three-dimensional (3D) and 4D CTA techniques have enhanced spatial appreciation of the perforator vessels, their vascular territory, and dynamic flow characteristics preoperatively (4, 5). However, current imaging modalities are limited by being displayed on a 2D surface, such as a computer screen. In contrast, a 3D-printed haptic biomodel allows both the surgeon and the patient to develop a superior understanding of the anatomy and the procedure with the goal of improved operative planning through the ability to interact directly with a model of the patient-specific anatomy. Historically, the technically challenging nature of 3D software and the high prices of early 3D printers usually meant that clinicians keen to exploit these advantages had to outsource 3D printing and the cost of outsourcing often precluded it from being implemented widely. In this review, we analyze how recent advancements have enabled 3D printing to transition from the research and development laboratory to the clinical 'bedside' potentially making it a ubiquitous application in plastic surgery.

3D Printing

3D printing, also known as rapid prototyping or additive manufacturing, describes a process by which a product derived from a computer-aided design (CAD) is built in a layer-by-layer fashion (**Figure 1**) (Video S1 in Supplementary Material) (6–8). In contrast to the conventional manufacturing processes like injection molding, 3D printing has introduced an era of design freedom and enabled rapid production of customized objects with complex geometries (9–11). One of the major advantages of 3D printing is the capacity to directly translate a concept into an end product in a convenient, cost-efficient manner. It eliminates the typical intermediary stages involved in a product development, such as development, production, assembly lines, delivery, and warehousing of parts (12), and the subsequent savings made from using fewer materials and labor lead to an overall reduction in the cost of production (13).

3D printing has been utilized in industrial design since the 1980s; however, it has only become adapted for medical application in the last decade (14). Imaging data from routine computed tomography (CT) or magnetic resonance imaging (MRI) can be converted into a CAD file using a variety of 3D software programs, such as Osirix (Pixmeo, Geneva, Switzerland) or 3D Slicer (Surgical Planning Laboratory, Boston, MA, USA) (**Figure 1**). These files are processed into data slices suitable for printing by proprietary softwares from the 3D printer manufacturers. While a range of 3D printing techniques have been developed for industrial use; stereolithography (SLA), multijet modeling (MJM), selective laser sintering (SLS), binder jetting, and fused deposition modeling (FDM) are the main approaches that have

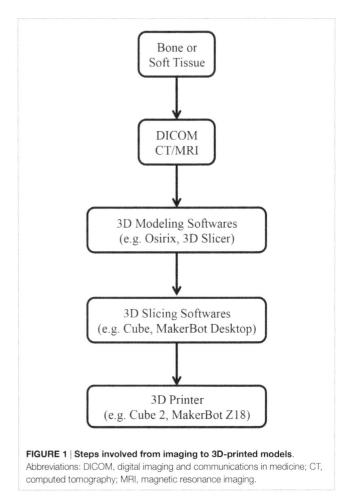

FIGURE 1 | Steps involved from imaging to 3D-printed models. Abbreviations: DICOM, digital imaging and communications in medicine; CT, computed tomography; MRI, magnetic resonance imaging.

been explored in the clinical setting (**Table 1**). We will explore each of these to evaluate their current and potential applications in clinical practice for both bony reconstruction and soft tissue reconstruction.

Types of 3D Printing
Stereolithography

Stereolithography is the earliest 3D printing technology described for fabricating biomodels, where a layer of liquid photopolymer or epoxy resin in a vat is cured by a low-power ultraviolet (UV) laser (15). Excess raw materials and the supporting structures must be manually removed from the final product and cured in a UV chamber (16–18). Currently, SLA is considered the gold standard in 3D biomodel production and can yield resolutions of up to 0.025 mm. Moreover, its efficiency increases when constructing larger objects and is able to faithfully reproduce internal structural details (19). However, the need for manual post-build handling makes it labor-intensive and it still takes more than a day to produce a large model. Furthermore, in comparison to other 3D printing techniques, it is considered more expensive due to the high cost of the raw materials and for the printer upkeep (20, 21). Recently, a novel modification to SLA has been developed called continuous liquid interface production (CLIP). This simplifies traditional SLA and increases the production speed by harnessing oxygen

TABLE 1 | A summary of the most commonly used 3D printing techniques in medical application.

3D printing techniques	Pros	Cons
SLA	Current gold standard High resolution Increased efficiency with increase in print size Detailed fabrication of internal structures	>1 day of printing time required Require extensive post-production manual handling High cost related to the materials, the printer, and the maintenance
MJM	High resolution Minimal post-production manual handling Multiple materials	High cost related to the material and printer Poorer surface finishing than SLA
SLS	Not require support structures Smooth surface finishing Print delicate structures Print in metal	Require post-production manual handling High cost related to the materials, the printer, and the maintenance Require expert handling of the printer
BJT	Not require support structures Multiple colors Multiple materials	Brittle Require extensive post-production manual handling Poor surface finish
FDM	Low cost Minimal maintenance High availability of printers	Require post-production manual removal of support structures Poor surface finish Mono-color and mono-material with the current technology

SLA, stereolithography; MJM, multijet modeling; SLS, selective laser sintering; BJT, binder jet technique; FDM, fused deposition modeling.

inhibition of UV-curable resin photopolymerization (22). This emerging modality has yet to be evaluated in plastic and reconstructive surgery but holds promise due to its combination of speed, structural integrity, and ability to fabricate complex structures.

MultiJet Modeling

Multijet modeling printing, also known as MultiJet Printing (3D Systems, Rock Hill, SC, USA) or Poly Jet Technology (Stratasys, Edina, MN, USA), is akin to SLA, but the liquid photopolymer is immediately cured by the UV light preventing the time-consuming post-processing in the UV chamber and the prototypes are built with gel-like support materials that are readily dissolvable in water (23). MJM can manufacture models with high resolution (16 μ) that is comparable to or better than SLA, with an added benefit of the capacity to print in multiple materials for the desired degree of tensile strength and durability. Furthermore, a MJM printer is easier to maintain than a SLA set-up. However, the high price of these printers makes MJM more suitable for large-scale productions than for office-based/bedside desktop application.

Selective Laser Sintering

Selective laser sintering describes a process where powdered forms of thermoplastic, metal, glass, or ceramic material are sintered by high-power laser beams in a layer-by-layer fashion (24, 25). Similar to SLA, the unsintered powders must be brushed away from the

final product; however, they provide support and eliminate the need for support structures. As a result, SLS yields models with smoother surface finish and facilitates the production of delicate structures with high accuracy. Furthermore, the unsintered powders can be reused leading to a reduction in cost compared to SLA (20, 26). However, SLS remains significantly more expensive than binder jet technique (BJT) (below) and FDM, due mainly to the cost of the printer. In addition, SLS printers can be potentially hazardous due to the presence of lasers, pistons, and gas chambers that can reach extremely high temperatures and hence, requires expert handling. These features have discouraged it from being widely implemented in non-industrial settings.

Binder Jet Technique

Binder jet technique, or powder bed technique, is the first 3D printing approach that reduced the cost of 3D printers, thereby enabling a widespread consumerization of 3D printing (27). Similar to the SLS process, printer heads eject a binder material along with colored dye onto a layer of powder, fusing them layer-by-layer into a plaster model (28). Unfused powders provide adequate support for the "overhanging" designs and hence, simultaneous deposition of support structures is rarely required. Moreover, binder jet 3D printers can print in multiple colors and materials, and have multiple printer heads for faster printing. One of the major drawbacks of binder jetting is that the final product usually lacks strength and has a poorer surface finish than SLA or SLS. Hence, all models require post-production strengthening with materials such as melted wax, cyanoacrylate glue, or epoxy.

Fused Deposition Modeling

Fused deposition modeling is the most commonly used consumer 3D printing technology available currently and is also the most affordable (21, 29, 30). A melted filament of thermoplastic material is extruded from a nozzle moving in the x-y plane and solidifies upon deposition on a build plate (31). After each layer, the build plate is lowered by 0.1 mm and the process is repeated until the final product is produced. Acrylonitrile-butadiene-styrene (ABS) and polylactic acid (PLA) are the most frequently used raw materials in FDM printers. A notable shortcoming for the use of FDM in medical applications is that most anatomical structures have complex shapes and hence, would require support structures. Although they are easy to remove manually, the aftermath generally leaves superficial damage to the model compromising its surface finish and esthetics. Hollow internal structures or blind-ended openings are particularly difficult to clean build material from. Furthermore, most household FDM printers are currently limited to fabricating in mono-color and mono-material. However, this can be overcome by recently developed dual-extruder technology, where two filaments of different color or material can be extruded from a common printer head. It is currently found in printers, such as MakerBot Replicator 2X Experimental (MakerBot Industries, New York, NY, USA), Cube 3 (3D Systems, Rock Hill, SC, USA), and Creatr x1 (Leapfrog, Emeryville, CA, USA). Moreover, the second extruder can be configured to build support structures using MakerBot Dissolvable Filament (MakerBot Industries), made up of high impact polystyrene (HIPS) (32). When the final product is immersed in water with limonene, a widely available citrus-scented solvent, the support structures selectively dissolve away within 8 to 24 h but these dual extruder printers have not yet become established in the mainstream.

3D Printing in Medicine

In the last decade or so, researchers have demonstrated a wide range of uses for 3D printing across numerous surgical disciplines. Clinically, 3D-printed haptic biomodels provide a tactile feedback and enable users to simulate complex anatomical movements, such as articulation at the temporomandibular joint, that are difficult to reproduce in a computer software (33). As a result, they facilitate an enhanced appreciation of the visuospatial relationship between anatomical structures for the surgeons (34). This can translate into shorter operative time, reduced exposure to general anesthesia, shorter wound exposure time and reduced intraoperative blood loss (18, 35, 36).

Preoperative Planning
In preoperative planning, 3D-printed biomodels have been beneficial in orbital and mandibular reconstruction in maxillofacial surgery (21, 37–41); craniofacial, skull base, and cervical spine reconstruction in neurosurgery (35); prefabrication of bony fixation plates and planning excision of bony lesions in orthopedic surgery (42, 43); mapping complex congenital heart defects and tracheobronchial variation in cardiothoracic surgery and cardiac transplantation (26, 44–52) (**Figure 2**); endovascular repair of abdominal aortic aneurysm and aortic dissection in vascular surgery (53–55); partial nephrectomy for renal tumors in urology (56); osteoplastic flap reconstruction of frontal sinus defects in ear, nose, and throat surgery (57, 58); and hepatectomy and liver transplantation in general surgery (59–61).

Intraoperative Guidance
Furthermore, 3D softwares have been used to fabricate patient-specific surgical templates and intraoperative guidance devices to aid surgeons in maxillofacial surgery (62–67), neurosurgery (68), orthopedic surgery (69), hand surgery (70), and general surgery (71).

Education
3D-printed haptic biomodels can be useful for educating patients during medical consultations and training surgical trainees (29, 45, 72–81).

Customized Prosthesis
Moreover, 3D printing has enabled rapid and convenient production of customized implants. Investigators have manufactured patient-specific mandibular implants in maxillofacial surgery (82–84), cranial vault implants for cranioplasty in neurosurgery (85, 86), hip implants in orthopedic surgery (87, 88), and a bioresorbable airway splint for complex tracheobronchomalacia in pediatric cardiothoracic surgery (89).

Allied Health
In other areas of medicine, 3D printing has revolutionized the manufacturing of hearing aids and currently 99% of all hearing aids in the world are 3D printed (90). Additionally, 3D printing

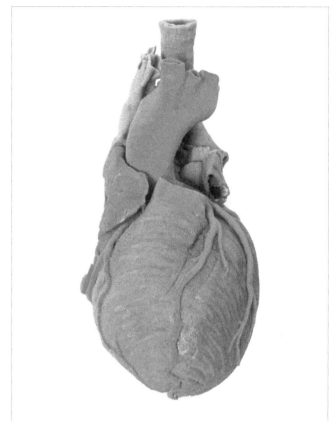

FIGURE 2 | 3D-printed haptic model of a heart and the great vessels fabricated using Projet x60 series 3D printers. Reproduced with permission from Centre for Human Anatomy and Education.

has helped in making complex diagnoses in forensic medicine (91); reformed anatomy education (92); helped in planning repairs of Charcot's foot in podiatry (93); permitted the fabrication of custom-made dental implants in dentistry (94–96); produced patient-specific 3D-printed medication in pharmaceutical industry (97, 98); and assembled custom-design tissue scaffolds in regenerative medicine (99, 100).

3D Printing at the Bedside

Despite a vast potential scope of 3D printing in clinical practice and significant media interest with frequent reports of the latest innovative advancements made using this technology (101). The incorporation of 3D printing as a clinical bedside application has not been widespread (102). One potential barrier is the perception amongst clinicians that 3D printing is technically sophisticated and is reserved for planning intricate operations and devising highly specialized implants (102). As a result, 3D printing is often outsourced to an external company, which compounds the cost and time. This demonstrates a lack of awareness of the increasing accessibility of the 3D softwares and the declining cost of the 3D printers (102).

3D Reconstruction Software
In order to fabricate a 3D biomodel, two types of software are required; firstly, a "3D modeling" software that translates the

DICOM (digital imaging and communications in medicine) files from CT/MRI scans into a CAD file, and secondly, a "3D slicing" software that divides the CAD file into thin data slices suitable for 3D printing (103).

3D Modeling Software

A range of 3D modeling softwares is available (**Table 2**); however, early ones, such as Mimics (Materialise NV, Leuven, Belgium), would incur a high cost for the initial purchase and for the ongoing software updates. Driven by the consumerization of 3D printing and an increasing number of both professional and community software developers, free open-source softwares, such as Osirix (104) and 3D Slicer (105–107), have become widely utilized. Our group prefers using them due to the latter's expansive developer community base, called the Slicer Community, a plethora of plug-in functions, and a user interface that is intuitive to an individual with no engineering background (108, 109). An ideal 3D modeling software should be free; capable of highlighting the region of interest and eliminate undesired areas using the threshold and the segmentation function, respectively; export the 3D model as a CAD file in a universally accepted 3D file format, such as STL (standard tessellation language); and possess an easy-to-use interface. Encouragingly, there are numerous 3D modeling softwares available in the market currently that fit all of the criteria (**Table 2**).

3D Slicing Software

3D slicing softwares digitally "slice" a CAD file into layers suitable for 3D printing. However, they are also useful for altering the orientation of the CAD file relative to the printer build plate to give an optimal direction, which minimizes the requirement for the support structures and, in turn, reduces the amount of material used and therefore also reduces the printing time. This process can be readily performed using proprietary softwares that accompany the 3D printers at no extra cost and usually possess a simple graphic user interface, such as Cube software (3D Systems) and MakerBot Desktop (MakerBot Industries).

3D Printers

The cost of early 3D printers, consisting of mostly the SLA type described above, precluded widespread adoption of 3D printing in the initial years; however, the expiration of key patents surrounding SLA and FDM in the last decade has fueled a surge in the number of commercial developers leading to an increase in the availability and a significant reduction of the cost (**Table 3**). Several affordable SLA 3D printers have entered the market since then, such as Form 1+ (Formlabs, Somerville, MA, USA) and ProJet 1200 (3D Systems). However, they are capable of building only small designs (i.e., 12.5 cm × 12.5 cm × 16.5 cm) and hence, remain unsuitable for many applications. Similarly, current MJM and SLS 3D printers are generally bulky and expensive, and require specialized skills for safe handling of the hardware and its maintenance. Binder jet 3D printers are gradually being avoided due to the brittle quality of the end-products and the large size of the printer. Currently, FDM 3D printers are the preferred option as a desktop application in medicine for their affordability and practicality. The accuracy and the quality of FDM products are comparable to SLA, SLS, and binder jet (110–112). Furthermore, FDM incurs the least cost in maintenance from ongoing print materials (**Table 4**).

3D Printing in Plastic and Reconstructive Surgery

In plastic and reconstructive surgery, 3D-printed haptic biomodels can potentially play a significant role in preoperative planning, intraoperative guidance, training and teaching, and fashioning patient-specific prosthesis (**Table 5**).

Preoperative Planning: Soft Tissue Mapping

Perforator flap surgery is routinely performed in the reconstruction of large soft tissue defects after trauma or an oncologic resection. Preoperative planning with CTA has revolutionized the field by enabling the reconstructive surgeon to identify an ideal donor site, flap, and perforator for a free flap transfer (3, 123), facilitating a greater flap success rate and an overall improvement in the

TABLE 2 | A summary of 3D modeling softwares that can convert a DICOM data from a standard CT/MRI scans into a CAD file.

Name	Company	Free	Threshold/ segmentation	Export STL	Easy user interface	OS platform
3D Slicer	Surgical Planning Laboratory	Y	Y	Y	Y	W, M
MITK	German Cancer Research Centre	Y	Y	Y	Y	W, M
Osirix	Pixmeo	Y	Y	Y	Y	M
MIPAV	NIH CIT	Y	Y	Y	N	W, M
MeVisLab	MeVis Medical Solutions AG	Y	Y	Y	N	W, M
InVesalius	CTI	Y	Y	Y	N	W, M
Mimics	Materialise NV	N	Y	Y	Y	W, M
Avizo/Amira	FEI Visualization Science Group	N	Y	Y	Y	W, M
3D Doctor	Able Software	N	Y	Y	Y	W
Dolphin Imaging 3D	Dolphin Imaging and Management	N	Y	Y	Y	W
Analyze	AnalyzeDirect	N	Y	Y	N	W, M
GuideMia	GuideMia	N	Y	Y	N	W, M
OnDemand3D	CyberMed	N	N	Y	N	W, M
VoXim	IVS Technology	N	Y	Y	N	W
ScanIP	Simpleware	N	Y	Y	N	W

STL, standard tessellation language; OS, operating system; Y, yes; N, no; W, Windows OS; M, Mac OS.

TABLE 3 | A summary of commercially available 3D printers from ten leading 3D printing companies in the world.

Type	Name	Company	Cost (USD)	Print area (cm)	Print resolution (nm)	Printer size (cm)	Printer weight (kg)
SLA	Form 1+	Formlabs	3,999	12.5 × 12.5 × 16.5	25	30.0 × 28.0 × 45.0	8
SLA	ProJet 1200	3D Systems	4,900	4.3 × 2.7 × 15.0	30.5	22.9 × 22.9 × 35.6	9
SLA	ProJet 6000	3D Systems	200,000	25.0 × 25.0 × 25.0	50	78.7 × 73.7 × 183.0	181
SLA	ProJet 7000	3D Systems	300,000	38.0 × 38.0 × 25.0	50	98.4 × 85.4 × 183.0	272
SLA	ProX 950	3D Systems	950,000	150.0 × 75.0 × 55.0	50	220.0 × 160.0 × 226.0	1,951
MJM	Objet 24 series	Stratasys	19,900	23.4 × 19.2 × 14.9	28	82.5 × 62.0 × 59.0	93
MJM	Objet 30 series	Stratasys	40,900	29.4 × 19.2 × 14.9	28	82.5 × 62.0 × 59.0	93
MJM	ProJet 3510 series	3D Systems	69,500	29.8 × 18.5 × 20.3	16	29.5 × 47.0 × 59.5	43.4
MJM	Objet Eden	Stratasys	123,000	49.0 × 39.0 × 20.0	16	132.0 × 99.0 × 120.0	410
MJM	ProJet 5000	3D Systems	155,000	53.3 × 38.1 × 30.0	32	60.3 × 35.7 × 57.1	53.8
MJM	ProJet 5500X	3D Systems	155,000	53.3 × 38.1 × 30.0	29	80.0 × 48.0 × 78.0	115.7
MJM	Connex series	Stratasys	164,000	49.0 × 39.0 × 20.0	16	140.0 × 126.0 × 110.0	430
MJM	Objet Connex series	Stratasys	164,000	49.0 × 39.0 × 20.0	16	142.0 × 112.0 × 113.0	500
MJM	Objet 1000	Stratasys	614,000	100.0 × 80.0 × 50.0	16	280.0 × 180.0 × 180.0	1,950
SLS	sPro series	3D Systems	300,000	55.0 × 55.0 × 46.0	80	203.0 × 160.0 × 216.0	2,700
SLS	ProX series	3D Systems	500,000	38.1 × 33.0 × 45.7	100	174.4 × 122.6 × 229.5	1,360
BJT	ProJet 160	3D Systems	40,000	23.6 × 18.5 × 12.7	100	74.0 × 79.0 × 140.0	165
BJT	ProJet 260C	3D Systems	40,000	23.6 × 18.5 × 12.7	100	74.0 × 79.0 × 140.0	165
BJT	ProJet 360	3D Systems	40,000	20.3 × 25.4 × 20.3	100	122.0 × 79.0 × 140.0	179
BJT	ProJet 460 Plus	3D Systems	40,000	20.3 × 25.4 × 20.3	100	122.0 × 79.0 × 140.0	193
BJT	ProJet 4500	3D Systems	40,000	20.3 × 25.4 × 20.3	100	162.0 × 80.0 × 152.0	272
BJT	ProJet 660 Pro	3D Systems	40,000	25.4 × 38.1 × 20.3	100	188.0 × 74.0 × 145.0	340
BJT	ProJet 860 Plus	3D Systems	40,000	50.8 × 38.1 × 22.9	100	119.0 × 116.0 × 162.0	363
FDM	Huxley Duo	RepRapPro	453	13.8 × 14.0 × 9.5	12.5	26.0 × 28.0 × 28.0	4.5
FDM	Mendel	RepRapPro	586	21.0 × 19.0 × 14.0	12.5	50.0 × 46.0 × 41.0	8
FDM	Ormerod 2	RepRapPro	702	20.0 × 20.0 × 20.0	12.5	50.0 × 46.0 × 41.0	6
FDM	Tricolor Mendel	RepRapPro	863	21.0 × 19.0 × 14.0	12.5	50.0 × 46.0 × 41.0	8
FDM	Cube 3	3D Systems	999	15.3 × 15.3 × 15.3	70	33.5 × 34.3 × 24.1	7.7
FDM	Buccaneer	Pirate 3D	999	14.5 × 12.5 × 15.5	85	25.8 × 25.8 × 44.0	8
FDM	Original +	Ultimaker	1,238	21.0 × 21.0 × 20.5	20	35.7 × 34.2 × 38.8	N/A
FDM	Replicator mini	MakerBot	1,375	10.0 × 10.0 × 12.5	200	29.5 × 31.0 × 38.1	8
FDM	Creatr	Leapfrog	1,706	20.0 × 27.0 × 20.0	50	60.0 × 50.0 × 50.0	32
FDM	Replicator 2	MakerBot	1,999	28.5 × 15.3 × 15.5	100	49.0 × 42.0 × 38.0	11.5
FDM	LulzBot TAZ 4	Aleph Objects	2,195	29.8 × 27.5 × 25.0	75	668.0 × 52.0 × 51.5	11
FDM	AW3D HDL	Airwolf 3D	2,295	30.0 × 20.0 × 28.0	100	61.0 × 44.5 × 46.0	17
FDM	Creatr HS	Leapfrog	2,373	29.0 × 24.0 × 18.0	50	60.0 × 60.0 × 50.0	40
FDM	Replicator 2x	MakerBot	2,499	24.6 × 15.2 × 15.5	100	49.0 × 42.0 × 53.1	12.6
FDM	Ultimaker 2	Ultimaker	2,500	23.0 × 22.5 × 20.5	20	35.7 × 34.2 × 38.8	N/A
FDM	Replicator 5th gen	MakerBot	2,899	25.2.19.9 × 15.0	100	52.8 × 44.1 × 41.0	16
FDM	AW3D HD	Airwolf 3D	2,995	30.0 × 20.0 × 30.0	60	61.0 × 44.5 × 46.0	17
FDM	Cube Pro	3D Systems	3,129	20.0 × 23 × 27.0	100	57.8 × 59.1 × 57.8	44
FDM	AW3D HDX	Airwolf 3D	3,495	30.0 × 20.0 × 30.0	60	61.0 × 44.5 × 46.0	17
FDM	AW3D HD2X	Airwolf 3D	3,995	27.9 × 20.3 × 30.5	60	61.0 × 45.7 × 45.7	18
FDM	Creatr xl	Leapfrog	4,988	20.0 × 27.0 × 60.0	50	75.0 × 65.0 × 126.0	37
FDM	Replicator Z18	MakerBot	6,499	30.5 × 30.5 × 45.7	100	49.3 × 56.5 × 85.4	41
FDM	Xeed	Leapfrog	8,705	35.0 × 27.0 × 60.0	50	101.0 × 66.0 × 100.0	115
FDM	Mojo	Stratasys	9,900	12.7 × 12.7 × 12.7	178	63.0 × 45.0 × 53.0	27
FDM	uPrint	Stratasys	13,900	20.3 × 15.2 × 15.2	254	63.5 × 66.0 × 94.0	94
FDM	Objet Dimension series	Stratasys	40,900	25.4 × 25.4 × 30.5	178	83.8 × 73.7 × 114.3	148
FDM	Fortus series	Stratasys	184,000	91.4 × 61.0 × 91.4	127	277.2 × 168.3 × 202.7	2,869

Where a 3D printer series is characterized, the lowest cost, largest print area, lowest print resolution, largest printer size, and greater printer weight are selected for comparison. SLA, stereolithography; MJM, multijet modeling; SLS, selective laser sintering; BJT, binder jet technique; FDM, fused deposition modeling; cm, centimeter; kg, kilograms; nm, nanometers; N/A, not available.

clinical outcomes (1, 2, 124). In addition to CTA, 3D biomodels can provide an additional layer of clinical information through visual and tactile examination.

In a recent report, our research group described a technique of fashioning a "reverse" model representing a soft tissue ankle defect that was utilized for planning a perforator flap-based reconstruction (**Figure 3**) (109). Routine CTA of the lower limbs (i.e., recipient site) and the forearms (i.e., donor site) were conducted and the DICOM data were converted into a CAD file using Osirix. The 3D image of the normal contralateral ankle was mirrored, superimposed over the image of the pathological side, and after digital subtraction using Magics software (Materialise

TABLE 4 | A summary of average raw material cost of each 3D printing technique.

Type of 3D printing	Average cost of print material (USD)
SLA	200 per L
MJM	300 per kg
SLS	500 per kg
BJT	100 per kg
FDM	50 per kg

SLA, stereolithography; MJM, multijet modeling; SLS, selective laser sintering; BJT, binder jet technique; FDM, fused deposition modeling; L, liter.

TABLE 5 | A summary of published application of 3D printing in Plastic and Reconstructive Surgery.

Application		Example	Reference
Preoperative planning	Soft tissue mapping	Breast reconstruction	(108)
		Ear reconstruction	(113, 114)
		Nasal reconstruction	(115)
		Mandibular soft tissue tumor resection	(116)
		"Reverse" model of ankle defect	(109)
		Sacral defect	(117)
	Vascular mapping	Internal mammary artery perforators	(118)
		DIEA perforators	(7)
	Bony mapping	Basal thumb osteoarthritis	(7)
	4D printing	Thumb movement	(119)
Intraoperative guidance		Bone reduction clamp	(70)
Surgical training		N/A	
Patient education		N/A	
Patient-specific prosthesis		Craniofacial implant	(120)
		"Ear and nose library"	(121, 122)

DIEA, deep inferior epigastric artery; 4D, four dimensional; N/A, not available.

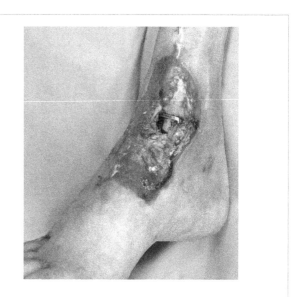

FIGURE 3 | Photograph of the soft tissue ankle defect showing the exposed metal hardware from a previous ankle reconstruction. Reproduced with permission from *Microsurgery* (109).

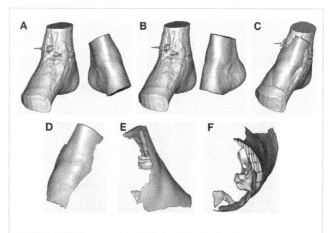

FIGURE 4 | 3D images of the right (pathological) ankle is juxtaposed to the left (normal) ankle (A). The left ankle is reflected **(B)** and superimposed on to the right ankle **(C)**. These images are subtracted from each other to produce a "reverse" model of the soft tissue defect **(D-F)**. Reproduced with permission from *Microsurgery* (109).

NV), a "reverse" model representing the wound defect is created (**Figure 4**). This mirroring function can also be performed in free open-source softwares, such as Osirix and 3D Slicer. This helped the surgeon preoperatively appreciate the length, width, and depth of the free flap that needed to be harvested in order to adequately cover the defect. Both the pathological ankle and the "reverse" model were fabricated in PLA filaments using a Cube 2 printer (3D Systems) (**Figures 5** and **6**) (Table S1 in Supplementary Material).

We also recently demonstrated the utility of a 3D-printed biomodel for planning perforator flap reconstruction of a sacral wound defect post-oncologic resection (117). Likewise, we used Osirix to translate the preoperative sacral CTA data into a CAD file. Due to the maximal build dimensions of the Cube 2 printer (i.e., 16 cm × 16 cm × 16 cm), the 3D image of the sacral defect was scaled down using the Cube software. The haptic model still accurately represented the shape and depth of the defect and its relationship with the surrounding anatomical structures.

3D printing can potentially be a valuable tool in the assessment of soft tissue volume. Volumetric analysis is an essential component of breast reconstructive surgery and currently surgeons rely on 2D photography or 3D scanning technology, such as VECTRA (Canfield Imaging Systems, Fairfield, NJ, USA) (125), and subjective visual assessment. One of the main limitations of 3D photography like VECTRA is the inability to account for an underlying chest wall asymmetry that may

incorrectly lead to an asymmetrical appearance despite equal breast parenchymal volumes. Moreover, the accuracy of each scan is reliant on the patients standing with their back flat against a wall, which may not be feasible in certain conditions, such as kyphosis or scoliosis. Recently, we reported the use of a 3D-printed model of a patient with post-mastectomy breast asymmetry for preoperative planning (**Figure 7**) (108). Despite being scaled down to fit the build size of the printer, having an accurate physical replica helped surgeons appreciate the difference in the breast shape and volume. Furthermore, using the segmentation function in Osirix we were able to quantify the breast parenchymal volume difference.

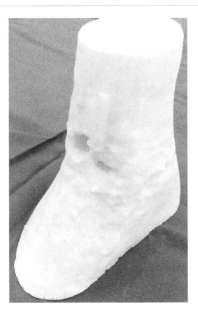

FIGURE 5 | 3D-printed haptic model of the soft tissue ankle defect. Reproduced with permission from *Microsurgery* (109).

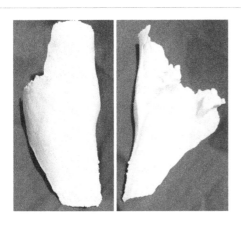

FIGURE 6 | 3D-printed haptic model of the "reverse" image representing the wound defect. Reproduced with permission from *Microsurgery* (109).

Preoperative Planning: Vascular Mapping

Understanding the vascular anatomy of perforators and their relationship with the regional anatomical structures is critical in perforator flap surgery and to this effect, CTA is currently the gold standard preoperative investigation (1, 2, 123, 126). Recently, Gillis and Morris reported a cadaveric study where a model of internal mammary artery perforators and the neighboring ribs was fabricated using a binder jet 3D printer (ProJet x60 series, 3D Systems) (118). The authors demonstrated the benefits of physically interacting with the model and the ability to visualize it in multiple planes to aid dissection and identification of the dominant perforator. However, they also noted a significant cost associated with outsourcing the 3D printing (USD 400–1,200) and the print material was too delicate for small-size blood vessels that required post-production strengthening with wax coating.

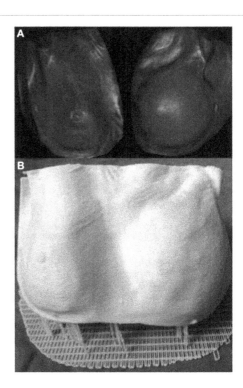

FIGURE 7 | 3D reconstructed CT images of a patient with breast asymmetry post-mastectomy (A) and the 3D printed breast model of the same patient (B). Reproduced with permission from *Breast Cancer Research and Treatment* (108).

Likewise, our group 3D printed the perforator anatomy for planning a deep inferior epigastric artery perforator (DIEP) flap breast reconstruction. From the preoperative CTA, we created a CAD file of the deep inferior epigastric artery (DIEA) with the surrounding bony landmarks using 3D Slicer and the Cube 2 printer. Despite having to scale down the model to fit the printer dimensions, surgeons could intuitively discern the arterial anatomy from the replica. Interestingly, the current technique impeded the perforators of DIEA to be 3D printed. Considering that the DICOM data of the CTA and the Cube 2 printer have a resolution of 0.625 and 0.200 mm, respectively, and the mean diameter of a DIEA perforator ranges between 1 and 1.4 mm (127), this may be most likely explained as a limitation of the 3D modeling software, 3D Slicer. This may be prevented in the future by installing free add-on software functions, such as Vascular Modeling Toolkit (VMTK, Orobix, Bergamo, Italy) in 3D Slicer, that are designed to specifically segment vascular structures. Currently, these are still early in the development phase and are difficult to manipulate without significant computer engineering proficiencies. As the field advances, we would naturally expect the user interface of these softwares to become easier to use.

Preoperative Planning: Bony Mapping

3D printing bony pathology in the forearm, wrist, and hand is another suitable utility of this technology in plastic and reconstructive surgery. CT scans have been the most commonly used imaging modality for medical 3D printing. Since they readily differentiate bones, 3D printing bony structures has become well established in various surgical disciplines, such as maxillofacial surgery (20, 21,

33, 128–130), neurosurgery (35, 68, 86), and orthopedic surgery (131–135). Using Osirix and Cube 2 printer, our research group 3D printed a model of a subluxed first carpometacarpal joint. Being able to visualize the model from various angles and the tactile feedback facilitated an intuitive understanding of the anatomical relationship between the first metacarpal and the trapezium. The information was useful for planning the optimal method of reduction.

A New Evolution: 4D Printing

Recently, we described for the first time the concept of applying 3D printing to 4D CT scans, or 4D printing, where time is added as the fourth dimension to the standard 3D printing (119). 4D CT is a novel imaging modality developed to remove motion artifacts from organs, such as lungs, in order to enhance the image quality and facilitate precise delivery of radiotherapy (136, 137). In plastic surgery, investigators have utilized 4D CTA to assess the vascular territories and the dynamic flow characteristics of an individual perforator (4, 5). Using Osirix and Cube 2 printer, our group 3D printed the carpal and metacarpal bones of a patient in life-size at various stages of the thumb movement, such as thumb abduction (**Figure 8**). In contrast to the 3D reconstructions on a 2D computer screen and 3D models, 4D-printed haptic models accurately depicted the position of the carpal bones during each movement and enabled an instinctive appreciation of the spatiotemporal relationship between them. One of the major disadvantages was the reliance on the clinician reviewing the 4D CT data to select the scans most representative of the carpal bone transition during each movement for 3D printing. This can be overcome as 3D printers become faster thus allowing more models to be fabricated.

Intraoperative Guidance

The convenience of 3D printing has propelled an innovation in custom designs of surgical templates and equipments that help guide the surgeon intraoperatively. In the literature, investigators have demonstrated the utility of 3D printing a modified army/navy surgical retractor (71); patient-specific orthognathic templates to guide osteotomy (66) and mandibular fracture reduction device (138) in maxillofacial surgery; screw fixation guide system in spinal neurosurgery (139); and drill templates to aid surgical correction of multilevel cervical spine instability in orthopedic surgery (69). In plastic and reconstructive surgery, Fuller et al. illustrated how 3D printing can expedite the

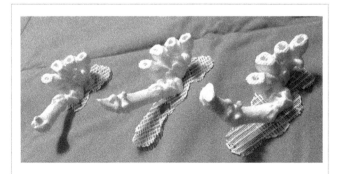

FIGURE 8 | 4D-printed haptic models of carpal and metacarpal bones demonstrating thumb abduction (from left to right). Reproduced with permission from *Journal of Reconstructive Microsurgery* (119).

development of a custom-made bone reduction clamp design for hand fractures, in comparison to the conventional processes that can become protracted and actually be discouraging to innovation (70). The authors collaborated with an engineer to produce 3D prototype designs and converted them into CAD files using free 3D softwares, such as SketchUp (Trimble Navigation, Sunnyvale, CA, USA) and MeshLab (ISTI-CNR, Pisa, Italy), respectively. 3D printing of the FDM prototypes was outsourced, costing USD 75 and 1–3 days for the delivery to arrive. The final design was manufactured in metal using an additive manufacturing technique, called direct metal laser sintering, and was again outsourced, costing USD 1,200 and 2 days for the delivery. The authors acknowledged that the 3D softwares for designing prototypes are currently not intuitive for clinicians with only basic computer proficiency. Furthermore, the final cost exceeded the cost of purchasing a standard equipment. However, as 3D printing technology advances and the 3D printing is performed "in-house", the difference may become minimal in the future.

Surgical Training

Detailed knowledge of anatomical structures and their spatial relationships are essential assets of a plastic surgeon and objectives of a surgical training program. Through the standard medical training, a surgical aspirant can gain procedural experiences from performing dissections on human cadavers as a medical student and assisting senior surgeons in the operating theater as a resident, leading toward a gradual acquisition of competence. However, human cadavers are becoming relatively scarce from the anatomical education curricula due to high maintenance costs, cultural and social controversies, and safety issues associated with the formalin-containing embalming fluids (92, 140). Furthermore, the operative experience gained as an assistant to a senior surgeon is secondary to a primary operator experience. To this end, 3D-printed anatomical models can serve as an accurate, tactile visualization tool and a surgical simulation device. Moreover, 3D-printed haptic biomodels can be utilized to reproduce complex, patient-unique pathologies that facilitate the surgical trainees to preoperatively predict potential intraoperative challenges and postoperative outcomes and aid in their learning. Subsequent improvement in the surgeon's competence may lead to enhanced clinical outcomes and a reduced risk of complications. Investigators from various surgical disciplines have demonstrated the utility of 3D printing in training, such as neurosurgery (72–77, 141, 142), cardiothoracic surgery (54, 78–80, 143–145), urology (81, 146), and general surgery (29) However, one of the major limitations currently is the ability to print in materials that closely mimic the biomechanical properties and modulus of real human tissue as well as possessing realistic colors. As more materials enter the scope of 3D printing, future 3D-printed biomodels will be able to more closely reproduce true anatomy (50, 72, 74, 79).

Patient Education

3D-printed replicas can be useful to facilitate the physician–patient interaction during a consultation with the aim of improved understanding of the intended procedure, its potential outcomes and complications and thus can form an important aspect of informed consent. Traditional CT/MRI scans are often difficult to comprehend for patients from a non-medical background. In recent times, plastic surgeons have utilized 3D scanning technology, such as

VECTRA (Canfield Imaging Systems), to accurately simulate potential outcomes from a cosmetic procedure on a computer screen (125). However, studies have consistently demonstrated that visual and tactile feedback from a 3D haptic model provides a superior understanding of anatomical details compared to 2D or 3D imaging techniques (34, 58, 147).

Patient-Specific Prosthesis

As modern medicine ultimately progresses toward individualized treatment approaches, customizability of 3D printing can transform the manufacturing of patient-specific prostheses to being widely accessible and affordable. In comparison to a standard implant, a custom-made one is more likely to yield superior functional and esthetic outcomes (148, 149). Typical 3D printing materials can be sterilized using chemicals, such as Food and Drug Administration approved glutaraldehyde protocols (71), steam (20), and gas (150) for intraoperative handling. In the last decade, investigators have reported 3D-printed prostheses of nose (121, 151), ears (122, 152–155), eyes (156, 157), face (158, 159), and hand (6, 160). Furthermore, an Italian research group led by De Crescenzio and Ciocca has established an "Ear and Nose Library" where CAD files of 3D scanned ears and noses of normal university students are stocked (121, 122). When patients have pathology affecting both ears or the entire nose that impedes mirroring of the normal contralateral side to reconstruct the defect, the clinicians can select the most suitable CAD file from this database to fashion a prosthesis. In plastic surgery, standard breast implants are available in different volumes, but in a limited number of shapes. To this effect, 3D-printed breast implants customized to conform to the individual variations in the chest wall anatomy and the patient's desired breast shape and size may lead to a more esthetic and satisfactory outcome.

Most reports have indicated that 3D-printed custom prostheses provide superior esthetics in comparison to the traditional wax-based handcrafted prosthetics (152, 154, 155). Furthermore, customized implants eschew the need to intraoperatively modify and adjust associated with the standard implants, which can directly lead to improved clinical outcomes, such as a reduction in the length of surgery, reduced exposure to anesthetics, and a decreased risk of complications like infection (161, 162). Currently, one of the major drawbacks is that most custom implants are manufactured using expensive 3D printing techniques, such as MJM (157) and SLS (151, 160). In contrast, the affordable FDM 3D printers are used to fabricate negative molds for silicone or wax-based casts, which ironically increases the overall production time and cost (121, 122, 152–154, 156, 158). This is mainly because at present,

only ABS and PLA filaments are available for FDM and their hard material characteristic makes them unsuitable for producing soft tissue prosthetics. However, as research and development in 3D printing continues to grow exponentially and more materials become available for FDM, we expect to be able to directly create a custom-made prosthesis affordably in the near future.

Future and Conclusion

In the last decade, image-guided 3D-printed haptic biomodels have proven to represent a valuable adjunct to the conventional 2D imaging modalities in plastic surgery for preoperative planning, producing intraoperative guidance tools, educating surgical trainees and patients, and fashioning patient-specific implants. In the early years, the technical complexity of 3D softwares and the prohibitive cost of 3D printers restricted accessibility of 3D printing in medicine. The expiration of key 3D printing patents has fueled an exponential development in the field and a significant reduction in the cost. Ultimately, we envision that 3D printing has the potential to become ubiquitous and function as an essential clinical bedside tool for a plastic surgeon.

Author Contributions

All authors contributed to the preparation of this manuscript. The manuscript has been seen and approved by all authors. The content of this article has not been submitted or published elsewhere.

Acknowledgments

The authors would like to acknowledge Dr. Alexandra Rizzitelli at Peninsula Health for her support.

Supplementary Material

TABLE S1 | A summary of the printing time and the amount of print material used to produce the 3D printed models in plastic and reconstructive surgery mentioned in the manuscript.

VIDEO S1 | A video demonstrating the binder jet 3D printing technique using a ProJet x60 series printer (3D Systems, Rock Hill, SC). After a layer of powder is deposited, a binder material mixed with colored dye is ejected on to the powder bed to fabricate a 3D haptic model in a layer-by-layer fashion. Filmed by PGM.

References

1. Rozen WM, Anavekar NS, Ashton MW, Stella DL, Grinsell D, Bloom RJ, et al. Does the preoperative imaging of perforators with CT angiography improve operative outcomes in breast reconstruction? *Microsurgery* (2008) **28**:516–23. doi:10.1002/micr.20526
2. Rozen WM, Ashton MW, Grinsell D, Stella DL, Phillips TJ, Taylor GI. Establishing the case for CT angiography in the preoperative imaging of abdominal wall perforators. *Microsurgery* (2008) **28**:306–13. doi:10.1002/micr.20496
3. Rozen WM, Ashton MW, Stella DL, Phillips TJ, Grinsell D, Taylor GI. The accuracy of computed tomographic angiography for mapping the perforators of the deep inferior epigastric artery: a blinded, prospective cohort study. *Plast Reconstr Surg* (2008) **122**:1003–9. doi:10.1097/PRS.0b013e3181845994
4. Colohan S, Wong C, Lakhiani C, Cheng A, Maia M, Arbique G, et al. The free descending branch muscle-sparing latissimus dorsi flap: vascular anatomy and clinical applications. *Plast Reconstr Surg* (2012) **130**:776e–87e. doi:10.1097/PRS.0b013e31826d9c5e
5. Nie JY, Lu LJ, Gong X, Li Q, Nie JJ. Delineating the vascular territory (perforasome) of a perforator in the lower extremity of the rabbit with four-dimensional computed tomographic angiography. *Plast Reconstr Surg* (2013) **131**:565–71. doi:10.1097/PRS.0b013e31827c6e49
6. Gerstle TL, Ibrahim AM, Kim PS, Lee BT, Lin SJ. A plastic surgery application in evolution: three-dimensional printing. *Plast Reconstr Surg* (2014) **133**:446–51. doi:10.1097/01.prs.0000436844.92623.d3
7. Chae MP, Hunter-Smith DJ, Rozen WM. Image-guided 3D-printing and haptic modeling in plastic surgery. In: Saba L, Rozen WM, Alonso-Burgos A, Ribuffo

D, editors. *Imaging in Plastic Surgery*. London: CRC Taylor and Francis Press (2014). p. 819–30.

8. Goiato MC, Santos MR, Pesqueira AA, Moreno A, dos Santos DM, Haddad MF. Prototyping for surgical and prosthetic treatment. *J Craniofac Surg* (2011) 22:914–7. doi:10.1097/SCS.0b013e31820f7f90

9. Levy GN, Schindel R, Kruth JP. Rapid manufacturing and rapid tooling with layer manufacturing (LM) technologies, state of the art and future perspectives. *CIRP Ann Manuf Technol* (2003) 52:589–609. doi:10.1016/S0007-8506(07)60206-6

10. Sealy W. Additive manufacturing as a disruptive technology: how to avoid the pitfall. *Am J Eng Technol Res* (2011) 11:86–93. doi:10.3727/194824 13X3608676060655

11. Hoy MB. 3D printing: making things at the library. *Med Ref Serv Q* (2013) 32:93–9. doi:10.1080/02763869.2013.749139

12. Srinivasan V, Bassan J. 3D printing and the future of manufacturing. *CSC Leading Edge Forum* (2012).

13. Schubert C, van Langeveld MC, Donoso LA. Innovations in 3D printing: a 3D overview from optics to organs. *Br J Ophthalmol* (2014) 98:159–61. doi:10.1136/bjophthalmol-2013-304446

14. Klein GT, Lu Y, Wang MY. 3D printing and neurosurgery – ready for prime time? *World Neurosurg* (2013) 80:233–5. doi:10.1016/j.wneu.2013.07.009

15. Hull CW. *Apparatus for Production of Three-Dimensional Objects by Stereolithography*. US Patent No. 4,575,330 (1986).

16. Hannen EJ. Recreating the original contour in tumor deformed mandibles for plate adapting. *Int J Oral Maxillofac Surg* (2006) 35:183–5. doi:10.1016/j.ijom.2005.07.012

17. Rozen WM, Ting JW, Baillieu C, Leong J. Stereolithographic modeling of the deep circumflex iliac artery and its vascular branching: a further advance in computed tomography-guided flap planning. *Plast Reconstr Surg* (2012) 130:380e–2e. doi:10.1097/PRS.0b013e31825903d1

18. Rozen WM, Ting JW, Leung M, Wu T, Ying D, Leong J. Advancing image-guided surgery in microvascular mandibular reconstruction: combining bony and vascular imaging with computed tomography-guided stereolithographic bone modeling. *Plast Reconstr Surg* (2012) 130:227e–9e. doi:10.1097/PRS.0b013e318255028e

19. Ono I, Gunji H, Suda K, Kaneko F. Method for preparing an exact-size model using helical volume scan computed tomography. *Plast Reconstr Surg* (1994) 93:1363–71. doi:10.1097/00006534-199406000-00005

20. Herlin C, Koppe M, Beziat JL, Gleizal A. Rapid prototyping in craniofacial surgery: using a positioning guide after zygomatic osteotomy – a case report. *J Craniomaxillofac Surg* (2011) 39:376–9. doi:10.1016/j.jcms.2010.07.003

21. Cohen A, Laviv A, Berman P, Nashef R, Abu-Tair J. Mandibular reconstruction using stereolithographic 3-dimensional printing modeling technology. *Oral Surg Oral Med Oral Pathol Oral Radiol Endod* (2009) 108:661–6. doi:10.1016/j.tripleo.2009.05.023

22. Tumbleston JR, Shirvanyants D, Ermoshkin N, Januszewicz R, Johnson AR, Kelly D, et al. Additive manufacturing. Continuous liquid interface production of 3D objects. *Science* (2015) 347:1349–52. doi:10.1126/science.aaa2397

23. Almquist TA, Smalley DR. *Thermal Stereolithography*. US Patent No. 5,141,680 (1992).

24. Deckard C. *Method and Apparatus for Producing Parts by Selective sintering*. US Patent No. 4,863,538 (1989).

25. Rengier F, Mehndiratta A, von Tengg-Kobligk H, Zechmann CM, Unterhinninghofen R, Kauczor HU, et al. 3D printing based on imaging data: review of medical applications. *Int J Comput Assist Radiol Surg* (2010) 5:335–41. doi:10.1007/s11548-010-0476-x

26. Mottl-Link S, Hubler M, Kuhne T, Rietdorf U, Krueger JJ, Schnackenburg B, et al. Physical models aiding in complex congenital heart surgery. *Ann Thorac Surg* (2008) 86:273–7. doi:10.1016/j.athoracsur.2007.06.001

27. McGurk M, Amis AA, Potamianos P, Goodger NM. Rapid prototyping techniques for anatomical modelling in medicine. *Ann R Coll Surg Engl* (1997) 79:169–74.

28. Sachs EM, Haggerty JS, Cima MJ, Williams PA. *Three-Dimensional Printing Techniques*. US Patent No. 5,204,055 (1993).

29. Watson RA. A low-cost surgical application of additive fabrication. *J Surg Educ* (2014) 71:14–7. doi:10.1016/j.jsurg.2013.10.012

30. Olszewski R, Szymor P, Kozakiewicz M. Accuracy of three-dimensional, paper-based models generated using a low-cost, three-dimensional printer. *J Craniomaxillofac Surg* (2014) 42(8):1847–52. doi:10.1016/j.jcms.2014.07.002

31. Crump SS. *Apparatus and Method for Creating Three-Dimensional Objects*. US Patent No. 5,121,329 (1992).

32. Dikovsky D, Napadensky E. *Three-Dimensional Printing Process for Producing a Self-Destructible Temporary Structure*. US Patent No. 8,470,231 (2013)

33. Chen Y, Niu F, Yu B, Liu J, Wang M, Gui L. Three-dimensional preoperative design of distraction osteogenesis for hemifacial microsomia. *J Craniofac Surg* (2014) 25:184–8. doi:10.1097/SCS.0000000000000391

34. Way TP, Barner KE. Automatic visual to tactile translation – part II: evaluation of the TACTile image creation system. *IEEE Trans Rehabil Eng* (1997) 5:95–105. doi:10.1109/86.559354

35. D'Urso PS, Barker TM, Earwaker WJ, Bruce LJ, Atkinson RL, Lanigan MW, et al. Stereolithographic biomodelling in cranio-maxillofacial surgery: a prospective trial. *J Craniomaxillofac Surg* (1999) 27:30–7. doi:10.1016/S1010-5182(99)80007-9

36. Guarino J, Tennyson S, McCain G, Bond L, Shea K, King H. Rapid prototyping technology for surgeries of the pediatric spine and pelvis: benefits analysis. *J Pediatr Orthop* (2007) 27:955–60. doi:10.1097/bpo.0b013e3181594ced

37. Liu YF, Xu LW, Zhu HY, Liu SS. Technical procedures for template-guided surgery for mandibular reconstruction based on digital design and manufacturing. *Biomed Eng Online* (2014) 13:63. doi:10.1186/1475-925X-13-63

38. Tsai MJ, Wu CT. Study of mandible reconstruction using a fibula flap with application of additive manufacturing technology. *Biomed Eng Online* (2014) 13:57. doi:10.1186/1475-925X-13-57

39. Lim CG, Campbell DI, Clucas DM. Rapid prototyping technology in orbital floor reconstruction: application in three patients. *Craniomaxillofac Trauma Reconstr* (2014) 7:143–6. doi:10.1055/s-0034-1371080

40. Engel M, Hoffmann J, Castrillon-Oberndorfer G, Freudlsperger C. The value of three-dimensional printing modelling for surgical correction of orbital hypertelorism. *Oral Maxillofac Surg* (2014). doi:10.1007/s10006-014-0466-1

41. Azuma M, Yanagawa T, Ishibashi-Kanno N, Uchida F, Ito T, Yamagata K, et al. Mandibular reconstruction using plates prebent to fit rapid prototyping 3-dimensional printing models ameliorates contour deformity. *Head Face Med* (2014) 10:45. doi:10.1186/1746-160X-10-45

42. Jeong HS, Park KJ, Kil KM, Chong S, Eun HJ, Lee TS, et al. Minimally invasive plate osteosynthesis using 3D printing for shaft fractures of clavicles: technical note. *Arch Orthop Trauma Surg* (2014) 134:1551–5. doi:10.1007/s00402-014-2075-8

43. Tam MD, Laycock SD, Bell D, Chojnowski A. 3-D printout of a DICOM file to aid surgical planning in a 6 year old patient with a large scapular osteochondroma complicating congenital diaphyseal aclasia. *J Radiol Case Rep* (2012) 6:31–7. doi:10.3941/jrcr.v6i1.889

44. Schmauss D, Haeberle S, Hagl C, Sodian R. Three-dimensional printing in cardiac surgery and interventional cardiology: a single-centre experience. *Eur J Cardiothorac Surg* (2014). doi:10.1093/ejcts/ezu310

45. Witschey WR, Pouch AM, McGarvey JR, Ikeuchi K, Contijoch F, Levack MM, et al. Three-dimensional ultrasound-derived physical mitral valve modeling. *Ann Thorac Surg* (2014) 98:691–4. doi:10.1016/j.athoracsur.2014.04.094

46. Schmauss D, Gerber N, Sodian R. Three-dimensional printing of models for surgical planning in patients with primary cardiac tumors. *J Thorac Cardiovasc Surg* (2013) 145:1407–8. doi:10.1016/j.jtcvs.2012.12.030

47. Schmauss D, Schmitz C, Bigdeli AK, Weber S, Gerber N, Beiras-Fernandez A, et al. Three-dimensional printing of models for preoperative planning and simulation of transcatheter valve replacement. *Ann Thorac Surg* (2012) 93:e31–3. doi:10.1016/j.athoracsur.2011.09.031

48. Sodian R, Weber S, Markert M, Loeff M, Lueth T, Weis FC, et al. Pediatric cardiac transplantation: three-dimensional printing of anatomic models for surgical planning of heart transplantation in patients with univentricular heart. *J Thorac Cardiovasc Surg* (2008) 136:1098–9. doi:10.1016/j.jtcvs.2008.03.055

49. Sodian R, Schmauss D, Markert M, Weber S, Nikolaou K, Haeberle S, et al. Three-dimensional printing creates models for surgical planning of aortic valve replacement after previous coronary bypass grafting. *Ann Thorac Surg* (2008) 85:2105–8. doi:10.1016/j.athoracsur.2007.12.033

50. Markert M, Weber S, Lueth TC. A beating heart model 3D printed from specific patient data. *Conf Proc IEEE Eng Med Biol Soc* (2007) 2007:4472–5. doi:10.1109/IEMBS.2007.4353332

51. Nakada T, Akiba T, Inagaki T, Morikawa T. Thoracoscopic anatomical subsegmentectomy of the right S2b + S3 using a 3D printing model with rapid prototyping. *Interact Cardiovasc Thorac Surg* (2014) 19(4):696–8. doi:10.1093/icvts/ivu174

52. Akiba T, Inagaki T, Nakada T. Three-dimensional printing model of anomalous bronchi before surgery. *Ann Thorac Cardiovasc Surg* (2014) **20**(Suppl):659–62. doi:10.5761/atcs.cr.13-00189

53. Tam MD, Laycock SD, Brown JR, Jakeways M. 3D printing of an aortic aneurysm to facilitate decision making and device selection for endovascular aneurysm repair in complex neck anatomy. *J Endovasc Ther* (2013) **20**:863–7. doi:10.1583/13-4450MR.1

54. Hakansson A, Rantatalo M, Hansen T, Wanhainen A. Patient specific biomodel of the whole aorta – the importance of calcified plaque removal. *Vasa* (2011) **40**:453–9. doi:10.1024/0301-1526/a000148

55. Sodian R, Schmauss D, Schmitz C, Bigdeli A, Haeberle S, Schmoeckel M, et al. 3-dimensional printing of models to create custom-made devices for coil embolization of an anastomotic leak after aortic arch replacement. *Ann Thorac Surg* (2009) **88**:974–8. doi:10.1016/j.athoracsur.2009.03.014

56. Silberstein JL, Maddox MM, Dorsey P, Feibus A, Thomas R, Lee BR. Physical models of renal malignancies using standard cross-sectional imaging and 3-dimensional printers: a pilot study. *Urology* (2014) **84**:268–72. doi:10.1016/j.urology.2014.03.042

57. Daniel M, Watson J, Hoskison E, Sama A. Frontal sinus models and onlay templates in osteoplastic flap surgery. *J Laryngol Otol* (2011) **125**:82–5. doi:10.1017/S0022215110001799

58. Suzuki M, Ogawa Y, Kawano A, Hagiwara A, Yamaguchi H, Ono H. Rapid prototyping of temporal bone for surgical training and medical education. *Acta Otolaryngol* (2004) **124**:400–2. doi:10.1080/00016480410016478

59. Igami T, Nakamura Y, Hirose T, Ebata T, Yokoyama Y, Sugawara G, et al. Application of a three-dimensional print of a liver in hepatectomy for small tumors invisible by intraoperative ultrasonography: preliminary experience. *World J Surg* (2014) **38**(12):3163–6. doi:10.1007/s00268-014-2740-7

60. Ikegami T, Maehara Y. Transplantation: 3D printing of the liver in living donor liver transplantation. *Nat Rev Gastroenterol Hepatol* (2013) **10**:697–8. doi:10.1038/nrgastro.2013.195

61. Zein NN, Hanouneh IA, Bishop PD, Samaan M, Eghtesad B, Quintini C, et al. Three-dimensional print of a liver for preoperative planning in living donor liver transplantation. *Liver Transpl* (2013) **19**:1304–10. doi:10.1002/lt.23729

62. Kang SH, Kim MK, Kim BC, Lee SH. Orthognathic Y-splint: a CAD/CAM-engineered maxillary repositioning wafer assembly. *Br J Oral Maxillofac Surg* (2014) **52**:667–9. doi:10.1016/j.bjoms.2014.01.023

63. Adolphs N, Liu W, Keeve E, Hoffmeister B. RapidSplint: virtual splint generation for orthognathic surgery – results of a pilot series. *Comput Aided Surg* (2014) **19**:20–8. doi:10.3109/10929088.2014.887778

64. Cousley RR, Turner MJ. Digital model planning and computerized fabrication of orthognathic surgery wafers. *J Orthod* (2014) **41**:38–45. doi:10.1179/1465313313Y.0000000075

65. Kim BC, Lee CE, Park W, Kim MK, Zhengguo P, Yu HS, et al. Clinical experiences of digital model surgery and the rapid-prototyped wafer for maxillary orthognathic surgery. *Oral Surg Oral Med Oral Pathol Oral Radiol Endod* (2011) **111**:278–85. doi:10.1016/j.tripleo.2010.04.038

66. Li B, Zhang L, Sun H, Yuan J, Shen SG, Wang X. A novel method of computer aided orthognathic surgery using individual CAD/CAM templates: a combination of osteotomy and repositioning guides. *Br J Oral Maxillofac Surg* (2013) **51**:e239–44. doi:10.1016/j.bjoms.2013.03.007

67. Metzger MC, Hohlweg-Majert B, Schwarz U, Teschner M, Hammer B, Schmelzeisen R. Manufacturing splints for orthognathic surgery using a three-dimensional printer. *Oral Surg Oral Med Oral Pathol Oral Radiol Endod* (2008) **105**:e1–7. doi:10.1016/j.tripleo.2007.07.040

68. D'Urso PS, Williamson OD, Thompson RG. Biomodeling as an aid to spinal instrumentation. *Spine (Phila Pa 1976)* (2005) **30**:2841–5. doi:10.1097/01.brs.0000190886.56895.3d

69. Spottiswoode BS, van den Heever DJ, Chang Y, Engelhardt S, Du Plessis S, Nicolls F, et al. Preoperative three-dimensional model creation of magnetic resonance brain images as a tool to assist neurosurgical planning. *Stereotact Funct Neurosurg* (2013) **91**:162–9. doi:10.1159/000345264

70. Fuller SM, Butz DR, Vevang CB, Makhlouf MV. Application of 3-dimensional printing in hand surgery for production of a novel bone reduction clamp. *J Hand Surg Am* (2014) **39**:1840–5. doi:10.1016/j.jhsa.2014.06.009

71. Rankin TM, Giovinco NA, Cucher DJ, Watts G, Hurwitz B, Armstrong DG. Three-dimensional printing surgical instruments: are we there yet? *J Surg Res* (2014) **189**:193–7. doi:10.1016/j.jss.2014.02.020

72. Waran V, Narayanan V, Karuppiah R, Owen SL, Aziz T. Utility of multimaterial 3D printers in creating models with pathological entities to enhance the training experience of neurosurgeons. *J Neurosurg* (2014) **120**:489–92. doi:10.3171/2013.11.JNS131066

73. Abla AA, Lawton MT. Three-dimensional hollow intracranial aneurysm models and their potential role for teaching, simulation, and training. *World Neurosurg* (2014). doi:10.1016/j.wneu.2014.01.015

74. Mashiko T, Otani K, Kawano R, Konno T, Kaneko N, Ito Y, et al. Development of three-dimensional hollow elastic model for cerebral aneurysm clipping simulation enabling rapid and low cost prototyping. *World Neurosurg* (2013). doi:10.1016/j.wneu.2013.10.032

75. Wurm G, Tomancok B, Pogady P, Holl K, Trenkler J. Cerebrovascular stereolithographic biomodeling for aneurysm surgery. Technical note. *J Neurosurg* (2004) **100**:139–45. doi:10.3171/jns.2004.100.1.0139

76. Wurm G, Lehner M, Tomancok B, Kleiser R, Nussbaumer K. Cerebrovascular biomodeling for aneurysm surgery: simulation-based training by means of rapid prototyping technologies. *Surg Innov* (2011) **18**:294–306. doi:10.1177/1553350610395031

77. Waran V, Narayanan V, Karuppiah R, Thambynayagam HC, Muthusamy KA, Rahman ZA, et al. Neurosurgical endoscopic training via a realistic 3-dimensional model with pathology. *Simul Healthc* (2014). doi:10.1097/SIH.0000000000000060

78. Costello JP, Olivieri LJ, Su L, Krieger A, Alfares F, Thabit O, et al. Incorporating three-dimensional printing into a simulation-based congenital heart disease and critical care training curriculum for resident physicians. *Congenit Heart Dis* (2014). doi:10.1111/chd.12238

79. Biglino G, Verschueren P, Zegels R, Taylor AM, Schievano S. Rapid prototyping compliant arterial phantoms for in-vitro studies and device testing. *J Cardiovasc Magn Reson* (2013) **15**:2. doi:10.1186/1532-429X-15-2

80. Bustamante S, Bose S, Bishop P, Klatte R, Norris F. Novel application of rapid prototyping for simulation of bronchoscopic anatomy. *J Cardiothorac Vasc Anesth* (2014) **28**:1134–7. doi:10.1053/j.jvca.2013.08.015

81. Cheung CL, Looi T, Lendvay TS, Drake JM, Farhat WA. Use of 3-dimensional printing technology and silicone modeling in surgical simulation: development and face validation in pediatric laparoscopic pyeloplasty. *J Surg Educ* (2014) **71**:762–7. doi:10.1016/j.jsurg.2014.03.001

82. Li J, Hsu Y, Luo E, Khadka A, Hu J. Computer-aided design and manufacturing and rapid prototyped nanoscale hydroxyapatite/polyamide (n-HA/PA) construction for condylar defect caused by mandibular angle ostectomy. *Aesthetic Plast Surg* (2011) **35**:636–40. doi:10.1007/s00266-010-9602-y

83. Klammert U, Gbureck U, Vorndran E, Rodiger J, Meyer-Marcotty P, Kubler AC. 3D powder printed calcium phosphate implants for reconstruction of cranial and maxillofacial defects. *J Craniomaxillofac Surg* (2010) **38**:565–70. doi:10.1016/j.jcms.2010.01.009

84. Saijo H, Igawa K, Kanno Y, Mori Y, Kondo K, Shimizu K, et al. Maxillofacial reconstruction using custom-made artificial bones fabricated by inkjet printing technology. *J Artif Organs* (2009) **12**:200–5. doi:10.1007/s10047-009-0462-7

85. Wurm G, Tomancok B, Holl K, Trenkler J. Prospective study on cranioplasty with individual carbon fiber reinforced polymer (CFRP) implants produced by means of stereolithography. *Surg Neurol* (2004) **62**:510–21. doi:10.1016/j.surneu.2004.01.025

86. D'Urso PS, Earwaker WJ, Barker TM, Redmond MJ, Thompson RG, Effeney DJ, et al. Custom cranioplasty using stereolithography and acrylic. *Br J Plast Surg* (2000) **53**:200–4. doi:10.1054/bjps.1999.3268

87. Bicanic G, Barbaric K, Bohacek I, Aljinovic A, Delimar D. Current concept in dysplastic hip arthroplasty: techniques for acetabular and femoral reconstruction. *World J Orthop* (2014) **5**:412–24. doi:10.5312/wjo.v5.i4.412

88. Koulouvaris P, Stafylas K, Sculco T, Xenakis T. Distal femoral shortening in total hip arthroplasty for complex primary hip reconstruction. A new surgical technique. *J Arthroplasty* (2008) **23**:992–8. doi:10.1016/j.arth.2007.09.013

89. Zopf DA, Hollister SJ, Nelson ME, Ohye RG, Green GE. Bioresorbable airway splint created with a three-dimensional printer. *N Engl J Med* (2013) **368**:2043–5. doi:10.1056/NEJMc1206319

90. Reeves P. Additive manufacturing & 3D printing medical & healthcare: a new industrial perspective. *The 3D Printing & Additive Manufacturing People.* Derbyshire (2014).

91. Wozniak K, Rzepecka-Wozniak E, Moskala A, Pohl J, Latacz K, Dybala B. Weapon identification using antemortem computed tomography with virtual 3D and rapid

prototype modeling – a report in a case of blunt force head injury. *Forensic Sci Int* (2012) 222:e29–32. doi:10.1016/j.forsciint.2012.06.012

92. McMenamin PG, Quayle MR, McHenry CR, Adams JW. The production of anatomical teaching resources using three-dimensional (3D) printing technology. *Anat Sci Educ* (2014) 7:479–86. doi:10.1002/ase.1475

93. Giovinco NA, Dunn SP, Dowling L, Smith C, Trowell L, Ruch JA, et al. A novel combination of printed 3-dimensional anatomic templates and computer-assisted surgical simulation for virtual preoperative planning in Charcot foot reconstruction. *J Foot Ankle Surg* (2012) 51:387–93. doi:10.1053/j.jfas.2012.01.014

94. Groth C, Kravitz ND, Jones PE, Graham JW, Redmond WR. Three-dimensional printing technology. *J Clin Orthod* (2014) 48:475–85.

95. Chen J, Zhang Z, Chen X, Zhang C, Zhang G, Xu Z. Design and manufacture of customized dental implants by using reverse engineering and selective laser melting technology. *J Prosthet Dent* (2014) 112:1088–95. doi:10.1016/j.prosdent.2014.04.026

96. Flugge TV, Nelson K, Schmelzeisen R, Metzger MC. Three-dimensional plotting and printing of an implant drilling guide: simplifying guided implant surgery. *J Oral Maxillofac Surg* (2013) 71:1340–6. doi:10.1016/j.joms.2013.04.010

97. Goyanes A, Buanz AB, Hatton GB, Gaisford S, Basit AW. 3D printing of modified-release aminosalicylate (4-ASA and 5-ASA) tablets. *Eur J Pharm Biopharm* (2014). doi:10.1016/j.ejpb.2014.12.003

98. Skowyra J, Pietrzak K, Alhnan MA. Fabrication of extended-release patient-tailored prednisolone tablets via fused deposition modelling (FDM) 3D printing. *Eur J Pharm Sci* (2014) 68C:11–7. doi:10.1016/j.ejps.2014.11.009

99. Lueders C, Jastram B, Hetzer R, Schwandt H. Rapid manufacturing techniques for the tissue engineering of human heart valves. *Eur J Cardiothorac Surg* (2014) 46:593–601. doi:10.1093/ejcts/ezt510

100. Chang JW, Park SA, Park JK, Choi JW, Kim YS, Shin YS, et al. Tissue-engineered tracheal reconstruction using three-dimensionally printed artificial tracheal graft: preliminary report. *Artif Organs* (2014) 38:E95–105. doi:10.1111/aor.12310

101. Lee Ventola C. Medical applications for 3D printing: current and projected uses. *P T* (2014) 39:704–11.

102. Fullerton JN, Frodsham GC, Day RM. 3D printing for the many, not the few. *Nat Biotechnol* (2014) 32:1086–7. doi:10.1038/nbt.3056

103. Hieu LC, Zlatov N, Vander Sloten J, Bohez E, Khanh L, Binh PH, et al. Medical rapid prototyping applications and methods. *Assemb Autom* (2005) 25:284–92. doi:10.1108/01445150510626415

104. Rosset A, Spadola L, Ratib O. OsiriX: an open-source software for navigating in multidimensional DICOM images. *J Digit Imaging* (2004) 17:205–16. doi:10.1007/s10278-004-1014-6

105. Fedorov A, Beichel R, Kalpathy-Cramer J, Finet J, Fillion-Robin JC, Pujol S, et al. 3D slicer as an image computing platform for the quantitative imaging network. *Magn Reson Imaging* (2012) 30:1323–41. doi:10.1016/j.mri.2012.05.001

106. Gering DT, Nabavi A, Kikinis R, Hata N, O'Donnell LJ, Grimson WE, et al. An integrated visualization system for surgical planning and guidance using image fusion and an open MR. *J Magn Reson Imaging* (2001) 13:967–75. doi:10.1002/jmri.1139

107. Golby AJ, Kindlmann G, Norton I, Yarmarkovich A, Pieper S, Kikinis R. Interactive diffusion tensor tractography visualization for neurosurgical planning. *Neurosurgery* (2011) 68:496–505. doi:10.1227/NEU.0b013e3182061ebb

108. Chae MP, Hunter-Smith DJ, Spychal RT, Rozen WM. 3D volumetric analysis for planning breast reconstructive surgery. *Breast Cancer Res Treat* (2014) 146(2):457–60. doi:10.1007/s10549-014-3028-1

109. Chae MP, Lin F, Spychal RT, Hunter-Smith DJ, Rozen WM. 3D-printed haptic "reverse" models for preoperative planning in soft tissue reconstruction: a case report. *Microsurgery* (2014). doi:10.1002/micr.22293

110. Ibrahim D, Broilo TL, Heitz C, de Oliveira MG, de Oliveira HW, Nobre SM, et al. Dimensional error of selective laser sintering, three-dimensional printing and PolyJet models in the reproduction of mandibular anatomy. *J Craniomaxillofac Surg* (2009) 37:167–73. doi:10.1016/j.jcms.2008.10.008

111. Silva DN, Gerhardt de Oliveira M, Meurer E, Meurer MI, Lopes da Silva JV, Santa-Barbara A. Dimensional error in selective laser sintering and 3D-printing of models for craniomaxillary anatomy reconstruction. *J Craniomaxillofac Surg* (2008) 36:443–9. doi:10.1016/j.jcms.2008.04.003

112. Fitzwater KL, Marcellin-Little DJ, Harrysson OL, Osborne JA, Poindexter EC. Evaluation of the effect of computed tomography scan protocols and freeform fabrication methods on bone biomodel accuracy. *Am J Vet Res* (2011) 72:1178–85. doi:10.2460/ajvr.72.9.1178

113. Bos EJ, Scholten T, Song Y, Verlinden JC, Wolff J, Forouzanfar T, et al. Developing a parametric ear model for auricular reconstruction: a new step towards patient-specific implants. *J Craniomaxillofac Surg* (2015) 43:390–5. doi:10.1016/j.jcms.2014.12.016

114. Nishimoto S, Sotsuka Y, Kawai K, Fujita K, Kakibuchi M. Three-dimensional mock-up model for chondral framework in auricular reconstruction, built with a personal three-dimensional printer. *Plast Reconstr Surg* (2014) 134:180e–1e. doi:10.1097/PRS.0000000000000263

115. Xu Y, Fan F, Kang N, Wang S, You J, Wang H, et al. Tissue engineering of human nasal alar cartilage precisely by using three-dimensional printing. *Plast Reconstr Surg* (2015) 135:451–8. doi:10.1097/PRS.0000000000000856

116. Cabalag MS, Chae MP, Miller GS, Rozen WM, Hunter-Smith DJ. Use of three-dimensional printed 'haptic' models for preoperative planning in an Australian plastic surgery unit. *ANZ J Surg* (2015). doi:10.1111/ans.13168

117. Garcia Tutor E, Romeo M, Chae MP, Hunter-Smith DJ, Rozen WM. 3D volumetric modeling and microvascular reconstruction of irradiated lumbosacral defects after oncologic resection. *J Reconstr Microsurg* (2015).

118. Gillis JA, Morris SF. Three-dimensional printing of perforator vascular anatomy. *Plast Reconstr Surg* (2014) 133:80e–2e. doi:10.1097/01.prs.0000436523.79293.64

119. Chae MP, Hunter-Smith DJ, De-Silva I, Tham S, Spychal RT, Rozen WM. Four-dimensional (4D) printing: a new evolution in computed tomography-guided stereolithographic modeling. Principles and application. *J Reconstr Microsurg* (2015). doi:10.1055/s-0035-1549006

120. Sutradhar A, Park J, Carrau D, Miller MJ. Experimental validation of 3D printed patient-specific implants using digital image correlation and finite element analysis. *Comput Biol Med* (2014) 52:8–17. doi:10.1016/j.compbiomed.2014.06.002

121. Ciocca L, De Crescenzio F, Fantini M, Scotti R. Rehabilitation of the nose using CAD/CAM and rapid prototyping technology after ablative surgery of squamous cell carcinoma: a pilot clinical report. *Int J Oral Maxillofac Implants* (2010) 25:808–12. doi:10.1080/10255840903251304

122. Ciocca L, De Crescenzio F, Fantini M, Scotti R. CAD/CAM bilateral ear prostheses construction for Treacher Collins syndrome patients using laser scanning and rapid prototyping. *Comput Methods Biomech Biomed Engin* (2010) 13:379–86. doi:10.1080/10255840903251304

123. Rozen WM, Chubb D, Grinsell D, Ashton MW. Computed tomographic angiography: clinical applications. *Clin Plast Surg* (2011) 38:229–39. doi:10.1016/j.cps.2011.03.007

124. Rozen WM, Garcia-Tutor E, Alonso-Burgos A, Acosta R, Stillaert F, Zubieta JL, et al. Planning and optimising DIEP flaps with virtual surgery: the Navarra experience. *J Plast Reconstr Aesthet Surg* (2010) 63:289–97. doi:10.1016/j.bjps.2008.10.007

125. Donfrancesco A, Montemurro P, Heden P. Three-dimensional simulated images in breast augmentation surgery: an investigation of patients' satisfaction and the correlation between prediction and actual outcome. *Plast Reconstr Surg* (2013) 132:810–22. doi:10.1097/PRS.0b013e3182a014cb

126. Rozen WM, Ashton MW. Modifying techniques in deep inferior epigastric artery perforator flap harvest with the use of preoperative imaging. *ANZ J Surg* (2009) 79:598–603. doi:10.1111/j.1445-2197.2009.05013.x

127. Rozen WM, Ashton MW, Le Roux CM, Pan WR, Corlett RJ. The perforator angiosome: a new concept in the design of deep inferior epigastric artery perforator flaps for breast reconstruction. *Microsurgery* (2010) 30:1–7. doi:10.1002/micr.20684

128. Lee JW, Fang JJ, Chang LR, Yu CK. Mandibular defect reconstruction with the help of mirror imaging coupled with laser stereolithographic modeling technique. *J Formos Med Assoc* (2007) 106:244–50. doi:10.1016/S0929-6646(09)60247-3

129. Cao D, Yu Z, Chai G, Liu J, Mu X. Application of EH compound artificial bone material combined with computerized three-dimensional reconstruction in craniomaxillofacial surgery. *J Craniofac Surg* (2010) 21:440–3. doi:10.1097/SCS.0b013e3181cfe9bc

130. Katsuragi Y, Kayano S, Akazawa S, Nagamatsu S, Koizumi T, Matsui T, et al. Mandible reconstruction using the calcium-sulphate three-dimensional model and rubber stick: a new method, 'mould technique', for more accurate, efficient and simplified fabrication. *J Plast Reconstr Aesthet Surg* (2011) 64:614–22. doi:10.1016/j.bjps.2010.08.010

131. Hsieh MK, Chen AC, Cheng CY, Chou YC, Chan YS, Hsu KY. Repositioning osteotomy for intra-articular malunion of distal radius with radiocarpal and/or distal radioulnar joint subluxation. *J Trauma* (2010) 69:418–22. doi:10.1097/TA.0b013e3181ca0834

132. Gan Y, Xu D, Lu S, Ding J. Novel patient-specific navigational template for total knee arthroplasty. *Comput Aided Surg* (2011) 16:288–97. doi:10.3109/1092908 8.2011.621214

133. Kunz M, Ma B, Rudan JF, Ellis RE, Pichora DR. Image-guided distal radius osteotomy using patient-specific instrument guides. *J Hand Surg Am* (2013) 38:1618–24. doi:10.1016/j.jhsa.2013.05.018

134. Kataoka T, Oka K, Miyake J, Omori S, Tanaka H, Murase T. 3-Dimensional prebent plate fixation in corrective osteotomy of malunited upper extremity fractures using a real-sized plastic bone model prepared by preoperative computer simulation. *J Hand Surg Am* (2013) 38:909–19. doi:10.1016/j.jhsa.2013.02.024

135. Minns RJ, Bibb R, Banks R, Sutton RA. The use of a reconstructed three-dimensional solid model from CT to aid the surgical management of a total knee arthroplasty: a case study. *Med Eng Phys* (2003) 25:523–6. doi:10.1016/S1350-4533(03)00050-X

136. Reinhardt JM, Ding K, Cao K, Christensen GE, Hoffman EA, Bodas SV. Registration-based estimates of local lung tissue expansion compared to xenon CT measures of specific ventilation. *Med Image Anal* (2008) 12:752–63. doi:10.1016/j.media.2008.03.007

137. Chang JY, Li QQ, Xu QY, Allen PK, Rebueno N, Gomez DR, et al. Stereotactic ablative radiation therapy for centrally located early stage or isolated parenchymal recurrences of non-small cell lung cancer: how to fly in a "no fly zone". *Int J Radiat Oncol Biol Phys* (2014) 88:1120–8. doi:10.1016/j.ijrobp.2014.01.022

138. Kontio R, Bjorkstrand R, Salmi M, Paloheimo M, Paloheimo KS, Tuomi J, et al. Designing and additive manufacturing a prototype for a novel instrument for mandible fracture reduction. *Surgery* (2012) S1:002. doi:10.4172/2161-1076.S1-002

139. Sugawara T, Higashiyama N, Kaneyama S, Takabatake M, Watanabe N, Uchida F, et al. Multistep pedicle screw insertion procedure with patient-specific lamina fit-and-lock templates for the thoracic spine: clinical article. *J Neurosurg Spine* (2013) 19:185–90. doi:10.3171/2013.4.SPINE121059

140. Lambrecht JT, Berndt DC, Schumacher R, Zehnder M. Generation of three-dimensional prototype models based on cone beam computed tomography. *Int J Comput Assist Radiol Surg* (2009) 4:175–80. doi:10.1007/s11548-008-0275-9

141. Kimura T, Morita A, Nishimura K, Aiyama H, Itoh H, Fukaya S, et al. Simulation of and training for cerebral aneurysm clipping with 3-dimensional models. *Neurosurgery* (2009) 65:719–25. doi:10.1227/01.NEU.0000354350.88899.07

142. Chueh JY, Wakhloo AK, Gounis MJ. Neurovascular modeling: small-batch manufacturing of silicone vascular replicas. *AJNR Am J Neuroradiol* (2009) 30:1159–64. doi:10.3174/ajnr.A1543

143. Sulaiman A, Boussel L, Taconnet F, Serfaty JM, Alsaid H, Attia C, et al. In vitro non-rigid life-size model of aortic arch aneurysm for endovascular prosthesis assessment. *Eur J Cardiothorac Surg* (2008) 33:53–7. doi:10.1016/j.ejcts.2007.10.016

144. Kalejs M, von Segesser LK. Rapid prototyping of compliant human aortic roots for assessment of valved stents. *Interact Cardiovasc Thorac Surg* (2009) 8:182–6. doi:10.1510/icvts.2008.194134

145. Armillotta A, Bonhoeffer P, Dubini G, Ferragina S, Migliavacca F, Sala G, et al. Use of rapid prototyping models in the planning of percutaneous pulmonary valved stent implantation. *Proc Inst Mech Eng H* (2007) 221:407–16. doi:10.1243/09544119JEIM83

146. Bruyere F, Leroux C, Brunereau L, Lermusiaux P. Rapid prototyping model for percutaneous nephrolithotomy training. *J Endourol* (2008) 22:91–6. doi:10.1089/end.2007.0025

147. Kim MS, Sbalchiero JC, Reece GP, Miller MJ, Beahm EK, Markey MK. Assessment of breast aesthetics. *Plast Reconstr Surg* (2008) 121:186e–94e. doi:10.1097/01.prs.0000304593.74672.b8

148. Chan YC, Qing KX, Cheng SW. Custom-made fenestrated stent grafts to preserve accessory renal arteries in patients with abdominal aortic aneurysms. *Acta Chir Belg* (2014) 114:183–8.

149. Hourfar J, Kanavakis G, Goellner P, Ludwig B. Fully customized placement of orthodontic miniplates: a novel clinical technique. *Head Face Med* (2014) 10:14. doi:10.1186/1746-160X-10-14

150. Lee SJ, Lee HP, Tse KM, Cheong EC, Lim SP. Computer-aided design and rapid prototyping-assisted contouring of costal cartilage graft for facial reconstructive surgery. *Craniomaxillofac Trauma Reconstr* (2012) 5:75–82. doi:10.1055/s-0031-1300964

151. Wu G, Zhou B, Bi Y, Zhao Y. Selective laser sintering technology for customized fabrication of facial prostheses. *J Prosthet Dent* (2008) 100:56–60. doi:10.1016/S0022-3913(08)60138-9

152. Sykes LM, Parrott AM, Owen CP, Snaddon DR. Applications of rapid prototyping technology in maxillofacial prosthetics. *Int J Prosthodont* (2004) 17:454–9.

153. Subburaj K, Nair C, Rajesh S, Meshram SM, Ravi B. Rapid development of auricular prosthesis using CAD and rapid prototyping technologies. *Int J Oral Maxillofac Surg* (2007) 36:938–43. doi:10.1016/j.ijom.2007.07.013

154. Karayazgan-Saracoglu B, Gunay Y, Atay A. Fabrication of an auricular prosthesis using computed tomography and rapid prototyping technique. *J Craniofac Surg* (2009) 20:1169–72. doi:10.1097/SCS.0b013e3181acdb95

155. De Crescenzio F, Fantini M, Ciocca L, Persiani F, Scotti R. Design and manufacturing of ear prosthesis by means of rapid prototyping technology. *Proc Inst Mech Eng H* (2011) 225:296–302. doi:10.1243/09544119JEIM856

156. Ciocca L, Scotti R. Oculo-facial rehabilitation after facial cancer removal: updated CAD/CAM procedures. A pilot study. *Prosthet Orthot Int* (2013). doi:10.1177/0309364613512368

157. Xie P, Hu Z, Zhang X, Li X, Gao Z, Yuan D, et al. Application of 3-dimensional printing technology to construct an eye model for fundus viewing study. *PLoS One* (2014) 9:e109373. doi:10.1371/journal.pone.0109373

158. Tsuji M, Noguchi N, Ihara K, Yamashita Y, Shikimori M, Goto M. Fabrication of a maxillofacial prosthesis using a computer-aided design and manufacturing system. *J Prosthodont* (2004) 13:179–83. doi:10.1111/j.1532-849X.2004.04029.x

159. Fantini M, De Crescenzio F, Ciocca L. Design and rapid manufacturing of anatomical prosthesis for facial rehabilitation. *Int J Interact Des Manuf* (2013) 7:51–62. doi:10.1007/s12008-012-0159-7

160. De Laurentis KJ, Mavroidis C. Mechanical design of a shape memory alloy actuated prosthetic hand. *Technol Health Care* (2002) 10:91–106.

161. Eppley BL. Craniofacial reconstruction with computer-generated HTR patient-matched implants: use in primary bony tumor excision. *J Craniofac Surg* (2002) 13:650–7. doi:10.1097/00001665-200209000-00011

162. Sammartino G, Della Valle A, Marenzi G, Gerbino S, Martorelli M, di Lauro AE, et al. Stereolithography in oral implantology: a comparison of surgical guides. *Implant Dent* (2004) 13:133–9. doi:10.1097/01.ID.0000127526.36938.4C

Tissue Engineered Materials in Cardiovascular Surgery: The Surgeon's Perspective

Andras P. Durko[1], Magdi H. Yacoub[2] and Jolanda Kluin[3]*

[1] Department of Cardiothoracic Surgery, Erasmus University Medical Center, Rotterdam, Netherlands, [2] Imperial College London, National Heart and Lung Institute, London, United Kingdom, [3] Department of Cardiothoracic Surgery, Amsterdam University Medical Center, Amsterdam, Netherlands

*Correspondence:
Jolanda Kluin
j.kluin@amsterdamumc.nl

In cardiovascular surgery, reconstruction and replacement of cardiac and vascular structures are routinely performed. Prosthetic or biological materials traditionally used for this purpose cannot be considered ideal substitutes as they have limited durability and no growth or regeneration potential. Tissue engineering aims to create materials having normal tissue function including capacity for growth and self-repair. These advanced materials can potentially overcome the shortcomings of conventionally used materials, and, if successfully passing all phases of product development, they might provide a better option for both the pediatric and adult patient population requiring cardiovascular interventions. This short review article overviews the most important cardiovascular pathologies where tissue engineered materials could be used, briefly summarizes the main directions of development of these materials, and discusses the hurdles in their clinical translation. At its beginnings in the 1980s, tissue engineering (TE) was defined as *"an interdisciplinary field that applies the principles of engineering and the life sciences toward the development of biological substitutes that restore, maintain, or improve tissue function"* (1). Currently, the utility of TE products and materials are being investigated in several fields of human medicine, ranging from orthopedics to cardiovascular surgery (2–5). In cardiovascular surgery, reconstruction and replacement of cardiac and vascular structures are routinely performed. Considering the shortcomings of traditionally used materials, the need for advanced materials that can "restore, maintain or improve tissue function" are evident. Tissue engineered substitutes, having growth and regenerative capacity, could fundamentally change the specialty (6). This article overviews the most important cardiovascular pathologies where TE materials could be used, briefly summarizes the main directions of development of TE materials along with their advantages and shortcomings, and discusses the hurdles in their clinical translation.

Keywords: tissue-engineering, bioengineering, cardiac surgery, heart surgery, *in-situ* tissue engineered, TEHV

CLINICAL NEED FOR ADVANCED MATERIALS IN CARDIOVASCULAR SURGERY

Congenital Heart Disease

Congenital heart defects affect ~9 of 1,000 newborns (7) and often require corrective surgery at an early age. Invasive treatment of congenital cardiac defects results in an increased life expectancy and can significantly improve quality-of-life (8).

Repair with a prosthetic patch is the cornerstone of reconstruction of diseased or defective cardiac and vascular structures in pediatric cardiac surgery. Patches are used for the closure of atrial or ventricular septal defects, for complex reconstructions in atrioventricular canal defects; in right ventricular outflow tract reconstruction in Tetralogy of Fallot; for aortic reconstruction in interrupted aortic arch or hypoplastic left heart syndrome; or when establishing cavo-pulmonary connection is required (9–13). As most of these operations are performed at very young or even neonatal age, repair must stay effective and durable in a rapidly changing physiological environment. Traditionally used materials—autologous or xenogeneic pericardium, or prosthetic materials like Dacron (DuPont, Wilmington, DE) or PTFE (polytetrafluoroethylene)—are suboptimal in this respect as they tend to calcify over time and cannot grow with the child (14–16).

As children will inevitably outgrow a prosthetic heart valve (PHV) implanted at young age, reconstruction of native valves is always preferred over replacement whenever feasible. However, if reconstruction fails or appears not possible, replacement of the dysfunctional valve with a PHV becomes necessary. In childhood, most commonly the pulmonary valve requires replacement, often using a right ventricle-to-pulmonary artery conduit (17). Unfortunately, none of the currently available allogenic or xenogeneic conduits can be considered ideal, as they cannot grow and degenerate on the long term (18–21). Besides pathologies of the pulmonary valve and right ventricular outflow tract, congenital aortic stenosis (AS) often necessitates valve replacement in the pediatric population. Although balloon palliation can buy some time until valve repair or replacement (22), patients with congenital AS often require a sequence of re-operations until they reach adulthood (23, 24), largely due to the absence of an optimal valve substitute.

Acquired Valvular Heart Disease

Parallel to aging of the adult population, degenerative valvular heart diseases are becoming increasingly prevalent in the western world (25). Additionally, in developing countries, rheumatic valvular heart disease causes a substantial and often underestimated burden (26). Although valve replacement with a PHV improves symptom status and long-term survival, currently available heart valve prostheses are also associated with certain complications (27, 28). Mechanical PHVs necessitate lifelong anticoagulation, which increases the risk of bleeding and thromboembolic events and is suboptimal for women in childbearing age (29, 30), while the limited long-term durability and inherent structural degeneration of bioprosthetic valves remain a major issue for the younger patient population (31, 32).

Vascular Grafts

In coronary artery bypass grafting, peripheral vascular reconstructions or when creating arteriovenous shunts for renal dialysis, small caliber vascular grafts are required. Although autologous vessels harvested from other parts of body are potentially ideal for this purpose, they are not always available or eligible for use. Traditionally used prosthetic grafts have numerous limitations due to their limited patency (33–35) and increased susceptibility for infections (36). This, together with the magnitude of the affected population necessitates intensive research for alternative solutions (37).

OVERVIEW OF TISSUE ENGINEERED SOLUTIONS

Tissue engineering, by providing advanced materials with physiological function and ability for growth and regeneration, could potentially fulfill these clinical needs. To create a TE product, the following are required: (i) a (biodegradable) scaffold to guide tissue formation; (ii) cells able to populate the scaffold; and (iii) (in the classical way of TE) a bioreactor, which simulates a physiological environment to augment tissue formation. Scaffolds used in cardiovascular TE can be from various origin. The most commonly used scaffold materials are summarized in (**Table 1**). Similarly, multiple cell-types might be used: among others, mesenchymal stem cells, endothelial progenitor cells or induced pluripotent stem cells can be utilized during the TE process (56). Bioreactors are specifically designed containers intended to provide an optimized, controlled environment where cell-scaffold interaction can take place (57). During "classical" TE, scaffolds are seeded with progenitor cells and incubated *in vitro* in a bioreactor. Following a period of maturation under controlled conditions, the TE product is implanted to the patient. Besides this "conventional" approach, various other, "incomplete" methods exist, where one or more steps of the "conventional" TE process are bypassed (58).

Some "TE" products are already cleared for clinical use: decellularized valves, porcine small intestinal submucosa and decellularized bovine pericardium (SynerGraft®, CryoLife Inc, Kennesaw, GA, United States; CorMatrix®, CorMatrix Cardiovascular, Roswell, GA, United States; CardioCel® Bioscaffold, LeMaitre Vascular, Burlington, MA, United States) are already parts of cardiovascular surgeon's armamentarium. Apart from decellularized allografts and porcine small intestinal submucosa, all other products are treated with glutaraldehyde (59) which can have a negative impact on cellular ingrowth following implantation (60). Furthermore, it is unclear if the above mentioned decellularized scaffolds degrade at all and whether they can truly be considered as TE products. Besides, all these products have inherent shortcomings. Allogenic tissues are generally cumbersome to procure and might still fail in the long term (61). Xenogeneic tissues can provoke inflammatory response leading to early degeneration and calcification. The first commercially available decellularized porcine valve dramatically failed due to a strong inflammatory response resulting in rapid degeneration and early structural

TABLE 1 | Most commonly used scaffold types in cardiovascular tissue engineering with examples.

Scaffold type	Examples			
	Implant type	Implant position	Species	Reference
Biological origin				
Decellularized vessels or valves				
Allogenic	Aortic root	Aortic	Human	(38)
Xenogeneic	Aortic root	Pulmonary	Ovine	(39)
Acellular or decellularized other xenogeneic tissues				
Pericardium	Patch	Various	Human	(40)
Small intestinal submucosa	Patch	Intracardiac	Human	(41)
	Valve	Tricuspid	Ovine	(42)
	Patch	Aortic arch	Human	(43)
	Patch	Right ventricular wall	Ovine	(44)
Allogenic or autologous engineered tissue				
	Valved conduit	Pulmonary	Canine	(45)
	Patch	Pulmonary	Human	(46)
	Vascular graft	A-V shunt	Human	(47–49)
	Valve	Aortic	Ovine	(50)
Synthetic origin				
	Valved conduit	Pulmonary	Ovine	(51, 52)
	Valve	Aortic	Ovine	(53)
	Vascular graft	Cavo-pulmonary connection	Human	(54)
	Valve	Pulmonary	Ovine	(55)

failure in pediatric patients (62). Although a promising concept, acellular porcine small intestinal submucosa patches can also provoke an inflammatory response and can demonstrate early degeneration or calcifications leading to valve insufficiency when used for aortic valve repair (63, 64), or aneurysm formation when used for aortic reconstruction in pediatric patients (65). Decellularized bovine pericardium, though treated with low concentrations of glutaraldehyde (66), was found to be safe and effective in the mid-term when used for patch repair of complex congenital cardiac anomalies (40) and exhibited greater strain resistance compared to porcine small intestinal submucosa (67). Nevertheless, the possibility of calcification of the decellularized bovine pericardium has also been raised recently (68) and the quest for the "ideal" tissue engineered material continues.

IN SITU TISSUE ENGINEERING WITH POLYMER SCAFFOLDS

During *in situ* TE, an unseeded biodegradable scaffold is implanted to the recipient. After implantation, the scaffold will be populated *in vivo* by cells scrambled from the circulation, with the recipient's own body acting as a bioreactor. This simplified approach saves substantial costs and prevents potential complications associated with incubating the scaffold in a bioreactor. Neo-tissue formation begins only after scaffold

implantation and can occur under completely physiological shear and pressure conditions (69).

Compared to biological materials, polymers materials are relatively easy to produce, handle, sterilize or store, and they can be manufactured in virtually any size or form. This creates the possibility of manufacturing directly off-the-shelf available TE cardiovascular implants and increases the interest in *in situ* TE using polymer scaffolds.

However, this technique also has certain shortcomings which have to be considered. During *in situ* TE, neo-tissue formation occurs in a less-controlled environment and cells repopulating the scaffold must be gathered from high blood flows which might not be ideal (70). Furthermore, a delicate balance between the pace of scaffold degeneration and neo-tissue formation is required to achieve an optimal result. Fortunately, in contrast to TE products from biological origin, the design of the prosthesis and the characteristics of the polymer material such as scaffold composition, scaffold or fiber thickness or fiber orientation can be relatively easily modified, if necessary (71–75).

Heart valve constructs from polymer scaffolds are currently under investigation in preclinical experiments. In sheep, these scaffolds have demonstrated satisfactory durability and function on mid- term when implanted in the pulmonary position as a surgical prosthesis (55) or as a valved conduit (76), or when used as a transcatheter aortic valve (53). Based on these encouraging results, the first-in-man investigations of the polymer scaffolds has recently been started (54).

CHALLENGES IN CLINICAL TRANSLATION

As any new technology awaiting clinical introduction (77), TE products in cardiovascular surgery must find a therapeutic gap, a "niche," where no ideal treatment option exists, and where the advantages of the new technology can be proven. Although the shortcomings of currently used materials are evident and some "TE" products are already approved and used in the clinical setting, there are many hurdles to overcome before TE materials can be routinely used in cardiovascular surgery (78).

Cardiovascular implants have to fulfill strict safety and performance criteria during their regulatory assessment before clinical introduction (79–81). During regulatory assessment, standards of the International Organization for Standardization (ISO) are widely used. The ISO 5840 standard on heart valve prostheses provides guidance on *in vitro* and *in vivo* hemodynamic and durability testing, as well as Objective Performance Criteria (OPC) for the assessment of complications after implantation (82). However, regulatory assessment of TE implants is complicated. During manufacturing, achieving consistence in the biological properties of cell-based products between batches is difficult, rendering TE products less reproducible than conventional cardiovascular implants. Furthermore, difficulties in sterilization, packaging and storage of cell-based TE products further limit their regulatory approval and widespread clinical use. On the other hand, *in situ* TE cardiovascular implants cannot be considered as "final products," as their properties are expected to change after implantation while they transform into normally functioning living tissue. Of note, this transformation might not be the same in all subjects receiving the same implant and tissue formation might occur differently in animals used for pre-clinical *in vivo* testing than in human recipients (83). These issues make the interpretation of the results derived from *in vitro* and *in vivo* testing cumbersome, and together with the plethora of approaches and techniques used for manufacturing, makes the regulatory assessment of TE cardiovascular implants difficult. To date, no specific ISO standard on TE heart valves exist and it is not clear how these products should be classified or assessed.

Besides, considering these unique properties of TE cardiovascular implants, important ethical issues might arise when it comes to *in human* testing or clinical introduction of these products (84). Irrespective of the local circumstances or the clinical need, the risk of implanting a prosthesis that might fail must always be carefully weighed against the perceived benefits (26, 85, 86).

Another important aspect of successful clinical introduction is the cost-effectiveness of the novel device or technique, compared to standard treatment (87). Although development of TE materials are expensive, *in-situ* TE valves constructed from biodegradable polymer scaffolds could be potentially cost effective, according to a recent early health technology assessment study (88).

PERSPECTIVES

Materials used in cardiovascular surgery must fulfill a few essential requirements: they must be hemostatic, hold sutures, be resistant to pressure and stress while being tissue-friendly and resistant to thrombosis. Additionally, an ideal material has normal tissue function and capability for growth and self-repair.

TE materials can potentially fulfill all of these essential requirements and *in situ* TE using polymer materials can offer a simplified and potentially cost-effective method to produce off-the-shelf available, TE cardiovascular implants. Although initial results are promising (55), future research is necessitated and there are still many obstacles to overcome before the use of these materials can become a part of the everyday practice of cardiovascular surgery (89). The use of novel cell free techniques to enhance the process of regeneration in TE include adding exosomes (90), hydrogels (91), direct (92, 93), or indirect induced pluripotent stem cell reprogramming using gene editing (94, 95) as well as stimulating myocardial cell division (96). Adding such strategies holds great promise in the future.

AUTHOR CONTRIBUTIONS

AD: drafting the first manuscript. MY and JK: critically revising the work for important intellectual content.

REFERENCES

1. Langer R, Vacanti JP. Tissue engineering. *Science.* (1993) 260:920–6. doi: 10.1126/science.8493529
2. Langer R, Vacanti J. Advances in tissue engineering. *J Pediatr Surg.* (2016) 51:8–12. doi: 10.1016/j.jpedsurg.2015.10.022
3. Vijayavenkataraman S, Lu WF, Fuh JY. 3D bioprinting of skin: a state-of-the-art review on modelling, materials, and processes. *Biofabrication.* (2016) 8:032001. doi: 10.1088/1758-5090/8/3/032001
4. Nie X, Wang DA. Decellularized orthopaedic tissue-engineered grafts: biomaterial scaffolds synthesised by therapeutic cells. *Biomater Sci.* (2018) 6:2798–811. doi: 10.1039/C8BM00772A
5. Bowles RD, Setton LA. Biomaterials for intervertebral disc regeneration and repair. *Biomaterials.* (2017) 129:54–67. doi: 10.1016/j.biomaterials.2017.03.013
6. Yacoub MH, Takkenberg JJ. Will heart valve tissue engineering change the world? *Nat Clin Pract Cardiovasc Med.* (2005) 2:60–1. doi: 10.1038/ncpcardio0112
7. van der Linde D, Konings EE, Slager MA, Witsenburg M, Helbing WA, Takkenberg JJ, et al. Birth prevalence of congenital heart disease worldwide: a systematic review and meta-analysis. *J Am Coll Cardiol.* (2011) 58:2241–7. doi: 10.1016/j.jacc.2011.08.025
8. Loup O, von Weissenfluh C, Gahl B, Schwerzmann M, Carrel T, Kadner A. Quality of life of grown-up congenital heart disease patients after congenital cardiac surgery. *Eur J Cardiothorac Surg.* (2009) 36:105–11; discussion 11. doi: 10.1016/j.ejcts.2009.03.023
9. Backer CL, Stewart RD, Bailliard F, Kelle AM, Webb CL, Mavroudis C. Complete atrioventricular canal: comparison of modified single-patch technique with two-patch technique. *Ann Thorac Surg.* (2007) 84:2038–46; discussion −46. doi: 10.1016/j.athoracsur.2007.04.129
10. Kaza AK, Lim HG, Dibardino DJ, Bautista-Hernandez V, Robinson J, Allan C, et al. Long-term results of right ventricular outflow tract reconstruction in neonatal cardiac surgery: options and outcomes. *J Thorac Cardiovasc Surg.* (2009) 138:911–6. doi: 10.1016/j.jtcvs.2008.10.058

11. Backer CL, Paape K, Zales VR, Weigel TJ, Mavroudis C. Coarctation of the aorta. Repair with polytetrafluoroethylene patch aortoplasty. *Circulation.* (1995) 92:II132–6. doi: 10.1161/01.CIR.92.9.132

12. Vitanova K, Cleuziou J, Pabst von Ohain J, Burri M, Eicken A, Lange R. Recoarctation after norwood i Procedure for hypoplastic left hea syndrome: impact of patch material. *Ann Thorac Surg.* (2017) 103:617–21. doi: 10.1016/j.athoracsur.2016.10.030

13. Stamm C, Friehs I, Mayer JE, Jr., Zurakowski D, Triedman JK, et al. Long-term results of the lateral tunnel fontan operation. *J Thorac Cardiovasc Surg.* (2001) 121:28–41. doi: 10.1067/mtc.2001.111422

14. Lee C, Lee CH, Hwang SW, Lim HG, Kim SJ, Lee JY, et al. Midterm follow up of the status of gore-Tex graft after extracardiac conduit fontan procedure. *Eur J Cardiothorac Surg.* (2007) 31:1008–12. doi: 10.1016/j.ejcts.2007.03.013

15. Kadowaki MH, Levett JM, Manjoney DL, Grina NM, Glagov S. Comparison of prosthetic graft materials as intracardiac right atrial patches. *J Surg Res.* (1986) 41:65–74. doi: 10.1016/0022-4804(86)90010-7

16. Giannico S, Hammad F, Amodeo A, Michielon G, Drago F, Turchetta A, et al. Clinical outcome of 193 extracardiac fontan patients: the first 15 years. *J Am Coll Cardiol.* (2006) 47:2065–73. doi: 10.1016/j.jacc.2005.12.065

17. The Society of Thoracic Surgeons. *Congenital Heart Surgery Database.* The Society of Thoracic Surgeons. (2019). Available online at: https://www.sts.org/registries-research-center/sts-national-database/congenital-heart-surgery-database.

18. Dearani JA, Danielson GK, Puga FJ, Schaff HV, Warnes CW, Driscoll DJ, et al. Late follow-up of 1095 patients undergoing operation for complex congenital heart disease utilizing pulmonary ventricle to pulmona artery conduits. *Ann Thorac Surg.* (2003) 75:399–410; discussion doi: 10.1016/S0003-4975(02)04547-2

19. Boethig D, Goerler H, Westhoff-Bleck M, Ono M, Daiber A, Haverich A, et al. Evaluation of 188 consecutive homografts implanted in pulmonary position after 20 years. *Eur J Cardiothorac Surg.* (2007) 32:133–42. doi: 10.1016/j.ejcts.2007.02.025

20. Homann M, Haehnel JC, Mendler N, Paek SU, Holper K, Meisner H, et al. Reconstruction of the RVOT with valved biological conduits: 25 years experience with allografts and xenografts. *Eur J Cardiothorac Surg.* (2000) 17:624–30. doi: 10.1016/S1010-7940(00)00414-0

21. Yong MS, Yim D, d'Udekem Y, Brizard CP, Robertson T, Galati JC, e al. Medium-term outcomes of bovine jugular vein graft and homograft conduits in children. *ANZ J Surg.* (2015) 85:381–5. doi: 10.1111/ans.13018

22. McCrindle BW, Blackstone EH, Williams WG, Sittiwangkul R, Spray TL Azakie A, et al. Are outcomes of surgical versus transcatheter balloon valvotomy equivalent in neonatal critical aortic stenosis? *Circulation.* (2001) 104(12 Suppl. 1):I152–8. doi: 10.1161/hc37t1.094837

23. Siddiqui J, Brizard CP, Galati JC, Iyengar AJ, Hutchinson D, Konstantinov IE, et al. Surgical valvotomy and repair for neonatal and infant congenital aortic stenosis achieves better results than interventional catheterization. *J Am Coll Cardiol.* (2013) 62:2134–40. doi: 10.1016/j.jacc.2013.07.052

24. d'Udekem Y, Siddiqui J, Seaman CS, Konstantinov IE, Galati JC, Cheung MM, et al. Long-term results of a strategy of aortic valve repair in the pediatric population. *J Thorac Cardiovasc Surg.* (2013) 145:461–7; discussion 7–9. doi: 10.1016/j.jtcvs.2012.11.033

25. Nkomo VT, Gardin JM, Skelton TN, Gottdiener JS, Scott CG, Enriquez-Sarano M. Burden of valvular heart diseases: a population-based study. *Lancet.* (2006) 368:1005–11. doi: 10.1016/S0140-6736(06)69208-8

26. Zilla P, Yacoub M, Zuhlke L, Beyersdorf F, Sliwa K, Khubulava G, et al. Global unmet needs in cardiac surgery. *Glob Heart.* (2018) 13:293–303. doi: 10.1016/j.gheart.2018.08.002

27. Kapadia SR, Leon MB, Makkar RR, Tuzcu EM, Svensson LG, Kodali S, et al. 5-year outcomes of transcatheter aortic valve replacement compared with standard treatment for patients with inoperable aortic stenosis (PARTNER 1): a randomised controlled trial. *Lancet.* (2015) 385:2485–91. doi: 10.1016/S0140-6736(15)60290-2

28. Brennan JM, Edwards FH, Zhao Y, O'Brien S, Booth ME, Dokholyan RS, et al. Long-term safety and effectiveness of mechanical versus biologic aortic valve prostheses in older patients: results from the society of thoracic surgeons

adult cardiac surgery national database. *Circulation.* (2013) 127:1647–55. doi: 10.1161/CIRCULATIONAHA.113.002003

29. Hammermeister K, Sethi GK, Henderson WG, Grover FL, Oprian C, Rahimtoola SH. Outcomes 15 years after valve replacement with a mechanical versus a bioprosthetic valve: final report of the veterans affairs randomized trial. *J Am Coll Cardiol.* (2000) 36:1152–8. doi: 10.1016/S0735-1097(00)00834-2

30. Steinberg ZL, Dominguez-Islas CP, Otto CM, Stout KK, Krieger EV. Maternal and fetal outcomes of anticoagulation in pregnant women with mechanical heart valves. *J Am Coll Cardiol.* (2017) 69:2681–91. doi: 10.1016/j.jacc.2017.03.605

31. Fatima B, Mohananey D, Khan FW, Jobanputra Y, Tummala R, Banerjee K, et al. Durability data for bioprosthetic surgical aortic valve: a systematic review. *JAMA Cardiol.* (2018) 4:71–80. doi: 10.1001/jamacardio.2018.4045

32. Saleeb SF, Newburger JW, Geva T, Baird CW, Gauvreau K, Padera RF, et al. Accelerated degeneration of a bovine pericardial bioprosthetic aortic valve in children and young adults. *Circulation.* (2014) 130:51–60. doi: 10.1161/CIRCULATIONAHA.114.009835

33. Desai M, Seifalian AM, Hamilton G. Role of prosthetic conduits in coronary artery bypass grafting. *Eur J Cardiothorac Surg.* (2011) 40:394–8. doi: 10.1016/j.ejcts.2010.11.050

34. Kashyap VS, Ahn SS, Quinones-Baldrich WJ, Choi BU, Dorey F, Reil TD, et al. Infrapopliteal-lower extremity revascularization with prosthetic conduit: a 20-year experience. *Vasc Endovascular Surg.* (2002) 36:255–62. doi: 10.1177/153857440203600402

35. Johnson WC, Lee KK. A comparative evaluation of polytetrafluoroethylene, umbilical vein, and saphenous vein bypass grafts for femoral-popliteal above-knee revascularization: a prospective randomized department of veterans affairs cooperative study. *J Vasc Surg.* (2000) 32:268–77. doi: 10.1067/mva.2000.106944

36. Kirkton RD, Prichard HL, Santiago-Maysonet M, Niklason LE, Lawson JH, Dahl SLM. Susceptibility of ePTFE vascular grafts and bioengineered human acellular vessels to infection. *J Surg Res.* (2018) 221:143–51. doi: 10.1016/j.jss.2017.08.035

37. Liyanage T, Ninomiya T, Jha V, Neal B, Patrice HM, Okpechi I, et al. Worldwide access to treatment for end-stage kidney disease: a systematic review. *The Lancet.* (2015) 385:1975–82. doi: 10.1016/S0140-6736(14)61601-9

38. Zehr KJ, Yagubyan M, Connolly HM, Nelson SM, Schaff HV. Aortic root replacement with a novel decellularized cryopreserved aortic homograft: postoperative immunoreactivity and early results. *J Thorac Cardiovasc Surg.* (2005) 130:1010–5. doi: 10.1016/j.jtcvs.2005.03.044

39. Paniagua Gutierrez JR, Berry H, Korossis S, Mirsadraee S, Lopes SV, da Costa F, et al. Regenerative potential of low-concentration sDS-decellularized porcine aortic valved conduits in vivo. *Tissue Engineer Part A.* (2015) 21:332–42. doi: 10.1089/ten.tea.2014.0003

40. Neethling WM, Strange G, Firth L, Smit FE. Evaluation of a tissue-engineered bovine pericardial patch in paediatric patients with congenital cardiac anomalies: initial experience with the aDAPT-treated cardioCel(R) patch. *Interact Cardiovasc Thorac Surg.* (2013) 17:698–702. doi: 10.1093/icvts/ivt268

41. Al Haddad E, LaPar DJ, Dayton J, Stephens EH, Bacha E. Complete atrioventricular canal repair with a decellularized porcine small intestinal submucosa patch. *Congenit Heart Dis.* (2018) doi: 10.1111/chd.12666

42. Zafar F, Hinton RB, Moore RA, Baker RS, Bryant R, 3rd, Narmoneva DA, et al. Physiological growth, remodeling potential, and preserved function of a novel bioprosthetic tricuspid valve: tubular bioprosthesis made of small intestinal submucosa-Derived extracellular matrix. *J Am Coll Cardiol.* (2015) 66:877–88. doi: 10.1016/j.jacc.2015.06.1091

43. Jacobsen RM, Mitchell ME, Woods RK, Loomba RS, Tweddell JS. Porcine small intestinal submucosa may be a suitable material for norwood arch reconstruction. *Ann Thorac Surg.* (2018) 106:1847–52. doi: 10.1016/j.athoracsur.2018.06.033

44. Baker RS, Zafar F, Kimura N, Knilans T, Osinska H, Robbins J, et al. In vivo remodeling of an extracellular matrix cardiac patch in an ovine model. *Asaio J.* (2018) doi: 10.1097/MAT.0000000000000864

45. Yamanami M, Yahata Y, Uechi M, Fujiwara M, Ishibashi-Ueda H, Kanda K, et al. Development of a completely autologous valved conduit with the sinus of valsalva using in-body tissue architecture technology: a pilot study in pulmonary valve replacement in a beagle model. *Circulation.* (2010) 122(11 Suppl.):S100–6. doi: 10.1161/CIRCULATIONAHA.109.922211

46. Kato N, Yamagishi M, Kanda K, Miyazaki T, Maeda Y, Yamanami M, et al. First successful clinical application of the *in vivo* tissue-Engineered autologous vascular graft. *Ann Thorac Surg.* (2016) 102:1387–90. doi: 10.1016/j.athoracsur.2016.06.095

47. McAllister TN, Maruszewski M, Garrido SA, Wystrychowski W, Dusserre N, Marini A, et al. Effectiveness of haemodialysis access with an autologous tissue-engineered vascular graft: a multicentre cohort study. *Lancet.* (2009) 373:1440–6. doi: 10.1016/S0140-6736(09)60248-8

48. Lawson JH, Glickman MH, Ilzecki M, Jakimowicz T, Jaroszynski A, Peden EK, et al. Bioengineered human acellular vessels for dialysis access in patients with end-stage renal disease: two phase 2 single-arm trials. *Lancet.* (2016) 387:2026–34. doi: 10.1016/S0140-6736(16)00557-2

49. Wystrychowski W, McAllister TN, Zagalski K, Dusserre N, Cierpka L, L'Heureux N. First human use of an allogeneic tissue-engineered vascular graft for hemodialysis access. *J Vasc Surg.* (2014) 60:1353–7. doi: 10.1016/j.jvs.2013.08.018

50. Syedain Z, Reimer J, Schmidt J, Lahti M, Berry J, Bianco R, et al. 6-month aortic valve implantation of an off-the-shelf tissue-engineered valve in sheep. *Biomaterials.* (2015) 73:175–84. doi: 10.1016/j.biomaterials.2015.09.016

51. Bennink G, Torii S, Brugmans M, Cox M, Svanidze O, Ladich E, et al. A novel restorative pulmonary valved conduit in a chronic sheep model: mid-term hemodynamic function and histologic assessment. *J Thorac Cardiovasc Surg.* (2018) 155:2591–601 e3. doi: 10.1016/j.jtcvs.2017.12.046

52. Brugmans M, Serrero A, Cox M, Svanidze O, Schoen FJ. Morphology and mechanisms of a novel absorbable polymeric conduit in the pulmonary circulation of sheep. *Cardiovasc Pathol.* (2018) 38:31–8. doi: 10.1016/j.carpath.2018.10.008

53. Miyazaki Y, Soliman OII, Abdelghani M, Katsikis A, Naz C, Lopes S, et al. Acute performance of a novel restorative transcatheter aortic valve: preclinical results. *EuroIntervention.* (2017) 13:e1410–e7. doi: 10.4244/EIJ-D-17-00554

54. Bockeria LA, Svanidze O, Kim A, Shatalov K, Makarenko V, Cox M, et al. Total cavopulmonary connection with a new bioabsorbable vascular graft: first clinical experience. *J Thorac Cardiovasc Surg.* (2017) 153:1542–50. doi: 10.1016/j.jtcvs.2016.11.071

55. Kluin J, Talacua H, Smits AI, Emmert MY, Brugmans MC, Fioretta ES, et al. *In situ* heart valve tissue engineering using a bioresorbable elastomeric implant - from material design to 12 months follow-up in sheep. *Biomaterials.* (2017) 125:101–17. doi: 10.1016/j.biomaterials.2017.02.007

56. Jover E, Fagnano M, Angelini G, Madeddu P. Cell sources for tissue engineering strategies to treat calcific valve disease. *Front Cardiovasc Med.* (2018) 5:155. doi: 10.3389/fcvm.2018.00155

57. Berry JL, Steen JA, Koudy Williams J, Jordan JE, Atala A, Yoo JJ. Bioreactors for development of tissue engineered heart valves. *Ann Biomed Eng.* (2010) 38:3272–9. doi: 10.1007/s10439-010-0148-6

58. Rabkin E, Schoen FJ. Cardiovascular tissue engineering. *Cardiovasc Pathol.* (2002) 11:305–17. doi: 10.1016/S1054-8807(02)00130-8

59. Pattar SS, Fatehi Hassanabad A, Fedak PWM. Acellular extracellular matrix bioscaffolds for cardiac repair and regeneration. *Front Cell Dev Biol.* (2019) 7:63. doi: 10.3389/fcell.2019.00063

60. Honge JL, Funder J, Hansen E, Dohmen PM, Konertz W, Hasenkam JM. Recellularization of aortic valves in pigs?. *Eur J Cardio-Thor Surg.* (2011) 39:829–34. doi: 10.1016/j.ejcts.2010.08.054

61. Horke A. Decellularization of aortic valves: only time will tell. *Eur J Cardiothorac Surg.* (2016) 49:707–8. doi: 10.1093/ejcts/ezv361

62. Simon P, Kasimir MT, Seebacher G, Weigel G, Ullrich R, Salzer-Muhar U, et al. Early failure of the tissue engineered porcine heart valve sYNERGRAFT in pediatric patients. *Eur J Cardiothorac Surg.* (2003) 23:1002–6; discussion 6. doi: 10.1016/S1010-7940(03)00094-0

63. Hofmann M, Schmiady MO, Burkhardt BE, Dave HH, Hubler M, Kretschmar O, et al. Congenital aortic valve repair using corMatrix((R)) : a histologic evaluation. *Xenotransplantation.* (2017) 24:12341. doi: 10.1111/xen.12341

64. Mosala Nezhad Z, Baldin P, Poncelet A, El Khoury G. Calcific degeneration of corMatrix 4 years after bicuspidization of unicuspid aortic valve. *Ann Thorac Surg.* (2017) 104:e431–e3. doi: 10.1016/j.athoracsur.2017.07.040

65. Erek E, Aydin S, Suzan D, Yildiz O, Demir IH, Odemis E. Early degeneration of extracellular matrix used for aortic reconstruction during the norwood operation. *Ann Thorac Surg.* (2016) 101:758–60. doi: 10.1016/j.athoracsur.2015.04.051

66. Strange G, Brizard C, Karl TR, Neethling L. An evaluation of admedus' tissue engineering process-treated (ADAPT) bovine pericardium patch (CardioCel) for the repair of cardiac and vascular defects. *Expert Rev Med Devices.* (2015) 12:135–41. doi: 10.1586/17434440.2015.985651

67. Neethling WML, Puls K, Rea A. Comparison of physical and biological properties of cardioCel(R) with commonly used bioscaffolds. *Interact Cardiovasc Thorac Surg.* (2018) 26:985–92. doi: 10.1093/icvts/ivx413

68. Salameh A, Greimann W, Vondrys D, Kostelka M. Calcification or not. This is the question. A 1-year study of bovine pericardial vascular patches (CardioCel) in minipigs. *Semin Thorac Cardiovasc Surg.* (2018) 30:54–9. doi: 10.1053/j.semtcvs.2017.09.013

69. Riem Vis PW, Kluin J, Sluijter JP, van Herwerden LA, Bouten CV. Environmental regulation of valvulogenesis: implications for tissue engineering. *Eur J Cardiothorac Surg.* (2011) 39:8–17. doi: 10.1016/j.ejcts.2010.05.032

70. Lichtenberg A, Cebotari S, Tudorache I, Sturz G, Winterhalter M, Hilfiker A, et al. Flow-dependent re-endothelialization of tissue-engineered heart valves. *J Heart Valve Dis.* (2006) 15:287–93; discussion 93–4.

71. Emmert MY, Schmitt BA, Loerakker S, Sanders B, Spriestersbach H, Fioretta ES, et al. Computational modeling guides tissue-engineered heart valve design for long-term *in vivo* performance in a translational sheep model. *Sci Transl Med.* (2018) 10:4587. doi: 10.1126/scitranslmed.aan4587

72. Van Lieshout M, Peters G, Rutten M, Baaijens F. A knitted, fibrin-covered polycaprolactone scaffold for tissue engineering of the aortic valve. *Tissue Eng.* (2006) 12:481–7. doi: 10.1089/ten.2006.12.481

73. Vaz CM, van Tuijl S, Bouten CV, Baaijens FP. Design of scaffolds for blood vessel tissue engineering using a multi-layering electrospinning technique. *Acta Biomater.* (2005) 1:575–82. doi: 10.1016/j.actbio.2005.06.006

74. Fioretta ES, Simonet M, Smits AI, Baaijens FP, Bouten CV. Differential response of endothelial and endothelial colony forming cells on electrospun scaffolds with distinct microfiber diameters. *Biomacromolecules.* (2014) 15:821–9. doi: 10.1021/bm4016418

75. Sohier J, Carubelli I, Sarathchandra P, Latif N, Chester AH, Yacoub MH. The potential of anisotropic matrices as substrate for heart valve engineering. *Biomaterials.* (2014) 35:1833–44. doi: 10.1016/j.biomaterials.2013.10.061

76. Soliman OI, Miyazaki Y, Abdelghani M, Brugmans M, Witsenburg M, Onuma Y, et al. Midterm performance of a novel restorative pulmonary valved conduit: preclinical results. *EuroIntervention.* (2017) 13:e1418–e27. doi: 10.4244/EIJ-D-17-00553

77. Dearani JA, Rosengart TK, Marshall MB, Mack MJ, Jones DR, Prager RL, et al. Incorporating innovation and new technology into cardiothoracic surgery. *Ann Thorac Surg.* (2018) 107:1267–74. doi: 10.1016/j.athoracsur.2018.10.022

78. Emmert MY, Fioretta ES, Hoerstrup SP. Translational challenges in cardiovascular tissue engineering. *J Cardiovasc Transl Res.* (2017) 10:139–49. doi: 10.1007/s12265-017-9728-2

79. *Council Directive 93/42/EEC.* (1993).

80. *Regulation (EU) 2017/745.* (2017).

81. US Food And Drug Administration. *Premarket Approval (PMA): US Department of Health and Human Services.* (2018). Available online at: https://www.fda.gov/MedicalDevices/DeviceRegulationandGuidance/HowtoMarketYourDevice/PremarketSubmissions/PremarketApprovalPMA/ucm2007514.htm#data.

82. ISO. *International Standard, ISO 5840:2015, Cardiovascular Implants - Cardiac Valve Prostheses.* International Organization for Standardization (ISO). (2015).

83. Klopfleisch R, Jung F. The pathology of the foreign body reaction against biomaterials. *J Biomed Mater Res A.* (2017) 105:927–40. doi: 10.1002/jbm.a.35958

84. Taylor DA, Caplan AL, Macchiarini P. Ethics of bioengineering organs and tissues. *Expert opinion on biological therapy.* (2014) 14:879–82. doi: 10.1517/14712598.2014.915308

85. Zilla P, Bolman RM, Yacoub MH, Beyersdorf F, Sliwa K, Zuhlke L, et al. The cape town declaration on access to cardiac surgery in the developing world. *Eur J Cardiothorac Surg.* (2018) 54:407–10. doi: 10.1093/ejcts/ezy272

86. Angell M. The ethics of clinical research in the third world. *N Engl J Med.* (1997) 337:847–9. doi: 10.1056/NEJM199709183371209

87. Antonides CFJ, Cohen DJ, Osnabrugge RLJ. Statistical primer: a cost-effectiveness analysis[†]. *Eur J Cardio-Thor Surg.* (2018) 54:209–13. doi: 10.1093/ejcts/ezy187

88. Huygens SA, Rutten-van Molken M, Noruzi A, Etnel JRG, Ramos IC, Bouten CVC, et al. What is the potential of tissue-engineered pulmonary valves in children? *Ann Thorac Surg.* (2018) doi: 10.1016/j.athoracsur.2018.11.066

89. Yacoub MH. In search of living valve substitutes. *J Am Coll Cardiol.* (2015) 66:889–91. doi: 10.1016/j.jacc.2015.07.007

90. Jing H, He X, Zheng J. Exosomes and regenerative medicine: state of the art and perspectives. *Transl Res.* (2018) 196:1–16. doi: 10.1016/j.trsl.2018.01.005

91. El-Sherbiny IM, Yacoub MH. Hydrogel scaffolds for tissue engineering: progress and challenges. *Glob Cardiol Sci Pract.* (2013) 2013:316–42. doi: 10.5339/gcsp.2013.38

92. Grath A, Dai G. Direct cell reprogramming for tissue engineering and regenerative medicine. *J Biol Eng.* (2019) 13:14. doi: 10.1186/s13036-019-0144-9

93. Ieda M, Fu JD, Delgado-Olguin P, Vedantham V, Hayashi Y, Bruneau BG, et al. Direct reprogramming of fibroblasts into functional cardiomyocytes by defined factors. *Cell.* (2010) 142:375–86. doi: 10.1016/j.cell.2010.07.002

94. Takahashi K, Tanabe K, Ohnuki M, Narita M, Ichisaka T, Tomoda K, et al. Induction of pluripotent stem cells from adult human fibroblasts by defined factors. *Cell.* (2007) 131:861–72. doi: 10.1016/j.cell.2007.11.019

95. Armstrong JPK, Stevens MM. Emerging technologies for tissue engineering: from gene editing to personalized medicine. *Tissue Eng Part A.* (2019) 25:688–92. doi: 10.1089/ten.tea.2019.0026

96. Yacoub MH. Bridge to recovery and myocardial cell division: a paradigm shift? *J Am Coll Cardiol.* (2015) 65:901–3. doi: 10.1016/j.jacc.2014.12.034

Permissions

The contributors of this book come from diverse backgrounds, making this book a truly international effort. This book will bring forth new frontiers with its revolutionizing research information and detailed analysis of the nascent developments around the world.

We would like to thank all the contributing authors for lending their expertise to make the book truly unique. They have played a crucial role in the development of this book. Without their invaluable contributions this book wouldn't have been possible. They have made vital efforts to compile up to date information on the varied aspects of this subject to make this book a valuable addition to the collection of many professionals and students.

This book was conceptualized with the vision of imparting up-to-date information and advanced data in this field. To ensure the same, a matchless editorial board was set up. Every individual on the board went through rigorous rounds of assessment to prove their worth. After which they invested a large part of their time researching and compiling the most relevant data for our readers.

The editorial board has been involved in producing this book since its inception. They have spent rigorous hours researching and exploring the diverse topics which have resulted in the successful publishing of this book. They have passed on their knowledge of decades through this book. To expedite this challenging task, the publisher supported the team at every step. A small team of assistant editors was also appointed to further simplify the editing procedure and attain best results for the readers.

Apart from the editorial board, the designing team has also invested a significant amount of their time in understanding the subject and creating the most relevant covers. They scrutinized every image to scout for the most suitable representation of the subject and create an appropriate cover for the book.

The publishing team has been an ardent support to the editorial, designing and production team. Their endless efforts to recruit the best for this project, has resulted in the accomplishment of this book. They are a veteran in the field of academics and their pool of knowledge is as vast as their experience in printing. Their expertise and guidance has proved useful at every step. Their uncompromising quality standards have made this book an exceptional effort. Their encouragement from time to time has been an inspiration for everyone.

The publisher and the editorial board hope that this book will prove to be a valuable piece of knowledge for researchers, students, practitioners and scholars across the globe.

List of Contributors

Elizabeth A. W. Sigston
Monash Institute of Medical Engineering, Monash University, Melbourne, VIC, Australia
Department of Surgery, School of Clinical Sciences at Monash Health, Monash University Melbourne, Melbourne, VIC, Australia
Department of Otolaryngology, Head and Neck Surgery, Monash Health, Melbourne, VIC, Australia

Juyong Chung
Department of Otolaryngology, Wonkwang University School of Medicine, Iksan, South Korea

Youngdo Jung, Shin Hur and Wan Doo Kim
Department of Nature-Inspired System and Application, Korea Institute of Machinery and Materials, Daejeon, South Korea

Jin Ho Kim and Sung June Kim
Nano-Bioelectronics & Systems Laboratory, Department of Electrical and Computer Engineering, Seoul National University, Seoul, South Korea

Yun-Hoon Choung
Department of Otolaryngology, Ajou University School of Medicine, Suwon, South Korea

Seung-Ha Oh
Department of Otorhinolaryngology, Sensory Organ Research Institute, Seoul National University Medical Research Center, Seoul National University College of Medicine, Seoul, South Korea

Michael Jiang, Jasmine Coles-Black and Jason Chuen
3dMedLab, Austin Health, The University of Melbourne, Parkville, VIC, Australia
Department of Surgery, Austin Health, The University of Melbourne, Heidelberg, VIC, Australia

Gordon Chen
3dMedLab, Austin Health, The University of Melbourne, Parkville, VIC, Australia

Matthew Alexander and Andrew Hardidge
Department of Surgery, Austin Health, The University of Melbourne, Heidelberg, VIC, Australia

Christopher David Roche
Northern Clinical School of Medicine, University of Sydney, Sydney, NSW, Australia
School of Biomedical Engineering, Faculty of Engineering and IT, University of Technology Sydney, Sydney, NSW, Australia
Department of Cardiothoracic Surgery, University Hospital of Wales, Cardiff, United Kingdom

Yiran Zhou and Liang Zhao
School of Mechanical and Mechatronic Engineering, Faculty of Engineering and IT, University of Technology Sydney, Sydney, NSW, Australia

Carmine Gentile
Northern Clinical School of Medicine, University of Sydney, Sydney, NSW, Australia
School of Biomedical Engineering, Faculty of Engineering and IT, University of Technology Sydney, Sydney, NSW, Australia

Alisha P. Pedersen, Pierre-Yves Mulon, Rebecca E. Rifkin and David E. Anderson
Department of Large Animal Clinical Sciences, College of Veterinary Medicine, University of Tennessee, Knoxville, TN, United States

Karrer M. Alghazali
Center for Integrative Nanotechnology Sciences, University of Arkansas at Little Rock, Little Rock, AR, United States
NuShores BioSciences LLC, Little Rock, AR, United States

Rabab N. Hamzah, Anwer Mhannawee, Zeid A. Nima, Christopher Griffin and Alexandru S. Biris
Center for Integrative Nanotechnology Sciences, University of Arkansas at Little Rock, Little Rock, AR, United States

Megan McCracken
Equine Hospital, Veterinary Health Center, University of Missouri College of Veterinary Medicine, Columbia, MO, United States

Robert L. Donnell
Department of Biomedical and Diagnostic Sciences, College of Veterinary Medicine, University of Tennessee, Knoxville, TN, United States

Yihui Song and Morgan Overmass
Save Sight Institute, Faculty of Medicine and Health, The University of Sydney, Sydney, NSW, Australia

Jiawen Fan
Key Laboratory of Myopia of State Health Ministry, Department of Ophthalmology and Vision Sciences, Eye and Ear, Nose and Throat (ENT) Hospital, Shanghai Medical College, Fudan University, Shanghai, China

Chris Hodge and Gerard Sutton
Save Sight Institute, Faculty of Medicine and Health, The University of Sydney, Sydney, NSW, Australia
New South Wales (NSW) Tissue Bank, Sydney, NSW, Australia
Vision Eye Institute, Chatswood, NSW, Australia

Frank J. Lovicu
Save Sight Institute, Faculty of Medicine and Health, The University of Sydney, Sydney, NSW, Australia
Discipline of Anatomy and Histology, School of Medical Sciences, The University of Sydney, Sydney, NSW, Australia

Jingjing You
Save Sight Institute, Faculty of Medicine and Health, The University of Sydney, Sydney, NSW, Australia
School of Optometry and Vision Science, University of New South Wales, Sydney, NSW, Australia

Ravikumar Vaghela, Andreas Arkudas, Raymund E. Horch and Maximilian Hessenauer
Department of Plastic and Hand Surgery, University Hospital of Erlangen, Friedrich–Alexander University Erlangen–Nürnberg (FAU), Erlangen, Germany

Damien Bolton
Department of Surgery, Austin Health, The University of Melbourne, Melbourne, VIC, Australia

Michael Y. Chen
Faculty, Queensland University of Technology, Brisbane, QLD, Australia
Herston Biofabrication Institute, Metro North Hospital and Health Service, Brisbane, QLD, Australia
Redcliffe Hospital, Metro North Hospital and Health Service, Brisbane, QLD, Australia

David Forrestal
Faculty, Queensland University of Technology, Brisbane, QLD, Australia
Herston Biofabrication Institute, Metro North Hospital and Health Service, Brisbane, QLD, Australia

Nicholas J. Rukin
Herston Biofabrication Institute, Metro North Hospital and Health Service, Brisbane, QLD, Australia
Redcliffe Hospital, Metro North Hospital and Health Service, Brisbane, QLD, Australia
School of Medicine, University of Queensland, Brisbane, QLD, Australia

Maria A. Woodruff
Engineering Faculty, Queensland University of Technology, Brisbane, QLD, Australia

Bronwyn L. Dearman
Skin Engineering Laboratory, Adult Burns Centre, Royal Adelaide Hospital, Adelaide, SA, Australia
Adult Burns Centre, Royal Adelaide Hospital, Adelaide, SA, Australia
Faculty of Health and Medical Science, The University of Adelaide, Adelaide, SA, Australia

Steven T. Boyce
Department of Surgery, University of Cincinnati, Cincinnati, OH, United States

John E. Greenwood
Skin Engineering Laboratory, Adult Burns Centre, Royal Adelaide Hospital, Adelaide, SA, Australia
Adult Burns Centre, Royal Adelaide Hospital, Adelaide, SA, Australia

Sebastian Blatt
Department of Oral and Maxillofacial Surgery, University Medical Center, Johannes Gutenberg University Mainz, Mainz, Germany
Platform for Biomaterial Research, BiomaTiCS Group, University Medical Center, Johannes Gutenberg University Mainz, Mainz, Germany

Daniel G. E. Thiem, Solomiya Kyyak, Bilal Al-Nawas and Peer W. Kämmerer
Department of Oral and Maxillofacial Surgery, University Medical Center, Johannes Gutenberg University Mainz, Mainz, Germany

Andreas Pabst
Department of Oral and Maxillofacial Surgery, Federal Armed Forces Hospital, Koblenz, Germany

Juan Su, Yanan Xing and Lihua Liu
Department of Gastrology Ward III, Xi'an International Medical Center Hospital, Xi'an, China

Huilin Zhang
Department of Digestive Endoscopy and Treatment Center, Xi'an International Medical Center Hospital, Xi'an, China

Maifang Ren and Yuefei Yin
Department of Gastrology Ward I, Xi'an International Medical Center Hospital, Xi'an, China

Babak Saravi, Gernot Lang and Rebecca Steger
Department of Orthopedics and Trauma Surgery, Faculty of Medicine, Medical Centre, Albert-Ludwigs-University of Freiburg, Freiburg, Germany

Andreas Vollmer
Department of Oral and Maxillofacial Surgery, Faculty of Medicine, Medical Centre, Albert-Ludwigs-University of Freiburg, Freiburg, Germany

Jörn Zwingmann
Department of Orthopedics and Trauma Surgery, St. Elisabeth Hospital Ravensburg, Ravensburg, Germany

Lena Mary Houlihan, David Naughton and Mark C. Preul
The Loyal and Edith Davis Neurosurgical Research Laboratory, Department of Neurosurgery, Barrow Neurological Institute, St. Joseph's Hospital and Medical Center, Phoenix, AZ, United States

Sahar Ahmed Abdalbary
Department of Orthopaedic Physical Therapy, Faculty of Physical Therapy, Nahda University, Beni Suef, Egypt

Sherif M. Amr
Department of Orthopaedic Surgery, Faculty of Medicine, Cairo University, Giza, Egypt

Khaled Abdelghany
Advanced Manufacturing Division, The Central Metallurgical Research and Development Institute, Helwan, Egypt

Amr A. Nssef
Department of Intervention Radiology, Radiology and Vascular Imaging, Faculty of Medicine, Cairo University, Giza, Egypt

Ehab A. A. El-Shaarawy
Department of Anatomy and Embryology, Faculty of Medicine, Cairo University, Giza, Egypt

Jennifer Fayad
In Silico Biomechanics Laboratory, National Center for Spinal Disorders, Buda Health Center, Budapest, Hungary
Department of Industrial Engineering, Alma Mater Studiorum, Universita di Bologna, Bologna, Italy
Department of Spine Surgery, Semmelweis University, Budapest, Hungary

Mate Turbucz and Ferenc Bereczki
Department of Industrial Engineering, Alma Mater Studiorum, Universita di Bologna, Bologna, Italy
School of PhD Studies, Semmelweis University, Budapest, Hungary

Benjamin Hajnal
Department of Industrial Engineering, Alma Mater Studiorum, Universita di Bologna, Bologna, Italy

Marton Bartos
Do3D Innovations Ltd., Budapest, Hungary

Andras Bank
National Center for Spinal Disorders, Buda Health Center, Budapest, Hungary

Aron Lazary
Department of Spine Surgery, Semmelweis University, Budapest, Hungary
National Center for Spinal Disorders, Buda Health Center, Budapest, Hungary

Peter Endre Eltes
Department of Industrial Engineering, Alma Mater Studiorum, Universita di Bologna, Bologna, Italy
Department of Spine Surgery, Semmelweis University, Budapest, Hungary

Khiem Tran Dang
Department of Research and Development for Innovative Medical Devices and Systems, Shiga University of Medical Science, Otsu, Japan
Department of Surgery, University of Medicine and Pharmacy at Ho Chi Minh City, Ho Chi Minh City, Vietnam

Shigeyuki Naka
Department of Surgery, Shiga University of Medical Science, Otsu, Japan
Department of Surgery, Hino Memorial Hospital, Hino, Japan

Atsushi Yamada and Tohru Tani
Department of Research and Development for Innovative Medical Devices and Systems, Shiga University of Medical Science, Otsu, Japan

Maoen Pan, Yuanyuan Yang, Tianhong Teng and Heguang Huang
Department of General Surgery, Fujian Medical University Union Hospital, Fuzhou, China

Chaoqian Zhao, Zeya Xu and Jinxin Lin
Key Laboratory of Optoelectronic Materials Chemical and Physics, Fujian Institute of Research on the Structure of Matter, Chinese Academy of Sciences, Fuzhou, China

Sarah Al-Himdani, Zita M. Jessop, Emman Combellack and Iain S. Whitaker
Reconstructive Surgery and Regenerative Medicine Research Group (ReconRegen), Institute of Life Science, Swansea University Medical School, Swansea, UK
The Welsh Centre for Burns and Plastic Surgery, Morriston Hospital, Swansea, UK

Ayesha Al-Sabah
Reconstructive Surgery and Regenerative Medicine Research Group (ReconRegen), Institute of Life Science, Swansea University Medical School, Swansea, UK

Amel Ibrahim
Reconstructive Surgery and Regenerative Medicine Research Group (ReconRegen), Institute of Life Science, Swansea University Medical School, Swansea, UK
The Welsh Centre for Burns and Plastic Surgery, Morriston Hospital, Swansea, UK
Institute of Child Health, University College London, London, UK

Shareen H. Doak
Reconstructive Surgery and Regenerative Medicine Research Group (ReconRegen), Institute of Life Science, Swansea University Medical School, Swansea, UK
In Vitro Toxicology Group, Institute of Life Science, Swansea University Medical School, Swansea, UK

Andrew M. Hart
Canniesburn Plastic Surgery Unit, Centre for Cell Engineering, University of Glasgow, Glasgow, UK

Charles W. Archer
Reconstructive Surgery and Regenerative Medicine Research Group (ReconRegen), Institute of Life Science, Swansea University Medical School, Swansea, UK
Cartilage Biology Research Group, Institute of Life Science, Swansea University Medical School, Swansea, UK

Catherine A. Thornton
Reconstructive Surgery and Regenerative Medicine Research Group (ReconRegen), Institute of Life Science, Swansea University Medical School, Swansea, UK
Human Immunology Group, Institute of Life Science, Swansea University Medical School, Swansea, UK

Michael P. Chae and Warren M. Rozen
3D PRINT Laboratory, Department of Surgery, Peninsula Health, Frankston, VIC, Australia

Monash University Plastic and Reconstructive Surgery Group (Peninsula Clinical School), Peninsula Health, Frankston, VIC, Australia

Paul G. McMenamin
Department of Anatomy and Developmental Biology, Centre for Human Anatomy Education, School of Biomedical Sciences, Faculty of Medicine, Nursing and Health Sciences, Monash University, Clayton, VIC, Australia

Michael W. Findlay
3D PRINT Laboratory, Department of Surgery, Peninsula Health, Frankston, VIC, Australia
Department of Surgery, Stanford University, Stanford, CA, USA

Robert T. Spychal
3D PRINT Laboratory, Department of Surgery, Peninsula Health, Frankston, VIC, Australia

David J. Hunter-Smith
3D PRINT Laboratory, Department of Surgery, Peninsula Health, Frankston, VIC, Australia
Monash University Plastic and Reconstructive Surgery Group (Peninsula Clinical School), Peninsula Health, Frankston, VIC, Australia

Andras P. Durko
Department of Cardiothoracic Surgery, Erasmus University Medical Center, Rotterdam, Netherlands

Magdi H. Yacoub
Imperial College London, National Heart and Lung Institute, London, United Kingdom

Jolanda Kluin
Department of Cardiothoracic Surgery, Amsterdam University Medical Center, Amsterdam, Netherlands

Index

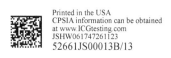

Printed in the USA
CPSIA information can be obtained
at www.ICGtesting.com
JSHW061747261123
52661JS00013B/13